Manual of I.V. Therapeutics

Manual of I.V. Therapeutics

Fourth Edition

Lynn Dianne Phillips, RN, MSN, CRNI

Faculty
Nurse Educator
Butte Community College
Oroville, California

F. A. DAVIS COMPANY ▪ Philadelphia

F. A. Davis Company
1915 Arch Street
Philadelphia, PA 19103
www.fadavis.com

Printed in the United States of America

Last digit indicates print number: 10 9 8 7 6 5 4 3 2 1

Acquisition Editor: Joanne P. DaCunha, RN, MSN
Developmental Editor: Alan Sorkowitz
Project Editor: Ilysa H. Richman
Manager, Art Department: Joan Wendt

Library of Congress Cataloging-in-Publication Data

Phillips, Lynn Dianne, 1947-
Manual of I.V. therapeutics / Lynn D. Phillips.—4th ed.
p. ; cm.
Includes bibliographical references and index.
ISBN 0-8036-1187-0 (pbk.)
1. Intravenous therapy—Handbooks, manuals, etc. I. Title: Manual of IV therapeutics. II. Title.
[DNLM: 1. Infusions, Intravenous—methods—Examination Questions. 2. Infusions, Intravenous—methods—Handbooks. 3. Infusions, Intravenous—nursing—Examination Questions. 4. Infusions, Intravenous—nursing—Handbooks. WB 39 P561m 2005]
RM170.P48 2005
615'.6—dc22 2004061785

This book is dedicated to
our first grandchild Makenzi Marie Allen
You light up our lives!
And as always
To my fabulous nursing students

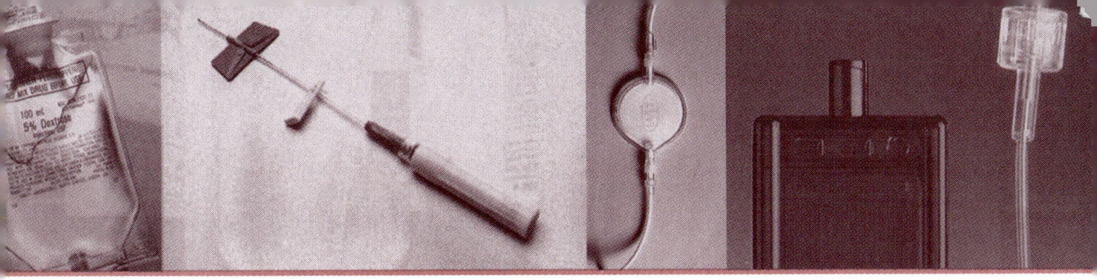

Preface

Manual of I.V. Therapeutics, Fourth Edition, provides comprehensive information on infusion therapy for the nursing student and the practicing nurse. New to this edition are nursing fast fact boxes that key out important information; boxed nursing points-of-care, which present nursing interventions; and a chapter on basic phlebotomy.

This self-paced, comprehensive text presents information ranging from a simple to complex format, incorporating theory into clinical application. The skills of recall, nursing process, critical thinking, and patient education is covered, along with detailed summaries, provide the foundation one needs to become a knowledgeable practitioner. The psychomotor skills associated with infusion therapy are presented in step-by-step recurring displays based on standards of practice.

Each chapter has accompanying objectives, defined glossary terms that are bolded within the text, a post-test, a key points summary, and a critical thinking case study. Icons and special boxes are used throughout each chapter to key the reader to Web sites, patient education, home care practice, cultural considerations, and standards of practice. Included in this new edition are step-by-step competency SkillChecks in the appendices. These SkillChecks can be used in the educational setting, as well as in agencies, for validating competencies of nurses in infusion skills. The icons used in this fourth edition are as follows:

NOTE > Identifies key points that are boxed within the text

Presents nursing interventions boxed within the text

Identifies Web Sites

Identifies Home Care Issues

Identifies Patient Education information

Identifies a media link, which refers to the book's accompanying CD–ROM, and is located in the critical thinking case study and post-test sections at the end of each chapter.

Identifies standards of practice throughout the text, including guidelines of the Infusion Nurses Society (INS), Occupational Safety and Health Administration (OSHA), Centers for Disease Control and Prevention (CDC), and Oncology Nurses Society (ONS).

This manual is divided into three units. Unit 1 lays the foundation for practice, Unit 2 provides basics of infusion therapy, and Unit 3 covers advanced practice.

Unit 1 consists of four chapters designed to give in-depth information to the reader on risk management, legal responsibilities, infection control practices, and fundamentals of fluid and electrolyte balance.

The six chapters in Unit 2 provide the essential solid foundation in infusion therapy practice. This fourth edition has incorporated recurring displays for procedures and for cultural and age-related issues. New to this unit is a chapter on basic phlebotomy practices. Unit 2 provides the reader with comprehensive information on infusion equipment for parenteral solutions, techniques for peripheral infusion therapy, complications, and the special needs of the geriatric and pediatric populations.

Unit 3 consists of five chapters encompassing the advanced topics of infusion medication delivery, management of central lines, transfusions therapy, antineoplastic theory, and nutritional support.

The appendices include a summary of the new CDC (2002) recommended procedures for maintenance for intravenous catheters and administration sets. The appendix also has a set of comprehensive competency SkillCheck forms.

The CD–ROM accompanying this textbook contains 300 questions based on standards of practice and follows the guidelines of the INS Core Curriculum for certification. The CD–ROM also includes guidelines for discussion and answers to the case studies.

I hope this new edition provides you, whether you are a practicing healthcare professional or student, with valuable insights into the safe practice of infusion therapy and a reference for this rapidly advancing field.

Lynn D. Phillips

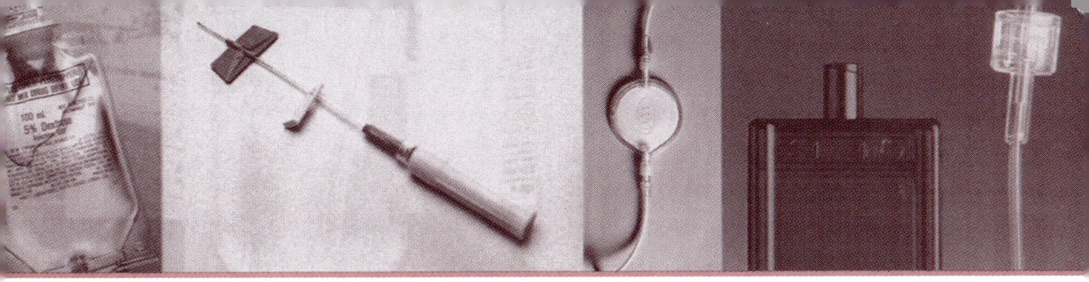

Acknowledgments

The author would like to acknowledge the following:

The nurses in the specialty practice of infusion therapy

The nursing department at Butte Community College for their support and encouragement during this revision

At F. A. Davis:

Joanne P. Da Cunha, Nursing Acquisitions Editor, who assisted in the final development of this manual

Alan Sorkowitz, of Alan Sorkowitz Editorial Services, who, as developmental editor, helped bring this vision to reality

Michael Bailey, Director of Production, for guiding this manuscript through the production process

Robert G. Martone, Publisher, *Nursing*, whose foresight brought the project to F. A. Davis

Berta Steiner, of Bermedica Production, Ltd., who assisted in the final editing and production of this manuscript

Appreciation is expressed to the following companies who provided product information, pictures and illustrations:

Abbott Laboratories Hospital Product Division, Abbott Park, Illinois

Alaris Medical Systems, San Diego, California

BARD Access Systems, Salt Lake City, Utah

Baxter International, Inc., Round Lake, Illinois

BD Medical Systems, Franklin Lakes, New Jersey

B. Braun Medical, Inc., Bethlehem, Pennsylvania

Cook Critical Care, Ellettsville, Indiana

Deltec, St. Paul, Minnesota

Enloe Medical Center, Chico, California

Infusion Nurses Society, Norwood, Massachusetts

Johnson and Johnson Endosurgery, Arlington, Texas

Medtronic, Inc., Northridge, California

Medi-Flex, Inc., Overland Park, Kansas

Medex, Inc., Carlsbad, California

Pall Biomedial Products Company, Port Washington, New York

Venetec International, Mission Viejo, California

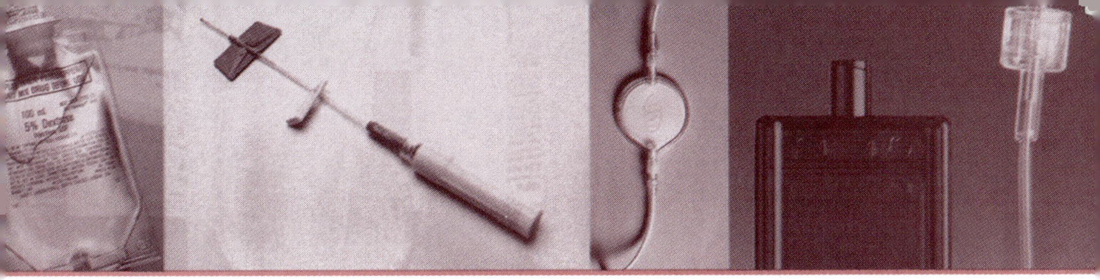

Contributors

Julie Eddins, RN, MSN, CRNI
Central Region Infusion Systems Specialist
Medex, Inc.
Fenton, Missouri
Central Venous Access

Pamela Hockett, RN, MSN, CNS, OCN
Vice President, Professional and Outpatient Services
Enloe Medical Center
Chico, California
Antineoplastic Therapy

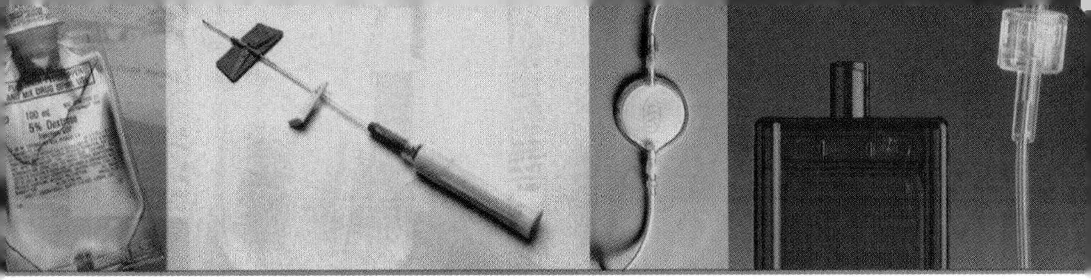

Consultants/Reviewers

Lynn Czaplewski, RN, C., BSN, CRNI, OCN
Infusion Specialist/Educator
Medical Consultants, Ltd.
Milwaukee, Wisconsin

Brenda Bradley Johansson, RN, C., MSN, CCRN
Faculty
Nurse Educator
Butte Community College
Oroville, California

Nancy K. Ledoyen, RN, BSN, OCN
Cancer Center Coordinator
Enloe Medical Center
Chico, California

Sue Masoorli, RN
CEO
Perivascular Nurse Consultants
Chila, Pennsylvania

Sally Miller, RN, MS
Nursing Faculty
Cabrillo College
Aptos, California

Nancy Moureau, BSN, CRNI
President
PICC Excellence, Inc.
Orange Park, Florida

Roxanne R. Perucca, MSN, CRNI
I.V. Therapy Nurse Manager
University of Kansas Hospital
Kansas City, Kansas

Ofelia Santigo, BSN, CRNI
Director of Clinical Services and Case Management Care IV, Inc.
Home Infusion and Disease Management Services
Wichita, Kansas

Mary Walsh, RN, BS, CRNI
Home Infusion Nurse Manager
South Shore Visiting Nurse Association
Braintree, Massachusetts

Katherine Werner, MSHA, BSN, CRNI
Vice President
National Home Infusion Association
Alexandria, Virginia

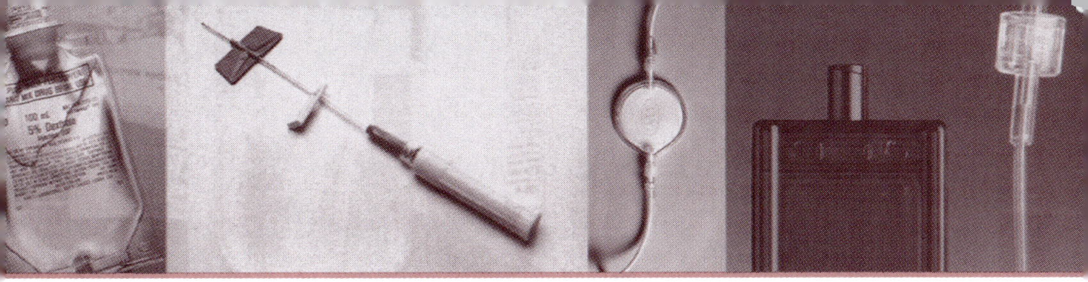

Contents

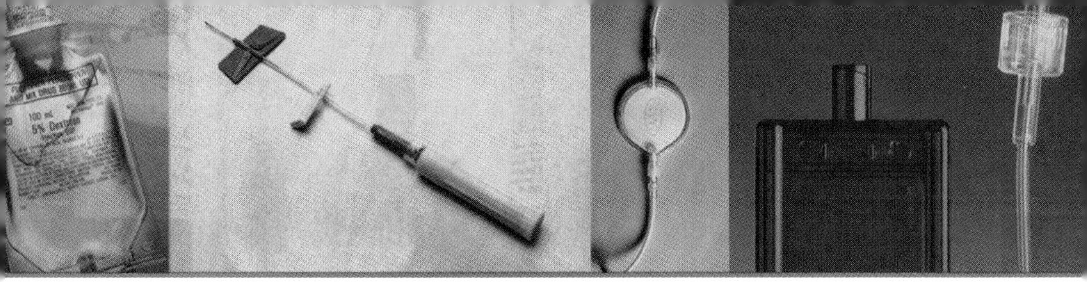

Tables

Unit 1

Fundamental Foundations of Practice

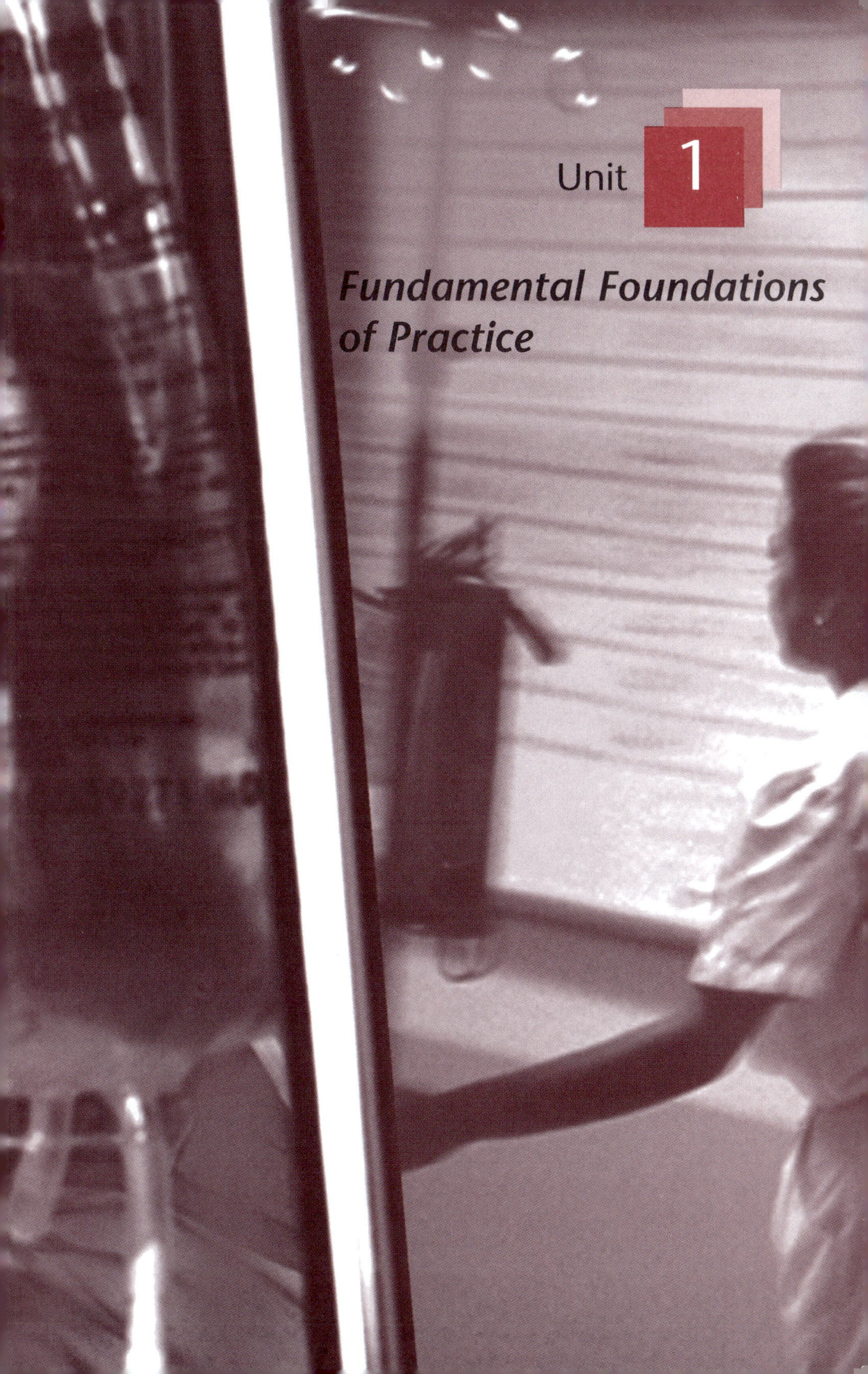

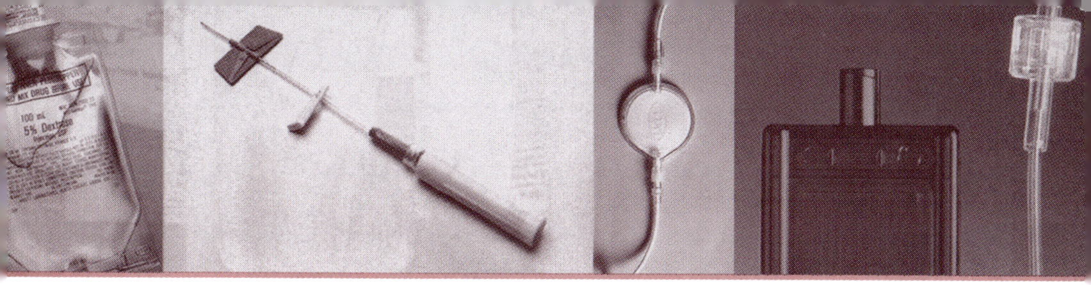

Chapter 1
Risk Management and Quality Patient Management

The world, more especially the hospital world, is in such a hurry, is moving so fast, that it is too easy to slide into bad habits before we are aware.
—Florence Nightingale, 1873

Chapter Contents

LEARNING OBJECTIVES

Upon completion of this chapter, the reader will be able to:

1. Define the terminology related to risk management and quality patient management.
2. Identify the sources of laws.
3. Differentiate between standards of care and standards of practice.
4. Identify the areas of breach of duty for the specialty of infusion nursing.
5. Define evidence-based practice, as it applies to infusion nursing.
6. State the key points in an unusual occurrence report.
7. State the definition of quality management.
8. State the three parts of a competency-based program.
9. Differentiate between performance improvement and total quality management.
10. Identify the role of the nurse as an expert witness.
11. Identify three occupational risks for the infusion nurse.

GLOSSARY

Audit A review of care using defined criteria

Benchmarking Structured, comparative trending of performances that represent "best-known" practices and the identification of goals against which all other levels of performance are measured

Civil law Laws that affect the legal rights of private persons or corporations

Competency Integrated behaviors derived from an explicit set of desired outcomes

Competency validation program **(CVP)** System developed by Clinical Center Nursing Department at the National Institutes of Health to identify, describe, validate, and document the nursing competencies required for safe and effective nursing practice

Competent Being capable or able; knowing how to function

Continuous quality improvement (CQI) Created to assist organizations in improving the quality of care.

Criminal law Offense against the general public; effects welfare of society as a whole

Criteria Elements necessary to define and measure quality

Data collection Gathering information through interviewing, observing, and inspecting

Dimensions of performance Characteristics of what is done and how well it is done

Documentation A recording, in written or printed form, containing original, official, or legal information

Evaluation Inspection, examination, and quality judgment

Evidence-based practice Process by which nurses make clinical decisions using the best available evidence, their clinical expertise, and patient preferences

Expert testimony Witness from the same professional specialty explaining to the court what the standard of care should be in the situation at hand

Goal Broad statement of a desired outcome

Implementation Carrying out a plan

Intervention Interference that may affect outcome

Liable Legally responsible for damages, answerable

Malpractice Negligent conduct of a professional person

Negligence Not acting in a reasonable or prudent manner

Nursing standard Specific statement about the quality of some facet of nursing care

Outcome The result of the performance (or nonperformance) of a function or process(es)

Performance improvement (PI) The continuous study and adaptation of functions and processes of a healthcare organization to increase the probability of achieving desired outcomes and to better meet the needs of patients and other users of services; the third segment of the performance measurement, assessment, and improvement system

Process A goal-directed, interrelated series of actions, events, mechanisms, or steps

Quality assurance (QA) The determination of the degree of excellence through monitoring and evaluating to detect and resolve problems

Quality management An ongoing, systematic process for monitoring, evaluating, and problem solving

Risk management Process that centers on identification analysis, treatment, and evaluation of real and potential hazards

Standards of care Focuses on the recipient of care and describes outcomes of care that patients can expect to receive

Standards of practice Focuses on the provider and defines the activities and behavior needed to achieve patient outcomes

Statutes Written laws enacted by the legislature
Structure Standard that refers to conditions and mechanisms that provide support for the delivery of care (e.g., policy and resources)
Tort Private wrong, by act or omission, that can result in a civil action by the harmed person
Total quality management (TQM) Management system fostering continuously improving performance at every level of every function by focusing on maximization of customer satisfaction; focus is on process
Unusual occurrence report Documentation of an incident that requires action because of potential or implied consequences

Legal and Ethical Issues in Infusion Therapy

Sources of Law

In the United States, there are four primary sources of law: (1) constitutional law, (2) statutory law, (3) administrative law, and (4) common law. In addition, law can be divided into two main branches: private law and public law. Constitutional law is a formal set of rules and principles that describe the powers of a government and the right of the people. Rights guaranteed in the Bill of Rights are consistent with the ethical principles of autonomy, confidentiality, respect for persons, and veracity. As participants in the healthcare system, nurses cannot be forced to forfeit any constitutionally guaranteed rights.

Formal laws written and enacted by federal, state, or local legislatures are known as statutory or legislative laws. Only a minimal number of **statutes** dealing with malpractice existed before the malpractice crisis of the mid-1970s. Changes in Medicare and Medicaid laws, statutory recognition of nurses in advanced practice, and proposed healthcare reform legislation are all examples of statutory or legislative law.

Administrative law is a form of law set by administrative agencies, such as the National Labor Relations Board and the Interstate Commerce Commission. State boards of nursing are examples of this type of legislative body.

The final source of law is common law, which is court-made law. Most law in the area of malpractice is court-made law. The courts are responsible for interpreting the statutes. Most malpractice law is not addressed by statute but is established by the courts (Burkhardt & Nathaniel, 2002).

Legal Terms

Legal terms that nurses should become familiar with are *criminal law, civil law, tort, malpractice*, and the *rule of personal liability*. **Criminal law** relates to an offense against the general public caused by the potential harmful effect to society as a whole. A government authority prosecutes criminal actions, and punishment includes imprisonment, fine, or both. The administration of I.V. therapy, if performed in an unlawful manner, can involve a nurse in a criminal offense. Violation of the Nurse Practice Act or the Medical Practice Act by an unlicensed person is considered a criminal offense.

Civil law or private law affects the legal rights of private persons and corporations. The branches of private law that are most applicable to nursing practice are contract law and tort law. Noncompliance with private law generally leads to a granting of monetary compensation to the injured party.

A private wrong, by act or omission, is referred to as a **tort**. Most tort law is found in common law. There are two types of tort: intentional and unintentional. Intentional torts include assault, battery, false imprisonment, restraints as a form of false imprisonment, defamation, and breach of confidentiality (Burkhart & Nathaniel, 2002). When dealing with a rational patient who refuses treatment, it is best to explain the treatment, verbally reassure the patient, and then notify the physician of refusal.

Negligence is the failure to do something that a reasonable person, guided by ordinary considerations, would do or doing something that a reasonable and prudent person would not do.

Malpractice is a type or subset of negligence, committed by a person in a professional capacity. Above simple negligence, malpractice is the form of negligence in which any professional misconduct, unreasonable lack of professional skill, or nonadherence to the accepted standard of care causes injury to a patient. Four components are required to prove liability for malpractice:

1. It must be established that the nurse had a duty to the patient.
2. A breach of standards of care or failure to carry out that duty must be proven.
3. The patient must suffer actual harm or injury.
4. There must be a causal relationship between the breach of duty and the injury suffered (O'Keefe, 2000).

NURSING FAST FACTS!

If an act of malpractice does not create harm, legal action cannot be initiated.

Coercion of a rational adult patient to place an intravenous catheter constitutes assault and battery.

The rule of personal liability is "every person is **liable** for his own tortuous conduct" (his own wrongdoing). A physician cannot protect a nurse from an act of negligence by bypassing this rule with verbal assurance.

Nurses are liable for their own wrongdoings in carrying out physicians' orders. This rule is relevant to nurses in the areas of medication errors (the most common cause of malpractice claims) and administration of I.V. fluids. Nurses have a legal and professional responsibility to be knowledgeable regarding the I.V. fluids, medications that are administered, and techniques for initiating and maintaining infusion devices.

The terms *assault* and *battery*, although usually used together, have different legal meanings. Both are intentional torts. Assault is defined as the unjustifiable attempt or threat to touch a person without consent that results in fear of immediately harmful or threatening contact. Touching need not actually occur. Battery is the unlawful, harmful, or unwarranted touching of another or the carrying out of threatened physical harm. Regardless of intent or outcome, touching without consent is considered battery. Even when the intention is beneficent and the outcome is positive, if the act is committed without permission, the nurse can be charged with battery.

Legal Causes of Action Related to Professional Practice

There are many causes of action involving nursing practice; however, the two most common are unprofessional practice and professional malpractice. Unprofessional practice or conduct is a departure from, or failure to conform to, the minimal standards of acceptable and prevailing nursing practices. In this case actual injury need not be established (NCSBN, 2003). In the infusion specialty examples would be breaches in duty to the patient, such as accepting the patient in assignment, and a deficiency in performing that duty, such as failing to perform a venipuncture according to reasonable and prudent standards of care. Unprofessional practice may result in the loss of license to practice.

Professional malpractice, a civil action, generally may be defined as professional misconduct or unreasonable lack of skill that results in harm. The four legal elements listed previously must be established in professional malpractice cases (Collins, 2001).

Breach of Duty

Nurses must be aware at all times that failure to observe, failure to intervene, and verbal rather than written orders are potential risks for all nursing areas. Nurses must assess each patient and formulate a nursing diagnosis to meet the specific patient's needs. At this time, the courts have not extended the concept of nursing diagnosis to the liability of a nurse's practice.

Malpractice cases are most frequently based on negligence in physical care. There are many documented cases of malpractice related to all procedures performed on patients. Sometimes the breach of duty occurs because a nurse fails to perform a procedure according to proper standards of care. A breach of application of standards of care can be the basis for negligence. Always ask what a reasonable and prudent nurse would do. In general, where employers and boards of nursing are concerned, the patient's outcome is a determining factor in deciding whether a nurse breached a standard of nursing practice or violated an employer's policy and therefore may be disciplined by either entity (Higginbotham, 2003). Medication errors are an area in which nurses have faced criminal charges for not following the five rights of medication administration (Institute for Safe Medication Practices, 1999).

Because of the risk of malpractice, policy and procedure manuals are vitally important in all aspects of physical nursing care. Practicing and performing specific physical care based on the policies and procedures ensure quality care.

NURSING FAST FACT!

The practice of using verbal orders rather than written orders potentially places nurses at higher liability risks.

INS Standard. Infusion therapy is initiated with a physician's order or on the order of a prescriber authorized by state Nurse Practice Acts using the nursing process. An order shall be complete and written in the patient's medical record. (INS 2000, 10)

Legal Perils of I.V. Therapy

Among the legal perils of infusion therapy, administering drugs is the major pitfall. Medication errors in general account for 2 in every 1,000 hospital deaths and are a frequent cause of malpractice suits. The most frequent medication errors are incorrect dose, wrong dose, and improper technique. Other risk factors for malpractice suits include:

- The average nurse doesn't get enough I.V. experience to become comfortable or proficient with all aspects of I.V. therapy.
- Entering the bloodstream with a foreign object and infusing medications and fluids have great potential to cause life-threatening complications.
- Litigation for nurses can result from
  - Infiltration and phlebitis
  - Fractured central venous catheters
  - Nerve injury, infiltration, and extravasations
  - Administering the wrong drug
  - Failure to document appropriately (Satarawala, 2000)

Standards of Care

The recipient of care, the patient, is the focus of standards of care. The Joint Commission on Accreditation of Healthcare Organizations (JCAHO) indicates that standards of care must be developed within organizations to measure quality based on expectations (JCAHO, 2000). Standards of care can be voluntary, such as those promulgated by professional groups, or they may be mandated legislatively. Nursing is regulated by these dual controls, both of which are aimed at providing quality patient care. The legal standards of care for I.V. nursing are derived from four sources: federal statutes and regulations, state statutes, professional standards, and institutional standards. Sources of standards of care relative to infusion nursing are listed in Table 1–1.

> Table 1–1 **SOURCES OF STANDARDS OF CARE**

Federal Regulations

Occupational Safety and Health Administration (OSHA)
Hazard communication standards; Guidelines for Antineoplastic Cytotoxic Drugs; Occupational Safe Exposure to Bloodborne Pathogens: Final Rule
Food and Drug Administration (FDA)
Safe Medical Device Act
Drug Enforcement Agency (DEA)
Regulated Controlled Substance Act
Centers for Disease Control and Prevention (CDC)
Guideline for Prevention of Intravascular Device-Related Infections

State Regulations

Department of Health and Human Services
Licensure of healthcare facilities

Professional Standards of Care

American Nurses Association (ANA)
Standards of Nursing Practice
National Association of Vascular Access Networks (NAVAN)
Position statements
Infusion Nurses Society (INS)
Standards of Practice, 2000, for infusion nursing
Oncology Nurses Society (ONS)
Access device guidelines
Association for Professionals in Infection Control and Epidemiology (APIC)
Guidelines for infection control practices
Joint Commission on Accreditation of Healthcare Organizations (JCAHO)
Nongovernmental accreditation body defines standards for healthcare organizations
American Association of Blood Banking (AABB)
Technical manual for blood banking
Environmental Protection Agency (EPA)
Hazardous materials and medical waste tracking
Emergency Care Research Institute (ECRI)
Independent nonprofit agency dedicated to improving the safety, efficacy, and cost-effectiveness of healthcare technology. Publishes monthly journal, Health Device System.

Sources: *Alexander & Webster (2001); Moreau & Maney (2003).*

Standards of nursing care reflect the missions, values, and philosophy of the agency. Nursing processes, professional accountability, fiscal responsibility, and other areas of care are included within these standards. **Standards of care** describe the results or outcomes of care and focus on the patient. These are called **performance standards** and should: (1) include the minimum acceptable behavior for the nurse congruent with department standards and standards of practice; (2) define performance in observable, measurable behaviors; (3) be specific to the staff nurse role and job description; (4) address all aspects of nurses' roles, including leadership and organizational expectations; and (5) serve as the basis for employee selection decisions and the performance appraisal system.

There are three types of standards in nursing:

1. Standards of structure, which consider the organizational framework
2. Standards of process, which encompass patient procedures in healthcare settings
3. Standards of outcome, which consider the objectives or goals of patient care

For nurses who practice predominantly in the area of infusion therapy, certification is advisable. Certification is the granting of special recognition to nurses who have practiced and pursued an advanced role in a particular area of nursing. A nongovernment agency or private organization confers certification on nurses who have a higher level of competency than that mandated by state licensure. Membership in the Infusion Nurses Society (INS) and certification (CRNI) by the Infusion Nurses Certification Corporation (INCC) are options to be considered.

Staying Current with Standards of Care for Infusion Therapy

Whenever nurses administer infusion therapy they must know and conform to acceptable nursing standards established by the facility as well as state and federal guidelines. The following list presents guidelines for safeguarding practice:

- Know venous anatomy and physiology and appropriate vein selection sites.
- Use infusion equipment appropriately.
- Clarify unclear orders and refuse to follow orders you know are not within the scope of safe nursing practice.
- Know the infusion indications, adverse responses, and special precautions or considerations for I.V. medications.
- Administer the medications or infusions at the proper or prescribed rate and within the ordered intervals.

- Assess the patient and monitor the I.V. site for complications; properly care for and maintain I.V. catheters. Promptly notify the physician of I.V. complications.
- Know and give appropriate treatments for complications.
- Provide proper patient education.
- Document all aspects of I.V. therapy, including patient teaching.
- Follow your institution's policies and procedures.
- Abide by your state's nurse practice act and national standards of I.V. practice, such as the Infusion Nurses Society Standards of Practice and guidelines for the Centers for Disease Control and Prevention and the Occupational Safety and Health Administration.
- Keep abreast of appropriate established research related to I.V. therapy (Satarawala, 2000).

Websites

JCAHO: *www.jcaho.org*
JCAHO perspectives on patient safety: *www.jcinc.com*
Intravenous Nurses Society: *www.ins1.org*
National Institutes of Health: *www.cc.nih.gov/nursing/nsgstand.html*
Medical Malpractice Resource Page: *www.helpquick.com/ medmal.htm*
Internet Legal Resource Guide: *www.ilrg.com*

Other sites:

Standards of Practice

Standards of practice focus on the provider of care and represent acceptable levels of practice in patient care delivery. Like the standards of care, practice standards address the clinical aspects of patient care services and imply patient outcomes. Standards of nursing practice define nursing accountability and provide a framework for evaluating professional competency. Standards of practice are consistent with research findings, national norms, and legal guidelines, and complement expectations of regulatory agencies. These standards reflect commitment to quality patient care and include generic and specialty standards of practice (Sierchio, 2001).

Standards of Nursing practice (ANA) are universal for all types of nursing; specialty standards are applicable to specific areas of practice such as the Infusion Nursing Standards of Practice by the Infusion Nurses Society (INS, 2000).

Ethics

Code of Ethics

A code of ethics acknowledges the acceptance by a profession of the responsibilities and trust that society has conferred and recognizes the duties and obligations inherent in that trust.

The Infusion Nursing Code of Ethics is based on the premise that infusion nurses both individually and collectively practice with awareness and that there are principles that guide the infusion nurse's actions. It is the purpose of the code to offer the infusion nurse a model for ethical decision making. The principles used in ethical and moral decision making are based on the following:

- Autonomy (right to self-determination, independence)
- Beneficence (doing good for patients)
- Nonmaleficence (doing no harm to patients)
- Veracity (truthfulness)
- Fidelity (obligation to be faithful)
- Justice (obligation to be fair to all people)

The infusion nurse should follow the ethical principles as stated in the Infusion Nursing Code of Ethics. This code of ethics is designed to serve as a helpful guide to assist the infusion nurse's practice. The code includes duties to the patient, duties to society, duties to the profession, and limitations of the infusion nurse's duties and obligations, while ensuring compassionate patient care (INS, 2000, S7; 2001).

HIPPA Privacy Rule

The U.S. Department of Health and Human Services (2003) issued the Standards for Privacy of Individually Identifiable Health Information (the Privacy Rule) under the Health Insurance Portability and Accountability Act of 1996 (HIPAA) to provide the first comprehensive federal protection for the privacy of personal health information. The final rule went into effect in April, 2003. The Privacy Rule requires healthcare providers to take reasonable actions to safeguard protected health information (PHI) and to discipline individuals who violate privacy policies. The Department of Health and Human Services is charged with enforcing the HIPAA legislation. External consequences can mean fines levied on the organization and the individual(s) involved and can include jail time for disclosing PHI maliciously or for personal gain. This new rule could potentially affect professional malpractice and has ethical as well as legal ramifications for infusion nurses.

Website

U.S. Department of Health and Human Services: *www.hhs.gov/ocr/hipaa/finalreg.html*

The I.V. Nurse's Role as Expert Witness

The role of expert witness is relatively new to the nursing profession. The nurse acting as an expert witness strengthens the argument that nursing is an autonomous profession in that no other profession can appropriately judge the practice of nurses.

Serving as an expert witness involves a complex and extensive process of examining evidence, reviewing pertinent nursing literature, giving depositions, and testifying in court (Burkhardt & Nathaniel, 2002). The role of the expert is *NOT* to establish standards of care. Rather, the expert's role is to educate the judge and jury regarding the standards already established by the profession. **Expert testimony** increases with the technical complexity of a case. Additional expertise, such as national I.V. certification or research experience, is also important.

The 2000 Revised Infusion Nursing Standards of Practice state that an expert nurse is certified in I.V. therapy: Certified Registered Nurse Intravenous (CRNI). An expert nurse gives advice and consultation throughout the litigation process.

NURSING FAST FACT!

The specialty area of I.V. therapy is a high-risk technical area.

Risk Management and Risk Assessment

The Revised Infusion Nursing Standards of Practice (INS, 2000) define **risk management** as "a process that centers on identification, analysis, treatment, and evaluation of real and potential hazards." Risk assessment is the scientific process of asking how risky something is. It is a process of collecting and analyzing scientific data "to describe the form, dimension, and characteristics of risk." Risk assessment and risk management are equally important but different processes, with different objectives, information content, and results.

Risk management concepts include the concerns that organizations face with exposure to losses. Organizations handle the chances of losses or risks by financing, purchasing insurance, or practicing loss control. Loss control consists of preventive and protective activities that are performed before, during, and after losses are incurred. Risk management involves all medical and facility staff. It provides for the review and analysis of risk and liability sources involving patients, visitors, staff, and facility property. Risk management consists of the following components:

- Identification and management of clinical areas of actual and high risk
- Identification and management of nonclinical (e.g., visitor, staff) areas of actual and high risk
- Identification and management of probable claims events
- Management of property loss occurrences
- Review and analysis of customer surveys and patient complaints
- Review and analysis of risk assessment surveys
- Operational linkages with hospital **quality management**, safety, and **performance improvement** programs
- Provision of risk management education
- Compliance with state risk management and applicable federal statutes, including the Safe Medical Devices Act (Clinical Orientation Manual, 1998)

Risk assessment is performed by government agencies such as the U.S. Environmental Protection Agency (EPA). Risk assessment takes different approaches depending on available information. Some assessments look back to try to assess effects after an event. They may also look ahead before a new product is approved for use.

JCAHO advocates establishing an integrated risk management and quality assurance program.

Risk management strategies combine the elements of both loss reduction and loss prevention. Risk management strategies that may decrease the risk of potential liability are as follows:

- Informed consent
- Unusual occurrence reports
- Sentinel events
- Documentation
- Professional liability insurance
- Patient relations
- Quality management (Alexander & Webster, 2001)

Informed Consent

One of the most effective proactive strategies taken in risk management is informed consent. The purpose of **informed consent** is to provide patients with enough information to enable them to make a rational decision regarding whether to undergo treatment. The focus is on a patient's understanding the procedure, not just signing consent to have the procedure performed.

The right of self-determination provides the basis for informed consent and is grounded in the bioethical principles of autonomy. A competent adult (competence to consent) is aware of the consequences of a decision and has the ability to make reasonable choices about health care, including the right to refuse health care.

There are categories of necessary elements for informed consent and informed refusal. The first category comprises the information elements. This involves the disclosure of appropriate information. Generally, this disclosure must include benefits and risks of procedure, alternative procedures, benefits and risk of the alternatives, and the qualifications of the provider.

The second category consists of the consent elements. The consent must be voluntary, not coerced. Consent can be manifested by conduct. For example, the infusion specialist states, "I am going to restart your I.V. now," and the patient holds out his or her arm.

There may be limits to consent, such as waiver of consent: the patient must know that options and risks exist even if he or she does not want to know what they are. Other limits to consent include verbal limits; for example, the patient may tell the infusion nurse, "Okay, I will let you try to restart my I.V., but only once."

The duty to obtain informed consent belongs to the person who will perform the procedure, but also may belong to the licensed person who is aware that the patient has not been informed, does not understand, or did not consent. A breach of this duty may result in discipline for unprofessional practice and/or a civil lawsuit for professional malpractice. If the infusion specialist knows that consent does not exist or the patient is not informed and has not waived that right, the infusion specialist must consult with the ordering provider, and go up the chain of command for assistance. Refer to Table 1–2 for elements necessary for informed consent (Collins, 2001).

INS Standard. The patient or a representative legally authorized to act on the patient's behalf shall be informed of potential complications associated with treatment or therapy. The nurse shall docu-

> Table 1–2 **ELEMENTS NECESSARY FOR INFORMED CONSENT**

Information Elements
Benefits and risks of the procedure
Alternative procedures
Benefits and risks of the alternatives
Qualifications of the provider

Consent Elements
Consent form on chart or waiver of consent
Consent is manifest by conduct; it is a voluntary process
Limits to consent
Waiver of consent: patient must know that options and risks exist even if he or she does not want to know what they are.

Note: Exceptions to requirement for consent are emergency situations, and other situations such as crimes, public safety, or healthcare worker safety (Collins, 2001).

ment the information given and patient's or legally authorized representative's response in the patient's medical record. (INS, 2000, 11)

Unusual Occurrence Reports

Unusual occurrence reports should be filed every time there is a deviation from the standard. These reports are simple records of an event and are considered an internal reporting mechanism for performance improvement. They should be reported to the superior staff member and the episode must be objectively charted, but reference to the report should not appear in the legal patient record.

The occurrence report should contain the following 10 key points:

1. Patient's admitting diagnosis
2. Date when the incident occurred
3. Patient's room number
4. Age of the patient
5. Location of the incident
6. Type of incident
7. Nature of incident (e.g., medication error, mislabeling, misreading, policy and procedure not followed, overlooked order on chart, patient identification not checked). It should be noted (on the unusual occurrence report) if a physician's order was needed after the occurrence.
8. Factual description of the incident
9. Patient's condition before the incident
10. Results of the incident or injury

NURSING FAST FACT!

Unusual occurrence reports are meant to be nonjudgmental, factual reports of the problem and its consequences.

Unusual occurrence reports are useful for identification of patterns of I.V. medication errors or potentially dangerous situations. Trend analysis monitors patterns of their occurrences. Nursing staff members must feel free to file reports; a report is not an admission of negligence. These reports have the potential to save lives by identifying unsafe practices. More than ever before, risk may be managed by prevention. In 1996, the JCAHO implemented five indicators on medication use for its Indicator Measurement System, a performance measurement system intended to help evaluate the performance of healthcare organizations as part of its survey and accreditation process.

INS Standard. An Unusual Occurrence Report shall document unusual or unanticipated occurrences or variances in practice. The report should be shared with appropriate departments, such as risk management and performance improvement teams. The report should result in specific quality and performance improvement measures as required by organizational policies and procedures. (INS, 2000, 16)

Documentation

Documentation provides legal accountability, communicates information to other healthcare workers, provides information for reimbursement, and assists with outcomes monitoring (Moureau & Maney, 2003). **Documentation** should be an accurate, timely, and complete written account of the care rendered to the patient. The healthcare record charts the patient's history, health status, and **goal** achievement. It should be objective and completed promptly. Documentation should be legible and include only standard abbreviations. Nurses and other healthcare providers should keep charts free of criticism or complaints. There should be no vacant lines in charts, and every entry should be signed. In an office or home care environment, dates of return visit, canceled or failed appointments, all telephone conversations, and all follow-up instructions should be recorded on the chart.

Since the 1990s, the emphasis has been on quality improvement, with a focus on evaluating organizational and clinical performance outcomes. Documentation is one way of evaluating **outcomes**. The many formats for charting include the problem-oriented medical record, pie charting, focus charting, narrative charting, and charting by exception. Regardless of the format developed for documenting infusion therapy, basic requirements of the plan of care exist, including goals, actual and potential problems, and nursing interventions and outcomes.

Documentation should include the number of attempts for each procedure, the patient's response to the procedure, adverse events, actions taken in the presence of complications, patient education provided, and descriptive information given for the informed consent and the patient's response (Moureau & Maney, 2003).

The Infusion Nurses Society (2000, 17) Standards of Practice recommend the following documentation guidelines:

- Type, length, and gauge of vascular access device
- Date and time of insertion, number and location of attempts, identification of site, type of dressing, and identification of the person inserting the device
- Patient's tolerance of insertion
- For midline (ML) and peripherally inserted central catheters (PICCs): external catheter length, midarm circumference, effective length of catheter inserted, and radiographic confirmation of the location of catheter tip if required
- Site condition and appearance using standardized assessment scales for phlebitis and/or infiltration/extravasation

- Care of site
- Specific safety or infection control precautions taken
- Patient or caregiver participation in and understanding of therapy and procedures
- Communication among healthcare professionals responsible for patient care and monitoring
- Type of therapy; drug; dose; and rate, time, and method of administration
- Patient's tolerance of therapy
- Pertinent diagnosis, assessment, and vital signs
- Client's symptoms, response to therapy, and/or laboratory test results
- Barriers to care or therapy and/or complications
- Discontinuation of therapy, including catheter length and integrity, site appearance, dressing applied, and patient tolerance

INS Standard. Documentation shall be legible, accessible to qualified personnel, and readily retrievable. The protocol for documentation should be established in organizational policies and procedures. (INS, 2000, 17)

Developing and Participating in Product Evaluation

Product Problem Reporting

In 1990, the Medical Device Act was amended to clearly place responsibility for ensuring that medical devices in domestic commercial distribution are safe and effective for their intended purposes.

The infusion nurse specialist plays an important role in the product selection and evaluation processes. Ongoing evaluation of products in use is important in the delivery of high-quality patient care. The infusion nurse specialist's participation with his or her colleagues from other departments enhances commitment to the specialty and to the facility (Alexander & Webster, 2001).

The Food and Drug Administration (FDA) regulates products in the United States, including over-the-counter and prescription drugs and pharmaceuticals, food, cosmetics, veterinary products, biologic devices, and medical devices. Nurses use many medical devices and are usually the primary reporters of device problems.

The following are examples of medical device problems related to I.V. therapy practice:

- Loose or leaking catheter hubs
- Occluded cannula
- Defective infusion pump tubing
- Contaminated infusates

- Misleading labeling
- Inadequate packaging
- Cracked or leaking I.V. solution bag

When to Report

Participation in product evaluation is an ongoing responsibility of professional practitioners. Inappropriate use of medical devices may contribute to pain and suffering. The FDA evaluates approximately 2000 medical devices each month. Devices are inspected on three levels:

1. Good manufacturing controls
2. Application for a device existing before 1976 and in common use
3. Implantable or hazardous devices

The simple act of "gerryrigging" or otherwise manipulating a device to overcome a small problem results in the liability for problems arising from use of that piece of equipment residing with the institution. The law states that the responsibility shifts to the institution when a practitioner interferes with the design of a piece of equipment.

What to Report

Report any problems with medical devices if the event observed involves, or has the potential to cause, a death, serious injury, or life-threatening malfunction. In 1992, a congressional hearing focused on needle safety, a needleless system, and safe medical devices. Since this hearing, the Occupational Safety and Health Administration (OSHA) and the Centers for Disease Control and Prevention (CDC), along with the FDA, have been collaboratively reviewing the issue of safe medical devices. OSHA expects hospitals to have an ongoing system in place to evaluate safer medical devices.

Report a complete description of the problem. Information regarding the device needs to be submitted, including:

- Product name
- Manufacturer's name and address
- Identification numbers of the device (lot number, model number, serial number, expiration date)
- Problem noted
- Name, title, and practice specialty of the device's user

How to Report

To report serious adverse events and problems with all medical products to MedWatch, complete their postage-paid form or contact them via telephone (800-FDA-1088), fax (800-FDA-1088), or their Website (*www.fda.gov/medwatch/report/hcp.htm*).

NURSING FAST FACT!

Use facilities under the Safe Medical Device Act (SMDA) of 1990 are legally required to report suspected medical device–related deaths to both the FDA and the manufacturer, if known, and serious injuries to the manufacturer or the FDA if the manufacturer is unknown. Health professionals within a user facility should familiarize themselves with their institution's procedures for SMDA reporting. The MedWatch form can be downloaded from the FDA's Website.

INS Standard. Infusion Nursing Standards of Practice (2000) address the nurse's role in product evaluation, product integrity, and product defect reporting. (Standard 18, 19, 20, 2000)

Performance Improvement and Quality Patient Management

Quality assurance (QA) may be defined as the determination of the degree of excellence through monitoring and evaluation to detect and resolve problems.

Risk Management + Quality Assurance = Quality Management

Quality management is a systematic process to ensure desired patient outcomes. A quality management program includes both risk management and quality assurance and is established to objectively identify, evaluate, and solve problems associated with I.V. patient treatment modalities.

Quality assurance requirements have always been a part of JCAHO's accreditation process, but introduction of the Agenda for Change in 1986 shifted the emphasis from problem-solving endeavors to continuous improvement of quality. With this shift, JCAHO initiated the transition from QA to **continuous quality improvement (CQI)**. The goal was to create **outcome** monitoring and evaluation processes to assist organizations in improving the quality of care. QA frequently focuses solely on the clinical aspects of care rather than on the interrelated managerial, governance, support, and clinical processes that affect patient care outcomes. Quality cannot be assured; it can only be assessed, managed, or improved. Dennis O'Leary, JCAHO president, has admitted that, in retrospect, quality assurance was an "unfortunate semantic selection because it does not accurately reflect JCAHO's vision of quality."

Beginning in the 1980s, healthcare consumers, third-party payers, and healthcare providers began looking at positive patient outcomes as a measure of quality. JCAHO was the driving force in this movement, along with peer review organizations (PROs), Medicare and Medicaid reimbursement regulations, federal and state laws, and court interpretations of liability and private health insurers' standards. In the early 1980s, guidelines initiated by JCAHO were formed to provide a nursing quality assurance (NQA) committee. This committee recognized that QA had to be ongoing to ensure high-quality patient care. The committee in each facility should include management, chief nursing officers, and staff members. NQA focuses on two endeavors: checking achievement of standards and solving patient care problems.

In 1995 JCAHO changed the wording of continuous quality improvement to **performance improvement (PI).** The goal of improving organization performance is to continuously improve patient health outcomes.

Approaches to Quality Management

Assessing the achievement of nursing care standards involves measuring the quality of care provided. This is part of the nursing process: observing care delivered, assessing patient satisfaction, documenting care received, and evaluating outcomes based on short- and long-term goals. Involving staff in quality assessments can increase their awareness of standards, as well as enhance their assessment skills. Three approaches to outcome are CQI; total quality management (TQM); and the newest approach, performance improvement (PI).

Continuous Quality Improvement

CQI is an approach to quality management that builds on the traditional QA models. This approach was first introduced in 1992 as an effective way to improve the quality of health care. In 1992, JCAHO first introduced standards that mandated CQI methodology from hospitals receiving accreditation surveys. CQI broadens the focus to all facets of an organization that affect patient outcomes, not just to those that affect the clinical aspects of care. An essential characteristic of CQI is that it is continuous; outcomes are never optimized but may be constantly improved. A distinctive feature of CQI is that it emphasizes improvement in the interdisciplinary processes involved in patient care delivery. CQI incorporates leadership principles from TQM and has become the central theme or standard in health care.

Performance Improvement

The use of outcomes and other performance measures complements the application of standards and completes the quality equation. Performance results usually validate the fact that an organization did the right things and provide the baseline stimulus for future quality improvement activities (JCAHO, 2000).

Performance is what is done and how well it is done to provide health care. Characteristics of what is done and how well it is done are called **dimensions of performance**.

Doing the right thing includes:

- The *efficacy* of the procedure or treatment in relation to the client's condition
- The *appropriateness* of a specific test, procedure, or service to meet the client's need

Doing the right thing well includes:

- The *availability* of a needed test, procedure, treatment, or service to the client who needs it
- The *timeliness* with which a needed test, procedure, treatment, or service is provided to the client
- The *effectiveness* with which tests, procedures, treatments, and services are provided.
- The *continuity* of the services provided to the client with respect to other services, practitioners, and providers over time
- The *safety* of the client and others to whom the care and services are provided
- The *efficiency* with which care and services are provided (JCAHO, 2000)
- The *respect and caring* with which care and services are provided

In 1998, JCAHO established standards, scoring, and aggregation rules for improving organization performance. The standards can be downloaded from their Website.

Website

JCAHO: *www.jcaho.org/standard/Itc-pi.html*

Other sites:

Total Quality Management

With the shift from QA to CQI and now to PI, healthcare organizations have recognized that quality is not a fixed commodity defined by healthcare professionals but is a strategic mission that must be shared by the entire organization. **Total quality management (TQM)** is an outgrowth of several healthcare organizations that have adopted a management system fostering continuous improvement at all levels and for all functions by focusing on maximizing customer satisfaction. TQM and CQI share many characteristics; however, unlike CQI, TQM is not unique to health care. It requires that those in top management be committed to the program and provide a clear vision for the organization; employees must participate actively in the quality improvement process. TQM contributes to a positive work environment, fosters collaboration, and promotes teamwork to enhance interdepartmental communication (Sierchio, 2001).

The quality improvement process may be performed by using lengthy studies, short-term sampling, or problem solving with documentation and reporting. Three categories are used to create a model for quality management, and each is linked as a measurement of quality patient care. The three categories are structure, process, and outcome.

Structure

Structure consists of the conditions and mechanisms that provide support for the actual provision of care. This is defined as evaluation of resources, both material and human. Material resources are classified as facilities, equipment, mission, philosophy, goals of organization, and financial resources. Human resources include the number and qualifications of nurses performing I.V.-related procedures.

Process

Process denotes what is actually done in giving and receiving care. Process is a goal-directed, interrelated series of actions, events, mechanisms, or steps. It includes a patient's activities in seeking care, **data collection**, and a practitioner's activities in making a nursing diagnosis, along with evaluation of actual performance of procedures. This link sets the standards by which evaluation can take place. Process standards focus on job descriptions, performance standards, procedures, and protocols.

Outcome

Outcome denotes the effect of care on the health status of patients. The result of the performance (or nonperformance) of a function or process is the outcome. Improvements in a patient's knowledge and changes in his or her health status are components of outcome criteria. The assessment of outcomes is a method by which quality of care is established. Outcome in the practice of I.V. therapy should reflect final results of the therapy, including patient recovery and rates of complications. Table 1–3 presents an example of a quality management model for catheter-related sepsis.

In summary, the goals of PI are to (1) prevent complications, (2) decrease morbidity and mortality, (3) decrease cost, (4) shorten hospital stays, (5) increase patient comfort, and (6) increase patient knowledge.

> Table 1–3 **EXAMPLE OF QUALITY MANAGEMENT MODEL: CATHETER-RELATED SEPSIS**

Structure (equipment)
- Aseptic equipment available for insertion of I.V. therapy
- Experience of clinician inserting line

Process
- Before line insertion, the site is prepared per policy and procedure by nurse
- I.V. lines are assessed for continued need after 72 hours

Outcome
- The rate of catheter-related sepsis will be less than X% *(Percentage determined by hospital, patient population, and experience of clinician inserting lines.)*

Helpful guidelines for evaluation of PI include the following:

- Centers for Disease Control (CDC), Guidelines for Prevention of Intravascular Infections
- Infusion Nurses Society (INS), Revised Infusion Nursing Standards of Practice, 2000
- Joint Commission on Accreditation of Healthcare Organizations (JCAHO) Performance Standards for I.V. Therapy
- American Association of Blood Banking (AABB)

Evidence-Based Practice

Current trends in nursing reflect an emphasis on **evidence-based practice.** The goal of evidence-based nursing (EBN) is to apply valid and reliable nursing research to clinical practice. A further goal is to bring the most current knowledge to clinicians. This is particularly important in light of the knowledge explosion in nursing and health care (Sisk, 2002).

Sources of information for clinical decision making include textbooks, journals, bibliographic databases, distilled information presented in the journal *Evidence-Based Nursing*, and Internet sites.

The methodology of EBN is comparable to that of evidence-based medicine, the problem-solving process. Evidence-based nursing is a five-step process:

1. Construct a relevant, answerable question from a clinical case.
2. Plan and carry out a search of the literature for the best external evidence.
3. Critically appraise the literature for validity and applicability.
4. Apply the evidence to your clinical practice.
5. Evaluate your performance.

Evidence-based practice has developed in the United States as a result of the emphasis on clinical research and the establishment of the National Institute for Nursing Research in the 1980s. EBN is an international movement, with leadership from nurses in the United Kingdom, the United States, Australia, New Zealand, and Germany.

Websites

Center for Evidence-Based Nursing: *www.york.ac.uk.healthsciences/centres/evidence/celon.htm*

Journal of Evidence-Based Nursing: *www.ebn.bmjjournals.com*

Evidence-based filters for Ovid CINAHL: *www.urmc.rochester.edu/Miner/Educ.ebnfilt.htm*

University of Minnesota: Evidence-Based Nursing: *www.evidence.ahc.umn.edu/ebn.htm*

Using I.V. therapy–related research studies to develop changes in procedure or policy, along with published standards such as Infusion Nurses Standards of Practice, is one way to apply evidence-based practice to infusion practice. The application of research to practice is important; however, it requires an investment of attention, methods, and resources to achieve the best outcomes for a specific patient population.

Benchmarking

Benchmarking is the collection and monitoring of key indicators that are reflective of a program's clinical performance (Galloway, 2002). Consumers are now more aware of healthcare organization quality indicators, such as morbidity and mortality. If an organization cannot demonstrate its own quality care measures, it risks losing patients and managed care contracts. This has propelled benchmarking into the realm of common business practice as a tool to enhance leverage within industry markets (Tran, 2003).

Problem-based benchmarking targets efforts toward improving specific concerns, such as improving medication error rate or decreasing patient waiting times. More recently, facilities are turning to process-based benchmarking, which entails targeting continuous improvement of key processes.

Managers can benchmark to help decide a variety of factors: where to allocate resources more efficiently, when to seek outside assistance, how to quickly improve current operations, and whether customer requirements are being adequately met.

Benchmarking can be used in infusion therapy to validate infusion therapy teams. By monitoring pertinent patient outcomes related to vascular access devices (VADs), facilities that use benchmarking can expect to see fewer problems with VADs, less difficulty starting catheters, less stress for patient and staff, less waiting time for central lines, less interruption of prescribed therapy, a shorter length of hospital stay, and increased patient and staff satisfaction (Galloway, 2002).

Barcoding

A new, advanced technological step to reduce and prevent medication administration errors is barcode-enabled point-of-care (BPOC) technology. It includes standard reports that reflect errors made, errors prevented, and reasons why nurses overrode warning messages. This quality improvement strategy to prevent medication errors is one step toward performance improvement (Douglas & Larrabee, 2003).

Developing Nursing Competency Standards

Competency Standards

JCAHO (2000) defines **competency** as "a determination of an individual's capability to perform expectations." A **competent** nurse in I.V. therapy is well qualified by education and capable of performing I.V. therapy in an exact and effective manner using the appropriate knowledge of nursing, technical expertise, and specialized skills (Dugger, 1997). Within the educational context, competency may be defined as a simultaneous integration of the knowledge, skills, and attitudes required for performance in a designated role and setting. In developing standards, it is important to have a clear understanding of terms such as *competent* and *competency*.

The practice setting for I.V. therapy delivery is as varied as the patient populations served by this specialty practice. In treatment of patients ranging from hospitalized neonates to elderly persons in extended care facilities or private homes, the competencies of nurses and the combination of knowledge, skills, and abilities necessary to fulfill the role of a nurse administering I.V. therapy span all ages and disease processes. Basic competencies are intended to serve as guidelines for practicing nurses and to assist in designing orientation and continuing education programs (Delisio, 2001).

I.V. nursing is defined as using the nursing process relating to technical and clinical application of fluids, electrolytes, infection control, oncology, pediatrics, pharmacology, quality assurance, technology and clinical applications, parenteral nutrition, and transfusion therapy (Delisio, 2001). The practice of I.V. nursing encompasses the nursing management and coordination of care to the patient in accordance with:

1. State statutes
2. INS standards of practice

3. Established institutional policy
4. JCAHO requirements

Elements

Elements of I.V. nursing competency include:

1. Accountability: The role of I.V. nurses implies that nurses are astute and knowledgeable enough to adjust their **interventions** (i.e., interference that may affect outcome) to accomplish short- and long-term care goals.
2. Communication: Exchange of information allows everyone involved in the patient's care to make intelligent decisions based on complete data and professional collaboration.
3. Collaboration: JCAHO demands multidisciplinary involvement at all levels of patient care. I.V. leaders must develop the skills of collaboration, consultation, and negotiation to achieve positive patient outcomes.
4. Autonomy: Nurses can have increased autonomy by being allowed to make certain decisions independently (Dugger, 1997).

Competency-Based Educational Programs

Competency-based educational programs establish specific goals, accountability, individualization, and behaviors for practitioners by defining clear expectations for levels of performance. The responsibility of ensuring a competent staff often falls to the institution in which a nurse is practicing. A framework for developing staff competencies and ensuring that the institution is delivering safe care includes:

- Development of standards
- Development of skills test
- Assessment of learning needs
- Establishment of a plan of educational programs
- Presentation of educational programs
- Evaluation of learning outcomes

Competencies should be directed toward essential mandatory aspects of performance, have measurable clinical behaviors, include **evaluation** mechanisms, and test cognitive performance **criteria**. A competency program can consist of self-assessment, skill checklist, self-study modules, written examinations, and program evaluation (Rudzik, 1999).

Three-Part Competency Model

A three-part competency model includes:

1. Competency statement: Statement that reflects a measurable goal
2. Domains of learning criteria: Cognitive criteria (knowledge base) and performance criteria (psychomotor skills: observed behaviors)

3. Evaluation and learning outcomes: Written tests, return demonstrations, and precepted clinical experience

This model will be used in each chapter of this book as a framework for assessing competency of I.V. practitioners.

All professional nurses are accountable and responsible for all parts of the tasks associated with I.V. therapy and for tasks that are delegated to the licensed practical nurse or technician for care rendered to the patient while under care (Dugger, 1997). The three-part competency model is an effective tool for ensuring competent practice. A competency-based educational model requires developing the three major parts of the model: the competency statement, the performance criteria, and the evaluation and learning options.

Competency Validation Program

The **competency validation program** (CVP) is based on current literature related to competency programs and reflects the work of Nursing Department Shared Governance Committees, the Nursing Department Education Center, and other Nursing Department staff. The CVP presumes that both professional and nonprofessional direct care providers are responsible and accountable for their practices and the outcomes of their patient care and other work (NIH, 2003). The CVP is available on the National Institute of Health's (NIH's) Website. Refer to Table 1–4 for Core Competency Guidelines.

Website

National Institute of Health: *wwwohrm.cc.nih.gov/train/competency*

> Table 1–4 **CORE COMPETENCY GUIDELINES**

Core competency (CC) must be written as a performance element.

Acceptable Methods of Assessing Competency

Direct observation by a supervisor, designated evaluator, instructor, or preceptor while the employee/student demonstrates the skill in the work setting

Observation by a supervisor, designated evaluator, instructor, or preceptor while the employee/student demonstrates the skills in simulated settings, such as skill labs and mock drills.

Direct observation and return demonstration may be supplemented with other forms of assessment such as tests. The testing should not be the primary means of assessment.

Documentation of Competency

Competency assessments will be documented

Assessment of core competencies will be documented on the CC Performance Enhancement Plan (PEP)

Use of department competency checklist or a department job/specific competency

Source: *NIH (2003).*

NURSING FAST FACT!

The NIH strongly recommends a "customer service" competency.

The core competencies for customer service as identified by the NIH (2003) apply to any setting; however, to provide for positive patient outcomes and avoid litigation, the following guidelines should be part of the nursing competencies for any facility: The nurse anticipates, assesses, and responds effectively to the needs of diverse customers both internal and external, making excellent customer service the first priority.

INS Standard. Clinical competencies should be in accordance with the state Nurse Practice Act and Infusion Nursing Standards of Practice. (INS, 2000, 5)

Occupational Risks

Two types of occupational hazards are associated with I.V. therapy: biologic and physical hazards. Inserting intravenous catheter lines, giving injections, handling and discarding sharps, and assisting with sterile procedures and many other high-risk procedures are an ordinary part of the daily practice regimen for nurses, especially those specializing in infusion therapy (Monarch, 2002).

Biologic Hazards

Hazards of bloodborne pathogens must be communicated to infusion nurses during training. Training should include information on bloodborne pathogens, as well as OSHA regulations and employers' exposure control plans. Healthcare employees face a significant risk as the result of occupational exposure to materials that may contain bloodborne pathogens, including hepatitis B virus (HBV), which causes hepatitis B (a serious liver disease) and human immunodeficiency virus (HIV), which causes acquired immunodeficiency syndrome (AIDS).

According to OSHA (2001), percutaneous injury with exposure to HIV- or HBV-infected blood in healthcare workers has accounted for 80 percent of occupational exposures, with 20 percent occurring before or during the use of needles and up to 70 percent after use and before disposal. Most needlestick injuries result from using unsafe needle devices rather than from carelessness by healthcare workers. Safer needle devices have been shown to significantly reduce needlestick injuries and exposures to potentially fatal bloodborne illnesses (CDC, 2001).

Factors that significantly increase infusion nurses' potential for exposure to HIV, HBV, and hepatitis C virus (HCV) include:

1. Use of hollow-bore catheters (over the needle catheters)
2. The increasing use of central line catheters in the hospital and home environment
3. The increasing number of nurses placing peripherally inserted central catheters (PICCs) in various settings
4. The expanding application of implantable vascular access catheters with manipulation of needles to access and de-access these devices

Exposure can be minimized or eliminated using a combination of engineering and work practice controls, personal protective clothing and equipment, training, medical surveillance, hepatitis B vaccination, signs and labels, and other provisions (OSHA, 2001).

Prevention of Exposure to Bloodborne Pathogens

STANDARD PRECAUTIONS

Nurses should follow standards established by OSHA regarding glove wearing and handwashing practices. All bodily secretions, and therefore fluids from patients, are potentially infectious. All personnel who have contact with patients must adhere to strict guidelines.

The National Institute for Occupational Safety and Health Rules for Occupational Exposure to Bloodborne Pathogens Standard enforces amended regulations regarding standard precautions (NIOSH, 2000b). OSHA's new standard makes universal (standard) precautions fully enforceable for the first time and spells out what inspectors will look for. Healthcare workers should be aware of how the rules are observed in each agency. The CDC established an additional system of isolation precautions. This new concept was adopted in 1996. Unlike universal precautions, which list "certain" body fluids as posing possible risks for transmission of bloodborne pathogens, standard precautions take a broader approach to the protection of medical staffs and patients. These new guidelines contain two tiers of precautions: standard and transmission based. Standard precautions combine the major features of universal precautions and body substance isolation (CDC, 2001).

For further information on infection control practices, see Chapter 2, Infection Control.

NEEDLELESS SYSTEMS

The Needlestick Safety and Prevention Act of November 2000, which took effect in April of 2001, reinforces the need to use safe needles to reduce injuries. Needleless systems and needle safety systems are the state-of-the-art technology of needle systems and are used to connect I.V. devices, administer infusates and medications, and sample blood. Estimates indicate that 600,000 to 800,000 needlestick and other percutaneous injuries occur annually in the United States (EPINet, 2000).

Needlestick injuries are associated with recapping the needle, improperly discarding the needle, carelessness, and accidents while performing tasks. Needlestick injuries can lead to exposure to HIV, HBV, HCV, and cytomegalovirus (CMV).

Properly designed safer needle devices provide:

- A barrier between the hands and the needle after use
- A means to allow or require the worker's hands to remain behind the needle at all times
- Safety features integral to the device itself rather than as accessories
- A feature that is in effect before disassembly
- Simple and easy operation with little or no training
- Minimum interference with the delivery of patient care

NOTE > Safety features for needleless and needle protection systems are discussed in detail in Chapter 6.

Exposure Prevention Information Network (EPINet) is a program that includes manuals and software, data collection tools, and tracking and reporting systems for surveillance of bloodborne exposures to track device injuries and evaluate the efficacy of safer needle devices.

Postexposure Prophylaxis (PEP)

Healthcare organizations should have a plan in place before an exposure occurs. This can be easily derived from the CDC updated guidelines of June 2001 (CDC, 2001). The following are essential elements in responding to an actual event:

1. Refer to the exposure plan for the organization.
2. Wash the wound or flush mucous membrane with water or saline.
3. Report the exposure to the appropriate department or individual ASAP.
4. Evaluate the risk of exposure.
5. Evaluate the source patient.
6. Evaluate the exposed person.
7. Make a decision about prophylaxis or therapy.
8. Make plans for follow-up (Tice, 2002).

Resources

EPINet: 800-528-9803
CDC Bloodborne pathogen PEP hotline: 800-893-0485
National Clinicians' Postexposure Prophylaxis hotline: 888-448-4911
Hepatitis Hotline: 888-443-7232

Websites

Needlestick information: UCLA Website: *www.needlestick.mednet.ucla.edu*
OSHA: *www.osha.gov* (See Safer Needle Devices, Protecting Health Care Workers)
National Clinicians' Postexposure Prophylaxis: *www.ucsf.edu.hivcntr*
CDC Hepatitis Branch: *www.cdc.gov/ncidod/disease/hepatitis/ hepatitis.htm*
EPINet: *www.med.virginia.edu*

Other sites:

Physical Hazards

Physical hazards associated with I.V. therapy include (but are not limited to) abrasions, contusions, chemical exposure, and latex allergy.

Abrasions and Contusions

Abrasions and contusions can be caused by needlesticks and contact with broken glass, sharp edges of containers, or any jagged-edge item. Small or undetected skin abrasions can be potential portals for microorganisms or viruses such as *Staphylococcus aureus*, herpes simplex, and HIV. Use caution when assembling and manipulating I.V. equipment. Excellent hand hygiene practices following CDC guidelines and use of barrier precautions prevent the invasion of microorganisms.

Chemical Exposure

OSHA published guidelines for the management of cytotoxic (antineoplastic) drugs in the workplace in 1986. Since that time, surveys indicated further clarification was needed in management of exposure to chemicals. OSHA revised its recommendations for hazardous drug handling in 1995. To provide recommendations consistent with current scientific knowledge, the information was expanded to cover hazardous drugs, in addition to the cytotoxic. The recommendations apply to all settings in which employees are occupationally exposed to hazardous drugs (OSHA, 2001).

Hazardous drugs (HDs) have demonstrated the ability to cause chromosome breakage in circulating lymphocytes and mutagenic activity in urine, along with causing skin necrosis after surface contacts with abraded skin or damage to normal skin. It is recommended that nurses preparing HDs wear surgical latex gloves (double gloves if these do not interfere with techniques) and wear a protective disposable gown made of lint-free, low-permeability fabrics with closed front, long sleeves, and elastic or knit-closed cuffs when indicated. Because surgical masks do not protect against inhalation of aerosols, a biologic safety cabinet or an air-purifying respirator should be used when preparing HDs. A plastic face shield or splash goggles should be worn if a biologic safety cabinet is not used (OSHA, 1999).

NOTE > Chapter 14 discusses steps in handling hazardous drugs.

Latex Allergy

Natural rubber latex allergy is a serious medical issue for healthcare workers. Latex allergy develops with exposure to natural rubber latex, a plant cytosol that is used extensively to manufacture medical gloves and other medical devices. Allergic reactions to latex range from asthma to anaphylaxis that can result in chronic illness, disability, career loss, and death. There is no treatment for latex allergy except complete avoidance of latex. Patients and healthcare providers must be assured of safety from sensitization and allergic reaction to latex (ANA, 1997).

Latex allergy affects between 8 percent and 12 percent of workers in all health disciplines who are regularly exposed to latex. In the healthcare industry, workers at risk of latex allergy from ongoing latex exposure include physicians, nurses, aides, dentists, dental hygienists, operating room employees, laboratory technicians, and housekeeping personnel (OSHA, 1999).

Latex allergy is a type I immunoglobulin E (IgE)–mediated hypersensitivity reaction that involves systemic antibody formation to proteins in products made of natural rubber latex. Natural rubber latex is harvested commercially from the rubber tree, *Hevea brasiliensis,* and used to manufacture rubber products. Natural rubber latex contains up to 240 potentially allergenic protein fragments.

Nurses working in infusion therapy are at risk because of the common routes of exposure. The routes of exposure for latex reaction for infusion specialists include aerosol and glove contact. Aerosolized latex exposure may be the greatest danger for those with type I latex allergy caused by respiratory distress (Gritter, 1999). For healthcare workers, the exposure route can be powder released in the air during the removal of powdered latex gloves. Latex proteins are carried on the powder from gloves and latex balloons and can remain airborne for as long as 5 to 12 hours. Frequent use of gloves during the insertion and maintenance of I.V. therapy increases the risk of sensitization. Radioallergosorbent testing (RAST) immunoassay is a blood test that measures the serum level of latex-specific IgE.

INS Standard. Latex exposure should be minimized. Healthcare workers and patients are provided education regarding latex allergy or sensitivity and methods to minimize risk of exposure. Nonlatex personal protective equipment is provided to latex-sensitive individuals. Nonlatex supplies and equipment shall be used on patients who have or may have latex allergy or sensitivity. (INS, 2000, 34)

Those sensitive to latex should take the following precautions:

- Avoid all contact with latex.
- Carry auto-injectable epinephrine.
- Wear a medical identification bracelet.
- Negotiate with hospitals and providers in advance for latex-safe healthcare delivery (NIOSH, 1999).

To reduce the risk of an allergic response, avoid using hand lotions or lubricants that contain mineral oil, petroleum salves, and other hydrocarbon-based gels or lotions to prevent the breakdown of the glove material and maintain barrier protection. Do not reuse disposable examination gloves because disinfecting agents can damage the barrier properties of gloves. Following hand hygiene guidelines is recommended after gloves are removed and before a new pair is applied. Gloves should not be stored where they will be subjected to excessive heat, direct ultraviolet or fluorescent light, or ozone (NIOSH, 2000a).

NONLATEX GLOVES

Nonlatex gloves made of alternative materials, with barrier protection equal to or better than that of latex gloves, are available. The protective characteristic of each material must be taken into consideration in relationship to the purpose for which the glove will be used (HealthCare Without Harm, 2001).

Information on how to select medical gloves and a list of nonlatex glove alternatives are available from the Sustainable Hospital Project (SHP) at University of Massachusetts Lowell.

More information about requirements for medical gloves can be found in the Medical Glove Guidance Manual (publication FDA 99–4257) formerly known as Guidance for Medical Gloves: A Workshop Manual (Center for Devices and Radiological Health, 1999). The manual is available in the July 30, 1999 *Federal Register*, or you can obtain the rules from the Center for Devices and Radiological Health's Fact on Demand system (800-899-0381). Further information can be obtained from HealthCare Without Harm (202-234-0091).

Websites

HealthCare Without Harm: *www.noharm.org*
Medical Glove Guidance Manual: *www.fda.gov/cdrh/manual/ glovmanl.pdf*

Latex Allergy: *wwwlatexallergyrn.com*
Latex Allergy: *wwwlatexalergyresources.org*
National Institute of Health: *www.nlm.nih.gov/medlineplus/latexallergy.html*
NIOSH alert: *www.cdc.gov/niosh/latexalt.html*
Sustainable Hospital Project (SHP) at University of Massachusetts Lowell: *www.sustainablehospital.org*

Other sites:

Patient Education

State nursing boards mandate patient education by including it in their rules and regulations. Failure to adhere to these stipulations constitutes a violation of state law. JCAHO also has measurement criteria for evaluation of hospitals and home care agencies on patient education practices.

Although detailed instructions and explanations are presented to a patient, the patient may refuse treatment.

Home Care Issues

Creating a safe home care environment for a nurse visiting a patient is part of the risk management for home care. Nurses in alternative settings must be aware that they have the same occupational risks as hospital-based nurses: biologic hazards, latex allergy, needlestick injury, and chemical exposure, as well as the increased risks of physical hazards. The home care setting places nurses at risk of exposure to a variety of external hazards.

The HIPAA privacy act pertains to all healthcare settings; therefore, confidentiality has the same legal boundaries in the home care setting as in the hospital.

There are four models of alternate–site infusion therapy:

1. The Home Infusion Model: A community-based provider licensed as a pharmacy that provides both pharmaceutical services and nursing services as well as equipment and supplies. The home infusion provider may also contract with a nursing agency to provide the home nursing visits.
2. The Physician's Office Model: A physician's office-based infusion center. The patient travels to the office to receive his or her infusion care. Sometimes a patient is taught to self-infuse by the nursing staff at the physician's office and may go home with extra medication to self-administer at home.

3. The Ambulatory Infusion Center (AIC): A facility that operates as a department of a hospital system or a free-standing infusion center that operates in conjunction with a pharmacy provider. (Free-standing AICs cannot be reimbursed by Medicare or Medicaid.)
4. The Specialty Pharmacy Provider Model: Pharmaceuticals are mailed to the patient from a centralized pharmacy provider. This model is often used for patients with chronic conditions who have learned to self-infuse. In some cases the specialty pharmaceutical provider also contracts with a local nursing agency to perform the infusion or to teach the patient to self-infuse.

Key Points

- Primary sources of law include constitutional statutes, administrative law, and common law. (Civil and criminal law are the two main classifications directly related to nursing practice.)
- Common torts in the nursing practice of I.V. therapy: Coercion of a rational adult patient to place an I.V. cannula device constitutes assault and battery.
- Nurses must understand the elements of malpractice (including duty, breach of duty, causation, and harm) to recognize situations of liability and litigation.
- Breaches of duty related to infusion therapy include:
  - Delay in administration of medication
  - Unfamiliarity with the drug
  - Inappropriate route of administration
  - Failure to qualify orders
  - Negligence in patient teaching
- I.V. nurses testifying as expert witnesses should be certified in infusion therapy (i.e., have their CRNI).
- Categories of risk management include:
  - Identifying patterns of risk through internal audits and tracking
  - Reporting individual risk-related incidents
  - Developing and participating in product evaluation systems
  - Monitoring patient care
  - Preventing events most likely to lead to liability
- Strategies for risk management include:
  - Understanding laws that govern practice
  - Establishing nursing standards of practice
  - Obtaining informed consent
  - Developing and participating in product evaluation
  - Developing nursing competency standards
  - Documentation
  - Competency standards

- Approaches to quality management include:
  - Performance improvement (PI)
  - Continuous quality improvement (CQI)
  - Total quality management (TQM)
- Competency-based educational programs establish goals, accountability, and behaviors for practitioners. The framework for developing staff competencies includes:
  - Developing standards
  - Developing skill lists
  - Assessing learning needs
  - Planning educational programs
  - Presenting educational programs
  - Evaluating learning outcomes
- Three-part model
  - Step 1: Critical behaviors are identified and competency standards written.
  - Step 2: Steps of performance criteria are made.
  - Step 3: Evaluation and remediation
- Occupational risks associated with infusion therapy include:
  - Biologic hazards of bloodborne pathogens
  - Needlestick injuries
  - Abrasions and contusions
  - Chemical exposure
  - Latex allergy

Critical Thinking: Case Study

A nurse in an outpatient infusion clinic discusses with a friend the admission of a woman community leader who is receiving treatment for cancer. The nurse's friend then talks to others, who talk to still others, until there is widespread knowledge of the patient's cancer in the community. The woman's daughter hears about her mother's cancer diagnosis at school and is very upset.

What recent act was violated in the initial conversation? What are the ramifications for this case. Who is at fault?

Media Link: Answers to the case study and more critical thinking activities are located on the CD–ROM.

Post-Test

1. The three parts of a competency-based program include:
  a. Competency statement, goal, and return demonstration
  b. Competency statement, criteria for learning, and evaluation
  c. Goal, evaluation, and feedback
  d. Assessment, problem statement, implementation

2. Occupational risks associated with I.V therapy include:
   - **a.** Malpractice, documentation errors, negligence
   - **b.** Latex allergy, exposure to bloodborne pathogens, burns
   - **c.** Exposure to bloodborne pathogens, latex allergy, exposure to hazardous drugs
   - **d.** Ingestion of chemicals, needlestick injuries, malpractice
3. The tool used to report critical incidents is:
   - **a.** Performance improvement sheet
   - **b.** Unusual occurrence report
   - **c.** Competency validation tool
   - **d.** Quality assurance report
4. The definition of standard of practice states that it:
   - **a.** Defines activities and behaviors of the practitioner needed to achieve patient outcomes
   - **b.** Focuses on the recipient of care and describes outcomes that the patient can expect to receive
   - **c.** Is an ongoing systematic process for monitoring and problem solving
   - **d.** Refers to conditions and mechanisms that provide support for the delivery of care
5. A nurse walks into a patient's room and finds the I.V. solution container dry. The bag had been hung 1 hour earlier. The nurse informs the charge nurse and the physician that this has occurred. The nurse is instructed to complete an unusual occurrence report. The report allows the analysis of adverse patient events by:
   - **a.** Evaluating quality care and the potential risks for injury to the patient
   - **b.** Determining the effectiveness of nursing interventions
   - **c.** Providing a method of reporting injuries to local, state, and federal agencies
   - **d.** Providing clients with necessary stabilizing treatments
6. A product evaluation is part of a nurse's responsibility to ensure product integrity. Examples of medical device problems related to I.V. therapy practice include all of the following **EXCEPT:**
   - **a.** Defective infusion pump tubing
   - **b.** Misleading labeling
   - **c.** Cracked or leaking I.V. solution bag
   - **d.** Outdated medication

7. The Safe Medical Device Act requires that medical device–related deaths be reported to:
   a. FDA
   b. OSHA
   c. JCAHO
   d. CDC
8. An agency that tracks and provides an avenue for reporting bloodborne exposures is:
   a. OSHA
   b. CDC
   c. EPINet
   d. NIOSH
9. Characteristics of performance improvement (doing the right thing well) include all of the following **EXCEPT**:
   a. Availability of a needed test
   b. Documenting the quality of care received
   c. Timeliness with which the test, procedure, and treatment are provided
   d. Continuity of the services provided
10. The definition of a tort is:
    a. A written law enacted by the legislature
    b. A private wrong, by act or omission, that can result in a civil action by the harmed person
    c. An offense against the general public
    d. Being capable or able; knowing how to function

Media Link: More test questions and rationales are located on the CD-ROM

References

Alexander, M., & Webster, H.K. (2001). Legal aspects of intravenous nursing. In Hankins, J., Lonsway, R.A., Hedrick, C., & Perdue, M. (eds.). *Infusion Nursing Society: Infusion Therapy in Clinical Practice* (2nd ed.). St. Louis: W.B. Saunders, pp. 50–64.

American Nurses Association (1997). Position statement: Latex allergy (Internet). Available: *www.nursingworld.org* (Sept. 15, 1977).

Burkhardt, M.A., & Nathaniel, A. (2002). *Ethics and Issues in Contemporary Nursing* (2nd ed.). New York: Delmar Thomson Learning.

Center for Devices and Radiological Health (1999). Letter to the medical glove industry (Internet). Available: *www.fda.gov/cdrh/dsma/glovelet.html* (July 30, 1999).

Centers for Disease Control and Prevention (2001). Updated US public health service guidelines for the management of occupational exposure to HBV, BCV, HIV and recommendations for postexposure prophylaxis. *MMWR Morbidity Mortality Weekly Report*, 50(11), 1–52.

Collins, S.E. (2001). Litigation risks for infusion specialists: Understanding the issues. *Journal of Infusion Therapy*, 24(6), 375–380.

Delisio, N.M. (2001). Intravenous nursing as a specialty. In Hankins, J., Lonsway, R.A., Hedrick, C., & Perdue, M. (eds.). In *The Infusion Therapy in Clinical Practice* (2nd ed.). Infusion Nurses Society, pp. 6–13.

Douglas, J., & Larrabee, S. (2003). Bring barcoding to the bedside. *Nursing Management*, 34(5), 37–40.

Dugger, B. (1997). Intravenous nursing competency: Why is it important? *Journal of Intravenous Nursing*, 6(20), 287–299.

EPINet (1999). Exposure prevention information network data reports. University of Virginia: International Health Care Worker Safety Center.

Galloway, M. (2002). Using benchmarking data to determine vascular access device selection. *Journal of Infusion Therapy*, 25(5), 320–325.

Gritter, M. (1999). Latex allergy: Prevention is the key. *Journal of Intravenous Nursing*, 22(5), 281–285.

HealthCare Without Harm (2001). Latex allergy in Health Care Fact Sheet. Washington, DC: HealthCare Without Harm.

Higginbotham, E. (2003). Does error+injury = negligence? *RN* 66(5), 67–68.

Infusion Nurses Society (2000). Revised Infusion Nursing Standards of Practice, 21(1S), 7–19.

Infusion Nurses Society (2001). Infusion Nursing Code of Ethics. *Journal of Infusion Nursing*, 24(4), 242–243.

Institute for Safe Medication Practices (1999). The five rights. Available: *www.ismp.org/msarticles/fiveright.html* (July 31, 2003).

Joint Commission on Accreditation of Healthcare Organizations (2000). *Comprehensive Accreditation Manual for Hospitals.* Oakbrook Terrace, IL: JCAHO, pp. 239–273, 397–404

Kansas University Medical Center (1998). Clinical Orientation Manual. *Risk Management*. Available: *www3.kumc.edu/comanual/risk.htm* (April 1998), 1–3.

Monarch, K. (2002). Legal aspects of infusion practice: Trends and issues. *Journal of Infusion Therapy*, 25 (6S), S21–S35.

Moureau, N., & Maney, S. (2003). Legal aspects of infusion nursing. *Journal of Vascular Access Devices*, 8(1), 8–12.

National Institute for Occupational Safety and Health (NIOSH) (1999). *Latex Allergy: A Prevention Guide.* Atlanta: CDC Pub 98-113-Latex.

National Institute for Occupational Safety and Health (NIOSH) (2000a). *Alert: Preventing Allergic Reactions to Natural Rubber Latex in the Workplace.* Washington, DC: National Institute for Occupational Safety and Health. Publication 97–135.

National Institute for Occupational Safety and Health (NIOSH) (2000b). *ALERT Preventing Needlestick Injuries in Health Care Settings*. US Department of Health and Human Services. Publication No. 2000–108.

National Institutes of Health (2003). Core competency guidelines. Available: *www.ohrm.cc.nih.gov/train/competency* (July 27, 2003).

Occupational Safety and Health Administration (OHSA) (1999). *OSHA Technical Manual Controlling Occupational Exposure to Hazardous Drugs.* U.S. Department of Labor Occupational Safety & Health Administration. Section VI: Chapter 2.

Occupational Safety & Health Administration (OSHA) (1999). *Technical Information Bulletin:* Potential for allergy to natural rubber latex gloves and other natural rubber products. U.S. Department of Labor. Washington, DC: OSHA.

Occupational Safety and Health Administration (OHSA) (2001). Occupational exposure to blood borne pathogens; Needlesticks and other sharps injuries; final rule. *Federal Register*, 66, 5317–5325.

O'Keefe, M.E. (2000). *Nursing Practice and the Law: Avoiding Malpractice and Other Legal Risks*. Philadelphia: F.A. Davis.

Rudzik, J. (1999). Establishing and maintaining competency. *Journal of Intravenous Nursing*, 22(2), 69–73.

Satarawala, R. (2000). Legal perils of IV therapy. *Nursing 2000*, 30(8), 44–47.

Sierchio, G.P. (2001). Quality management. In Hankins, J., Lonsway, R.A., Hedrick, C., & Perdue, M. (eds.). *Infusion Nurses Society: Infusion Therapy in Clinical Practice* (2nd ed.). Philadelphia: W.B. Saunders, pp. 26–49.

Sisk, B. (2002). Evidence-based nursing. Clinical Nursing Resources newsletter. Available: *www.nursescribe.com*

Tice, A.D. (2002). Bloodborne pathogen exposure and recommendations for management. *Journal of Infusion Nursing*, 25(6S), S5–S9.

Tran, M.N. (2003). Take benchmarking to the next level. *Nursing Management*, 34 (1), 19–23.

U.S. Department of Health and Human Services (2003). The HIPAA Privacy Rule and Research. Available: *www.hhs.gov/ocr/hipass/finalreg.html* (July 2003).

Answers to Chapter 1 Post-Test

1. **b**
2. **c**
3. **b**
4. **a**
5. **a**
6. **d**
7. **a**
8. **c**
9. **b**
10. **b**

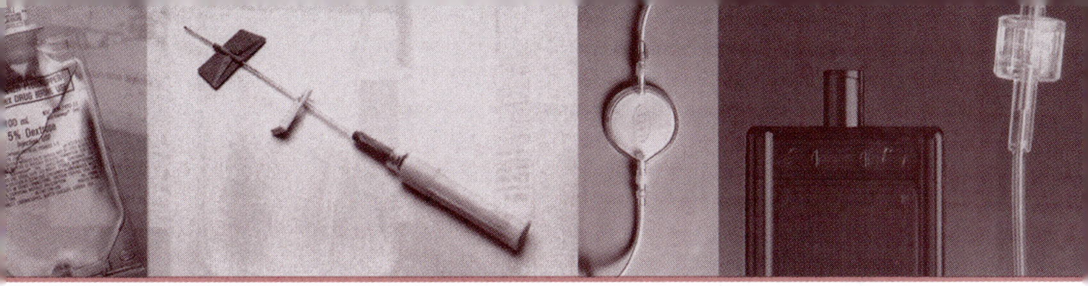

Chapter 2
Infection Control Measures

It may seem a strange principle to enunciate as the very first requirement in a hospital that it should do the sick no harm. It is quite necessary to lay down such a principle.
—Florence Nightingale, 1859

Chapter Contents

LEARNING OBJECTIVES

Upon completion of this chapter, the reader will be able to:

1. State the definitions of the glossary terms.
2. Discuss the function of the immune system.
3. Identify the organs involved in the immune system.
4. Identify the factors important for maintaining the well-being of the host.
5. State the four clinical symptoms of an impaired host.
6. State the causes of secondary immune deficiencies.
7. Identify the three carrier states.
8. Discuss the links in the chain of infection.
9. Identify strategies to prevent infection.
10. State the factors that influence formation of infusion phlebitis.
11. State the Infusion Nursing Standards of Practice for preventing infection.
12. Discuss sources of intravenous (I.V.) cannula-related infections.
13. State the most prevalent microorganisms found in I.V.-related infections.
14. Discuss the point of care for infection control practices related to infusion therapy.

GLOSSARY

Antigens Microbic invaders that bombard the body and trigger an immune response

Asepsis Freedom from infection or infectious material; absence of viable pathogenic organisms

Bloodborne pathogens Pathogenic microorganisms that are present in human blood and can cause disease in humans

Colonization Growth of microorganisms in a host without producing overt clinical symptoms or detected immune reaction

Contamination Microorganisms present on a body surface without tissue invasion or physiologic reaction

Dissemination Movement of microorganisms from an individual into the immediate environment or movement of microorganisms from a confined site (e.g., skin, kidney) to the bloodstream to other parts of the body

Endogenous Produced within or caused by factors within the organism

Epidemiology Branch of science concerned with the study of the factors determining and influencing the frequency and distribution of disease, injury, and other health-related events and their causes in a defined human population for the purpose of establishing programs to prevent and control their development and spread

Exogenous Developed or originating outside the organism

Extrinsic contamination Of external origin

Hand hygiene A general term that applies to either handwashing, antiseptic handwash, antiseptic hand rub, or surgical hand antisepsis

Hematogenous Produced by or derived from the blood; disseminated through the bloodstream or by the circulation

Host The organism from which a microorganism obtains its nourishment

Immunosuppression Inhibition of the formation of antibodies to antigens that may be present

Intrinsic contamination Contamination during manufacture

Leukopenia Reduction of the number of leukocytes in the blood to a count of 5000 or less

Nosocomial infection Hospital-acquired infection, which was not present or incubating at the time of admission

Passive acquired immunity Transient immunity that develops from a person-to-person passage of immune cells or from gamma-globulin infusion

Pathogen Any disease-producing agent or microorganism

Phlebitis Inflammation of a vein

Reservoir The place where the organism maintains its presence, metabolizes, and replicates

Resident flora Microorganisms that are indigenous to each individual and are present mainly on the skin and in the respiratory, gastrointestinal, and reproductive systems

Septicemia The presence of pathogenic microorganisms or their toxins in the blood or other tissues; the condition associated with such a presence

Transient flora Microorganisms that are picked up, usually on the skin, that can be removed fairly easily with hand hygiene.

Transmission The movement of an organism from the source to the host

Virulence Relative power and degree of pathogenicity possessed by organisms to produce disease

The intravenous system provides a direct access into the vascular system, and thus an understanding of basic epidemiology principles and common causative organisms due to infusion therapy is imperative. In the United States, the following organizations set standards and guidelines for infection control related to infusion therapy:

- U.S. Centers for Disease Control and Prevention (CDC), which is a division of the Department of Health and Human Services and establishes guidelines for infection control practices
- U.S. Occupational Safety and Health Administration (OSHA), which is the enforcing agency that provides the mandates to protect employees of all fields
- Infusion Nurses Society (INS), which sets standards for practice and provides a framework for the development of infusion policies and procedures in all practice settings
- Association of Vascular Access Network (NAVAN)
- Association of Practitioners in Infection Control and Epidemiology, Inc.

Websites

NAVAN: *www.navan.org*
APIC: *www.apic.org*
CDC: *www.cdc.org*
INS: *www.ins1.org*
National Nosocomial Infection Surveillance (NNIS): *www.cdc.gov/ncidod/hip/surveill/NNIS*

Other sites:

To be a competent practitioner, it is important to have an understanding of the functioning of the immune system, the principles of epidemiology, infectious disease processes, and infections caused by infusion therapy.

Immune System Function

The immune system provides the body with a way of distinguishing itself from foreign invaders. These invaders constantly bombard the body and trigger immune responses. They are termed **antigens** and can include microbes such as viruses, bacteria, and parasites. The appropriate immune response occurs when the immune system recognizes and destroys invading antigens.

The immune system also acts as a "clean-up crew" that disposes of used, mutant, or damaged cells that result from catabolism, growth, and injury (Smeltzer & Bare, 2004).

Organs

The organs and cells involved in the immune system form a complex when antigens and immune system cells are constantly moving through the lymph system, blood circulation, and lymphatic organs. The primary organs of the immune system are the thymus and bone marrow. Secondary organs include lymph nodes, spleen, liver, Peyer's patches, appendix, tonsils and adenoids, and lungs. Table 2–1 shows the locations and functions of these organs.

Mechanisms of Defense

A mutual compatibility exists between a healthy host (human) and environmental microbes. The factors most important in maintaining the well being of the host are nonspecific responses and specific immune

> Table 2–1 **ORGANS OF THE IMMUNE SYSTEM**

Organs	Location	Function
	Primary	
Thymus	Mediastinal cavity	Provides immune function in early years: T-cell development
Bone marrow	Ribs, sternum, long bones	Produces stem cells, which are precursors to leukocytes and lymphocytes
	Secondary	
Lymph nodes	Interconnected system of vessels and modes; chains of pathway of lymph drainage	Stores T cells, B cells, macrophages; circulates leukocytes; drains and filters waste products (cellular debris)
Spleen	Left upper abdominal quadrant beneath diaphragm	Stores red cells, leukocytes, platelets, lymphocytes; serves as hematopoietic organ; filters out antigens
		Kupffer's cells filter out antigens
Liver	Right upper abdominal quadrant Small intestine	Areas of lymphoid tissue that contain B cells and T cells
Peyer's patches, appendix	Right lower abdominal quadrant Pharynx	Unknown Filter antigenic material and cellular debris
Tonsils and adenoids	Thoracic cavity	
Lungs		

responses. The natural immune response consists of nonspecific defenses present at birth. These mechanisms function without prior exposure to an antigen. Nonspecific mechanisms include:

- First-line mechanisms
  - Physical: Skin, mucous membranes, epiglottis, respiratory tract cilia, sphincters
  - Chemical: Tears, gastric acidity, vaginal secretions
  - Mechanical: Lacrimation, intestinal peristalsis, urinary flow
- Second-line mechanisms
  - Phagocytosis, complement cascade

Nonspecific Immune Responses

Physical nonspecific mechanisms of defense against infections include intact skin and mucosal barriers. The skin forms the first barrier against infection; it is a physical barrier that contains secretions with antibacterial actions. This tight network of cells provides an impenetrable physical barrier against invasion by microbes that reside on the external or internal environment (Brachman, 1998).

Chemical barriers inhibit growth and invasion by environmental microbes. Chemical barriers include acid secretion by mucus, urine acidity, and a variety of lipids secreted in the skin. There are also physiologic mechanisms. The large airway of the lungs secretes mucus that traps inspired particles; the inspired debris is removed by epithelium and expectorated.

Through mechanical action, peristalsis in the gastrointestinal (GI) tract and urinary tract expels organisms from the internal environment of the host (Hudak et al., 1998).

Age influences nonspecific factors and is associated with decreased resistance at either end of the age spectrum—the very young and the very old. Factors such as surgery and the presence of chronic disease (e.g., diabetes, blood disorders, certain lymphomas, and collagen diseases) alter host resistance, which influences nonspecific factors.

Specific Immune Response

Acquired or specific host defense mechanisms function most efficiently when there has been prior exposure to invading antigens. Passive acquired immunity is transient and develops by passage of immune cells from one person to another or by gamma-globulin infusion. Active acquired immunity develops from direct contact with antigens by disease. The key players in specific immune response are leukocytes, T-cell lymphocytes, B lymphocytes, immunoglobulin, and the complement cascade.

Leukocytes make up one of the most important components of the immune system. A differential white blood cell (WBC) count provides specific information related to infections and disease. **Leukopenia** is defined as a reduction of the number of leukocytes in the blood to a count of less than 5000/mm^3. Normal WBC counts range from 5000 to 10,000/mL. Other components of the immune system are the B and T lymphocytes, which form the specific immune response system. Lymphocytes have specific antigen recognition and can neutralize toxin and phagocytize invading bacteria and viruses. Lymphocytes recognize a specific antigen because of the presence in the antigens of genes known as human leukocyte antigen (HLA) genes.

Immunoglobulin (Ig) circulates throughout the body, aiding in the destruction of microorganisms and neutralizing toxin. Immunoglobulins are divided into five major classes: IgA, IgD, IgE, IgG, and IgM. The absence of one or more of these substances has been linked to infection or disease processes.

The phagocytic cells provide a first line of defense against invasion by bacteria and selected fungi. These cells circulate in the bloodstream until summoned by chemical mediators to sites of infections. The immune system provides a surveillance network that enables the host to monitor and identify foreign material and generate specific protection against invading pathogens. Immunologic responses are mediated through the production of antibodies that circulate in the plasma.

The complement system consists of a complex of about 17 different proteins that are responsible for several steps in the inflammatory process, including summoning phagocytic cells to the site of infection. Complement also attaches to the infectious agent and promotes ingestion by the phagocyte. The complement proteins are numbered C1 through C9 and act in a cascade fashion to initiate action of the next protein. These proteins are part of the nonspecific and specific response systems. As a nonspecific immune response, C3 and C5 increase vascular permeability and chemically attract granulocytes. As part of the specific response, the normally inactive proteins are activated by specific antibodies in two pathways: the classic pathway requires interaction of C1 with the antigen–antibody complex, or the alternative pathway occurs in the absence of a specific antibody (Smeltzer & Bare, 2004).

Impaired Host Resistance

Many factors can result in impaired host defense. Persons who acquire an infection because of a deficiency in any of their multifaceted host defenses are referred to as compromised hosts. Persons with major defects related to specific immune responses are referred to as **immunosuppressed** hosts. These two terms often are used interchangeably.

The following is a general clinical picture of immune dysfunction:

- Infections occur frequently.
- Infections are more severe than usual.

- Unusual infecting agents or infections with opportunistic organisms occur.
- There is an incomplete response to treatment without complete elimination of the infecting agent.

Primary immunodeficiency disorders are congenital or inherited. B-cell immunodeficiencies account for about 50 percent of primary immunodeficiencies, and T-cell immunodeficiencies account for about 40 percent (Smeltzer & Bare, 2004).

Secondary immunodeficiencies arise from disease processes or therapies that decrease immune system organ or cell function. These deficiencies are acquired. Causes of secondary immune deficiency are age, stress, trauma, poor nutritional status, and drug therapy. Often these types of immunodeficiencies are transient and respond well to antibody therapy with IgG or a removal of the cause (Swenson, 2000).

Basic Principles of Epidemiology

Epidemiology is the "study of things that happen to people." Historically, it involves the study of epidemics. Epidemiology is the study of determinants, occurrence, and distribution of health and disease in a population (Carlson, Perdue, & Hankins, 2001).

Colonization

Infection is the replication of organisms in the tissue of a host and development of clinical signs and symptoms. **Colonization** is the presence of a microorganism in or on a host, with growth and multiplication of the microorganisms with no clinical symptoms or detected immune reaction at the time of isolation.

A carrier (or colonized person) is an individual colonized with a specific microorganism and from whom the organism can be recovered but who shows no signs or symptoms of the presence of the microorganism. A carrier may have a history of previous disease. The carrier state may be transient (short term), intermediate (on occasion), or chronic (long term, permanent, or persistent).

Dissemination

Dissemination is the shedding of microorganisms into the immediate environment from a person carrying them. Cultures of air samples, surfaces, and objects reveal dissemination or shedding of microorganisms. Some facilities routinely culture all or selected asymptomatic staff in an attempt to identify carriers of certain organisms; however, such surveys lack practical relevance unless related to a specific outbreak of disease.

Usually only a fraction of colonized persons are disseminating; therefore, nondisseminators are not associated with the actual spread of infection.

The risk of dissemination is generally greater from individuals with disease caused by that organism than from individuals with subclinical infection or who are colonized with the organism.

Nosocomial Infections

Nosocomial infections develop within a hospital or are produced by organisms acquired during hospitalization. Infections incubating at the time of a patient's admission to the hospital are not nosocomial; rather, they are community acquired unless they are from a previous hospitalization. Community-acquired infections, however, can be a source of infection for other patients or personnel and must be considered in the total scope of hospital-related infections (Brachman, 1998). These infections may involve anyone in contact with the hospital environment, including staff, volunteers, visitors, and workers. Nosocomial infections are preventable, and their sources can be endogenous or exogenous.

Endogenous infections are caused by a person's own flora. **Exogenous infections** are from sources outside a person's body.

Chain of Infection

Infections result from interaction between infectious agents and susceptible hosts. This interaction is called **transmission.** The chain of infection refers to six links that make up the chain: the causative agent or microorganism; the place where the organism naturally resides (reservoir); a method (mode) of transmission; a portal of entry into a host; and the susceptibility of the host. To control infection, the chain of infection must be attacked at its weakest link (Fig. 2–1).

First Link: Causative Agent

The first link in the chain of infection is the microbial agent or source, which may be a bacterium, fungus, virus, or parasite. The ability of an organism to induce disease is called its **virulence** or invasiveness.

Second Link: Reservoir

All organisms have a reservoir, or source of microorganisms. Common sources include other humans, the client's own microorganisms, plants, animals, or the general environment. People themselves are the most common source of infection for others. The reservoir is the place where the organism maintains its presence, metabolizes, and replicates. Viruses

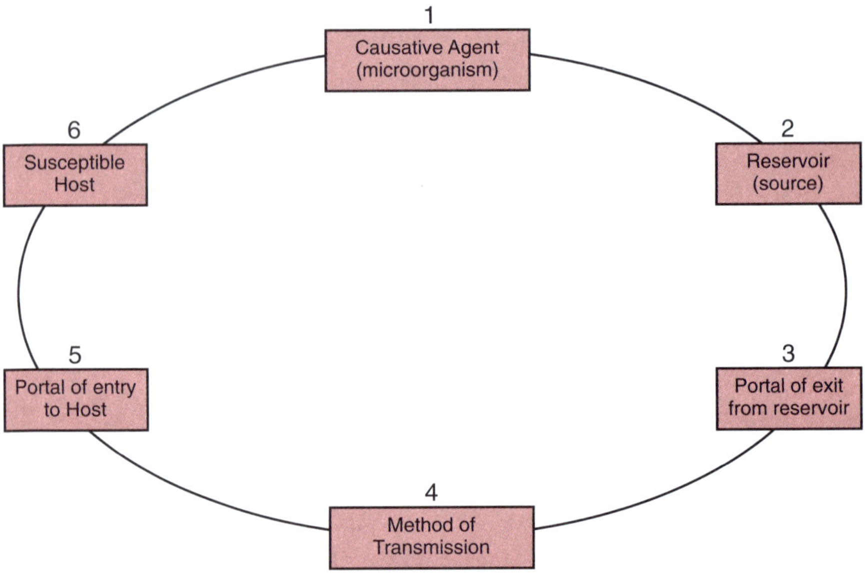

Figure 2–1 ■ Chain of infection.

survive better in human reservoirs, whereas the reservoir of gram-negative bacteria may have either a human or animal reservoir or an inanimate reservoir is usually a human **transmission**.

Third Link: Portal of Exit from Reservoir

The exit site is important in transmission of infection. Organisms from humans usually have a single portal of exit. The major portals of exit are the respiratory tract, gastrointestinal (GI) tract, and skin (e.g., in wounds). In addition, blood may be a portal of exit and is a concern for infusion nurses.

Fourth Link: Method (Mode) of Transmission

After a microorganism leaves its source or reservoir, it requires a means of transmission to reach another person or host through a receptive portal of entry. There are three mechanisms of transmission:

1. Direct transmission. Direct transmission involves direct transfer of organisms from person to person through touching, biting, kissing, or sexual intercourse. Droplet spread is also a form of direct transmission but can occur only if the source and host are within three feet of each other. (Refer to Transmission-Based Precautions.)

2. Indirect transmission. Indirect transmission can either be vehicle-borne or vector-borne.
   a. Vehicle-borne transmission. A vehicle is any substance that serves as an intermediate means to transport and introduce an infectious agent into a susceptible host. Examples are toys, handkerchiefs, soiled linen, or clothes.
   b. Vector-borne transmission. A vector is an animal or flying or crawling insect that serves as an intermediate means for transporting an infectious agent. An example is the mosquito carrying the West Nile virus.
3. Airborne transmission. Airborne transmission involves droplets or dust. Droplet nuclei, the residue of evaporated droplets, is transmitted by air currents to a suitable portal of entry. Examples are tuberculosis or dust particles containing *Clostridium difficile* spores from soil.

Fifth Link: Portal of Entry to the Susceptible Host

A person can become infected once the organism enters the body. The skin is a barrier to infectious agents; however, any break in the skin can readily serve as a portal of entry. Microorganisms often enter the body of the host by the same route they used to leave the source.

Sixth Link: Susceptible Host

A susceptible host is any person who is at risk for infection. Intact skin is the best defense against infection; for this manner of transmission, you must have a portal of reentry with non-intact skin. A compromised host is a person who has impaired natural defense mechanisms. Examples include the very young or very old, and those receiving immune suppression treatment for cancer, chronic illness, or following a successful organ transplant (Kozier, Erb, & Berman, 2004).

Breaking the Chain of Infection

New Microbiologic Methods

New laboratory methods can determine strains of bacterial organisms at the molecular level. Current standard nosocomial outbreak investigations often involve some type of molecular analysis.

Advancement of Epidemiologic Methods

At one time, epidemiologic methodology was descriptive and analytical; now sophisticated methods include relative risk, risk ratios, regression analysis, and correlation coefficients to study nosocomial infections.

Computerization of infection control surveillance has expanded epidemiology databases.

Continuous Quality Improvement Programs

The linking of hospital reimbursement to quality of care and assessment has been a strong incentive to expand the model and methods of hospital epidemiology to continuous quality improvement surveillance. Quality assessment of noninfectious risks requires risk and outcome definitions.

Risk Management

Formal programs have been established to deal with poor outcome evaluation and control in patients with liability-centered and malpractice-related risk management programs.

Antibiotic Use

The Joint Commission on Accreditation of Healthcare Organizations (JCAHO) requires medical staffs to develop a systematic process for evaluating empiric, therapeutic, and prophylactic uses of drugs; this process includes programs for review of antibiotic use. Each hospital should provide support for a group concerned with the appropriate use of antibiotics. This team should be headed by an infectious disease physician. Strategies to improve antibiotics use include education, ordering policies, drug utilization review, restriction policies, control of laboratory susceptibility testing, and limitation of contact time between physician and pharmaceutical company representatives.

To break the chain of infection, antimicrobial therapy is used in three stages. Stage 1 therapy is used when an infection is diagnosed or suspected and broad-spectrum therapy by I.V. route is initiated. Stage 1 is guided by a report of sample microscopy (e.g., morphology or Gram stain). Stage 1 patients are usually unstable from the standpoint of the infection process. The causative organisms should be cultured before the patient is treated with antibiotics. Table 2–2 presents a list of antibiotics and their effectiveness against certain pathogens at this stage.

Stage 2 therapy is adjusted to antimicrobial agents active against the isolated organism. Results of antibiotic sensitivity testing are used to guide therapy. Antimicrobial agents with a narrower spectrum of activity are often used. A third and final stage is reached when the patient shows signs of successful treatment and is converted to oral therapy before he or she is discharged.

Pharmacoepidemiology

The JCAHO requires that hospitals have the capacity to document and evaluate adverse drug reactions in their patients. The link between antibiotic use issues and adverse drug reactions has involved epidemiologists

> Table 2–2 **ANTIMICROBIAL AGENTS EFFECTIVE AGAINST CERTAIN NOSOCOMIAL PATHOGENS**

Organism	Antimicrobial Agents
Gram-Positive	
Staphylococci (methicillin sensitive)	First-generation cephalosporin, nafcillin
Staphylococci (methicillin resistant)	Vancomycin
Enterococci	Ampicillin or vancomycin with or without aminoglycoside
Clostridium difficile (diarrhea, colitis)	Oral vancomycin, oral metronidazole
Gram-Negative	
Klebsiella spp.	Cephalosporin, quinolone
Escherichia coli	Imipenem or third-generation cephalosporin with or without aminoglycoside
Enteric bacilli (*Enterobacter, Citrobacter, Serratia* spp.)	Ceftazidime, aztreonam, or extended-spectrum penicillin with or without aminoglycoside, ciprofloxacin
Pseudomonas aeruginosa	
Acinebacter spp.	Imipenem, ciprofloxacin
Legionella spp.	Erythromycin with or without imipenem
Other	
Candida spp.	Amphotericin B, fluconazole, ketoconazole
Aspergillus spp.	Amphotericin B, itraconazole
Anaerobes	Clindamycin, metronidazole, ticarcillin/clavulanate, ampicillin/sulbactam

Source: *Carlson, B., Perdue, M., & Hankins, J. (2001). Infection control. In Terry, J., Baranowski, L., Lonsway, R., & Hedrick, C. (eds.). Intravenous Therapy: Clinical Principles and Practice, (2nd ed.). Philadelphia: W.B. Saunders, p. 132, with permission.*

in pharmacoepidemiology (i.e., study of both the beneficial and adverse effects of drugs).

Emporiatrics

Physicians involved in infection control are often asked for travel advice. It is relevant for hospital epidemiologists to stay apprised of current infectious disease events worldwide. This study of disease in travelers is called emporiatrics.

Infusion-Related Infections

Epidemiology

Each year in the United States, hospitals and clinics purchase approximately 150 million intravascular devices. Most are peripheral venous catheters; however, in the United States more than 5 million central venous devices of various types are inserted annually. More than 200,000 nosocomial bloodstream infections occur each year in the United States; most are related to different types of intravascular devices (Maki & Mermel, 1998). Since 1970, CDC's National Nosocomial Infection Surveillance (NNIS) System has been collecting data on the incidence and etiologies of hospital-acquired infections, including CVC-associated bloodstream infections (BSIs). Rates of CVC-associated BSI vary considerably by hospital size. During 1992–2001, NNIS reported ICU rates of CVC-associated BSI ranging from 2.9 to 11.3 BSIs per 1000 CVC days.

The types of organisms that most commonly cause hospital-acquired BSIs change over time and are as follows:

- 1986–1989: Coagulase-negative staphylococci, followed by *Staphylococcus aureus*
- 1992–1999: Coagulase-negative staphylococci, followed by enterococci, are now the most frequently isolated causes of hospital-acquired BSIs.

In the 1992–1999 statistics, coagulase-negative staphylococci accounted for 37 percent and *S. aureus* 12.6 percent of reported hospital-acquired BSIs. Enterococci accounted for 13.5 percent of BSIs, an increase from 8 percent reported in the 1986–1989 statistics. *Candida* spp. caused 8 percent of hospital-acquired BSIs reported in both data collection periods. Resistance of *Candida* spp. to commonly used antifungal agents is increasing. Gram-negative bacilli accounted for 19 percent of catheter-associated BSIs in 1986–1989 as compared with 14 percent in 1992–1999. An increasing percentage of ICU-related isolates are caused by Enterobacteriaceae (CDC, 2002b).

Pathogenesis

The important pathogenic determinants of catheter-related infection are (1) the material of which the device is made and (2) the intrinsic virulence factors of the infecting organism. Catheters made of polyvinyl chloride or polyethylene are more likely to cause adherence of microorganisms than are catheters made of Teflon, silicone elastomer, or polyurethane. The majority of catheters sold in the United States are no longer made of polyvinyl chloride or polyethylene. Certain catheter materials are more thrombogenic than others, a characteristic that also might predispose to catheter colonization and catheter-related infection.

The adherence properties of a given microorganism also are important in the pathogenesis of catheter-related infection. Certain strains of coagulase-negative staphylococci produce an extracellular polysaccharide often referred to as "slime." In the presence of glucose-containing fluids, certain *Candida* spp. might produce slime similar to that of bacterial counterparts. This slime potentiates the pathogenicity by allowing organisms to withstand host defense mechanisms (Branchini et al., 1994).

Catheter-Related Infections

In the United States, 15 million CVC days occur in ICUs each year. The average rate of CVC-associated BSIs is 5.3 per 1000 catheter days in ICU; approximately 80,000 CVC-associated BSIs occur in ICUs each year (CDC, NISS, 2001). A total of 250,000 cases of CVC-associated BSIs have been estimated to occur annually if entire hospitals are assessed. The attributed mortality is an estimated 12 percent to 25 percent for each infection, and the cost to the healthcare system is a minimum of $25,000 per episode (Kluger & Maki, 1999).

Website

Nosocomial Surveillance System: *www.ncbi.nlm.nih.gov*

Infections related to CVADs generally are categorized as early and delayed infections. Early infections are those occurring within the first 2 to 3 weeks after CVAD implantation. Early infections generally are caused by bacterial contamination during the initial catheter insertion. These infections are most commonly caused by skin flora (*Streptococcus* and *Staphylococcus*).

Delayed infections occur more than 2 to 3 weeks after catheter implantation because of poor wound care, migration of organisms along the catheter tract, or seeding of the CVAD from a secondary source.

Clinical manifestations of infection are variable and depend on the type of infection present. Local infection may present as cellulitis with erythema, induration, pain, and inflammation. Serosanguineous or purulent discharge may be present from the skin exit site, indicating inflammation around the catheter.

Sources of Catheter-Related Infections

Microorganisms that colonize the skin of hospitalized patients cause the majority of intravascular catheter–related bloodstream infections: staphylococci (both coagulase-negative and coagulase-positive *S. aureus*), *Candida* spp., *Corynebacterium* spp., and *Bacillus* spp. (Maki & Mermel, 1998). The major sources of cannula-related infections are the skin flora, contamination of the catheter hub, contamination of infusate, and hematogenous colonization of the device (Fig. 2–2).

Primary risk factors associated with central infusion line infections include duration of catheterization (number of catheter days), multiple

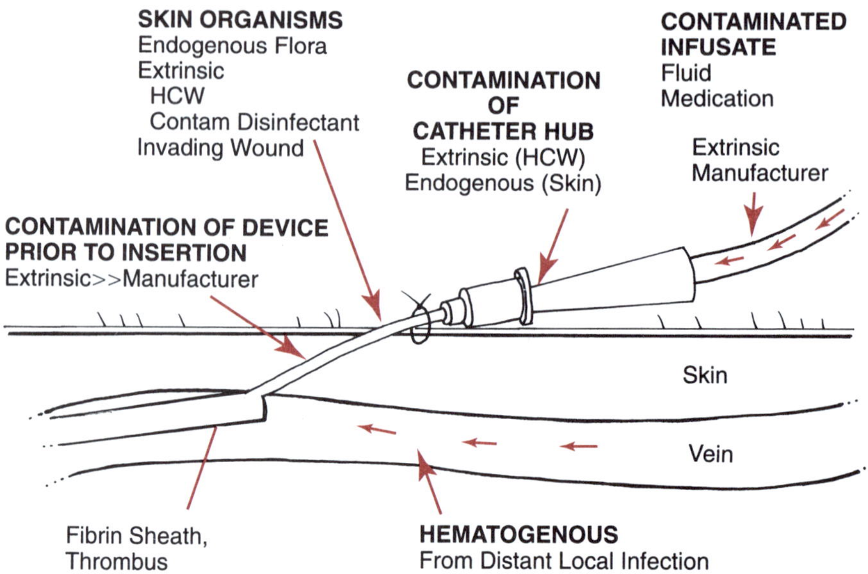

Figure 2–2 ■ Sources of I.V. cannula-related infections.

lines, colonization of catheter insertion site by skin organisms, location of catheter subclavian placement, aseptic dressing changes, and aseptic insertion technique. Factors contributing to a lesser degree to central line infections include secondary bacteremia, host defense status, contaminated infusate, and number of catheter lumen (single versus triple lumen). The CDC guidelines for changing catheters, administration sets, and catheter site care are presented in Appendix A.

Factors that predispose patients with CVADs to infection include longer durations of catheter placement, catheters with multiple lumens, catheters made of polyvinyl chloride, catheters that develop fibrin sheaths at the distal catheter tip, port systems that accumulate sludge or blood products within the port reservoir, and a compromised immune status in patients (Ray, 1999). Implantable devices are associated with the lowest rate of infectious complications of all CVAD systems (Maki & Mermel, 1998).

Phlebitis

The presence of phlebitis connotes a substantially increased risk of infection and indicates the need for immediate removal of the catheter to reduce the severity of phlebitis, for symptomatic relief, and to prevent catheter colonization from progressing to bloodstream infection. A few of the risk factors for increased phlebitis rates include: phlebitis exceeds 50 percent by the fourth day after catheterization, female gender, and

> Table 2–3 RISK FACTORS FOR INFUSION PHLEBITIS

- Catheter material
  - Polypropylene > Teflon
  - Silicone elastomer > polyurethane
  - Teflon > polyetherurethane
  - Teflon > steel needle
- Catheter size
  - Large bore > smaller bore
  - 8-inch Teflon > 2-inch Teflon
- Insertion in emergency room > inpatient units
- Disinfection of skin with antiseptic before catheter insertion
  - None > chlorhexidine-alcohol
- Experience, skill of person inserting catheter
  - House offices, nurses > hospital I.V. team
  - House officers, nurses > decentralized unit I.V. nurse educator
- Increasing duration of catheter placement in site
- Subsequent catheters beyond the first infusate
  - Low-pH solutions (e.g., dextrose-containing solutions)
  - Potassium chloride
  - Hypertonic glucose, amino acids, lipid for parenteral nutrition
  - Antibiotics (especially β-lactams, vancomycin, metronidazole)
  - High rate of flow of I.V. fluid (>90 mL/h)
- Frequent I.V. dressing changes
  - Daily >every 48 hours
- Catheter-related infection
- Host factors
  - "Poor quality" peripheral veins
  - Insertion site
  - Upper arm, wrist > hand
- Age
  - Children: older > younger
  - Adults: younger > older
- Gender
  - Female > male
- Ethnicity
  - European American > African American
- Underlying medical disease
- Individual biologic vulnerability

NOTE: The > symbol denotes a significantly greater risk of phlebitis.

***Source:** Maki, D.G. & Mermel, L.A. (1998). Infections due to infusion therapy. In Bennett, J., & Brachman, P. (eds.). Hospital Infections (4th ed.). Philadelphia: Lippincott-Raven, p. 690, Adapted with permission.*

catheter materials. Refer to Table 2–3 for a complete list of risk factors (Maki & Mermel, 1998).

Treatment of Catheter-Related Infections

Antibiotic therapy for catheter-related infection is often initiated with speculative antibiotic therapy. Vancomycin is usually recommended when an increased number of methicillin-resistant staphylococci is present. In the absence of methicillin-resistant *S. aureus*, penicillinase-resistant penicillins, such as nafcillin or oxacillin, should be used. Third- or fourth-generation cephalosporins are used for *Pseudomonas aeruginosa*. Amphotericin B or I.V. fluconazole should also be considered for treatment when fungemia is suspected. The initial choice of antibiotics depends on the patient's clinical presentation.

Patients should be separated into those with complicated infections, in which there is septic thrombosis, endocarditis, osteomyelitis or possible metastatic seeding, and those with uncomplicated bacteremia in which there is no evidence of such complications. Refer to Table 2–4 for approaches to management of patient with bloodstream infections.

If there is prompt response to initial antibiotic therapy, most patients who are not immunocompromised, and without underlying valvular heart disease or an intravascular prosthetic device, should receive antimi-

> Table 2–4 **MANAGEMENT OF PATIENTS WITH CENTRAL VENOUS CATHETER–RELATED BLOODSTREAM INFECTIONS**

Nontunneled CVCs			
Complicated		**Uncomplicated**	
Cause	**Treatment**	**Cause**	**Treatment**
Septic thrombosis or endocarditis	Remove CVC. Treat with systemic antibiotic for 4–6 weeks.	Coagulase-negative *Staphylococcus*	Remove CVC. Treat with systemic antibiotic for 5–7 days.
Osteomyelitis	Remove CVC. Treat with systemic antibiotic for 6–8 weeks.	*Staphylococcus aureus*	Remove CVC. Treat with systemic antibiotic for 14 days.
		Gram-negative bacilli	Remove CVC. Treat with systemic antibiotic for 10–14 days.
		Candida spp.	Remove CVC. Treat with antifungal therapy for 14 days.

Tunneled Catheters and Implanted Devices			
Complicated		**Uncomplicated**	
Cause	**Treatment**	**Cause**	**Treatment**
Tunnel infection Port abscess	Remove CVC/ID. Treat with systemic antibiotic for 10–14 days.	Coagulase-negative *Staphylococcus*	■ May retain CVC/ID. Use systemic antibiotic for 7 days plus antibiotic lock therapy for 10–14 days. ■ Remove CVC/ID if there is clinical deterioration or persisting or relapsing bacteremia.

(Continued on following page)

Cause	Treatment	Cause	Treatment
Septic thrombosis or Endocarditis	Remove CVC/ID. Treat with antibiotics for 4–6 weeks	*Staphylococcus aureus*	■ Remove CVC/ID. Treat with systemic antibiotic for 14 days if TEE(–). ■ For CVC/ID salvage therapy, if TEE(–) use systemic and antibiotic lock therapy for 14 days. ■ Remove CVC/ID if there is clinical deterioration or persisting or relapsing bacteremia.
Osteomyelitis	Remove CVC/ID. Treat with systemic antibiotic for 6–8 weeks.	Gram-negative bacilli	■ Remove CVC/ID. Treat with systemic antibiotic for 10–14 days. ■ For CVC/ID salvage, use systemic and antibiotic lock therapy for 14 days. ■ If no response, remove and treat with systemic antibiotic therapy for 10–14 days.
		Candida spp.	■ Remove CVC/ID. Treat with antifungal therapy for 14 days after last positive blood culture.

TEE = Transesophageal echocardiography.

Source: *Mermel, L.A., Farr, B., Sherertz, R.J., et al. (2001). Guidelines for the management of intravascular catheter-related infections. Journal of Intravenous Nursing, 24(3), 180–205.*

crobial therapy for 10 to 14 days. A more prolonged course of antibiotic therapy (4 to 6 weeks) should be considered if there is persistent bacteremia or fungemia (Mermel et al., 2001).

AGE-RELATED CONSIDERATIONS 2–1

Most nosocomial bloodstream infections in pediatric patients are related to the use of an intravascular device. The rate of CVC-related infections is 1.7 to 2.4 infections per 1000 catheter-days, depending on the type of device use (Strovroff & Teague, 1998). The pediatric population is diverse, and the risk of infection varies with age, birthweight, underlying disease, host factors, medications, type of device, and nature of the infusate (Baltimore, 1998).

Infusate-Related Infections

The proliferation of microbes in 5 percent dextrose in water is most commonly related to tribe *Klebsiella* spp., *Pseudomonas cepacia, Acinetobacter* spp., and *Serratia* spp. Most bacteria grow in 0.9 percent sodium chloride fluids, but *Candida* species flourish in synthetic amino acids and 25 percent dextrose solutions (Maki & Mermel, 1998).

Mechanisms of Fluid Contamination

Parenteral fluids can become contaminated during administration owing to the duration of uninterrupted infusion through the same administration set and to the frequency with which the set is manipulated. Microorganisms gain access from air entering bottles, from entry points into the administration set, from the I.V. device through the line, or at the junction between the administration set and the catheter hub.

Molds gain access into glass I.V. bottles through microscopic cracks long before the bottle is hung for use; visible cloudiness or filmy precipitates and "ungus balls" in an I.V. bottle are visible to nurses.

Total parenteral nutrition fluids should be used as soon as possible after preparation and stored at 4°C for growth of *C. albicans* to be suppressed.

NURSING FAST FACT!

Manipulations of the delivery system, especially the administration set, provide means for access of microorganisms to in-use infusate (Maki & Mermel, 1998).

Before use, containers of fluid should be examined against light and dark backgrounds for cracks, defects, turbidity, and particulate matter. Any glass container lacking a vacuum when opened should be considered contaminated.

Nursing Points-of-Care: Preventing Infusate-Related Infections

- Inspect all infusates before administering.
- Observe stringent asepsis during preparing and compounding admixtures in the central pharmacy or on individual patient care units.
- Follow good aseptic techniques when handling infusions, such as when injecting medications or changing bags or bottles of fluids.
- Replace the administration set at periodic intervals to prevent the buildup of dangerous introduced contaminants and to further reduce the risk of related septicemia.

Additional factors that contribute to contamination of infusion-related infection include:

1. *Faulty handling.* Glass containers can become cracked or damaged and plastic bags punctured; bacteria and fungi may invade a hairline crack in an I.V. container.
2. *Admixtures.* The risk of contamination when admixtures are prepared is decreased when trained personnel prepare mixtures under laminar flow hoods. The use of a strict aseptic technique is vital.
3. *Manipulation of in-use I.V. equipment.* Faulty technique in handling equipment can lead to contamination.
4. *Injection ports.* Aseptic technique must be maintained when injection ports are used for "piggyback" or secondary infusions. The injection port located at the distal end of the tubing can expose the patient to excreta and drainage.

INS Standard. Latex injection and access ports should be aseptically cleansed before access. (INS, 2000, 41)

5. *Three-way stopcocks.* These adjunct devices are potential sources of transmission of bacteria because their ports, unprotected by sterile covering, are open to moisture and contaminants. These devices are usually connected to central venous catheters (CVCs) and arterial lines and are frequently used for drawing blood. Using an aseptic technique is vital.

NURSING FAST FACTS!

Whenever fluid is seen leaking at injection sites, connections, or vents, the I.V. set should be replaced.

If intrinsic contamination of a commercially distributed product is identified or even strongly suspected, especially if clinical infections have occurred as a consequence, the local, state, and federal (e.g., CDC and FDA) public health authorities must be contacted immediately. The unopened lot or lots should be quarantined and saved for analysis (Maki & Mermel, 1998).

Refer to Table 2–5 for microorganisms most frequently encountered in catheter-related, central venous catheter–related, infusate-related, and blood product–related infections.

Culturing Techniques

If the I.V. catheter is in any way compromised, it should be cultured. The recommended method for culturing a catheter is the semiquantitative culture technique (Procedures Display 2–1). Semiquantitative culture technique involves thoroughly cleaning the area around the insertion site with

> Table 2–5 **MICROORGANISMS MOST FREQUENTLY ENCOUNTERED**

Source	Pathogens
Catheter related	Coagulase-negative staphylococci*
Peripheral I.V. catheter	*Staphylococcus aureus*
	Candida spp.*
Central venous catheters	Coagulase-negative staphylococci
	Staphylococcus aureus
	Candida spp.
	Corynebacterium spp. (especially JK-1)
	Klebsiella and *Enterobacter* spp.
	Mycobacterium spp.
	Trichophyton beigelii
	Fusarium spp.
	*Malassezia furfur**
Contaminated I.V. infusate	Tribe *Klebsiella*
	Enterobacter cloacae
	Enterobacter agglomerans
	Serratia marcescens
	Klebsiella spp.
	Burkholderia cepacia
	Bukrholderia acidovorans, Burkholderia picketti
	Stenotrophomonas maltophilia
	Citrobacter freundii
	Flavobacterium spp.
	Candida tropicalis
Contaminated blood products	*E. cloacae*
	S. marcescens
	Ochrobactrum anthropi
	Flavobacterium spp.
	Burkholderia spp.
	Yersinia spp.
	Salmonella spp.

**Also seen with peripheral I.V. catheters in association with the administration of lipid emulsion for parenteral nutritional support.*

Source: *Maki, D.G. & Mermel, L.A. (1998). Infections due to infusion therapy. In Bennett, J., & Brachman, P. (eds.). Hospital Infections (4th ed.). Philadelphia: Lippincott-Raven, p. 690. Adapted with permission.*

70 percent alcohol and permitting the area to air dry. Alcohol is recommended because the residual antimicrobial activity of iodine-containing solutions may kill organisms on the catheter when it is removed. After the catheter is withdrawn, at least 5 cm of the tip and the catheter segment, beginning 1 to 2 mm inside the skin–catheter junction point, is clipped off with sterile scissors and dropped into a sterile specimen tube or cup. Purulent drainage at the site should be cultured before the site is cleaned.

The following are disadvantages of this semiquantitative method: (1) this method may fail to detect bacteremia of the internal lumens of the catheter tip and (2) the catheter must be removed for culturing and may not actually be the source of infection.

PROCEDURES DISPLAY 2–1

Steps in Catheter Culturing

When an I.V.-related infection is suspected, obtain culture from suspected source.

Patient Assessment:

- Verify patient identity.
- Obtain physician's order.
- Place patient in a comfortable position.
- Assess I.V. site.

Equipment needed:

- Sterile scissors
- Sterile gloves
- 70 Percent alcohol swab
- Sterile specimen container
- Label

Instructions to Patients:

- Inform patient of purpose of culture.
- Inform patient that there is no discomfort or pain associated with this procedure.

Procedure:

1. Explain procedure to patient.
2. Remove dressing over I.V. site.
3. Wash hands and put on sterile gloves.
4. Wipe skin around puncture site with 70 percent alcohol to cleanse area of any blood or antimicrobial ointment.
5. Withdraw catheter carefully. Be sure to direct the removed portion of the catheter upward to keep it away from the patient's skin.
6. Hold catheter over specimen container; with sterile scissors, cut half the length of the catheter and drop it into the container.
7. Close container and label.

Documentation:

Document all relevant information:

- Record on the patient's chart the taking of the specimen and source.
- Include the date and time; the appearance of the exudate; the color, consistency, amount, and odor of any drainage; and any discomfort experienced by the patient.

NURSING FAST FACT!

A positive, semiquantitative culture of 15 or more colony-forming units (CFUs) confirms a local cannula infection (Maki & Mermel, 1998).

Culture any purulent drainage from the site. If the I.V. solution is the suspected source of infection, send the fluid container and tubing to a laboratory for analysis.

Blood cultures drawn through a peripheral vein and through the I.V. cannula can be a helpful alternative to culturing the cannula. If the results of the catheter blood sample are five times the peripheral blood sample, a catheter-related infection is suspected and the catheter should be removed.

Strategies for Preventing/Treating Infection

Nurses involved in maintaining vascular access devices must have the knowledge base and competency to initiate infusion-related protocols to prevent infection. The principles of infection control provide the foundation for the delivery of infusion therapy. Prevention begins with knowledge regarding the techniques used to prevent infection.

1. Follow CDC Standard Precautions Guidelines

In 1996, the Hospital Infection Control Practice Advisory Committee (HICPAC) of the CDC developed new isolation guidelines that better addressed the growing concerns of the transmission of resistant organisms. The new system for isolation blends body substance isolation, category isolation, and disease-specific isolation into a two-tiered approach.

Tier One: Standard Precautions

Standard precautions incorporate the fundamentals of universal precautions (designed to reduce exposure risks to bloodborne pathogens) and body substance isolation (designed to reduce risk of exposures to pathogens residing in moist body fluids) and require consistent use for all patients regardless of their infection status.

Standard precautions are imposed when (1) there is risk of exposure to blood; (2) there is risk of exposure to all other body fluids, including secretions and excretions (not including sweat), whether or not evidence of blood is present; (3) nonintact skin is present; and (4) there will be contact with any mucous membranes.

NURSING FAST FACT!

The primary barriers to protect healthcare workers from blood and/or body fluid exposures are gloves in conjunction with appropriate hand hygiene

(Continued on following page)

practices, eye protection, and mucous membrane protection (i.e., face shield or goggles and mask).

Tier Two: Transmission-Based Precautions

Transmission-based precautions are the second tier of the isolation precautions. These additional precautions are based on the known or suspected infectious state of the patient and the possible routes of transmission. There are three categories of transmission-based precautions:

1. Airborne precautions, which require special air handling and ventilation to prevent the spread of these organisms. They also require additional respiratory protection (HEPA or N95 respirators for patients with tuberculosis). Examples of infections are tuberculosis, varicella, and measles.
2. Droplet precautions, which require the use of mucous membrane protection (eye protection and masks) to prevent infectious organisms from contacting the conjunctivae or mucous membranes of the nose or mouth. Examples of infections are mumps, rubella, influenza, and pertussis.
3. Contact precautions, which require the use of gloves and gowns when direct skin-to-skin contact or with contaminated environment is anticipated. Examples of infections are *Clostridium difficile* enteritis, methicillin-resistant *Staphylococcus aureus,* and vancomycin-resistant *Enterococcus* spp. (CDC, 1996).

NURSING FAST FACT!

Implementation of standard precautions has implications for infusion therapy nurses: Use of I.V. therapy carts and trays may be limited for patients who are on contact transmission precautions.

2. Follow Hand Hygiene Procedure

Skin Function/Barrier Protection

The primary function of the skin is to reduce water loss, provide protection against abrasive action and microorganisms, and act as a permeability barrier to the environment. Barrier function arises from the dying, degeneration, and compaction of underlying epidermis and from the process of synthesis of the stratum corneum occurring at the same rate as loss. The barrier to percutaneous absorption lies within the stratum corneum, the thinnest and smallest compartment of the skin. The formation of the skin barrier is under homeostatic control, which is illustrated by the epidermal response to barrier disturbance by skin stripping or solvent extraction.

The goal of using specific products for **hand hygiene** is to maintain normal barrier function. The normal barrier function is biphasic: 50 percent to 60 percent of barrier recovery typically occurs within 6 hours, but complete normalization of barrier function requires 5 to 6 days (CDC, 2002a).

Transmission of Pathogens on Hands

Transmission of healthcare-associated pathogens from one patient to another via the hands of healthcare workers (HCWs) requires the following sequence of events:

1. Organisms present on the patient's skin or that have been shed onto inanimate objects must be transferred to the hands of HCWs.
2. These organisms must then be capable of surviving for at least several minutes on the hands of personnel.
3. Hand washing or hand antisepsis by the worker was inadequate or omitted entirely, or the agent used for hand hygiene was inappropriate.
4. The contaminated hands of the HCW must come in direct contact with another patient (CDC, 2002a).

NURSING FAST FACT!

Studies have documented contamination of HCWs hands with potential healthcare-associated pathogens. Serial cultures revealed that 100 percent of HCWs carried gram-negative bacilli at least once, and 64 percent carried S. aureus at least once (CDC, 2002a).

Preparations Used for Hand Hygiene

Hand hygiene reduces nurses' and patients' risks of infection. Good hand hygiene with plain ordinary soap has only minimal antimicrobial activity. However, it can remove loosely adherent dirt, organic material, and **transient flora.** A vigorous 10- to 15-second scrub with antiseptics (alcohols, chlorhexidine, chlorine, hexachlorophene, iodine, chloroxylenol [PCMX], quaternary ammonium compounds, and triclosan) has excellent in vitro germicidal activity against gram-positive and gram-negative bacteria.

Alcohol-based products are more effective for standard handwashing or hand antisepsis by HCWs than soap or antimicrobial soaps. Applying friction removes most microbes and should be used when placing invasive devices, when persistent antimicrobial activity is desired, and when it is important to reduce the numbers of **resident skin flora** in addition to transient microorganisms (CDC, 2002a).

Alcohol-based hand rubs intended for uses in hospitals are available as low-viscosity rinses, gels, and foams. Alcohols are not appropriate for use when hands are visibly dirty or contaminated.

CDC RECOMMENDATIONS FOR HAND HYGIENE IN HEALTH-CARE SETTINGS

Indications for hand washing and hand antisepsis:

- When hands are visibly dirty or contaminated with blood or other body fluids, wash hands with either a non-antimicrobial soap or water or an antimicrobial soap and water.
- If hands are not visibly soiled use an alcohol-based hand rub for routinely decontaminating hands in all other clinical situations.
- Decontaminate hands before having direct contact with patients.
- Decontaminate hands before donning sterile gloves when inserting a central intravascular catheter.
- Decontaminate hands before inserting a peripheral vascular catheter.
- Decontaminate hands after contact with patient's intact skin (taking pulse, blood pressure).
- Decontaminate hands after contact with body fluids or excretions, mucous membranes, non-intact skin, and wound dressing if hands are not visibly soiled.
- Decontaminate hands if moving from a contaminated body site to a clean body site during patient care.
- Decontaminate hands after removing gloves.
- Before eating and after using a restroom, wash hands with a non-antimicrobial soap and water or with an antimicrobial soap and water.
- Antimicrobial-impregnated wipes (towelettes) may be considered as an alternative to washing hands with non-antimicrobial soap and water.

NURSING FAST FACTS!

- *It is recommended that healthcare agencies provide personnel with efficacious hand-hygiene products that have a low irritancy potential, particularly when these products are used multiple times per shift.*
- *Using gloves should not replace handwashing and does not provide complete protection*
- *For insertion of peripheral catheters good hand hygiene before catheter insertion or maintenance, combined with proper aseptic technique during catheter manipulation, provides protection against infection. Central venous catheter (CVC) insertion carries a substantially greater risk for infection; therefore, the level of barrier precautions needed to prevent infection during insertion of CVC should be more stringent (CDC, 2002b).*

OTHER HAND HYGIENE RECOMMENDATIONS (CDC, 2002A)

- Do not wear artificial fingernails or extenders when having direct contact with patients at high risk.
- Keep natural nail tips less than $\frac{1}{4}$ inch long.
- Wear gloves when in contact with blood or potentially infectious materials, mucous membranes, and non-intact skin.
- Remove gloves after caring for a patient. Do not wear the same pair of gloves for the care of more than one patient, and do not wash gloves between uses with different patients.
- Change gloves during patient care if moving from a contaminated body site to a clean body site.

3. Use Appropriate Skin Antisepsis

The Infusion Nurses Society (2000) Standards of Practice and CDC (2002) support the use of the following antiseptic solutions to prepare the site prior to venipuncture:

- 10 Percent povidone-iodine
- 70 Percent isopropyl alcohol
- 2 Percent aqueous chlorhexidine gluconate
- 2 Percent tincture of chlorhexidine (Approved July 2000 FDA)

Povidone-iodine has been the most widely used antiseptic for cleansing insertion sites; however, recent studies support the use of 2 percent aqueous chlorhexidine gluconate as a superior solution to lower BSI rates. The 2 percent chlorhexidine gluconate has also been shown to decrease the skin irritations reported from use of other skin preparation agents (Hibbard et al. 2002; Maki, 1991).

Practice criteria for insertion of peripheral, midline, arterial, central, and peripherally inserted central catheter (PICC) include the use of aseptic technique and site preparation with antimicrobial solutions (INS, 2000, 47). In addition, the following guidelines should be used to maintain integrity of the infusion site (INS, 2000, 47):

- Powder-free gloves should be used.
- Clipping should be performed to remove excess hair at the intended vascular access site when necessary.
- Antimicrobial solutions in a single-unit use configuration should be used.
- Alcohol should not be applied after the application of 10 percent povidone-iodine preparation because alcohol negates the effect of 10 percent povidone-iodine.
- The antimicrobial preparation solution should be allowed to air-dry completely before proceeding with the vascular access device insertion procedure.
- Maximum barrier precautions including sterile gown, gloves, cap, masks, protective eyewear, surgical scrub, and large sterile drapes

and towels should be used for midline, arterial, central, and peripherally inserted central catheters.

NURSING FAST FACT!

After initial site preparation, sterile gloves should be changed prior to midline, arterial, central, and peripherally inserted central catheter placement.

4. Use Catheter Site Dressing Regimens

Transparent, semipermeable polyurethane dressing is used in many clinical settings. These dressings reliably secure the infusion device, permit continuous visual inspection of the catheter site, permit patients to bathe and shower without saturating the dressing, and require less frequent changes than do standard gauze and tape dressings.

Data from studies suggest that colonization among catheters dressed with transparent dressings (5.7 percent) is comparable to that of those dressed with gauze (4.6 percent) and that no clinically substantial differences exist in the incidences of either catheter colonization or phlebitis (Maki & Ringer, 1987; CDC, 2002).

In a multicenter study (Maki, 2000) a chlorhexidine-impregnated sponge (Biopatch™) placed over the site of short-term arterial and CVDs reduced the risk of catheter colonization and catheter-related BSIs. No adverse systemic effects resulted from use of this device (CDC, 2002b).

5. Use Catheter Securement Devices

Sutureless devices are available and can be advantageous over sutures in preventing catheter-related BSIs. One study compared sutureless device with sutures for the securement of PICCs; in this study, catheter-related bloodstream infections were reduced in the group of patients receiving the sutureless device (Yamamoto, Solomon, & Soulen, 2001).

6. Use Topical Antimicrobial Ointments

Povidone-iodine ointment applied at the site of insertion of hemodialysis catheters has been studied as a prophylactic intervention to reduce the incidence of catheter-related infections. Other antibiotic ointments applied to the catheter insertion site also have been studied and have yielded conflicting results. The risk of catheter colonization with *Candida* spp. might be increased with the use of antibiotic ointments that have no fungicidal activity (CDC, 2002b).

NURSING FAST FACT!

Any ointment that is applied to the catheter insertion site should be checked against the catheter and ointment manufacturers' recommendations regarding compatibility.

7. Use Antimicrobial/Antiseptic-Impregnated Catheters and Cuffs

Catheters and cuffs that are coated or impregnated with antimicrobial or antiseptic agents can decrease the risk for catheter-related bloodstream infections. Several different types of materials are used to coat catheters and cuffs. They include:

- Chlorhexidine/silver sulfadiazine: Newest generation available with coating over both the internal and external luminal surfaces. More expensive than standard catheters.
- Minocycline/rifampin: Available impregnated on both the external and internal surfaces. May increase the risk of resistance among pathogens, especially staphylococci.
- Platinum/silver: Ionic metals have a broad antimicrobial activity and are being used in catheters and cuffs.
- Silver cuffs: Ionic silver has been used in subcutaneous collagen cuffs attached to CVCs. Provides antimicrobial activity and cuff provides a mechanical barrier to the migration of microorganisms (CDC, 2002b).

8. Use Anticoagulants

Anticoagulant flush solutions are used widely to prevent catheter thrombosis. Thrombi and fibrin deposits on catheters may serve as a focal point for microbial colonization of intravascular catheters and the use of anticoagulants might have a role in the prevention of CRBSIs (CDC, 2002b).

9. Use Antibiotic Locks

The purpose of antibiotic lock therapy is to sterilize the lumen of the catheter. Most frequently the therapy is over a 2-week period of time. Antibiotic lock therapy for catheter-related bloodstream infections is often used in conjunction with systemic antibiotic therapy and involves instilling in the catheter lumen a high concentration of an antibiotic to which the causative microbe is susceptible. The antibiotic is mixed with 50 to 100 U of heparin or normal saline in sufficient volume to fill the catheter lumen and installed or "locked" into the catheter lumen during periods when the catheter is not being used (Mermel et al., 2001).

NURSING PLAN OF CARE

INFECTION CONTROL

Focus Assessment

Subjective

- History of risk factors: Fever, diarrhea

Objective

- Baseline immunologic studies: T-cell count, WBC count, differential
- Vital signs, especially temperature
- Redness, inflammation, purulent drainage, tenderness, and warmth of insertion site

Patient Outcome/Evaluation Criteria

Patient will:

- Be free from nosocomial infection.
- Maintain adequate oxygenation.
- Verbalize understanding of precautions for catheter care.
- Report any need for additional dressing changes.
- Not contaminate healthcare team, other patients, or family.

Nursing Diagnoses

- Risk for infection related to immunodeficiency and malnutrition
- Risk for impaired gas exchange related to alveolar capillary membrane changes with infection
- Risk for altered thought processes related to HIV or opportunistic infection of central nervous system
- Risk for knowledge deficit related to illness and impact on patient's future
- Risk for infection transmission

Nursing Management

1. Use standard precautions.
2. Use aseptic technique and follow appropriate protocols when changing catheter dressing, I.V. tubing, and solutions.
3. Use sterile technique when inserting and removing catheter and when maintaining system.
4. Ensure complete skin preparation before insertion.
5. Ensure peripheral catheter removal within 72 and 96 hours.
6. Change insertion site dressing when wet, soiled, or nonocclusive.
7. Secure proximal I.V. connections with a Luer locking set, if possible.

(Continued on following page)

NURSING PLAN OF CARE

INFECTION CONTROL *(Continued)*

8. Monitor for:
   a. Signs and symptoms of sepsis (fever, hypotension, positive blood cultures).
   b. Oxygen saturation with oximetry.
9. Observe hand hygiene techniques between patients.
10. Use proper insertion and maintenance of invasive devices.
11. Use sterile equipment and aseptic technique appropriately.
12. Give attention to proper skin care.
13. Use needleless I.V. systems.

Pediatric infection control practices are covered in Chapter 10; infection control issues related to blood products are covered in Chapter 13; CVC infections are discussed further in Chapter 12; and issues of infection control related to parenteral nutrition are covered in Chapter 15.

Patient Education

In all healthcare environments, patient education is an important component in preventing catheter-related complications. Education regarding vascular access management is crucial. Information regarding catheter management should be individualized to meet the patient's needs but remain consistent with established policies and procedures for infection control.

Education should include:

- Instructions on hand hygiene; aseptic technique; and concept of dirty, clean, and sterile
- Proper methods for handling equipment
- Judicious use of antibiotics, which is a major nursing role to slow an epidemic of drug-resistant infections
- Importance of complying with directions for prescribed antibiotics
- Written information on steps for dressing changes
- Assessment of the site and the key signs and symptoms to report to the home care agency, hospital healthcare worker, or physician.

Home Care Issues

It is generally believed that at-home risk factors for developing a catheter-related infection should be somewhat lower than risk factors in a hospital setting. Research and study are needed to describe infection risks in the home setting.

The Environmental Protection Agency (EPA) has developed many advisory committees regarding infectious waste disposal in the home care setting. The Medical Waste Tracking Act of 1988 mandated to the EPA the investigation and development of guidelines for handling home-generated medical waste. The home care provider should establish policies and procedures for handling waste. Prepackaged kits are available from a number of manufacturers and include sharps disposal systems and the CHemBLOC spill kit.

Each home healthcare nurse or aide needs appropriate equipment and supplies related to infection control. OSHA requires that hand hygiene and eyewash stations are available to employees who are exposed to blood and body fluids. The stations may not be available in the home setting; it is important to provide an alternative until the employee has access to them. It is important to have antiseptic wipes to clean hands, a spill kit in event of a large amount of blood or body fluid is spilled on the floor or a surface, and appropriate containers for disposal and transport of medical waste and contaminated sharps.

Rubbermaid® tubs with a sealing lid work well for transporting medical waste from homes to the home healthcare agency. Sharps containers must be used for all contaminated sharps.

Healthcare workers should use an alcohol-based hand rinse or foam, rubbing vigorously to cover all parts of the hands until dry. If hands are visibly soiled, the nurse may have to go out of the way to find a source of running water because alcohol does not remove soil or organic matter (CDC, 2002a).

Key Points

- In the United States, the CDC, a division of the Department of Health and Human Services, is the agency that investigates, develops, recommends, and sets standards for infection control practices.
- The purpose of the immune system is to recognize and destroy invading antigens. Organs include primary (thymus and bone marrow) and secondary (lymph nodes, spleen, liver, Peyer's patches, appendix, tonsils and adenoids, and lungs).
- Impaired host resistance includes:
  - B-cell immunodeficiencies (50 percent of primary immunodeficiencies)
  - T-cell immunodeficiencies (40 percent of primary immunodeficiencies)
  - The epidemiologic triangle consists of:
    - The host: The living person or animal that provides the atmosphere in which organisms are able to live

  - The agent: The organism that is capable of eliciting a disease process
  - The environment: The interacting group of conditions, surroundings, and influences in which the host and agent coexist
- A nosocomial infection is one that develops in a patient during or after, but as a result of, his or her stay in a healthcare setting.
- One of the main complications of infusion therapy is sepsis (septicemia), a pathologic state, usually accompanied by fever, which results from the presence of microorganisms in the bloodstream. Staphylococci are responsible for the majority of nosocomial I.V.-related infections.
- Risk factors for infection include:
  - Percutaneously inserted, noncuffed CVCs used for hemodialysis (highest risk)
  - Peripherally inserted CVCs (lower risk)
  - Surgically implanted CVCs (lowest risk)
  - CVCs in all forms pose the greatest risk of septicemia; the skin site is the most common source of organism colonization.
- Strategies for prevent/treat infection include:
  - Following CDC Standard Precautions guidelines
  - Using the correct hand hygiene procedure
  - Use of appropriate skin antisepsis
  - Catheter site dressing regimens
  - Using catheter securement devices
  - Using antibiotic ointments
  - Using antimicrobial/antiseptic-impregnated catheters and cuffs
  - Using anticoagulants
  - Antibiotic lock therapy.

Critical Thinking: Case Study

A patient is admitted with uncontrolled diabetes mellitus. She has a saline lock in place in her left wrist area. A symptomatic drop in blood sugar to 38 mg/dl requires she receive 50 mL of 50 percent dextrose infused at 3 mL/min via the peripheral infusion site. She responds well, but the next day needs another dose of dextrose via the same infusion site for a second drop in BS. At discharge, she complains of burning and pain at the site. The nurse documents that the catheter is intact upon discontinuation of the peripheral catheter, but no assessment data or subjective patient complaints are recorded. The patient is admitted three days later with purulent drainage from the left wrist infusion site, temperature of 101, and pulse rate of 100.

What is the probable cause of the second admission? What are contributing factors? What breach of standards of practice occurred? What are the legal ramifications of this case?

Media Link: Answers to the case study and more critical thinking activities are located on the CD–ROM.

Post-Test

1. Which of the following constitute the first line of nonspecific defense mechanisms?
   a. Phagocytosis, complement cascade
   b. Leukocytes, proteins
   c. Physical and chemical barriers
   d. Immune system and phagocytes
2. The complement system consists of 17 different:
   a. Glucose molecules
   b. Proteins
   c. Fatty acids
   d. Immune responses
3. The most common immunodeficiency disorders are:
   a. B-cell immunodeficiencies
   b. T-cell immunodeficiencies
   c. Induced by drug therapy
   d. Caused by poor nutritional status
4. All of the following are carrier states **EXCEPT:**
   a. Transient
   b. Intermediate
   c. Chronic
   d. Acute
5. Which of the following describes dissemination?
   a. Shedding of microorganisms into the environment from a person carrying them
   b. Infections that develop within a hospital or are produced by organisms during a patient's hospitalization
   c. Infections caused by a patient's own flora
   d. The first link in the chain of infections
6. All of the following describe the movement of organisms from source to host **EXCEPT:**
   a. Contact spread
   b. Airborne
   c. Dissemination
   d. Vector borne

7. Microorganisms frequently found in contaminated blood products include all of the following **EXCEPT:**
   a. *Pseudomonas* spp.
   b. *Salmonella* spp.
   c. *Enterobacter cloacae*
   d. *Staphylococcus aureus*
8. All of the following can contribute to the contamination of I.V. equipment and lead to sepsis **EXCEPT:**
   a. Electronic infusion devices
   b. Faulty handling of equipment
   c. Injection ports
   d. Three-way stopcocks
9. Which of the following is the *best* intervention to prevent a central venous catheter bloodstream infection?
   a. Change administration set every 24 hours.
   b. Avoid using the catheter for lab draws.
   c. Change transparent dressing every 72 hours.
   d. Follow standard precautions.
10. Which of the following is the recommended method of culture for purulent drainage?
    a. Agar
    b. Semiquantitative
    c. Semiqualitative
    d. Broth culture

Media Link: Use the enclosed CD–ROM for more practice questions, answers, and rationales .

References

Baltimore, R.S. (1998). Neonatal nosocomial infections. *Seminars in Perinatology*, 22, 25–32.

Brachman, P.S. (1998). Epidemiology of nosocomial infections. In Bennett, J.V., & Brachman, P.S., (eds.). *Hospital Infections* (4th ed.). Philadelphia: Lippincott-Raven, pp. 3–16.

Branchini, M.L., Pfaller, M.A., Rhine-Chalberg, J., et al. (1994). Genotypic variation and slime production among blood and catheter isolates of *Candida parapsilosis*. *Journal of Clinical Microbiology*, 32, 452–456.

Carlson, K., Perdue, M.B., & Hankins, J. (2001). Infection control. In Hankins, J.,

Lonswy, R.A., Hedrick, C., & Perdue, M.B. (eds.). *Infusion Therapy in Clinical Practice* (2nd ed.). Infusion Nurses Society, pp. 126–140.

Chang, L., Tsai, J., Huang, S., & Shih, C. (2003). Evaluation of infection complications of the implantable venous access system in a general oncologic population. *American Journal of Infection Control*, 31(1), 34–39.

Hibbard, J.S., Mulberry, G.K, & Brady, A.R. (2002). A clinical study comparing the skin antisepsis and safety of chloraPrep, 70% isopropyl alcohol, and 2% percent aqueous chlorhexidine. *Journal of Infusion Therapy*, 25(4), 244–249.

Hudak, C.M., Gallo, B.M., & Morton, P.G. (1998). *Critical Care Nursing: A Holistic Approach* (7th ed.). Philadelphia: Lippincott-Raven, pp. 863–867.

Humar, A., Ostromecki, A., Direnfeld, J., et al. (2000). Prospective randomized trial of 10% povidone-iodine versus 0.5% tincture of chlorhexidine as cutaneous antisepsis for prevention of central venous catheter infection. *Clinical Infectious Diseases*, 31, 1001–1007.

Infusion Nurses Society (2000). Intravenous Nursing Standards of Practice. *Journal of Intravenous Nursing* 23(6S), 1–81.

Intravenous Nurses Society (2002). *Policies and Procedures for Infusion Nursing* (2nd ed.). Intravenous Nurses Society.

Kluger, D.M., & Maki, D.G. (1999). The relative risk of intravascular device related bloodstream infections in adults. In Abstracts of the 39th Interscience Conference on Antimicrobial Agents and Chemotherapy, San Francisco, CA. American Society for Microbiology, Abstr. 524.

Kozier, B., Erb, G., Berman, A., et al. (2004). *Fundamentals of Nursing Concepts: Process and Practice* (7th ed.). Upper Saddle River, NJ: Pearson-Prentice Hall, pp. 632–633.

Maki, D.G., & McCormack, K.N. (1987). Defatting catheter insertion sites in total parenteral nutrition is of no value as an infection control measure. *American Journal of Medicine*, 83, 833–840.

Maki, D.G., & Mermel, L.A. (1998). Infection due to infusion therapy. In Bennett, J.V., & Brachman, P.S., (eds.). *Hospital Infections* (4th ed.). Philadelphia: Lippincott-Raven.

Mermel, L.A., Farr, B.M., Sherertz, R.J., et al. (2001). Guidelines for the management of intravascular catheter-related infection. *Journal of Intravenous Nursing*, 24(3), 180–205.

National Kidney Foundation (2001). III. NKF-K/DOQI Clinical practice guidelines for vascular access: Update 2000. *American Journal of Kidney Disease*, 37(Suppl), S137–181.

Occupational Safety and Health Administration. Occupational exposure to bloodborne pathogens; needlesticks and other sharps injuries; final rule. *Federal Register* 2001; 66 (12): 5318–5325.

Ray, C.E. (1999). Infection control principles and practices in the care and management of central venous access devices. *Journal of Intravenous Therapy*, 22(6S), S18–25.

Smeltzer, S.C., & Bare, B.G. (2004). *Brunner & Suddarth's Textbook of Medical–Surgical Nursing* (10th ed.). Philadelphia: Lippincott Williams & Wilkins, pp. 1522–1535.

Strovroff, M., & Teague, W.G. (1998). Intravenous access in infants and children. *Pediatric Clinics of North America*, 45, 1373–1393.

Swenson, M.R. (2000). Autoimmunity and immunotherapy. *Journal of Intravenous Nursing*, 23(5S), S8–S13.

U.S. Centers for Disease Control and Prevention (1996). Guidelines for isolation precautions in hospitals. Part II. Recommendations for isolation precautions in hospitals. *American Journal of Infection Control*, 24(1), 32–52.

U.S. Centers for Disease Control and Prevention. National Noscocomial Infections Surveillance (2001). System report, day summary from January 1995–June 2001. *American Journal of Infection Control*, 29(6), 405.

U.S. Centers for Disease Control and Prevention (2002a). Guideline for hand hygiene in health-care settings. *MMWR Morbidity Mortality Weekly Report*, 51(No. RR-16), 1–44.

U.S. Centers for Disease Control and Prevention. (2002b). Guidelines for prevention of intravascular catheter-related infections. *MMWR Morbidity Mortality Weekly Report*, 51(No. RR-10), 1–28.

U.S. Occupational Safety and Health Administration (2001). Occupational exposure to bloodborne pathogens; needlesticks and other sharps injuries; final rule. *Federal Register*, 66(12), 5318–5325.

Yamamoto, A.J., Solomon J.A., Soulen, M.C., et al. (2002). Sutureless securement device reduces complications of peripherally inserted central venous catheters. *Journal of Vascular Intervention Radiology 29(2), 10–14.*

Answers to Chapter 2 Post-Test

1. **c**
2. **b**
3. **a**
4. **d**
5. **a**
6. **d**
7. **d**
8. **a**
9. **d**
10. **b**

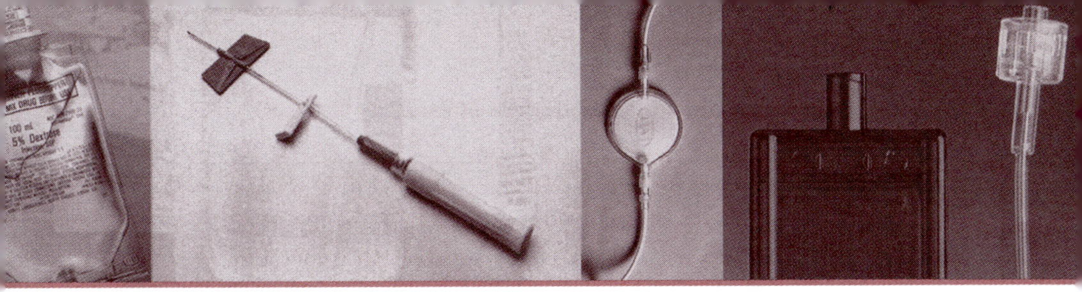

Chapter 3
Fundamentals of Fluid Balance

Chinese say that water is the most powerful element, because it is perfectly nonresistant. It can wear away rock and sweep all before it.
—Florence Scovel Shinn

Chapter Contents

LEARNING OBJECTIVES

Upon completion of this chapter, the reader will be able to:

1. Define terminology related to fluids and electrolytes.
2. Identify the three fluid compartments within the body.
3. Identify the mechanisms of daily intake and daily output.
4. State the functions of body fluids.
5. Differentiate between active and passive transport.
6. Define the concept of osmosis and give examples of this concept.
7. State the average insensible loss for a 24-hour period.
8. Describe the homeostatic organs.
9. Compare and contrast the movement of water in hypotonic, hypertonic, and isotonic solutions.
10. Summarize the major fluid balance disorders.
11. List the six major body systems assessed for fluid balance disturbances.
12. Identify patients at risk for fluid volume deficit and fluid volume excess using the nurses' quick assessment guide.
13. Determine the nursing diagnoses appropriate for care of patients experiencing fluid balance disturbances.

GLOSSARY

Active transport The passage of a substance across a cell membrane by an energy-consuming process that permits diffusion to take place

Antidiuretic hormone (ADH) A hormone secreted from the pituitary mechanism that causes the kidney to conserve water; sometimes referred to as the "water-conserving hormone"

Atrial natriuretic peptide (ANP) ANP is a cardiac hormone found in the atria of the heart that is released when atria are stretched by high blood volume.

Body fluid Body water in which electrolytes are dissolved

Diffusion The passage of molecules of one substance between the molecules of another to form a mixture of the two substances

Extracellular fluid (ECF) Body fluid located outside the cells

Filtration The process of passing fluid through a filter using pressure

Fingerprinting edema A condition in which imprints are made on the hands, sternum, or forehead when pressed firmly by the fingers

Homeostasis The ability to restore equilibrium under stress

Hypertonic Having an osmotic pressure greater than that of the solution with which it is compared

Hypotonic Having an osmotic pressure less than that of the solution with which it is compared

Insensible loss Output that is difficult to measure, such as perspiration

Interstitial fluid Body fluid between the cells

Intracellular fluid (ICF) Body fluid inside the cells

Intravascular fluid The fluid portion of blood plasma

Isotonic Having an osmotic pressure equal to that of blood; equivalent osmotic pressure

Oncotic pressure The osmotic pressure exerted by colloids (proteins), as when albumin exerts oncotic pressure within the blood vessels and helps to hold the water content of the blood in the intravascular compartment

Osmolarity A measure of solute concentration; the concentration of a solution in terms of osmoles of solutes per liter of solution

Osmosis The movement of water from a lower concentration to a higher concentration across a semipermeable membrane

Sensible loss Output that is measurable

Solute The substance that is dissolved in a liquid to form a solution

Syndrome of inappropriate antidiuretic hormone (SIADH) secretion A condition in which excessive ADH is secreted, resulting in hyponatremia.

Body Fluid Composition

Body fluid is body water in which electrolytes are dissolved. Water is the largest single constituent of the body. Body water, the medium in which cellular reactions take place, constitutes approximately 60 percent of total body weight (TBW) in young men and 50 percent to 55 percent in women. Table 3–1 provides percentages of total body fluids in relation to age and gender. Fat tissue contains little water, and the percentage of total body water varies considerably based on the amount of body fat present. In addition, total body water progressively decreases with age, making up about 50 percent of body weight in elderly people (Metheny, 2000). Figure 3–1 gives the values of total body fluids in relation to age and gender.

AGE-RELATED CONSIDERATIONS 3–1

Infants have proportionately more body fluid (70 to 80 percent of body weight) than any other age group. Infants are at higher risk for fluid volume deficit during times of increased external temperatures (NSNA, 1997).

> Table 3–1 **PERCENTAGES OF TOTAL BODY FLUID IN RELATION TO AGE AND GENDER**

Age	% of Water = Body Weight
Full-term newborn	70 to 80
1-year-old	64
Puberty to 39 years	Men: 60 Women: 55
40 to 60 years	Men: 55 Women: 47
Over 60 years	Men: 52 Women: 46

Source: *Metheny, N.M. (2000). Fluid and electrolyte balance. In Metheny, N.M. (ed.). Nursing Considerations (4th ed). Philadelphia: Lippincott-Williams & Wilkins. Copyright 2000 by Lippincott-Williams & Wilkins. Reprinted with permission.*

CULTURAL AND ETHNIC CONSIDERATIONS 3–1

A person's age, gender, ethnic origin, and weight can influence the amount and distribution of body fluid. For example, African Americans often have larger numbers of fat cells compared with other groups and therefore have less body water (Lee, Barrett, & Ignatavicius, 1996; Giger & Davidhizar, 1999).

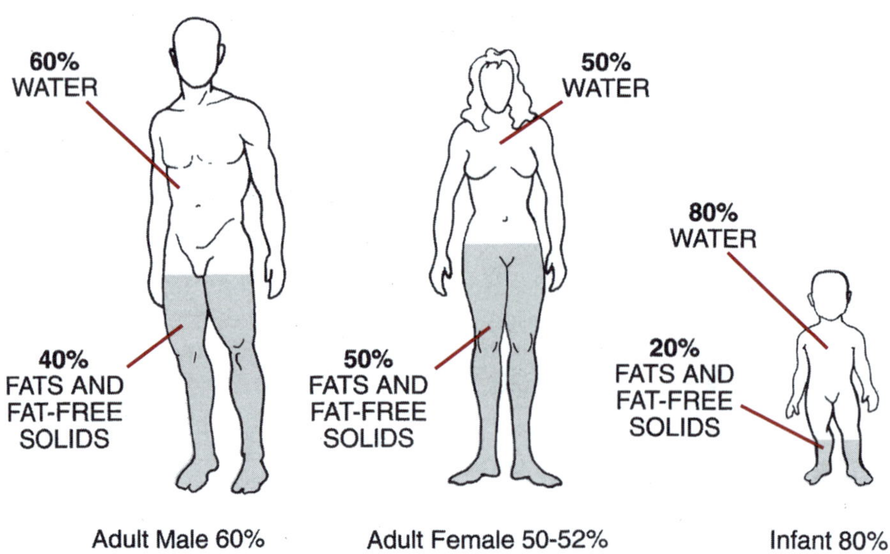

Figure 3–1 ■ Percentages of body water.

Fluid Distribution

Homeostasis is dependent on fluid and electrolyte intake, physiologic factors (e.g., organ function, hormones, age, gender), disease state factors (e.g., respiratory, renal, or metabolic disorders), external environmental factors (e.g., temperature, humidity), and pharmacologic interventions.

Water is a neutral polar molecule in which one part is negative and one part is positive. Body water is distributed within cells and outside cells. The body water within the cells is referred to as **intracellular fluid** (ICF); fluid outside the cells is referred to as **extracellular fluid** (ECF) and consists of two compartments, interstitial and intravascular. Approximately 40 percent of the TBW is composed of the fluid inside the cell (ICF). Another 20 percent is fluid outside the cell (ECF) and is divided between **interstitial** and **intravascular** spaces, with 15 percent in the tissue (interstitial) space and only 5 percent represented in the plasma (intravascular) space. The interstitial fluid lies outside of the blood vessels in the interstitial spaces between the body cells. Lymph and cerebrospinal fluids, although highly specialized, are usually regarded as interstitial fluid. Figure 3–2 gives a representation of body water distribution.

An exchange of fluid occurs continuously among the intracellular, plasma, and interstitial compartments. Of these three spaces, the intake or elimination of fluid from the body directly influences only the plasma. Changes in the intracellular and interstitial fluid compartments occur in response to changes in the volume or concentration of the plasma.

The internal environment needs to remain in homeostasis; therefore, the intake and output of fluid must be relatively equal, as in healthy individuals. In those who are ill, this balance is frequently upset, and intake of fluid may become diminished or even cease. Output may vary with the influences of increased temperature, increased respiration, draining wounds, or gastric suction.

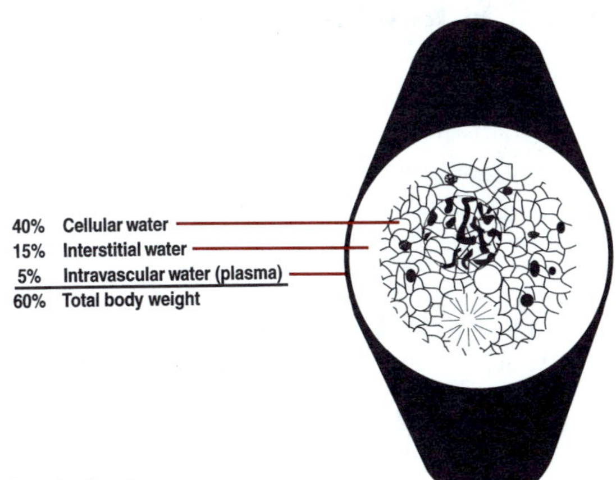

Figure 3–2 ■ Percentages of body fluid.

Normal sources of water per day include liquids, water-containing foods, and metabolic activity. In healthy adults, the intake of fluids varies from 1000 to 3000 mL/day, and 200 to 300 mL is produced from oxidation.

NURSING FAST FACT!

Normally intake and output will approximately balance only every 72 hours; thus, an appropriate target date would be 3 days (Cox, 2003).

The elimination of fluid is considered either **sensible** (measurable) loss or **insensible** (not measurable) loss. Water is eliminated from the body by the skin, kidneys, bowels, and lungs. Approximately 300 to 500 mL of water are eliminated through the lungs every 24 hours, and the skin eliminates about 500 mL/day of water in the form of perspiration. The amount of insensible loss in an adult is considered to be approximately 500 to 1000 mL/day. Losses through the gastrointestinal (GI) tract are only about 100 to 200 mL per day because of the reabsorption of most of the fluid in the small intestines. Increased losses of GI fluids can occur from diarrhea or intestinal fistulas (Metheny, 2000).

Significant sweat losses occur if a patient's body temperature exceeds 101°F (38.3°C) or if the room temperature exceeds 90°F. Insensible loss is also increased if respirations are increased to more than 20 per minute.

The formula to use in calculating a patients insensible water loss is 300 to 400 mL/m^2 per day. For example, for a patient with renal failure, fluid requirements could be estimated by calculating the patient's body surface area times the insensible water loss (Adelman & Solhung, 1996).

Fluid Function

Fluids within the body have several important functions. The ECF transports nutrients to the cells and carries waste products away from the cells by means of the capillary bed. Body fluids are in constant motion, maintaining living conditions for body cells (Metheny, 2000). The fluid within the body also has the following functions:

1. Maintains blood volume.
2. Regulates body temperature.
3. Transports material to and from cells.
4. Serves as an aqueous medium for cellular metabolism.
5. Assists digestion of food through hydrolysis.
6. Acts as a solvent in which solutes are available for cell function.
7. Serves as a medium for the excretion of waste.

Fluid Transport

Body fluids are in constant motion, maintaining healthy living conditions for body cells. The ECF interfaces with the outside world and is modified by it, but the ICF remains stable. Nutrients are transported by the ECF to the cells and wastes are carried away from the cells by means of the capillary bed (Metheny, 2000).

Movement of particles through the cell membrane occurs through four transport mechanisms: passive transport consisting of diffusion, osmosis, and filtration; and active transport. Materials are transported between the ICF and the extracellular compartment by these four mechanisms.

Passive Transport

Passive transport is also referred to as non–carrier-mediated transport. It is the movement of solutes through membranes without the expenditure of energy. It includes passive diffusion, osmosis, and filtration.

Passive Diffusion

Passive diffusion is the passive movement of water, ions, and lipid-soluble molecules randomly in all directions from a region of high concentration to an area of low concentration. Diffusion occurs through semipermeable membranes by the substance either passing through pores, if small enough, or dissolving in the lipid matrix of the membrane wall. If there is no force opposing diffusion, particles distribute themselves evenly. Many substances can diffuse through the cell membrane, and these substances diffuse in both directions. Influencing factors in the diffusion process are concentration differences, electrical potential, and pressure differences across the pores. The greater the concentration, the greater the rate of diffusion. An increase in the pressure on one side of the membrane increases the molecular forces striking the pores, thus creating a pressure gradient. Other factors that increase diffusion include:

- Increased temperature
- Increased concentration of particles
- Decreased size or molecular weight of particles
- Increased surface area available for diffusion
- Decreased distance across which the particle mass must diffuse

Osmosis

Osmosis is the passage of water from an area of lower particle concentration toward one with a higher particle concentration across a semipermeable membrane. For a membrane to be semipermeable, it has to be more permeable to water than to solutes. This process tends to equalize the concentration of two solutions.

Osmosis governs the movement of body fluids between the intracellular and ECF compartments, therefore influencing the volumes of fluid within each. Through the process of osmosis, water flows through semipermeable membranes toward the side with the higher concentration of particles (thus from lower to higher).

PRESSURE GRADIENTS

Osmotic pressure develops as solute particles collide against each other. Osmotic pressure is the amount of hydrostatic pressure needed to draw a solvent (water) across a membrane and develops as a result of a high concentration of particles colliding with one another. As the number of solutes increases, there is less space for them to move; therefore, they come in contact with one another more frequently. This results in increased osmotic pressure, which causes the movement of fluid. The concentration of a solution containing more solute particles increases the collisions, creating a greater osmotic pressure. Osmotic pressure is measured in milliosmoles (mOsm). Whereas osmolality is the total number of osmotically active particles per liter of solution, osmolarity refers to the concentration of a solute in a volume of solution. The two terms are very similar and are often used interchangeably. The term osmolarity will be used within this text. The normal osmolarity of body fluids is between 280 and 295 mOsm/L, and the osmolarity of ICF and ECF is always equal.

Filtration

Filtration is the transfer of water and a dissolved substance from a region of high pressure to a region of low pressure; the force behind it is hydrostatic pressure (i.e., the pressure of water at rest). The pumping heart provides hydrostatic pressure in the movement of water and electrolytes from the arterial capillary bed to the interstitial fluid. Diffusion moves in either direction across a membrane; filtration moves in one direction only because of the hydrostatic, osmotic, and interstitial fluid pressure. Filtration is likened to pouring a solution through a sieve: the size of the opening in the sieve determines the size of the particle to be iltered.

The plasma compartment contains more protein than the other compartments. Plasma protein, composed of albumin, globulin, and fibrinogen, creates an osmotic pressure at the capillary membrane, preventing fluid from the plasma from leaking into the interstitial spaces. Osmotic pressure created within the plasma by the presence of protein (mainly albumin) keeps the water in the vascular system.

Starling's Law of the Capillaries maintains that under normal circumstances, fluid filtered out of the arterial end of a capillary bed and reabsorbed at the venous end is exactly the same, creating a state of near-equilibrium. However, it is not exactly the same because of the difference in hydrostatic pressure between the arterial and venous capillary beds. The pressure that moves fluid out of the arterial end of the network amounts to a total of 28.3 mm Hg. The pressure that moves fluid back into circulation at the venous capillary bed is 28 mm Hg. The small amount of excess remaining in the interstitial compartment is returned to the circulation by way of the lymphatic system (Craven and Himle, 2003).

Active Transport

Active transport is similar to diffusion except that it acts against a concentration gradient. Active transport occurs when it is necessary for ions (electrolytes) to move from an area of low concentration to an area of high concentration. By definition, active transport implies that energy expenditure must take place for the movement to occur against a concentration gradient. Adenosine triphosphate (ATP) is released from the cell to enable certain substances to acquire the energy needed to pass through the cell membrane. For example, sodium concentration is greater in ECF; therefore, sodium tends to enter by diffusion into the intracellular compartment. This tendency is offset by the sodium–potassium pump, which is located on the cell membrane. In the presence of ATP, the sodium–potassium pump actively moves sodium from the cell into the ECF. Active transport is vital for maintaining the unique composition of both the extracellular and intracellular compartments (Lee, 1996).

Tonicity of Solutions

Tonicity reflects the concept and effects of hypotonic, hypertonic, and isotonic solutions on body cells. Figure 3–3 shows the movement of water by osmosis in hypotonic, isotonic, and hypertonic solutions.

Isotonic solutions, such as 0.9 percent sodium chloride (NaCl) and 5 percent dextrose in water, have the same osmolarity as that of normal body fluids. Solutions that have an osmolarity of 250 to 375 mOsm/L are considered isotonic solutions and have no effect on the volume of fluid within the cell; the solution remains within the ECF space. Isotonic solutions are used to expand the ECF compartment.

Hypotonic solutions contain less salt than the intracellular space, and when infused, have an osmolarity below 250 mOsm/L, and move water into the cell, causing the cell to swell and possibly burst. By lowering the serum osmolarity, the body fluids shift out of the blood vessels into the interstitial tissue and cells. Hypotonic solutions hydrate cells and can deplete the circulatory system. An example of a hypotonic solution is 2.5 percent dextrose in water.

Hypertonic solutions, conversely, cause the water from within a cell to move to the ECF compartment, where the concentration of salt is greater, causing the cell to shrink. Hypertonic solutions have an osmolarity of 375 mOsm/L and above. These solutions are used to replace elec-

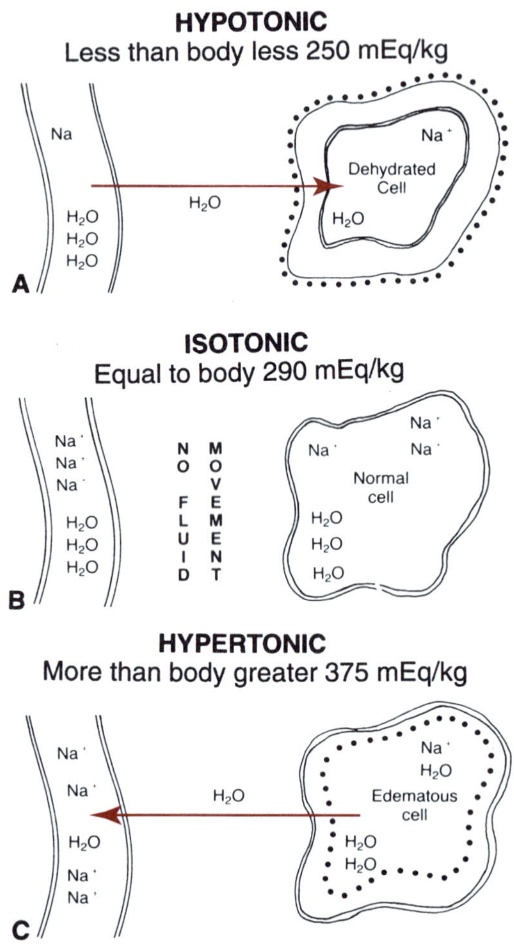

Figure 3–3 ■ Effects of fluid shifts in isotonic, hypertonic, and hypotonic states. (From Kuhn, M. [1998]. *Pharmacotherapeutics: A Nursing Process Approach,* [4th ed.]. Philadelphia: F.A. Davis, p. 128, with permission.)

trolytes. When hypertonic dextrose solutions are used alone, they also are used to shift ECF from interstitial tissue to plasma. Examples of hypertonic solutions are 5 percent dextrose and 0.9 percent NaCl, or 5 percent dextrose and Normosol M. Figure 3–4 illustrates tonicity (osmolarity) ranges.

The osmotic pressure exerted by plasma colloids (or solutes) is called the colloid osmotic pressure, or oncotic pressure. For example, albumin, a plasma protein, exerts oncotic pressure within the blood vessels and helps to hold the water content of the blood in the intravascular space. Proteinates are concentrated in the intracellular (55 mEq/L) and intravascular (16 mEq/L) spaces.

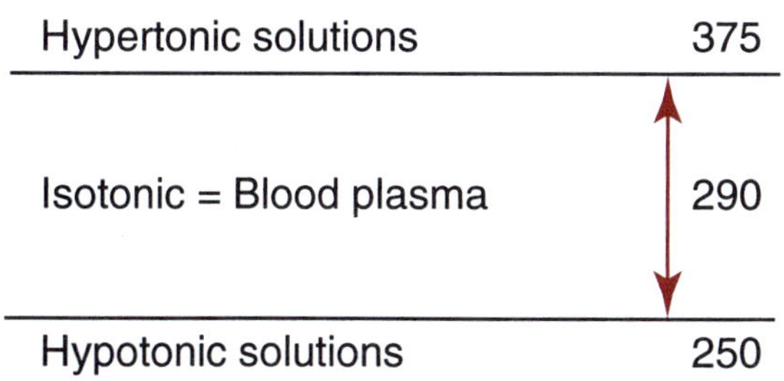

Figure 3–4 ■ Tonicity/osmolarity ranges of solutions.

Homeostatic Mechanisms

Regulation of body water is maintained through exogenous sources, such as the intake of food and fluids, and endogenous sources that are produced within the body through chemical oxidation process. Several homeostatic mechanisms are responsible for the balance of fluid and electrolytes within the body. When homeostasis is compromised and imbalance occurs, the nurse is responsible for managing the exogenous source of fluid replacement via the intravenous route. The endogenous sources of balancing fluid and electrolytes is through various body systems such as the renal, cardiovascular, lymphatic, respiratory, nervous, and endocrine systems.

Renal System

The kidneys are vital to the regulation of fluid and electrolyte balance. They normally filter 170 L of plasma per day in the adult, and excrete only 1.5 L of urine (Metheny, 2000). They act in response to bloodborne messengers such as aldosterone and antidiuretic hormone (ADH).

Renal failure can result in multiple fluid and electrolyte imbalances.

Functions of the kidneys in fluid balance are:

- Regulation of fluid volume and osmolarity by selective retention and excretion of body fluids
- Regulation of electrolyte levels by selective retention of needed substances and excretion of unneeded substances
- Regulation of pH of ECF by excretion or retention of hydrogen (H^+) ions
- Excretion of metabolic wastes (primarily acids) and toxic substances (Metheny, 2000).

Cardiovascular System

The pumping action of the heart provides circulation of blood through the kidneys under pressure, which allows urine to form. Renal perfusion makes renal function possible. Blood vessels provide plasma to reach the kidneys in sufficient volume (20 percent of circulating blood volume) to permit regulation of water and electrolytes. Baroreceptors located in the carotid sinus and aortic arch respond to the degree of stretch of the vessel wall, which has been generated by the body's reaction to hypovolemia. The response is to stimulate fluid retention.

Atrial natriuretic peptides (ANPs) are produced by the cardiac atria, ventricles, and other vessels in response to changes in ECF volume. When atrial pressure is increased, ANP released by the atrial and ventricular myocytes acts on the nephron to increase sodium excretion. Low atrial pressures inhibit release of ANP (Levin, Gardner, & Samson, 1998).

Lymphatic System

The lymphatic system serves as an adjunct to the cardiovascular system by removing excess interstitial fluid (in the form of lymph) and returning it to the circulatory system. Fluid overload in the interstitial compartment would result if it were not for the lymphatic system. The lymphatic system carries the excess fluid, proteins, and large particulate matter that cannot be reabsorbed by the venous capillary bed out of interstitial compartment. This minute excess (0.3 mm Hg) accounts for 1.7 mm/min of fluid. If the lymphatic system were not continually removing this small amount of fluid, there would be a buildup of 2,448 mL in the interstitial compartment over a 24-hour period of time (Guyton & Hall, 2000).

Respiratory System

The lungs are vital for maintaining homeostasis and constitute one of the main regulatory organs of fluid and acid–base balance. The lungs regulate acid–base balance by regulation of the hydrogen (H^+) ion concentration. Alveolar ventilation is responsible for the daily elimination of approximately 13,000 mEq of H^+ ions. The kidneys excrete only 40 to 80 mEq of hydrogen daily. Under influence from the medulla, the lungs act promptly to correct metabolic acid–base disturbances by regulating the level of carbon dioxide (a potential acid) in the ECF. Functions of the lungs in body fluid balance are:

- Regulation of metabolic alkalosis by compensatory hypoventilation, resulting in carbon dioxide (CO_2) retention and increased acidity of the ECF
- Regulation of metabolic acidosis by causing compensatory hyperventilation, resulting in CO_2 excretion and thus decreased acidity of the ECF
- Removal of 300 to 500 mL of water daily through exhalation (i.e., insensible water loss)

Nervous System

The nervous system is the master controller in fluid and electrolyte balance through the regulation of sodium and water. It does this by stimulating various endocrine glands.

Endocrine System

The glands responsible for aiding in homeostasis are the adrenal, pituitary, and parathyroid glands. The endocrine system responds selectively to the regulation and maintenance of fluid and electrolyte balance through hormonal production.

Antidiuretic Hormone

The pituitary hormone influencing water balance is ADH. This hormone, which affects renal reabsorption of water, is also referred to as the "water-conserving" hormone. Functions of ADH are to maintain osmotic pressure of the cells by controlling renal water retention or excretion and control of blood volume. Excessive secretion of ADH results in the syndrome of inappropriate antidiuretic hormone secretion (SIADH).

Numerous drugs (e.g., alcohol, narcotic antagonists) can block ADH activity or reduce tubular responsiveness to ADH (e.g., lithium, demeclocycline), which results in increased water loss, causing dehydration and hypernatremia. Increased ADH secretion may be the result of disease (hormone-secreting tumor, head injury) or may be related to administration of drugs such as chlorpropamide, Vinca alkaloids, carbamazepine, cyclophosphamide, tricyclic antidepressants, and narcotics (Metheny, 2000).

Factors that affect ADH production include pathologic changes such as head trauma and tumors of the brain or lung, anesthesia and surgery in general, and certain drugs (e.g., barbiturates, antineoplastics, and nonsteroidal anti-inflammatory agents [NSNA, 1997]).

Parathyroid Hormone

The parathyroid gland is embedded in the corners of the thyroid gland and regulates calcium and phosphate balance. The parathyroid gland influences fluid and electrolytes, increases serum calcium levels, and lowers serum phosphate levels. A reciprocal relationship exists between extracellular calcium and phosphate levels. When the serum calcium level is low, the parathyroid gland secretes more parathyroid hormone. The parathyroid hormone can increase the serum calcium level by promoting calcium release from the bone as needed. Calcitonin from the thyroid gland increases calcium return to the bone, thus decreasing the serum calcium level.

Aldosterone

The adrenal cortex is important in fluid and electrolyte homeostasis. The primary adrenocortical hormone influencing the balance of fluid is aldosterone. Aldosterone is responsible for the renal reabsorption of sodium, which results in the retention of chloride and water and the excretion of potassium. Aldosterone also regulates blood volume by regulating sodium retention.

Epinephrine

Epinephrine, another adrenal hormone, increases blood pressure, enhances pulmonary ventilation, dilates blood vessels needed for emergencies, and constricts unnecessary vessels.

Cortisol

When produced in large quantities, the adrenocortical hormone cortisol can produce sodium and fluid retention and potassium deficit.

Physical Assessment

A body systems approach is the best method for assessing fluid and electrolyte imbalances related to I.V. therapy. The I.V. nurse should begin by assessing vital signs, infusion rate of any I.V. infusions, and intake and output. Nurses should follow this with assessing body systems at the beginning of each shift and as needed to monitor the patient's reactions to infusions.

Neurologic

There is a progressive loss of central nervous system (CNS) cells with advancing age, along with decreases in the sense of smell and tactile sense. The thirst mechanism in elderly people may be diminished and is a poor guide for fluid needs in older patients. An ill patient may not be able to verbalize thirst or to reach for a glass of water. Sensation of thirst depends on excitation of the cortical centers of consciousness. The use of antianxiety agents, sedatives, or hypnotic agents can lead to confusion and disorientation, causing the patient to forget to drink fluid. Changes in orientation can also be an indicator of fluid volume deficit.

Fluid volume changes, along with serum sodium levels, affect the CNS cells, resulting in irritability, lethargy, confusion, seizures, or coma. CNS cells shrink in sodium excess and expand when serum sodium levels decrease. Assessment of neuromuscular irritability is particularly important when imbalances in calcium, magnesium, and sodium are suspected.

Cardiovascular

The quality and rate of the pulse are indicators of how the patient is tolerating the ECF volume. The peripheral veins in the extremities provide a way of evaluating plasma volume. Examination of hand veins can evaluate the plasma volume. Peripheral veins empty in 3 to 5 seconds when the hand is elevated and fill in the same amount of time when the hand is lowered to a dependent position. Peripheral vein filling takes longer than 3 to 5 seconds in patients with sodium depletion and extracellular dehydration (Metheny, 2000). Slow emptying of the peripheral veins indicates overhydration and excessive blood volume (Fig. 3–5).

A 20-mm Hg fall in systolic blood pressure when shifting from the lying to the standing position (postural hypotension) usually indicates fluid volume deficit. The jugular vein provides a built-in manometer for evaluation of central venous pressure (CVP). Changes in fluid volume are reflected by changes in neck vein filling.

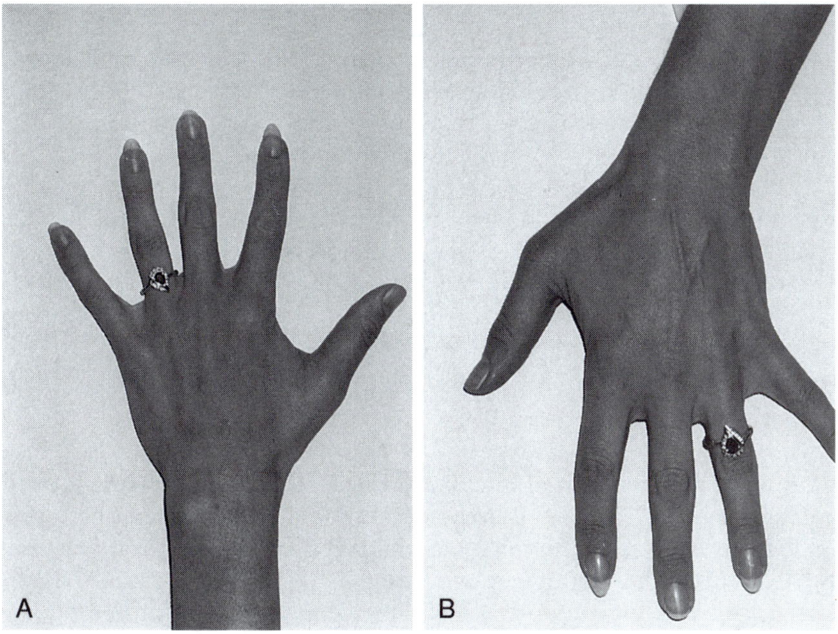

Figure 3–5 ■ Hand vein assessment. Peripheral vein takes longer than 3 to 5 seconds in patients with sodium depletion and dehydration. Slow emptying of hand veins indicates overhydration and excessive blood volume.

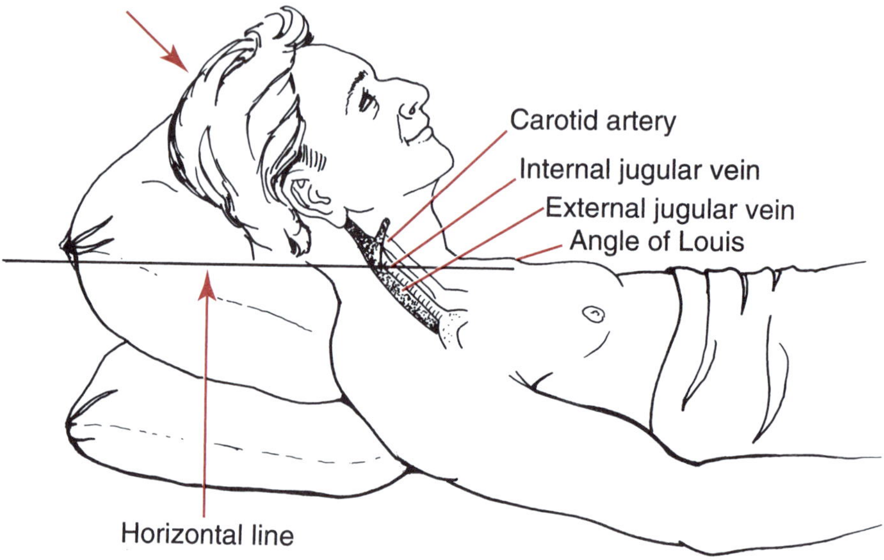

Figure 3–6 ■ Jugular venous distention.

The external jugular veins, with the patient supine, fill to the anterior border of the sternocleidomastoid muscle. Flat neck veins in the supine position indicate a decreased plasma volume. When the patient is in a 45-degree position, the external jugular distends no higher than 2 cm above the sternal angle. Neck veins distending from the top portion of the sternum to the angle of the jaw indicate elevated venous pressure (Fig. 3–6).

Edema indicates expansion of interstitial volume. Edema can be localized (usually caused by inflammation) or generalized (usually related to capillary hemodynamics). Edema should be assessed over bony surfaces of the tibia or sacrum and rated according to severity from 1+ to 4+ (Fig. 3–7; Horne & Swearingen, 1993). The presence of periorbital edema suggests significant fluid retention.

Respiratory

A key to the assessment of circulatory overload is an assessment of the lung fields. Changes in respiratory rate and depth may be a compensatory mechanism for acid–base imbalance. Tachypnea (>20 respirations/min) and dyspnea indicate fluid volume excess (FVE). Moist crackles in the absence of cardiopulmonary disease indicate fluid volume excess. Shallow, slow breathing may indicate metabolic alkalosis or respiratory acidosis. Deep, rapid breathing may indicate respiratory alkalosis or metabolic acidosis. See Chapter 4 for further information on acid–base imbalances.

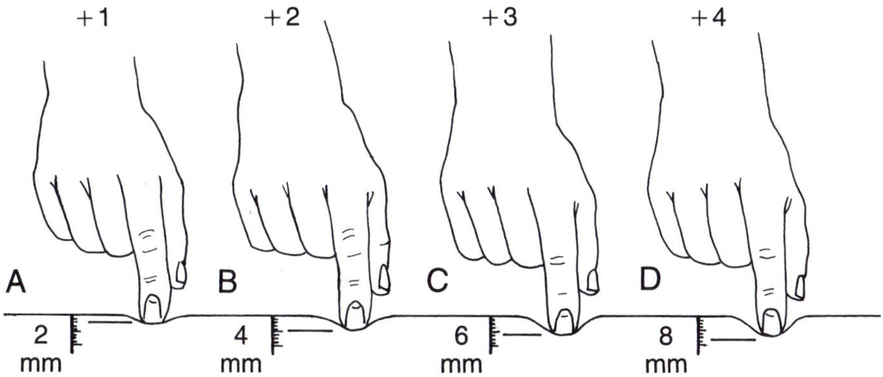

Figure 3–7 ■ Edema scale.

Skin Appearance and Temperature

Assessments of temperature and skin surface are key in determining fluid volume changes. Pinching the area over the hand, inner thigh, sternum, or forehead can assess skin turgor. In a well-hydrated person, the pinched skin immediately falls back to its normal position when released. This elastic property, referred to as turgor, is partially dependent on interstitial fluid volume. In a person with a fluid volume deficit, the skin may remain slightly elevated for many seconds. In persons older than age 55 years, skin turgor is generally reduced because of loss of elasticity, particularly in areas that have been exposed to the sun. A more accurate assessment can be made on the skin over the sternum. A condition in which placement of fingers firmly on the patient's skin leaves finger imprints is called fingerprinting and is associated with fluid volume excess. Fingerprint edema is demonstrated by pressing a finger firmly over the sternum or other body surface for a period of 15 to 30 seconds. Upon removal of the finger, a positive sign is a visible fingerprint similar to that seen when a fingerprint is made on paper with ink.

AGE-RELATED CONSIDERATIONS 3–2

In infants (children less than 18 months of age) sunken or depressed fontanels can indicate fluid volume deficit (FVD) and bulging fontanels can indicate FVE.

Special Senses

The eyes, mouth, lips, and tongue are also key indicators of fluid volume imbalances. The absence of tearing and salivation in a child is a sign of fluid volume deficit. In a healthy person, the tongue has one longitudinal furrow. In the person with fluid volume deficit, the tongue has additional longitudinal furrows and is smaller because of fluid loss (Metheny, 2000).

Mucous membranes often show the first sign of dehydration; as fluid volume decreases, the mouth becomes dry and sticky and the lips dry and cracked. In fluid volume deficit, the patient's eyes tend to appear sunken; in significant fluid volume excess, periorbital edema is present.

NURSING FAST FACT!

Good oral hygiene is imperative with mouth-breathing patients. If the patient is receiving good oral care and the crusted, dry, furrowed tongue is not improving, fluid volume deficit must be restored to aid in solving this problem.

Body Weight

Taking daily weights of patients with potential fluid imbalances is an important clinical tool. Accurate body weight measurement is a better indicator of gains or losses than intake and output records. A loss or gain of 1 kg (2.2 lb.) reflects a loss or gain of 1 L of body fluid. Generally, fluid volume deficit or excess is considered severe when body weight fluctuates 15 percent higher or lower than the person's normal body weight. Table 3–2 provides a summary of assessment findings that indicate altered fluid status.

Fluid Volume Imbalances

Fluid volume imbalances may reflect an increase or a decrease in total body fluid or an altered distribution of body fluids. There are two major alterations in ECF balance: fluid volume deficit (FVD) and fluid volume excess (FVE).

Fluid Volume Deficit

Extracellular fluid volume deficit reflects a contracted vascular compartment caused by either a significant ECF loss or by an accumulation of fluid in the interstitial space. ECF deficit is also referred to as dehydration. It may be caused by an actual decrease in body water; excessive fluid loss or inadequate fluid intake; or a relative decrease in which fluid (plasma) shifts from the intravascular compartment to the interstitial space, a process called "third spacing" (Lee, 1996).

> Table 3–2 **QUICK ASSESSMENT GUIDE FOR FLUID IMBALANCES**

Area of Clinical Assessment	Signs and Symptoms of Fluid Volume Deficit (Hypovolemia)	Signs and Symptoms of Fluid Volume Excess (Hypervolemia)
Neurologic	Irritability, restlessness, lethargy, and confusion (seizures and coma) Thirst	
Cardiovascular	Frank or postural hypotension Tachycardia Weak, thready pulses Decreased pulse volume Cool extremities with delayed capillary refill Flat neck veins Poor peripheral vein filling CVP <4 cm	Galloping heart rhythm (heart S_3 sound) in adults Distended neck veins Slow emptying hand veins CVP >11 cm Bounding full pulse Peripheral edema
Respiratory	Lungs clear Respirations may be rapid and shallow	Tachypnea (>20) and dyspnea Irritated cough Hacking cough – becoming moist and productive Labored breathing Wet lung sounds (moist crackles) Decreased O_2 saturation Cyanosis
Skin appearance and temperature	Low-grade fever Dry skin "tenting" Sunken or depressed fontanels in infants	Bulging fontanels in children under 18 months Edematous skin (1+ to 4+)
Eyes	Decreased tearing and dry conjunctiva Sunken eyeballs	Periorbital edema
Lips	Dry lips, cracked	No change
Oral cavity	Dry Increased tongue furrows, tongue coated Sticky mucous membranes	No change
Urine volume and concentration	Concentrated urine and low volume <30 mL/h Specific gravity high: >1.035	Polyuria Specific gravity <1.010
Body weight	Weight loss 5%: Mild deficit 5–10%: Moderate deficit >15%: Severe deficit (especially important in children)	Weight gain (acute and rapid) 5%: Mild excess 5–10%: Moderate excess >15%: Severe excess
Diagnostic lab findings	Normal or high HCT and BUN Serum osmolarity elevated: >300 Serum sodium >150 mEq Serum glucose elevated >120 mg/dL	HCT and BUN decreased Serum osmolality is low <275 Serum sodium low <125 mEq

Sources: *Hogan & Wane (2003); Metheny (2000); Hudak (1998).*

Etiology and Pathophysiology

Fluid volume deficit occurs when there is either an excessive loss of body water or an inadequate compensatory intake. The ECF consists predominantly of the electrolytes sodium and chloride, both of which tend to attract water; loss of these electrolytes also leads to loss of water.

Gastrointestinal dysfunction is the most common cause of ECF deficit. Other common causes include overzealous use of diuretics and diaphoresis.

Fluid volume deficit also occurs in third spacing, which is caused by peritonitis, intestinal obstruction, postoperative conditions, thrombophlebitis, acute pancreatitis, ascites, fistula drainage, and burns. Third spaces are extracellular body spaces in which fluid is not normally present in large amounts, but in which fluid can accumulate. Fluid that accumulates in third spaces is physiologically useless because it is not available for use. Common sites for collection of third space fluid include tissue spaces, abdomen, pleural spaces, and pericardial space (Hogan & Wave, 2003).

Common Causes of Isotonic Dehydration

- Hemorrhage resulting in loss of fluid, electrolytes, proteins, and blood cells in proportional amounts, resulting in inadequate vascular volume
- Gastrointestinal losses: Vomiting, diarrhea, nasogastric suction, drainage from fistulas and tubes. Tend to be lost in proportional amounts
- Fever, environmental heat, and diaphoresis result in profuse sweating, causing water and sodium loss.
- Burns initially damage skin and capillary membranes allow fluid, electrolytes, and proteins to escape into the burned tissue, resulting in inadequate vascular volume.
- Diuretics cause excessive loss of fluid and electrolytes in proportional amounts.
- Third space fluid shifts occur when fluid moves from the vascular space into physiologically useless extracellular spaces.

Common Causes of Hypertonic Fluid Dehydration

- Inadequate fluid intake: Patients who are unable to respond to thirst independently (bedridden, infants, elderly who have nausea, and anorexia, those who are NPO without adequate fluid replacement)
- Decreased water intake results in ECF solute concentration and leads to cellular dehydration (Hogan & Wane, 2003).

AGE-RELATED CONSIDERATIONS 3–3

Infants and small children are prone to dehydration. In addition, in children, skin turgor begins to diminish after 3 percent to 5 percent of body weight is lost.

Clinically, ECF deficit is characterized by acute weight loss, altered cardiovascular function that reflects the underlying ECF volume deficit, and complaints of nausea and vomiting. The cardiovascular assessment is the most important part of the process to determine plasma volume changes. In a patient who is hypovolemic, the heart rate increases, the blood pressure decreases, and the peripheral pulses are weak. Symptoms reflect a dehydrated state with sunken eyeballs, poor skin turgor, and oliguria commonly seen.

Laboratory findings in fluid volume deficit reflect hemoconcentration with the serum hemoglobin, hematocrit, and proteins increased. Blood urea nitrogen is elevated above 20 mg/100 mL. The urine specific gravity reflects high solute concentration of more than 1.030.

Treatment

Treatment for patients with an ECF volume deficit entails fluid replacement (orally or intravenously) until the oliguria is relieved and the cardiovascular and neurologic systems stabilize. Isotonic electrolyte solutions such as 0.9 percent NaCl or lactated Ringer's solution are used to treat hypotensive patients with a fluid volume deficit. A hypotonic electrolyte solution (0.45 percent NaCl) is often used to provide electrolyte and free water for renal excretion of metabolic wastes (Metheny, 2000).

NURSING FAST FACT!

Extreme caution must be exercised in fluid replacement therapy to avoid fluid overload.

Fluid Volume Excess

Extracellular fluid volume excess causes an expansion of the ECF compartment. The primary cause of ECF excess is cardiovascular dysfunction. Fluid volume excess is always secondary to an increase in total body sodium content, which causes total body water increase. Normally, the posterior pituitary decreases secretion of the ADH when excess water moves into the cells. This causes the kidney to eliminate excess fluid. However, if a patient has an excessive secretion of ADH, the water will be retained, placing the patient at risk for fluid volume excess. Excessive secretion of ADH can be caused by fear, pain, postoperative reaction 12 to 24 hours after surgery, and acute infections.

Etiology and Pathophysiology

Conditions that cause isotonic overhydration include excessive administration of oral or I.V. fluids, excessive irrigation of body cavities or organs, and use of hypotonic fluids to replace isotonic fluid losses (Lee, 1996).

Hypotonic fluid overload is also called water intoxication. Conditions that cause hypotonic overload are SIADH, excessive water intake, and congestive heart failure.

AGE-RELATED CONSIDERATIONS 3–4

If a person has poor cardiac function, fluid overload can occur rapidly and lead to congestive heart failure. This is a common issue for older persons, who often have poor cardiac reserve and a history of cardiovascular disease.

Clinically, ECF volume excess has distinct signs and symptoms, the most prominent being weight gain. Edema is usually not apparent until 2 to 4 kg of fluid has been retained. Alterations in respiratory and cardiovascular function are present and include hypertension and tachycardia. In addition to common assessment findings, some patients also experience confusion, altered levels of consciousness, skeletal muscle weakness, and increased bowel sounds.

In fluid volume excess, the hematocrit may be decreased because of hemodilution. The serum sodium and serum osmolarity will be decreased if hypervolemia occurs as a result of excessive retention of water.

COMMON CAUSES OF ISOTONIC OVERHYDRATION

- Renal failure leading to decreased excretion of water and sodium
- Heart failure leading to stasis of blood in the circulation and venous congestion
- Excess fluid intake of isotonic I.V. solutions
- High corticosteroid levels due to therapy, stress response, or disease results in sodium and water retention
- High aldosterone levels (stress response adrenal dysfunction, liver damage, and metabolic problems)

COMMON CAUSES OF HYPOTONIC OVERHYDRATION (WATER INTOXICATION)

- More fluid is gained than solute.
- Serum osmolality falls, causing cells to swell (cerebral cells most sensitive).
- Repeated plain water enemas.
- Overuse of hypotonic I.V. fluids
- In young children or infants, ingestion of inappropriately prepared formula and/or excess water (use of water bottle as pacifier)
- SIADH causes kidneys to retain large amounts of water without sodium.

NURSING FAST FACT!

Severe or prolonged isotonic fluid volume excess in a person with a healthy heart and kidneys is usually compensated through increasing urinary output.

Treatment

Treatment of ECF volume excess is directed toward sodium and fluid restriction, administration of diuretics, and the treatment of the underlying cause (Hudak, 1998). Evaluate the patient for potential fluid and electrolyte imbalances as a consequence of corrective therapy.

NURSING PLAN OF CARE

FLUID VOLUME DEFICIT

Focus Assessment

Subjective

- History of contributing factors and cause, such as diabetes mellitus, cardiac disease, or GI disorder
- Recent weight changes
- History of laxative, enema, or diuretic overuse
- Fluid intake (amount and type)

Objective

- Present weight
- Changes in mentation
- Dry skin and mucous membranes
- Poor skin turgor
- Decreased pulse rate
- Decreased blood pressure
- Slow vein filling
- Decreased urine output
- Increased urine specific gravity

Patient Outcome/Evaluation Criteria

Patient will:

- Increase fluid intake to a minimum of 2000 mL/d unless contraindicated.
- Maintain adequate urine output and urine specific gravity within normal range.
- Be free of injury.
- Verbalize adequate knowledge of condition as well as therapeutic and preventive measures.

Nursing Diagnoses

- Fluid volume deficit related to failure of regulatory mechanisms
- Fluid volume deficit related to loss of body fluid and inadequate fluid intake

(Continued on following page)

NURSING PLAN OF CARE

FLUID VOLUME DEFICIT *(Continued)*

- Fluid volume deficit related to high-solute tube feedings
- Altered oral mucous membrane related to dehydration
- Altered tissue perfusion: Cardiopulmonary, renal, and peripheral related to hypovolemia
- Risk of injury related to altered sensorium and/or dizziness
- Knowledge deficit related to risk factors and therapeutic interventions

Nursing Management

1. Monitor specific assessment parameters related to management of FVD including:
   a. Fluid status, including intake and output
   b. Specific gravity
   c. Trends of daily weights
   d. Hemodynamic status (central venous pressure when appropriate)
   e. Signs of dehydration: Skin turgor, delayed capillary refill, weak or thready pulse, severe thirst, dry mucous membranes, decreased urine output, and hypotension
2. Monitor fluid loss (e.g., bleeding, vomiting, diarrhea, and perspiration tachypnea).
3. Administer isotonic solutions for extracellular rehydration, if appropriate.
4. Administer hypotonic solutions for intracellular rehydration, if appropriate.
5. Monitor laboratory data:
   a. Hemoglobin and hematocrit
   b. Serum sodium levels
   c. Serum osmolarity
   d. Blood urea nitrogen (BUN)
   e. Serum electrolytes
6. Encourage oral fluid intake.
7. Promote skin integrity.
8. Provide comfort measures:
   a. Good oral hygiene (rinse with equal parts of peroxide and water)
   b. Avoid glycerin and lemon or alcohol-based mouthwashes, which can be drying.
   c. Avoid sucking on hard candy or chewing gum, both of which can further dry oral mucous membranes.
   d. Apply lip moisturizer.
   e. Apply skin moisturizer.

(Continued on following page)

9. Listen to client's concerns, answer questions, and implement teaching.
10. Implement measures to control nausea, vomiting, diarrhea, and high fever.
11. Administer medication therapy according to orders:
    a. Antiemetics to prevent fluid losses due to nausea and vomiting
    b. Antidiarrheals to prevent fluid losses for the GI tract
    c. ADH vasopressin used to corrrect diabetes insipidus
    d. Antipyretics used to control fever and minimize fluid losses.

Sources: *Sparks & Taylor (1998), Hogan & Wane (2003), Metheny (2000).*

Patient Education

Teach patient risk factors for development of FVD or FVE.

Explain to client and family the reasons for intake and output records. Teach the client to keep track of oral liquids consumed.

Assess patient's understanding of the type of fluid loss being experienced.

Give verbal and written instructions for fluid replacement (drink at least 3 quarts of liquid).

Teach to increase the fluid intake during hot days, in the presence of fever or infection and to decrease activity during extreme weather.

Teach how to observe for dehydration (especially in infants).

Instruct to seek medical consultation for continued dehydration.

Teach appropriate use of laxatives, enemas, and diuretics.

Inform patient to notify physician if he or she has excessive edema or weight gain (more than 2 lbs) or increased shortness of breath.

Provide literature concerning low-salt diets; consult with dietitian if necessary.

Provide dietary education.

Teach to avoid adding salt while cooking.

Teach to avoid caffeine because it acts as a mild diuretic.

Home Care Issues

Consider home care visit to follow up with patients with diabetes mellitus, cardiovascular disorders, and severe GI disorders.

Follow up with home care for patients taking drug therapy (diuretics) for edema.

Consider home care visit to follow up on diet and instructions on use of pressure stockings.

Key Points

- Fluid is distributed in three compartments: intracellular (40 percent), intravascular (5 percent), and interstitial (15 percent); total body weight in water is 60 percent for an average adult.
- Fluid is transported passively by filtration, diffusion, and osmosis.
- Electrolytes are actively transported by ATP on cell membranes and the sodium–potassium pump.
- Osmosis is the movement of water from a lower concentration to a higher concentration across a semipermeable membrane.
- The osmolarity of I.V. solutions has the following ranges:
  - Isotonic solutions: 250 to 375 mOsm/L
  - Hypotonic solutions: less than 250 mOsm/L
  - Hypertonic solutions: greater than 375 mOsm/L
- The homeostatic organs that regulate fluid and electrolyte balance include the kidneys; heart and blood vessels; lungs; and adrenal, parathyroid, and pituitary glands
- There are six areas to assess for fluid balance: neurologic status, cardiovascular, respiratory, integumentary, special senses, and body weight
- Fluid imbalances fall into two categories:
  - Fluid volume deficit caused primarily by disorders of the GI system; signs and symptoms reflect a dehydrated individual. Treatment is aimed at rehydration with isotonic sodium chloride.
  - Fluid volume excess caused primarily by cardiovascular dysfunction, renal or endocrine dysfunction, and too-rapid administration of I.V. fluids; signs and symptoms reflect fluid overload. Treatment is aimed at decreasing the sodium level, using diuretics to increase the excretion of fluids, and treating the underlying cause.

Critical Thinking: Case Study

A 28-year-old woman was admitted to the hospital after 3 days of severe diarrhea and poor intake. She weights 120 lbs on admission (preillness weight, 132 lbs). Her BUN was 40 mg/dL and serum creatinine was 1.3 mg/dL, potassium was 3.2 mEq/mL, sodium 133 mEq/mL. Skin turgor was poor and urine output was 15 mL/h (specific gravity 1.030). Blood pressure was 120/80 mm Hg recumbent and fell to 98/60 mm Hg when erect. Pulse was 110, weak and regular.

What percent of body weight did she lose? What concerns would the nurse have regarding her laboratory work? What nursing diagnoses would apply to this woman? What I.V. fluids would you anticipate the physician to order? What nursing interventions would be implemented?

Media Link: Use the enclosed CD–ROM for more critical thinking activities, and the answers to this case study.

Post-Test

1. A solution of 5 percent dextrose and 0.9 percent NaCl has an osmolarity of 559. By administering this, you know that fluid will move from the ____ space to the ___ space.
   a. Intracellular, vascular
   b. Vascular, interstitial
   c. Interstitial, cellular
2. A solution of 0.45 percent NaCl has an osmolarity of 154. By administering this, you know that fluid will move from the ___ space to the ___ space.
   a. Intracellular, vascular
   b. Vascular, intracellular
   c. Interstitial, cellular
3. Lactated Ringer's solution has an osmolarity of 273. By administering this, you know that fluid will:
   a. Move from the intracellular space to the vascular space.
   b. Move from the vascular space to the cellular space.
   c. Stay in the vascular space.
4. Water is transported passively by:
   a. Diffusion
   b. Osmosis
   c. Filtration
   d. All of the above
5. You have just completed a physical assessment of a 68-year-old man. He knows who he is but is unsure of where he is (previous orientation normal). His eyes are sunken, his mouth is coated with an extra longitudinal furrow, and his lips are cracked. Hand vein filling takes more than 5 seconds, and tenting of the skin appears over the sternum. His vital signs are blood pressure of 128/60 mm Hg, pulse of 78, and respiratory rate of 16 (previously 150/78, 76, 16, respectively). Your assessment would lead you to suspect:
   a. Fluid volume deficit
   b. Fluid volume excess
6. If the external temperature is 101°F, which of the following age groups is at highest risk for fluid volume deficit?
   a. Infants
   b. School-age children
   c. Adolescents
   d. Middle-aged adults

7. All of the following could be the etiology for a nursing diagnosis of fluid volume excess **EXCEPT:**
   - a. Excessive infusion of 0.9 percent sodium chloride solution
   - b. Suppression of parathyroid function
   - c. SIADH
   - d. Congestive heart failure
8. Which of the following lab values are consistent with fluid volume deficit?
   - a. Urine specific gravity 1.010
   - b. Blood urea nitrogen 6
   - c. Hemoglobin 13
   - d. Serum osmolarity 305 mOsm/kg
9. All of the following conditions produce excess antidiuretic hormone **EXCEPT:**
   - a. Head trauma
   - b. Anesthesia
   - c. Ovarian cancer
   - d. Brain tumor
10. All of the following should be part of a focused assessment if a patient presents with peripheral edema **EXCEPT:**
    - a. Assessment of cardiovascular system
    - b. Laboratory assessment of specific gravity
    - c. Assessment of respiratory system
    - d. Laboratory assessment of blood sugar

Media Link: Use the enclosed CD–ROM for more practice questions, answers, and rationales.

References

Adelman, R.D., & Solhung, M.J. (1996). Pathophysiology of body fluids and fluid therapy. In Behrman, R.E., Kliegman, R.M., & Arvin, A.M. (eds.). *Nelson's Textbook of Pediatrics* (15th ed.). Philadelphia: W.B. Saunders, pp. 185–222.

Craven, R.F, & Hirnle, C.J. (2003). *Fundamentals of Nursing: Human Health and Function* (4th ed.). Philadelphia: Lippincott-Williams & Wilkins, pp. 910–938.

Giger, J.N., & Davidhizar, R.E. (1999). *Transcultural Nursing: Assessment and Intervention*. St. Louis: Mosby.

Guyton, A.C., & Hall, J.C. (2000). *Textbook of Medical Physiology* (10th ed.). Philadelphia: W.B. Saunders, pp. 110–114.

Hogan, M.A. & Wane, D. (2003). *Fluids, Electrolytes, and Acid–Base Balance: Reviews and Rationales.* Upper Saddle River, NJ: Prentice-Hall, pp. 17–27.

Hudak, C.M, Gallo, B.M., & Morton, P.G. (1998). *Critical Care Nursing: A Holistic Approach.* Philadelphia: Lippincott-Williams & Wilkins, pp. 544–547.

Lee, C.A., Barrett, C., & Ignatavicius, D.D. (1996). *Fluid and Electrolytes: A Practical Approach* (4th ed.). Philadelphia: F.A. Davis.

Levin, E.R., Gardner, D.G., & Samson, W.K. (1998). Natriuretic peptides. *New England Journal of Medicine*, 339(5), 321–328.

Metheny, N.M. (2000). Fluid and electrolyte balance. In Metheny N.M. (ed.). *Nursing Considerations* (4th ed.). Philadelphia: Lippincott-Williams & Wilkins.

National Student Nurses Association, Inc. (1997). *Fluids and Electrolytes.* Albany, NY: Delmar.

Sparks, S.M., & Taylor, C.M. (1998). *Nursing Diagnosis Reference Manual* (4th ed.). Springhouse, PA: Springhouse Corporation.

Answers to Chapter 3 Post-Test

1. **a**
2. **b**
3. **c**
4. **b**
5. **a**
6. **a**
7. **b**
8. **d**
9. **c**
10. **d**

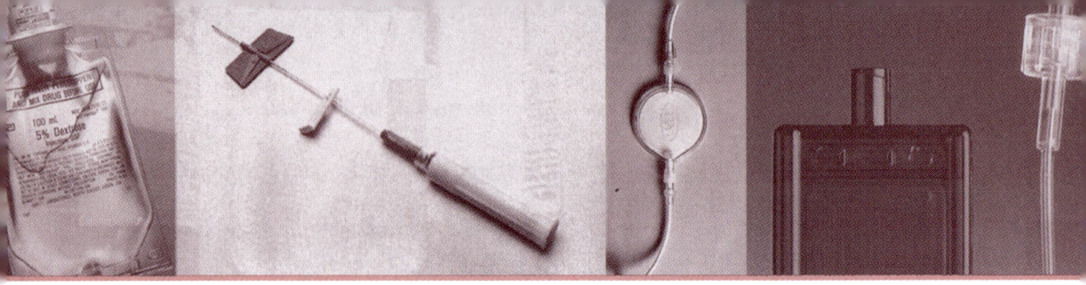

Chapter 4
Fundamentals of Electrolyte Balance

When they went ashore the animals that took up a land life carried with them a part of the sea in their bodies, a heritage which they passed on to their children and which even today links each land animal with its origin in the ancient sea.
—Rachel Carson, 1961

Chapter Contents

LEARNING OBJECTIVES

Upon completion of this chapter, the reader will be able to:

1. Define terminology related to electrolytes.
2. State the seven major electrolytes within the body fluids.
3. Differentiate between cations and anions.
4. Contrast each of the seven electrolytes and their major roles in body fluids.
5. Identify signs and symptoms of deficits of sodium, potassium, calcium, magnesium, chloride, and phosphate.
6. Identify signs and symptoms of excesses of sodium, potassium, calcium, magnesium, chloride, and phosphate.
7. Recognize patients at risk for electrolyte imbalances.
8. State the normal pH range of body fluids.
9. Compare clinical manifestations of metabolic acidosis and alkalosis.
10. Identify regulatory organs of acid–base balance.
11. Identify nursing diagnoses and interventions related to electrolyte balance.

GLOSSARY

Acidosis Blood pH below normal (less than 7.35)

Alkalosis Blood pH above normal (greater than 7.45)

Anion Negatively charged electrolyte

Antidiuretic hormone (ADH) A hormone secreted from the pituitary mechanism that causes the kidney to conserve water; sometimes referred to as the "water-conserving hormone"

Cation Positively charged electrolyte

Chvostek's sign A sign elicited by tapping the facial nerve about 2 cm anterior to the earlobe, just below the zygomatic process; the response is a spasm of the muscles supplied by the facial nerve

pH Hydrogen ion (H^+) concentration

Syndrome of inappropriate antidiuretic hormone (SIADH) secretion A condition in which excessive ADH is secreted, resulting in hyponatremia

Tetany Continuous tonic spasm of a muscle

Trousseau's sign A spasm of the hand elicited when the blood supply to the hand is decreased or the nerves of the hand are stimulated by pressure; elicited within several minutes by applying a blood pressure cuff inflated above systolic pressure

Basic Principles of Electrolyte Balance

Chemical compounds in solution behave in one of two ways: they separate and combine with other compounds, or they remain intact. One group of compounds remains intact; these are called nonelectrolytes (e.g., urea, dextrose, and creatinine). These compounds do not separate from their complex form when added to a solution. The second group of compounds, electrolytes, dissociates or separates in solution. These compounds break up into separate particles known as ions in a process called ionization. The major electrolytes in body fluid include sodium, potassium, calcium, magnesium, chloride, phosphorus, and bicarbonate.

Ions, which are the dissociated particles of an electrolyte, each carry an electrical charge, either positive or negative. Negative ions are called **anions** and positive ions are called **cations.**

Electrolytes are active chemicals that unite. The ions are expressed in terms of milliequivalents (mEq) per liter rather than milligrams. A milliequivalent measures chemical activity or combining power rather than weight. For example, when a hostess creates a guest list for a party, she does not invite 1000 pounds of boys per 1000 pounds of girls; rather, she invites the same number of boys and girls. In total, the milliequivalents of cations in a given compartment is equal to the milliequivalents of anions. There are 154 mEq of anions and 154 mEq of cations in the plasma. Each water compartment of the body contains electrolytes. The concentration and composition of electrolytes vary from compartment to compartment. See Table 4–1 for a diagrammatic comparison of electrolyte composition in the fluid compartments.

Most of the electrolytes have more than one physiologic role; often several electrolytes work together to mediate chemical events. The physiologic roles of electrolytes include:

> Table 4–1 **COMPARISON OF ELECTROLYTE COMPOSITION IN FLUID COMPARTMENTS**

Intracellular Water (approx. mEq/liter)		*Extracellular Water (approx. mEq/liter)*			
		PLASMA		**m INTERSTITIAL FLUID**	
Cations 205 mEq	Anions 205 mEq	Cations 154 mEq	Anions 154 mEq	Cations 154 mEq	Anions 154 mEq

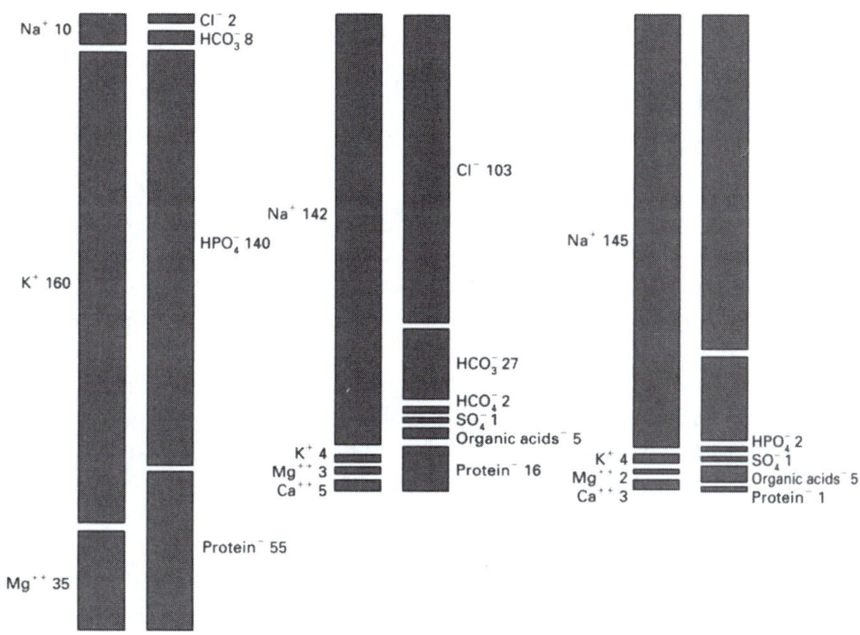

- Maintaining electroneutrality in fluid compartments
- Mediating enzyme reactions
- Altering cell membrane permeability
- Regulating muscle contraction and relaxation
- Regulating nerve impulse transmission
- Influencing blood clotting time

The electrolyte content of intracellular fluid (ICF) differs from that of extracellular fluid (ECF). Usually only ECF plasma electrolytes are measured because of the special techniques required to measure the concentration of electrolytes in ICF. The serum plasma levels of electrolytes are important in the assessment and management of patients with electrolyte imbalances.

Sodium (Na^+)

Normal Reference Value: 135 to 145 mEq/L

Physiologic Role

The physiologic role of sodium includes:

- Regulation of fluid distribution in the body: Water follows sodium.
- Maintenance of body fluid osmolarity
- Promotion of neuromuscular response: Transmission of nerve and muscle impulses depends on sodium, gradient between ECF and ICF.
- Regulation of acid–base balance: Sodium combines with chloride and bicarbonate to alter pH (NSNA, 1997).

The major function of sodium is to maintain ECF volume. Extracellular sodium level has an effect on the cellular fluid volume based on the principle of osmosis. Sodium represents about 90 percent of all the extracellular cations. Sodium does not easily cross the cell wall membrane and is therefore the most abundant cation of ECF.

A low serum sodium level results in dilute ECF, therefore allowing water to be drawn into the cells (lower to higher concentration). Conversely if the serum sodium is high, water is drawn out of the cells, leading to cellular dehydration. Figure 4–1 shows the relationship between sodium and cellular fluid. The normal daily requirement for sodium in adults is approximately 100 mEq.

The kidneys are extremely important in the regulation of sodium. This regulation is primarily accomplished through the action of the hormone aldosterone. Hyponatremia is a common complication of adrenal insufficiency because of aldosterone and cortisol deficiencies. Elderly persons have a slower rate of aldosterone secretion, which places them at risk for sodium imbalances.

NURSING FAST FACT!

The cerebral cells are very sensitive to changes in serum sodium levels and exhibit adaptive changes to sodium imbalances (Hogan & Wane, 2003).

Three factors can create a sodium imbalance:

1. Change in the sodium content of the ECF such as a deficit caused by excessive vomiting
2. Change in the chloride content, which can affect both the sodium concentration and the amount of water in the ECF; when the ratio

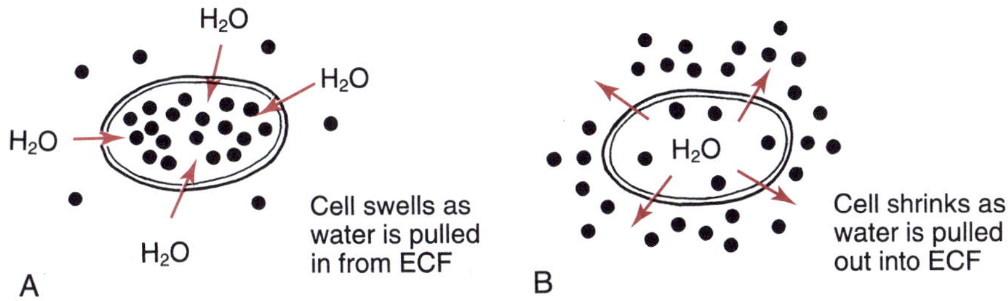

Figure 4–1 ■ Sodium and cellular fluid relationship. *(A)* Hyponatremia. The cell swells as water is pulled in from the extracellular fluid. *(B)* Hypernatremia. The cell shrinks as water is pulled out into the extracellular fluid.

of chloride to sodium deviates from normal, it is reflected as an acid–base imbalance (Lee, Barrett, & Ignatavicius, 1996)

3. Change in the quantity of water in the ECF

Serum Sodium Deficit: Hyponatremia

Hyponatremia is a condition in which the sodium level is below normal (less than 135 mEq/L). A low sodium level can be the result of an excessive loss of sodium or an excessive gain of water; in either event, hyponatremia is caused by a relatively greater concentration of water than of sodium. Sodium deficit is usually associated with hypervolemia states.

Pathophysiology and Etiology

The pathophysiology that contributes to sodium deficit (hyponatremia) is often a sign of a serious underlying disease; there are also many causes of hyponatremia.

All gastrointestinal (GI) secretions contain sodium; therefore, any abnormal loss of GI secretions can cause a sodium deficit. GI disorders such as vomiting, diarrhea, drainage from suction or fistulas, and excessive tap water enemas may also cause hyponatremia.

Other causes of hyponatremia are losses from skin in excessive sweating, combined with excessive water consumption and the use of thiazide diuretics (especially dangerous with low-salt diets).

Hormonal factors such as labor induction with oxytocin and the syndrome of inappropriate antidiuretic syndrome (SIADH) cause the amount of sodium per volume to be reduced, in turn causing a dilutional hyponatremia. Oxytocin has been shown to have an intrinsic antidiuretic hormone effect, acting to increase water reabsorption from the glomerular filtrate. Adrenal insufficiency (aldosterone deficiency) also can cause sodium loss (Metheny, 2000). Other factors include excessive parenteral hypo-osmolar fluids such as dextrose in water solutions.

NURSING FAST FACT!

SIADH has progressed from a rare occurrence to the most common cause of hyponatremia seen in general hospitals. It occurs in patients with inflammatory disorders such as pneumonia; tuberculosis; abscess; oat cell cancer of the lung; and central nervous system (CNS) disorders such as meningitis, trauma, stroke, and degenerative diseases (Metheny, 2000).

Chemical agents may also impair renal water excretion, leading to sodium deficit. Pharmacologic agents that contribute to sodium deficit include nicotine, chlorpropamide (Diabinese), cyclophosphamide (Cytoxan), morphine, barbiturates, and acetaminophen.

Signs and Symptoms

Hyponatremia affects cells of the CNS. Patients with chronic hyponatremia may experience impaired sensation of taste, anorexia, muscle cramps, feeling of exhaustion, apprehension, feeling of impending doom (Na^+ less than 115), and focal weaknesses (e.g., hemiparesis, ataxia). Patients with acute hyponatremia caused by water overload experience the same symptoms as well as fingerprint edema (sign of intracellular water excess). Patients undergoing operative procedures involving irrigations may develop hyponatremia (such as transurethral resection of prostate [TURP] and endometrial ablation).

AGE-RELATED CONSIDERATIONS 4–1

Dehydration and chronic hyponatremia can lead to confusional states that interfere with fluid intake in elderly people, who are very susceptible to dehydration.

Because of the differences in cerebral metabolism, women (especially premenopausal women) seem to be at substantially greater risk than men for developing severe neurologic symptoms and irreversible brain damage related to hyponatremia. Young women account for most of the reported cases of fatalities secondary to hyponatremia.

Diagnostic Tests

- Serum sodium: Less than 135 mEq/L
- Serum osmolarity: Less than 280 mOsm/L
- Urine specific gravity: Less than 1.010 (except in SIADH)
- Urine sodium: Decreased (usually less than 20 mEq/L)
- Hematocrit: Above normal when fluid volume deficit (FVD) exists
- Decreased blood urea nitrogen (BUN)

Treatment and Management

Treatment of patients with hyponatremia aims to provide sodium by the dietary, enteral, or parenteral route. Patients able to eat and drink can easily replace sodium by ingesting a normal diet. Those unable to take sodium orally must take the electrolyte by the parenteral route. An isotonic saline or Ringer's solution may be ordered, such as 0.9 percent sodium chloride (NaCl), or lactated Ringer's solution.

NURSING FAST FACT!

When the primary problem is water retention, it is safer to restrict water than to administer sodium. An I.V. solution that can contribute to hyponatremia is excessive administration of 5 percent dextrose in water.

General treatment guidelines for patients with hyponatremia are:

1. Replace sodium and fluid losses through diet or parenteral fluids. (If serum sodium level is lower than 125 mEq/L, it is important to quickly bring the level up to more than 125 mEq/L, then to gradually continue to return the sodium to a normal level.)
2. Restore normal ECF volume.
3. Correct any other electrolyte losses such as potassium or bicarbonate.

Nursing Points-of-Care: Hyponatremia

Nursing assessments include:

1. Obtain a patient history of high-risk factors for hyponatremia (vomiting, diarrhea, eating disorders, low-sodium diet).
2. Obtain a history of medications with emphasis on those predisposing patients to hyponatremia (i.e., diuretics).
3. Assess for signs of hyponatremia.
4. Obtain baseline laboratory tests (e.g., serum sodium, serum osmolarity, serum potassium, serum chloride, and urinary specific gravity).

Key nursing interventions include:

1. Monitoring laboratory tests with emphasis on serum sodium
2. Monitoring GI losses
3. Keeping accurate records of fluid intake and output
4. Monitoring for changes in central venous system symptoms
5. Weighing the patient daily

Serum Sodium Excess: Hypernatremia

The serum level of sodium is elevated to above 145 mEq/L in patients with hypernatremia. This elevation can be caused by a gain of sodium without water or a loss of water without loss of sodium.

Pathophysiology and Etiology

Increased levels of serum sodium can occur with deprivation of water, occurring when a person cannot respond to thirst; during hypertonic tube feeding with inadequate water supplements; with excessive parenteral administration of sodium-containing solutions; and when a person is drowning in seawater. Sodium is lost with watery diarrhea (a particular problem in infants), increased insensible loss, ingestion of sodium in unusual amounts, profuse sweating, heat stroke, and diabetes insipidus when water intake is inadequate. Cerebral cells adapt to high sodium levels by shrinking as the osmotic pressure drives fluid out of the cells, leading to decreased brain volume (Hogan & Wane, 2003).

AGE-RELATED CONSIDERATIONS 4–2

In aging adults, there is a diminished thirst response that may lead to inadequate fluid intake. Infants are unable to obtain fluid independently and may be at risk of inadequate fluid intake, especially in warmer weather.

Signs and Symptoms

Patients with hypernatremia may experience marked thirst; elevated body temperature; swollen tongue; red, dry, sticky mucous membranes; severe hypernatremia; disorientation; and irritability or hyperactivity when stimulated.

Diagnostic Tests

- Serum sodium: Greater than 145 mEq/L
- Chloride may be elevated.
- Serum osmolarity: Greater than 295 mOsm/kg
- Urine specific gravity: Greater than 1.015 (except for those with diabetes insipidus)
- Dehydration test: Water is withheld for 16 to 18 hours; serum and urine osmolarity are checked 1 hour after administration of antidiuretic hormone (ADH); this test is used to identify the cause of polyuric syndromes (central versus nephrogenic diabetes insipidus).

Treatment and Management

The goal of treatment of patients with hypernatremia is to gradually lower the serum sodium level, infusing a hypotonic electrolyte solution such as 0.45 percent normal saline or 5 percent dextrose in water. Gradual reduction is necessary to decrease the risk of cerebral edema. The sodium level should not be lowered more than 15 mEq/L in an 8-hour period of time for adults (Weldy, 1996).

Generally, treatment guidelines for hypernatremia are:

1. Infusion of an isotonic solution (0.9 percent NaCl) or hypotonic electrolyte solution (0.45 percent NaCl or 5 percent dextrose in water)
2. Sodium levels can also be decreased by use of diuretics, which induce excretion of water and sodium.

Nursing Points-of-Care: Hypernatremia

Nursing assessment includes:

1. Obtain a patient history of high-risk factors for hypernatremia (e.g., increased sodium intake, water deprivation, increased adrenocortical hormone production, use of sodium-retaining drugs).
2. Assess for signs of hypernatremia.
3. Obtain baseline values of laboratory tests, especially serum sodium.

Key nursing interventions include:

1. Monitoring laboratory test results with emphasis on serum sodium and serum osmolarity
2. Keeping accurate fluid intake and output records
3. Monitoring for signs of pulmonary edema when the patient is receiving large amounts of parenteral sodium chloride

Potassium (K^+)

Normal Reference Value: 3.5 to 5.5 mEq/L

Physiologic Role

The physiologic role of potassium includes:

- Regulation of fluid volume within the cell
- Promotion of nerve impulse transmission
- Contraction of skeletal, smooth, and cardiac muscle
- Control of hydrogen ion (H^+) concentration, acid–base balance; when potassium moves out of the cell, hydrogen ions move in, and vice versa
- Role of enzyme action for cellular energy production.

Potassium is an intracellular electrolyte with 98 percent in the ICF and 2 percent in the ECF. Potassium is a dynamic electrolyte. Cellular potassium replaces ECF potassium if it becomes depleted. Potassium is acquired through diet and must be ingested daily because the body has no effective method of storage. The daily requirement is 40 mEq. Potassium influences both skeletal and cardiac muscle activity. Alterations in the concentration of plasma potassium change myocardial irritability and rhythm. Potassium moves easily into the intracellular space when the body is metabolizing glucose. It moves out of the cells during strenuous exercise, when cellular metabolism is impaired, or when the cell dies. Potassium, along with sodium, is responsible for transmission of nerve impulses. During nerve cell innervation, these ions exchange places, creating an electrical current (Metheny, 2000).

There is a relationship between acid–base imbalances and potassium balance. Hypokalemia can cause alkalosis, which in turn can further decrease serum potassium. Hyperkalemia can cause acidosis, which in turn can further increase serum potassium.

The regulation of potassium is related to several other processes, including:

- Sodium level: Enough sodium must be available for exchange with potassium.
- Hydrogen ion excretion: When there is an increase in hydrogen ion excretion, there is a decrease in potassium excretion.
- Aldosterone level: An increased level of aldosterone stimulates and increases excretion of potassium.
- Potassium imbalances are common in clinical practice because of their association with underlying disease, injury, or ingestion of certain medications.

Serum Potassium Deficit: Hypokalemia

Hypokalemia is a serum potassium level below 3.5 mEq/L. It usually reflects a real deficit in total potassium stores; however, it may occur in patients with normal potassium stores when alkalosis is present. Hypokalemia is a common disturbance; many factors are associated with this deficit, and many clinical conditions contribute to it.

Pathophysiology and Etiology

Many conditions can lead to potassium deficit, including GI and renal loss, increased use of increased perspiration, shifting of extracellular potassium into the cells, and poor dietary intake.

Gastrointestinal loss includes diarrhea or laxative overuse, prolonged gastric suction, and protracted vomiting.

Renal loss includes potassium-wasting diuretic therapy; excessive use of glucocorticoids; ingestion of drugs such as sodium penicillin, carbenicillin, or amphotericin B; excessive ingestion of European licorice (which mimics the action of aldosterone); and excessive steroid administration.

Sweat loss includes heavy perspiration in persons acclimated to the heat.

Shifting into the cells can occur with total parenteral nutrition therapy without adequate potassium supplementation, alkalosis, and excessive administration of insulin.

Poor dietary intake can occur with anorexia nervosa, bulimia, and alcoholism.

Signs and Symptoms

Patients with hypokalemia may experience neuromuscular changes such as fatigue, muscle weakness, diminished deep tendon reflexes, and flaccid paralysis (late). Other symptoms include anorexia, nausea, vomiting, irritability (early), increased sensitivity to digitalis, electrocardiographic (ECG) changes, and death (in those with severe hypokalemia) caused by cardiac arrest.

Diagnostic Tests

- Serum potassium: Less than 3.5 mEq/L
- Arterial blood gas (ABG): May show metabolic alkalosis (increased pH and bicarbonate ion).
- Elevated serum glucose levels (increased insulin secretion and increased osmotic pressure)
- ECG: ST-segment depression, flattened T wave, presence of U wave, and ventricular dysrhythmias (Fig. 4–2)
- Potential for decreased serum chloride levels
- Potential for decreased magnesium levels (because hypomagnesemia can potentiate hypokalemia)

NURSING FAST FACT!

Clinical signs and symptoms rarely occur before the serum potassium level has fallen below 3 mEq/L.

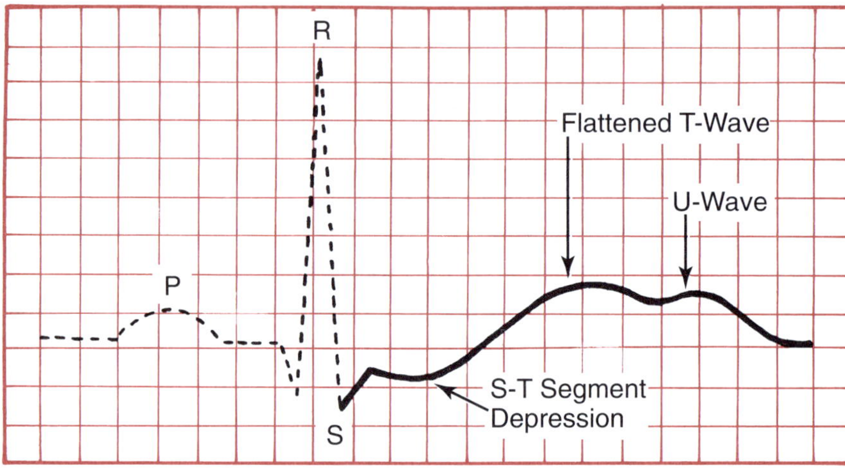

Figure 4–2 ■ Sample ECG tracing: Hypokalemia. The ECG tracing for hypokalemia has ST-segment depression, flattened T wave, and the presence of a U wave.

Potassium replacement must take place slowly to prevent hyperkalemia. Extreme caution should be used when potassium chloride replacement exceeds 120 mEq in 24 hours. The patient must be monitored for dysrhythmias.

Treatment and Management

Replacement of potassium is the key concept in treating patients with potassium deficit. General treatment guidelines include:

1. Mild hypokalemia is usually treated with dietary increases of potassium or oral supplements.
2. Salt substitutes (e.g., Morton Salt Substitute, Co-Salt, Adolph's Salt Substitute) contain potassium and can be used to supplement potassium intake.
3. If the serum potassium is below 2 mEq/L, monitor the patient's ECG and administer potassium by means of a secondary piggyback set in a volume of 100 mL (Metheny, 2000).

Table 4–2 gives critical guidelines for nursing in I.V. administration of potassium.

> Table 4–2 **CRITICAL GUIDELINES FOR ADMINISTRATION OF POTASSIUM**

Never give a potassium I.V. push.

Potassium chloride (KCl) should be added to a nondextrose solution such as isotonic saline to treat severe hypokalemia because administration of KCl in a dextrose solution may cause a small reduction in the serum potassium level.

Never administer concentrated potassium solutions without first diluting them as directed.

KCl preparations greater than 60 mEq/L **should not** be given in a peripheral vein. Concentrations greater than 8 mEq/100 mL can cause pain and irritation of peripheral veins and lead to postinfusion phlebitis.

When adding KCl to infusion solutions, especially plastic systems, make sure the KCl mixes with the solution thoroughly. Invert and agitate the container to ensure mixing. ***Do not add KCl to a hanging container!***

For patients with any degree of renal insufficiency or heart block, Zull (1989) recommends reducing the infusion by 50 percent. For example, 5 to 10 mEq/h rather than 10 to 20 mEq/h.

Administer potassium at a rate not to exceed 10 mEq/h through peripheral veins.

For patients with extreme hypokalemia, rates should be no more than 40 mEq/h while ECG is constantly monitored.

If KCl is administered into the subcutaneous tissue (infiltration), it is extremely irritating and can cause serious tissue loss. Use extravasation protocol in this situation.

Nursing Points-of-Care: Hypokalemia

Nursing assessment includes:

1. Obtain history of high-risk factors for hypokalemia such as vomiting, renal disease, and diuretic use.
2. Assess for signs of hypokalemia.
3. Obtain baseline laboratory test values such as ECG reading, serum potassium, and serum osmolarity.

Key nursing interventions include:

1. Monitoring the laboratory test results, especially serum potassium
2. Keeping accurate intake and output records
3. Monitoring for changes in cardiac response
4. Monitoring for signs of phlebitis (potassium irritates veins) when given by I.V. route

Serum Potassium Excess: Hyperkalemia

Hyperkalemia occurs less frequently than hypokalemia, but it can be more dangerous. It seldom occurs in patients who have normal renal function. Hyperkalemia is defined as a serum plasma level of potassium above 5.5 mEq/L. The main causes of hyperkalemia are (1) increased intake of potassium (oral or parenteral), (2) decreased urinary excretion of potassium, and (3) movement of potassium out of the cells and into the extracellular space.

Pathophysiology and Etiology

High levels of serum potassium can be caused by either a gain of potassium body or shift of potassium from the ICF to the ECF (NSNA, 1997). Hyperkalemia can be caused by excessive administration of potassium parentally or orally; severe renal failure resulting in reduced potassium excretion; release of potassium from altered cellular function, such as with burns or crush injuries; and acidosis.

Drugs that can cause a predisposition to hyperkalemias include potassium penicillin, indomethacin, amphetamines, nonsteroidal anti-inflammatory drugs, alpha agonists, beta blockers, succinylcholine, cyclophosphamide, and potassium-sparing diuretics. Pseudohyperkalemia can occur with prolonged tourniquet application during blood withdrawal.

Signs and Symptoms

Patients with hyperkalemia may experience changes shown on ECGs, vague muscle weakness, flaccid paralysis, anxiety, nausea, cramping, and diarrhea.

Diagnostic Tests

- Serum potassium: Greater than 5.5 mEq/L
- ABG values: Metabolic acidosis (decreased pH and bicarbonate ion)
- ECG: Widened QRS, prolonged PR, and ventricular dysrhythmias (Fig. 4–3)
- If dehydration is causing hyperkalemia, then hematocrit, hemoglobin, and sodium and chloride levels should be drawn.
- If associated with renal failure, creatinine and BUN levels should be drawn.

Treatment and Management

The following are guidelines for the treatment of patients with hyperkalemia:

1. Restrict dietary potassium in mild cases.
2. Discontinue supplements of potassium.
3. Administer I.V. calcium gluconate if necessary for cardiac symptoms.
4. Administer I.V. sodium bicarbonate, which alkalinizes the plasma and causes a temporary shift of potassium into the cells.

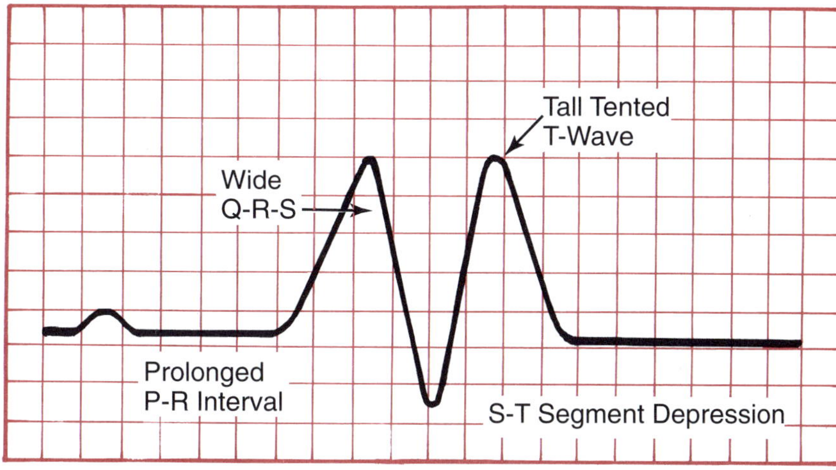

Figure 4–3 ■ Sample ECG tracing: Hyperkalemia. The ECG tracing for hyperkalemia shows progressive changes; tall, thin T waves; prolonged PR intervals; ST-segment depression; widened QRS; and loss of P wave.

5. Administer regular insulin (10 to 25 U) and hypertonic dextrose (10%), which causes a shift of potassium into the cells.
6. Peritoneal dialysis or hemodialysis may be ordered.

Nursing Points-of-Care: Hyperkalemia

Nursing assessment includes:

1. Obtain client history relative to high-risk factors for hyperkalemia (renal disease, potassium-sparing diuretics, excessive salt substitute use).
2. Assess for signs of hyperkalemia.
3. Obtain baseline ECG; assess for altered T waves.
4. Obtain baseline serum potassium.

Key nursing interventions include:

1. Monitoring the laboratory test results, especially serum potassium
2. Keeping accurate intake and output records
3. Monitoring for changes in cardiac response
4. Monitoring vital signs, with special attention to tachycardia and bradycardia

> Table 4–3 **CRITICAL GUIDELINES FOR REMOVAL OF POTASSIUM**

Treatment Guidelines
■ **Sodium polystyrene sulfonate** is a cation exchange resin that removes potassium from the body by exchanging sodium for potassium in the intestinal tract. This method should not be the sole treatment for severe hyperkalemia because of its slow onset.
Oral sodium polystyrene sulfonate (15 to 30 g); may repeat every 4 to 6 hours as needed; it removes potassium 1 to 2 hours.
Rectal sodium polystyrene sulfonate (50 g) as retention enema; when administered, use an inflated rectal catheter to ensure retention of the dissolved resin for 30 to 60 minutes; it removes potassium in 30 to 60 minutes; each enema can lower the plasma potassium concentration by 0.5 to 1.0 mEq/L
■ **Dialysis** is used when more aggressive methods are needed. Peritoneal dialysis is not as effective as hemodialysis. Whereas peritoneal dialysis can remove approximately 10 to 15 mEq/h, hemodialysis can remove 25 to 35 mEq/h.
■ **Glucose and insulin**
Insulin facilitates potassium movement into the cells, reducing the plasma potassium level. Glucose administration in nondiabetic patients may cause a marked increase in insulin release from the pancreas, producing desired plasma potassium-lowering effects.
500 mL of 10 percent dextrose with 10 to 15 U of regular insulin over 1 hour: The potassium-lowering effects are delayed about 30 minutes but are effective for 4 to 6 hours (Zull, 1989).
■ **Emergency measures**
Calcium gluconate: 10 mL of 10 percent calcium gluconate administered slowly over 2 to 3 minutes. Administer only to patients who need immediate myocardial protection against toxic effects of severe hyperkalemia. Protective effect begins within 1 to 2 minutes and lasts only 30 to 60 minutes.
Sodium bicarbonate: 45 mEq (1 ampule of 7.5% sodium bicarbonate) infused slowly over 5 minutes. This temporarily shifts potassium into the cells and is helpful in patients with metabolic acidosis.

Table 4–3 provides critical guidelines for nursing in treatment of patients with potassium excess.

Calcium (Ca^{2+})

Normal Reference Value: 8.5 to 10.5 mg/dL

Physiologic Role

The physiologic role of calcium includes:

- Maintaining skeletal elements; calcium is needed for strong, durable bones and teeth
- Regulating neuromuscular activity
- Influencing enzyme activity
- Converting prothrombin to thrombin, a necessary part of the material that holds cells together

The calcium ion is most abundant in the skeletal system, with 99 percent residing in the bones and teeth. Only 1 percent is available for rapid exchange in the circulating blood bound to protein. The parathyroid hormone (PTH) is responsible for transfer of calcium from the bone to plasma. PTH also augments the intestinal absorption of calcium and enhances net renal calcium reabsorption. Calcium is acquired through dietary intake. Adults require approximately 1 g of calcium daily, along with vitamin D and protein, which are required for absorption and utilization of this electrolyte.

Calcium is instrumental in activating enzymes and stimulating essential chemical reactions. It plays an important role in maintaining the normal transmission of nerve impulses and has a sedative effect on nerve cells. Calcium plays its most important role in the conversion of prothrombin to thrombin, a necessary sequence in the formation of a clot.

Calcium and phosphate have a reciprocal relationship; that is, an increase in calcium level causes a drop in the serum phosphorus concentration, and a drop in calcium causes an increase in phosphorus level.

Calcium is present in three different forms in the plasma: (1) ionized (50 percent of total calcium); (2) bound (less than 50 percent of total calcium); and (3) complexed (small percentage that combines with phosphate). Only ionized calcium (i.e., calcium affected by plasma pH, phosphorus, and albumin levels) is physiologically important. A relationship between ionized calcium and plasma pH is reciprocal; an increase in pH decreases the percentage of calcium that is ionized. The relationship between plasma phosphorus and ionized calcium is also reciprocal. Albumin does not affect ionized calcium, but it does affect the amount of calcium bound to proteins.

Serum Calcium Deficit: Hypocalcemia

A reduction of total body calcium levels or a reduction of the percentage of ionized calcium causes hypocalcemia.

Pathophysiology and Etiology

Total calcium levels may be decreased because of increased calcium loss, reduced intake secondary to altered intestinal absorption, and altered regulation, as in those with hypoparathyroidism.

The most common cause of hypocalcemia is inadequate secretion of PTH caused by primary hypoparathyroidism or surgically induced hypoparathyroidism. It can also result from calcium loss through diarrhea and wound exudate, acute pancreatitis, hyperphosphatemia usually associated with renal failure, inadequate intake of vitamin D or minimal sun exposure, prolonged nasogastric tube suctioning resulting in metabolic alkalosis, and infusion of citrated blood (citrate–phosphate–dextrose).

Many drugs can lead to the development of hypocalcemia, including potent loop diuretics dioxin, dilantin, and phenobarbital, antineoplastic drugs, some radiographic contrast media, large doses of corticosteroids, heparin, and antacids (Hogan & Wane, 2003).

Signs and Symptoms

Patients with hypocalcemia may experience neuromuscular symptoms such as numbness of the fingers, cramps in the muscles (especially the extremities), hyperactive deep tendon reflexes, and a positive **Trousseau's sign** (Fig. 4–4) and **Chvostek's sign** (Fig. 4–5).

Other symptoms include irritability, memory impairment, delusions, seizures (late), prolonged QT interval, and altered cardiovascular hemodynamics that may precipitate congestive heart failure. In patients with hypocalcemia caused by citrated blood transfusion, the cardiac index, stroke volume, and left ventricular stroke work values have been found to be lower.

The most dangerous symptom associated with hypocalcemia is the development of laryngospasm and tetany-like contractions. A low magnesium level and a high potassium level potentiate the cardiac and neuromuscular irritability produced by a low calcium level. However, a low potassium level can protect patients from hypocalcemic tetany (Lee et al., 1996).

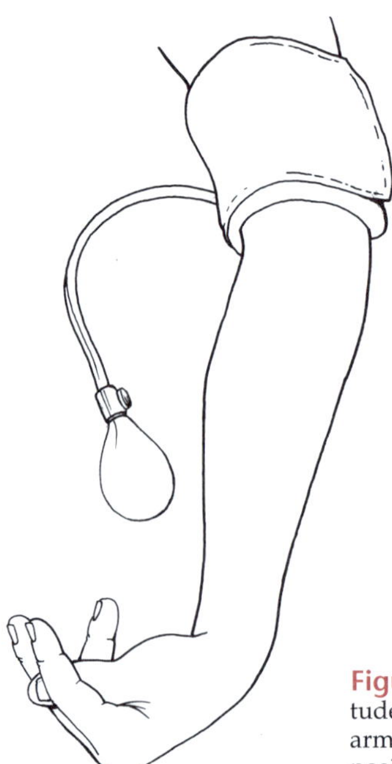

Figure 4–4 ■ Positive Trousseau's sign. Carpopedal attitude of the hand when blood pressure cuff is placed on the arm and inflated above systolic pressure for 3 minutes. A positive reaction is the development of carpal spasm.

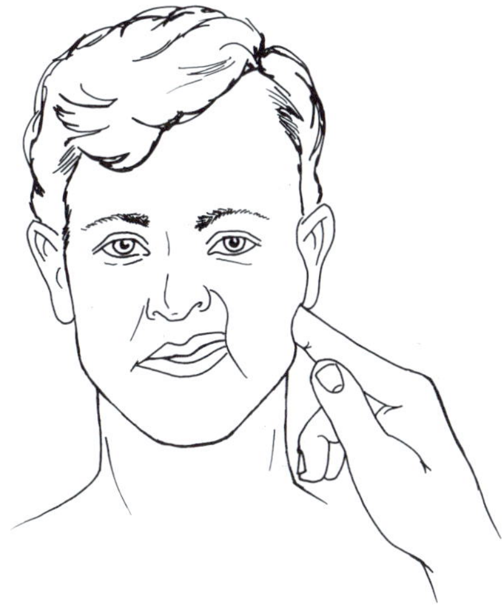

Figure 4–5 ■ Positive Chvostek's sign, which occurs after tapping the facial nerve approximately 2 cm anterior to the earlobe. Unilateral twitching of the facial muscle occurs in some patients with hypocalcemia or hypomagnesemia.

Diagnostic Tests

- Total serum calcium less than 8.5 mg/dL
- Ionized calcium level less than 4.0 mg/dL
- X-ray films detect bone fractures and thinning
- Bone mass density tests for signs of osteoporosis
- Potential for hypomagnesemia (1 mg/dL)
- Potential for hypokalemia (less than 3.5 mEq/mL)
- Hyperphosphatemia (greater than 2.6 mEq/mL)
- Potential for elevated creatinine from renal insufficiency

Treatment and Management

The goal of treatment is to alleviate the underlying cause.

Treatment of patients with hypocalcemia consists of administration of calcium gluconate, either orally (preferred) with calcium supplements, 1000 mg/day, to raise the total serum calcium level by 1 mg/dL, or intravenously, 10 to 20 mL of a 10 percent solution in 5 percent dextrose in water for 20 minutes.

AGE-RELATED CONSIDERATIONS 4–3

There are two types of hypocalcemia in newborn infants. The first occurs early after birth during the first 3 days of life; this is attributed to parathyroid immaturity or maternal hyperparathyroidism. This resolves within the first week of life (Metheny, 2000). The second type of neonatal hypocalcemia occurs about 1 week after birth and is associated with hyperphosphatemia and hypomagnesemia. Providing milk with a high phosphorus level can lead to hyperphosphatemia and then hypocalcemia (Narins, 1994).

Nursing Points-of-Care: Hypocalcemia

Nursing assessments include:

1. Obtain history relative to potential causes of hypocalcemia, such as low-calcium diet, lack of vitamin D, low-protein diet, chronic diarrhea, or hormonal disorders.
2. Obtain history of drugs that could predispose the patient to hypocalcemia, such as furosemide (Lasix) or cortisone.
3. Assess for signs of hypocalcemia.
4. Obtain baseline values for serum calcium, ionized calcium serum albumin, and acid–base status.

Key nursing interventions include:

1. Taking safety precautions and preparing to adopt seizure precautions if hypocalcemia is severe
2. Monitoring laboratory test results with emphasis on serum and ionized calcium
3. Monitoring ECGs for changes in pattern
4. Monitoring for irritation of subcutaneous tissue and tissue sloughing when calcium is given parenterally
5. Monitoring for signs of cardiac arrhythmias in patients receiving digitalis and calcium supplements
6. Monitoring for hypocalcemia in patients receiving massive transfusion of citrated blood

Serum Calcium Excess: Hypercalcemia

Hypercalcemia is caused by excessive release of calcium from bone, almost always from malignancy, hyperparathyroidism, thiazide-diuretic use, or excessive calcium intake.

Pathophysiology and Etiology

Most symptoms of hypercalcemia are present only when the serum calcium level is greater than 12 mg/dL and tend to be more severe if hypercalcemia develops quickly. Causes of hypercalcemia include hyperparathyroidism, Paget's disease, multiple fractures, and overuse of calcium-containing antacids. Patients with solid tumors that have metastasized, such as breast, prostate, and malignant melanomas, and hematologic tumors, such as lymphomas, acute leukemia, and myelomas, are also at risk for developing hypercalcemia.

Drugs that predispose an individual to hypercalcemia include calcium salts, megadoses of vitamin A or D, thiazide diuretics (potentiate the action of PTH), androgens or estrogen for breast cancer therapy, I.V. lipids, lithium, and tamoxifen.

Signs and Symptoms

Patients with hypercalcemia may experience neuromuscular symptoms such as muscle weakness, incoordination, lethargy, deep bone pain, flank pain, and pathologic fractures (caused by bone weakening). Other symptoms include constipation, anorexia, nausea, vomiting, polyuria or polydipsia leading to uremia if not treated, and renal colic caused by stone formation. Patients taking digitalis must take calcium with extreme care because it can precipitate severe dysrhythmias.

Diagnostic Tests

- Total serum calcium: May be more than 10.5 mg/dL.
- Serum ionized calcium: Greater than 5.5 mg/dL
- Serum parathyroid hormone: Increased levels in primary or secondary hyperparathyroidism
- Radiography: May reveal osteoporosis, bone cavitation, or urinary calculi.

Treatment and Management

Hypercalcemia should be treated according to the following guidelines:

1. Treat the patient's underlying disease.
2. Administer saline diuresis. Fluids should be forced to help eliminate the source of the hypercalcemia. A solution of 0.45 percent NaCl or 0.9 percent NaCl I.V. dilutes the serum calcium level. Rehydration is important to dilute the Ca^{2+} ion and promote renal excretion.
3. Give inorganic phosphate salts orally (Neutra-Phos) or rectally (Fleet Enema).
4. Provide hemodialysis or peritoneal dialysis to reduce serum calcium levels in life-threatening situations.
5. Use furosemide, 20 to 40 mg every 2 hours, to prevent volume overloading during saline administration.
6. Administer calcitonin, 4 to 8 U/kg intramuscularly or subcutaneously every 6 to 12 hours. This will temporarily lower the serum calcium level by 1 to 3 mg/100 mL.
7. Give bisphosphonates to inhibit bone reabsorption. Pamidronate is effective, 60 to 90 mg in 1 L of 0.9 percent NaCl or 5 percent dextrose in water is infused over 24 hours.
8. Administer plicamycin (mithramycin), which inhibits bone reabsorption and reliably lowers serum calcium. It is used only in those with malignant hypercalcemia because of its toxicity. A single dose of 25 g/kg in 500 mL of 5 percent dextrose in water is infused intravenously over 4 to 6 hours (Phillips & Kuhn, 1999).

Nursing Points-of-Care: Hypercalcemia

Nursing assessment includes:

1. Obtain a patient history of probable cause of hypercalcemia, such as cancer; excessive use of calcium supplements, antacids, or thiazide diuretics; or steroid therapy.
2. Assess for signs of hypercalcemia.
3. Obtain baseline values for serum calcium and serum phosphate.
4. Obtain baseline ECG.
5. Assess client's fluid volume status and mental alertness.

Key nursing interventions include:

1. Monitoring changes in vital signs and laboratory tests
2. Encouraging the patient to drink 3 to 4 L of fluid per day
3. Encouraging the patient to consume fluids (e.g., cranberry or prune juice) that promote urine acidity to help prevent formation of renal calculi
4. Keeping accurate fluid intake and output records
5. Monitoring for digitalis toxicity
6. Handling the patient gently to prevent fractures
7. Encouraging the patient to avoid high-calcium foods

Magnesium (Mg^{2+})

Normal Reference Value: 1.5 to 2.5 mEq/L

Physiologic Role

The physiologic role of magnesium includes:

- Enzyme action
- Regulation of neuromuscular activity (similar to calcium)
- Regulation of electrolyte balance, including facilitating transport of sodium and potassium across cell membranes, influencing the utilization of calcium, potassium, and protein

Magnesium is a major intracellular electrolyte. The normal diet supplies approximately 25 mEq of magnesium. Approximately one third of serum magnesium is bound to protein; the remaining two thirds exists as free cations. The same factors that regulate calcium balance have an influence on magnesium balance. Magnesium balance is also affected by many of the same agents that decrease or influence potassium balance.

Magnesium acts directly on the myoneural junction and affects neuromuscular irritability and contractility, possibly exerting a sedative effect. Magnesium acts as an activator for many enzymes and plays a role in both carbohydrate and protein metabolism. Magnesium affects the cardiovascular system, acting peripherally to produce vasodilation. Imbalances in magnesium predispose the heart to ventricular dysrhythmias (Metheny, 2000).

Serum Magnesium Deficit: Hypomagnesemia

Hypomagnesemia is often overlooked in critically ill patients. This imbalance is considered to be one of the most underdiagnosed electrolyte deficiencies (Metheny, 2000). Symptoms of hypomagnesemia tend to occur when the serum level drops below 1.0 mEq/L.

Pathophysiology and Etiology

Hypomagnesemia can result from chronic alcoholism; malabsorption syndrome, especially if the small bowel is affected; prolonged malnutrition or starvation; prolonged diarrhea; acute pancreatitis; administration of magnesium-free solutions for more than one week; and prolonged nasogastric tube suctioning.

Drugs that predispose an individual to hypomagnesemia include aminoglycosides, diuretics, cortisone, amphotericin, digitalis, cisplatin, and cyclosporine. Infusion of collected blood preserved with citrate can also cause hypomagnesemia (Lee et al., 1996).

Signs and Symptoms

Patients with hypomagnesemia often experience neuromuscular symptoms, such as hyperactive reflexes, coarse tremors, muscle cramps, positive Chvostek's and Trousseau's signs (see Figs. 4–4 and 4–5), seizures, paresthesia of the feet and legs, and painfully cold hands and feet. Other symptoms include disorientation, dysrhythmias, tachycardia, and increased potential for digitalis toxicity.

Diagnostic Tests

- Serum magnesium: Less than 1.5 mEq/L
- Urine magnesium: Helps to identify renal causes of magnesium depletion.
- Serum albumin: A decrease may cause a decreased magnesium level resulting from the reduction in protein-bound magnesium.

- Serum potassium: Decreased because of failure of the cellular sodium–potassium pump to move potassium into the cell and because of the accompanying loss of potassium in the urine
- Serum calcium: May be reduced because of a reduction in the release and action of PTH.
- ECG: Findings of tachydysrhythmias, prolonged PR and QT intervals, widening of the QRS, ST segment depression, and flattened T waves. A form of ventricular tachycardia (i.e., torsades de pointes) associated with all three electrolyte imbalances (i.e., magnesium, calcium, and potassium) may develop.

Treatment and Management

Treatment of patients with hypomagnesemia includes:

1. Administering oral magnesium salts
2. Administering 40 mEq (5 g) of magnesium sulfate added intravenously to 1 L of 5 percent dextrose in water or 5 percent dextrose/NaCl
3. Administering 1 to 2 g of 10 percent solution of magnesium sulfate by direct I.V. push at a rate of 1.5 mL/min (Phillips & Kuhn, 1999)

Table 4–4 provides critical guidelines for nurses who are administering magnesium.

NURSING FAST FACT!

Be aware that other CNS depressants could cause further depressed sensorium when magnesium sulfate is being administered. Therefore, be prepared to deal with respiratory arrest if hypermagnesemia inadvertently occurs during administration of magnesium sulfate.

> Table 4–4 **CRITICAL GUIDELINES FOR ADMINISTRATION OF MAGNESIUM**

- Double check the order for magnesium administration to ensure that it stipulates the concentration of the solution to be used. Do not accept orders for "amps" or "vials" without further clarification.
- Use caution in patients with impaired renal function; watch urine output.
- Reduce other CNS depressants when given concurrently with magnesium preparations.
- Therapeutic doses of magnesium can produce flushing and sweating, which occur most often if the administration rate is too fast.
- Closely assess patients receiving magnesium.

Nursing Points-of-Care: Hypomagnesemia

Nursing assessment includes:

1. Obtain a patient history, being alert to factors that predispose to hypomagnesemia such as alcoholism, laxative abuse, total parenteral nutrition (TPN), and potassium-wasting diuretic use.
2. Assess for signs and symptoms of hypomagnesemia.
3. Obtain baseline values for laboratory tests, serum magnesium, serum calcium, and serum potassium.
4. Obtain baseline ECG.

Key nursing interventions include:

1. Monitoring vital signs
2. Monitoring closely for digitalis toxicity
3. Keeping accurate intake and output records
4. Taking safety precautions if a patient is mentally confused

Serum Magnesium Excess: Hypermagnesemia

Hypermagnesemia occurs when a person's serum level is greater than 2.5 mEq/L. The most common cause of hypermagnesemia is renal failure in patients who have an increased intake of magnesium.

Pathophysiology and Etiology

Renal factors that lead to hypermagnesemia include renal failure, Addison's disease, and inadequate excretion of magnesium by kidneys.

Other causes include hyperparathyroidism; hyperthyroidism; and iatrogenic causes such as excessive magnesium administration during treatment of patients with eclampsia, hemodialysis with excessively hard water with a dialysate inadvertently high in magnesium, or ingestion of medications high in magnesium, such as antacids and laxatives.

Signs and Symptoms

Patients with hypermagnesemia may experience neuromuscular symptoms such as flushing and sense of skin warmth, lethargy, sedation, hypoactive deep tendon reflexes, depressed respirations, and weak or absent cry in newborn. Other symptoms include hypotension, sinus bradycardia, heart block, and cardiac arrest (serum level greater than 15 mEq/L) and increased susceptibility to digitalis toxicity, nausea, vomiting, and seizures.

Diagnostic Tests

- Serum magnesium: Greater than 2.5 mEq/L
- ECG: Findings of QT interval and atrioventricular block may occur (at levels greater than 2.5 mEq/L).

Treatment and Management

Guidelines for treatment of patients with hypermagnesemia are:

1. Decrease oral magnesium intake.
2. Administer calcium gluconate to antagonize the action of magnesium.
3. Support respiratory function.
4. Order peritoneal or hemodialysis in severe cases of hypermagnesemia.

Nursing Points-of-Care: Hypermagnesemia

Nursing assessment includes:

1. Evaluate possible causes of hypermagnesemia, including renal insufficiency and chronic laxative use.
2. Assess for signs of hypermagnesemia.
3. Obtain baseline values for serum magnesium and serum calcium.
4. Obtain baseline ECG.

Key nursing interventions include:

1. Monitoring vital signs
2. Monitoring laboratory test values
3. Monitoring for ECG changes
4. Encouraging fluid intake if not contraindicated
5. Being prepared to provide ventilatory assistance or resuscitation

Phosphorus (HPO_4^-)

Normal Reference Value: 3.0 to 4.5 mg/dL

Physiologic Role

The physiologic role of phosphorus is:

- Phosphorus is essential to all cells.
- Role in metabolism of proteins, carbohydrates, and fats
- Essential to energy, necessary in the formation of high-energy compounds adenosine triphosphate (ATP) and adenosine diphosphate (ADP)
- As a cellular building block, it is the backbone of nucleic acids and is essential to cell membrane formation.
- Delivery of oxygen; functions in formation of red blood cell enzyme.

Approximately 80 percent of phosphorus in the body is contained in the bones and teeth, and 20 percent is abundant in the ICF. PTH plays a major role in homeostasis of phosphate because of its ability to vary phosphate reabsorption in the proximal tubule of the kidney. PTH also allows for the shift of phosphate from bone to plasma.

Phosphorus plays an important role in delivery of oxygen to tissues by regulating the level of 2,3-diphosphoglycerate (2,3-DPG), a substance in red blood cells that decreases the affinity of hemoglobin for oxygen.

NURSING FAST FACT!

Phosphorus and calcium have a reciprocal relationship: an increase in the phosphorus level frequently causes hypocalcemia.

Serum Phosphate Deficit: Hypophosphatemia

Phosphorus is a critical constituent of all the body's tissues. Hypophosphatemia occurs when the serum level is below the lower limit of normal (less than 2.5 mg/dL). This imbalance may occur in the presence of total body phosphate deficit or may merely reflect a temporary shift of phosphorus into the cells.

Pathophysiology and Etiology

Hypophosphatemia can result from overzealous refeeding, total parenteral nutrition administered without adequate phosphorus, malabsorption syndromes, or alcohol withdrawal. GI losses include vomiting, chronic diarrhea, and malabsorption syndromes.

Hormonal influences such as hyperparathyroidism enhance renal phosphate excretion. Drugs that predispose an individual to hypophosphatemia include aluminum-containing antacids (which bind phosphorus, thereby lowering serum levels), diuretics, androgens, corticosteroids, glucagon, epinephrine, gastrin, and mannitol. Other causes include treatment of patients with diabetic ketoacidosis (dextrose with insulin causes a shift of phosphorus into cells).

Signs and Symptoms

Hypophosphatemia can affect the CNS, neuromuscular and cardiac status, and the blood. An affected patient may experience disorientation, confusion, seizures, paresthesia (early), profound muscle weakness, tremor, ataxia, incoordination, dysarthria, dysphagia, and congestive cardiomyopathy. Hypophosphatemia affects all blood cells, especially red cells. It causes a decline in 2,3-DPG levels in erythrocytes. 2,3-DPG in red cells normally interacts with hemoglobin to promote the release of oxygen. With reduced 2,3-DPG, oxygen delivery to peripheral tissues is impaired.

Diagnostic Tests

- Serum phosphorus: Less than 2.5 mg/dL (1.7 mEq/L)
- Serum PTH: Elevated
- Serum magnesium: Decreased because of increased urinary excretion of magnesium
- Serum alkaline phosphate: Increased with increased osteoblastic activity
- Radiography: Skeletal changes of osteomalacia or rickets

Treatment and Management

Treatment should include the following regimen:

1. For mild to moderate deficiency, oral phosphate supplements, such as Neutra-Phos or Phospho-Soda, can be administered.
2. For severe hypophosphatemia, administer I.V. phosphorus solutions.

NURSING FAST FACT!

In treating patients, be aware that calcium levels should be monitored closely.

Serum Phosphate Excess: Hyperphosphatemia

A variety of conditions can lead to hyperphosphatemia, but the major disorder is renal disease.

Nursing Points-of-Care: Hypophosphatemia

Nursing assessment includes:

1. Obtain a patient history with focus on factors that put patients at high risk for hypophosphatemia, such as alcoholism, use of TPN, and diabetic ketoacidosis.
2. Assess for signs of hypophosphatemia.
3. Obtain baseline laboratory values of serum phosphate and serum calcium.

Key nursing interventions include:

1. Monitoring for cardiac, GI, and neurologic abnormalities
2. Monitoring for changes in laboratory test values
3. Keeping accurate intake and output records
4. Taking safety precautions when a patient is confused
5. Being alert to signs when feeding is restarted after prolonged starvation (refeeding syndrome)
6. Being alert to complications of I.V. administration of phosphorus (hypocalcemia, hyperphosphatemia)

Pathophysiology and Etiology

Hyperphosphatemia can result from renal insufficiency, hypoparathyroidism, or increased **catabolism.** It is also seen in patients with cancer states such as myelogenous leukemia and lymphoma.

Drugs that can predispose an individual to hyperphosphatemia include oral phosphates, I.V. phosphates, phosphate laxatives, and excessive vitamin D, tetracyclines, and methicillin. Other causes include massive blood transfusions caused by phosphate leaking from the blood cells.

Signs and Symptoms

Patients with hyperphosphatemia may experience many symptoms, including hypocalcemia; tetany (short-term); soft tissue calcification (long-term); mental changes, such as apprehension, confusion, and coma; and increased 2,3-DPG levels in red blood cells.

Diagnostic Tests

- Serum phosphorus: Greater than 4.5 mg/dL (2.6 mEq/L)
- Serum calcium: Useful in assessing potential consequences of treatment

- Serum PTH: Decreased in those with hypoparathyroidism
- BUN: To assess renal function
- Radiography: Skeletal changes of osteodystrophy

Treatment and Management

Treatment should include the following regimen:

1. Identify the underlying cause of hyperphosphatemia.
2. Restrict dietary intake.
3. Administer the intake of phosphate-binding gels (e.g., Amphojel, Basaljel, and Dialume).

Nursing Points of Care: Hyperphosphatemia

Nursing assessment includes:

1. Obtain a patient history for factors that place patients at high risk for hyperphosphatemia, including renal insufficiency and laxative use.
2. Assess for signs and symptoms of hyperphosphatemia.
3. Obtain baseline laboratory values for serum phosphate.
4. Check urinary output; less than 600 mL/day increases serum phosphate levels.

Key nursing interventions include:

1. Monitoring for cardiac, GI, and neuromuscular abnormalities
2. Monitoring changes in laboratory test values
3. Keeping accurate intake and output records
4. Observing the patient for signs and symptoms of hypocalcemia; when phosphate levels increase, calcium levels decrease.

Chloride (Cl^-)

Normal Reference Value: 95 to 108 mEq/L

Physiologic Role

The physiologic role of chloride is:

- Regulation of serum osmolarity
- Regulation of fluid balance; when sodium is retained chloride is also retained, causing water retention and increased fluid volume.
- Control of acidity of gastric juice

- Regulation of acid–base balance
- Role in oxygen–carbon dioxide exchange (chloride shift)

Chloride is the major anion in the ECF. Changes in serum chloride concentration are usually secondary to changes in one or more of the other electrolytes. Chloride has a reciprocal relationship with bicarbonate (HCO_3). For example, a decrease in HCO_3 concentrations results in a reciprocal rise in chloride level; when chloride level decreases, HCO_3 level increases in compensation. Chloride exists primarily combined as sodium chloride or hydrochloric acid. Measurement of serum chloride is most frequently done for its inferential value.

Reabsorption of chloride by the renal tubules is one of the major regulatory functions of the kidneys. As sodium chloride is reabsorbed, water follows through osmosis. It is through this function that vascular blood volume is maintained.

Chloride plays its most important role in acid–base balance. Its role in the pH balance of the ECF is referred to as the "chloride shift." The chloride shift is an ionic exchange that occurs within red blood cells. This shift preserves the electrical neutrality of the red blood cells and maintains a 1:20 ratio of carbonic acid and HCO_3 that is essential for pH balance of the plasma.

Serum Chloride Deficit: Hypochloremia

Loss of chloride ions occurs mainly through GI losses and significantly alters acid–base balance because of the reciprocal relationship with HCO_3.

Pathophysiology and Etiology

Hypochloremia results primarily from severe vomiting and diarrhea, pyloric obstruction, acute infection, and use of chlorothiazide diuretics. Other causes of hypochloremia include the prolonged use of I.V. 5 percent dextrose in water, which dilutes serum electrolytes.

Signs and Symptoms

Patients with hypochloremia may experience neuromuscular symptoms such as tetany and hypertonic reflexes. Other symptoms include depressed respiration and excessive loss of chloride, resulting in alkalosis because of an increase in HCO_3 level.

NURSING FAST FACT!

A deficiency in chloride reflects a deficiency in potassium. When replacing potassium, use potassium chloride solution. When the serum level drops to 80 mEq/L or below there is severe impaired mentation, hypotension and cardiac dysrhythmias. Correct the underlying disorder.

Diagnostic Tests

- Serum chloride: Less than 96 mEq/L (less than 80 mEq/L indicates serious imbalance)
- ABG values: Consistent with alkalosis
- ECG: May show dysrhythmias related to associated hyperkalemia.

Treatment and Management

The principles of treating patients with hypochloremia are twofold: (1) treat the underlying cause (alkalosis) and (2) administer NaCl solutions.

Nursing Points-of-Care: Hypochloremia

Nursing assessment includes:

1. Obtain a patient history of conditions that predispose an individual to hypochloremia, such as continuous vomiting.
2. Assess for signs and symptoms of hypochloremia.
3. Assess for signs of metabolic alkalosis.
4. Obtain baseline laboratory test values for serum chloride.

Key nursing interventions include:

1. Monitoring changes in laboratory test values for serum chloride and potassium
2. Monitoring for increased signs of hypochloremia
3. Monitoring serum carbon dioxide or arterial bicarbonate for metabolic alkalosis
4. Keeping accurate records of gastric secretions

Serum Chloride Excess: Hyperchloremia

Excessive Cl^- ions result from any condition that causes a decrease in HCO_3 and can also influence the acid–base balance.

Pathophysiology and Etiology

Trauma such as head injury causes retention of sodium and chloride ions. Hormonal factors affecting retention of chloride include excessive secretion of adrenal cortical hormone. Severe dehydration elevates levels of serum electrolytes, including chloride. As bicarbonate ions decrease, chloride ions increase in metabolic acidosis.

Signs and Symptoms

Patients with hyperchloremia may experience symptoms related to acidosis, such as drowsiness, lethargy, headache, weakness, tremors, dyspnea, tachypnea, Kussmaul respirations (with pH less than 7.20), hyperventilation, and dysrhythmias. If the serum chloride is above 115 mEq/L serious mentation, hypo- or hypertension, and cardiac dysrhythmias may occur. Correct the underlying disorder.

Diagnostic Tests

- Serum chloride: Greater than 106 mEq/L
- Serum carbon dioxide: Less than 22 mEq/L when associated with acidosis
- Serum pH: Less than 7.35 when associated with metabolic acidosis
- ECG: Presence of dysrhythmias

Table 4–5 summarizes common electrolyte imbalances that can occur in a variety of clinical settings.

Nursing Points-of-Care: Hyperchloremia

Nursing assessment includes:

1. Obtain history of predisposing conditions such as head injury or cortisone use.
2. Assess for signs and symptoms of hyperchloremia.
3. Obtain baseline laboratory test values for serum chloride and potassium.

Key nursing interventions include:

1. Monitoring changes in laboratory test values, especially serum chloride and serum potassium
2. Monitoring for increased signs of hyperchloremia
3. Monitoring serum carbon dioxide or arterial bicarbonate levels for metabolic acidosis
4. Keeping an accurate record of 24-hour urinary output

Acid–Base Balance

The regulation of the hydrogen ion concentration of body fluids is actually the key component of acid–base balance. The pH of a fluid reflects the

> Table 4–5 **PATIENTS AT RISK FOR ELECTROLYTE IMBALANCE**

Patient Care Unit	Conditions That Can Lead to Imbalance	Potential Electrolyte Imbalances
Geriatric	Prolonged diarrhea	Fluid volume deficit
	Prolonged malnutrition	Hypernatremia
	Diuretic therapy	Hypokalemia
Medical	Anorexia nervosa	Fluid volume deficit
	Profuse sweating	Hyponatremia
	Overuse of antacids	Hypomagnesemia
	Gastroenteritis	Hypocalcemia
	Hyperparathyroidism	Hypokalemia
	Diabetic ketoacidosis	Hyperkalemia
	Alcoholism	Hypermagnesemia
	Renal failure	
	SIADH	
Surgical	Infections	Fluid volume deficit
	Surgical hypoparathyroidism	Fluid volume excess
	Nasogastric suction	Hypokalemia
	Postoperative complications	Hypomagnesemia
	Use of pharmacologic agents: morphine,	Hypocalcemia
	penicillin, and carbenicillin	Hypochloremia
	Ileus	Hyponatremia
Oncologic	Myelogenous leukemia	Hypomagnesemia
	Lymphoma	Hyponatremia
	Cytoxan	Hypercalcemia
	Hypertonic tube feeding	Hypernatremia
	Neoplastic disease	Hypermagnesemia
	Solid tumors: Breast and prostate	Hypocalcemia*
	Malignant melanoma	Hyperkalemia*
		Hyperphosphatemia*
Critical care	Crushing injuries	Hypomagnesemia
	Total parenteral nutrition administration	Hypophosphatemia
	Hypertonic tube feedings	Hyponatremia
	Burns	Hypercalcemia
	Drowning in sea water	Hypernatremia
	Head injuries	Hyperkalemia

**Components of tumor lysis syndrome.*

hydrogen ion concentration of that fluid. The normal pH of arterial blood ranges from 7.35 to 7.45. A solution is either basic or acidic on the basis of the concentration of hydrogen ions in the solution, and the pH scale is used to describe the hydrogen ion concentration. The pH scale is a logarithmic scale with values from 0.00 to 14.00. A neutral solution (i.e., neither acidic nor basic) has a pH of 7.00 (Lee et al., 1996).

The inverse proportion of the pH to the concentration of hydrogen ions is reflected in the concept that the higher the pH value, the lower the hydrogen ion concentration. Conversely, the lower the pH value, the higher the hydrogen ion concentration. Therefore, a pH below 7.35 reflects an acidic state, but a pH greater than 7.45 indicates alkalosis and a lower hydrogen ion concentration. A variation from 7.35 to 7.45 of 0.4 in either direction can be fatal. Figure 4–6 shows the pH scale.

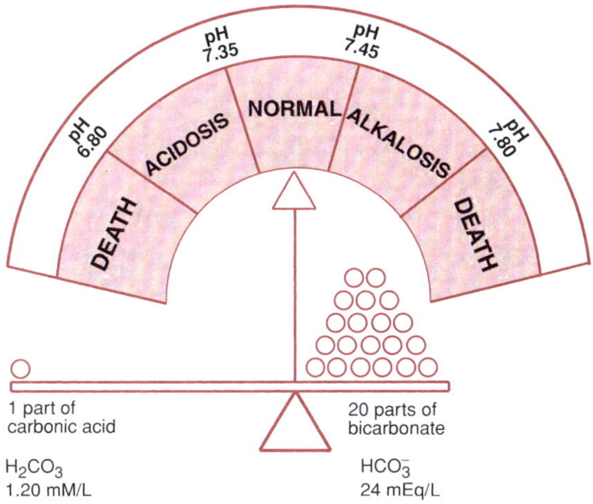

Figure 4–6 ■ Acid–base scale.

Three mechanisms operate to maintain the appropriate pH of the blood:

1. Chemical buffer systems in the ECF and within the cells
2. Removal of carbon dioxide by the lungs
3. Renal regulation of the hydrogen ion concentration

Chemical Buffer Systems

The buffer systems are fast-acting defenses that provide immediate protection against changes in the hydrogen ion concentration of the ECF. The buffers also serve as transport mechanisms that carry excess hydrogen ions to the lungs.

A buffer is a substance that reacts to minimize **pH** changes when either acid or base is released into the system. There are three primary buffer systems in the ECF: the hemoglobin system, the plasma protein system, and the bicarbonate system. The capacity of a buffer is limited; therefore, after the components of a buffer system have reacted, they must be replenished before the body can respond to further stress.

The hemoglobin and deoxyhemoglobin found in red blood cells, together with their potassium salts, act as buffer pairs. The electrolyte chloride shifts in and out of the red blood cells according to the level of oxygen in the blood plasma. For each chloride ion that leaves a red blood cell, a bicarbonate ion enters the cell; for each chloride ion that enters a red blood cell, a bicarbonate ion is released.

Plasma proteins are large molecules that contain the acid (or base) and salt form of a buffer. Proteins then have the ability to bind or release hydrogen ions.

The bicarbonate buffer system maintains the blood's pH in the range of 7.35 to 7.45 with a ratio of 20 parts bicarbonate to 1 part carbonic acid by a process that is called hydration of carbon dioxide and is a means of buffering the excess acid in the blood. If a strong acid is added to the body, the ratio is upset. In this acid imbalance, the largest amount of carbon dioxide diffuses in the plasma to the red blood cells; carbon dioxide then combines with plasma protein. Carbon dioxide that is dissolved in the blood combines with water to form carbonic acid (Lee et al., 1996).

Respiratory Regulation

In healthy individuals, the lungs form a second line of defense in maintaining the acid–base balance. When carbon dioxide combines with water, H_2CO_3 is formed. Therefore, an increase in the acid carbon dioxide lowers the pH of blood, creating an acidotic state; a decrease in the carbon dioxide level increases the pH, causing the blood to become more alkaline. After H_2CO_3 is formed, it dissociates into carbon dioxide and water. The carbon dioxide is transferred to the lungs, where it diffuses into the alveoli and is eliminated through exhalation. Therefore, the rate of respiration affects the hydrogen ion concentration. An increase in respiratory rate causes carbon dioxide to be blown off by the lungs, resulting in an increase in pH. Conversely, a decrease in respiratory rate causes retention of carbon dioxide and thus a decrease in pH. This means that the lungs can either hold the hydrogen ions until the deficit is corrected or inactivate the hydrogen ions into water molecules to be exhaled with the carbon dioxide as vapor, thereby correcting the excess. It takes from 10 to 30 minutes for the lungs to inactivate the hydrogen molecules by converting them to water molecules (Lee et al., 1996).

Renal Regulation

The kidneys regulate the hydrogen ion concentration by increasing or decreasing the HCO_3 ion concentration in the body fluid by a series of complex chemical reactions that occur in the renal tubules. The regulation of acid–base balance by the kidneys occurs chiefly by increasing or decreasing the HCO_3 ion concentration in body fluids. Hydrogen is secreted into the tubules of the kidney, where it is eliminated in the urine. At the same time, sodium is reabsorbed from the tubular fluid into the ECF in exchange for hydrogen and combines with HCO_3 ions to form the buffer, $NaHCO_3$.

The kidneys help to regulate the extracellular concentration of HCO_3. Two buffer systems help the kidney to eliminate excess hydrogen in the urine: the phosphate buffer system and the ammonia buffer system. With each of these, an excess of hydrogen is secreted and HCO_3 ions are formed; sodium is reabsorbed, thus forming $NaHCO_3$. The time it takes for a change to occur in the acid–base balance can range from a fraction of a second to more than 24 hours. Although the kidneys are the most powerful regulating mechanism, they are slow to make major changes in the acid–base balance (Metheny, 2000).

Major Acid–Base Imbalances

There are two types of acid–base imbalances: (1) metabolic (base bicarbonate deficit and excess) **acidosis** and **alkalosis** and (2) respiratory (carbonic acid deficit and excess) acidosis and alkalosis. The balanced pH of the arterial blood is 7.4, and only small variations of up to 0.05 can exist without causing ill effects. Deviations of more than five times the normal concentration of H^+ in the ECF are potentially fatal (Horne & Derrico, 1999).

Metabolic Acid–Base Imbalance

Normal Reference Value: 22 to 26 mEq/L

Metabolic Acidosis: Base Bicarbonate Deficit

Metabolic acidosis (HCO_3 deficit) is a clinical disturbance characterized by a low pH and low plasma HCO_3 level. This condition can occur by a gain of hydrogen (H^+) ion or a loss of HCO_3.

Pathophysiology and Etiology

Metabolic acidosis occurs with loss of HCO_3 from diarrhea, draining fistulas, and administration of TPN. Diabetes mellitus, alcoholism, and starvation cause ketoacidosis. Respiratory or circulatory failure, ingestion of certain drugs or toxins (e.g., salicylates, ethylene glycol, or methyl alcohol), some hereditary disorders, and septic shock cause lactic acidosis. It can also result when renal failure results in excessive retention of hydrogen ions.

NURSING FAST FACT!

Hyperkalemia is usually present in clinical cases of acidosis (Metheny, 2000).

Signs and Symptoms

Patients with metabolic acidosis may experience CNS-related symptoms such as headache, confusion, drowsiness, increased respiratory rate, and Kussmaul respirations. Other symptoms include nausea, vomiting, decreased cardiac output, and bradycardia (when serum pH is less than 7.0).

Diagnostic Tests

- ABG values: pH less than 7.35, HCO_3 less than 22 mEq/L
- $Paco_2$: Less than 38 mm Hg
- Serum HCO_3: Less than 22 mEq/L
- Serum electrolytes: Elevated potassium possible, because of exchange of intracellular potassium for hydrogen ions in the body's attempt to normalize acid–base environment
- ECG: Dysrhythmias caused by hyperkalemia

Treatment and Management

Patients with metabolic acidosis are treated by (1) reversing the underlying cause (e.g., diabetic ketoacidosis, alcoholism related to ketoacidosis, diarrhea, acute renal failure, renal tubular acidosis, poisoning, or lactic acidosis); (2) eliminating the source (if the cause is excessive administration of sodium chloride); and (3) administering $NaHCO_3$ (7.5 percent 44.4 mEq/50 mL or 8.4 percent 50 mEq/50 mL I.V. when pH is equal to or less than 7.2). Concentration depends on severity of acidosis and presence of any serum sodium disorders.

NURSING FAST FACT!

Give $NaHCO_3$ cautiously to avoid patients' developing metabolic alkalosis and pulmonary edema secondary to sodium overload.

Potassium replacement: hyperkalemia is usually present, but potassium deficit can occur. If a deficit of less than 3.5 mEq/L is present, the potassium deficit must be corrected before $NaHCO_3$ is administered because the potassium shifts back into the ICF when the acidosis is correct.

Metabolic Alkalosis: Base Bicarbonate Excess

Metabolic alkalosis (i.e., HCO_3 excess) is a clinical disturbance characterized by a high pH and a high plasma HCO_3 concentration and can be produced by a gain of HCO_3 or a loss of hydrogen ion.

Nursing Points-of-Care: Metabolic Acidosis

Nursing assessment includes:

1. Obtain a patient history of health problems that relate to metabolic acidosis such as diabetes or renal disease.
2. Obtain baseline vital signs with focus on the respiration and cardiac functioning.
3. Assess for symptoms of metabolic acidosis.
4. Obtain baseline values for ABGs and laboratory tests. Note the serum electrolytes, serum CO_2 content, HCO_3 and blood sugar level.

Key nursing interventions include:

1. Providing safety precautions when a patient is confused
2. Monitoring the patient's dietary and fluid intake and output record
3. Monitoring laboratory results for changes
4. Monitoring the patient for changes in vital signs, especially changes in respiration, cardiac function, and CNS signs

Pathophysiology and Etiology

Metabolic alkalosis occurs with GI loss of hydrogen ions from gastric suctioning and vomiting. Renal loss of hydrogen ions occurs from potassium-losing diuretics, excess of mineralocorticoid, hypercalcemia, and hypoparathyroidism. In patients with hypokalemia and carbohydrate refeeding after starvation, hydrogen ions shift from ECF into the cells, depleting serum levels. This also occurs when excessive ingestion of alkalis (e.g., antacids such as Alka-Seltzer), parenteral administration of $NaHCO_3$ during cardiopulmonary resuscitation, and massive blood transfusions increase serum levels of HCO_3.

Signs and Symptoms

Patients with metabolic alkalosis may experience dizziness and depressed respirations in addition to impaired mentation, tingling of fingers and toes, circumoral paresthesia, and hypertonic reflexes. Other symptoms include hypotension, cardiac dysrhythmias, hyperventilation, hypokalemia, and decreased ionized calcium (i.e., carpopedal spasm).

Diagnostic Tests

- ABG values: pH greater than 7.45; HCO_3 greater than 26 mEq/L
- $Paco_2$: Greater than 42 mm Hg
- Serum HCO_3: Greater than 26 mEq/L
- Serum electrolytes: Low serum potassium (less than 4 mEq/L) and low serum chloride
- ECG: Assess for dysrhythmias (Horne & Swearingen, 1993).

NURSING FAST FACT!

Hypokalemia is often present in patients with alkalosis.

Treatment and Management

Patients with metabolic alkalosis are treated by (1) reversing the underlying cause, (2) administering sufficient chloride for the kidney to excrete the excess HCO_3, and (3) replacing potassium if a chloride deficit is also present.

Nursing Points-of-Care: Metabolic Alkalosis

Nursing assessment includes:

1. Obtain history of health problems related to metabolic alkalosis (e.g., peptic ulcer, vomiting, adrenocortical hormone abnormalities).
2. Obtain baseline vital signs.
3. Assess for signs and symptoms of metabolic alkalosis.
4. Obtain baseline values for ABGs and serum electrolyte, serum CO_2 content, and HCO_3

Key nursing interventions include:

1. Providing safety precautions for hyperexcitability states
2. Monitoring the patient's fluid intake and output
3. Monitoring laboratory results for changes
4. Monitoring the patient for changes in vital signs, with particular attention to respirations and CNS
5. Monitoring for changes in cardiac rhythm, especially in patients taking cardiac glycosides

Respiratory Acid–Base Imbalance

Normal Reference Value: Partial pressure of carbon dioxide ($Paco_2$): 38 to 42 mm Hg.

Respiratory Acidosis: Carbonic Acid Excess

Respiratory acidosis is caused by inadequate excretion of carbon dioxide and inadequate ventilation, resulting in an increase of serum levels or carbon dioxide and H_2CO_3. Acute respiratory acidosis is usually associated with emergency situations.

Pathophysiology and Etiology

Acute respiratory acidosis can result from pulmonary, neurologic, and cardiac causes, such as pulmonary edema; aspiration of a foreign body; pneumothorax; severe pneumonia; severe, prolonged exacerbation of acute asthma; overdose of sedatives; cardiac arrest; and massive pulmonary embolism.

Chronic respiratory acidosis results from emphysema, bronchial asthma, bronchiectasis, postoperative pain, obesity, and tight abdominal binders.

Signs and Symptoms

Acute signs and symptoms include tachypnea; dyspnea; dizziness; seizures; warm, flushed skin, and ventricular fibrillation. Chronic signs and symptoms occur if $PaCO_2$ exceeds the body's ability to compensate, and include respiratory symptoms.

Diagnostic Tests

- ABG values: *Acute:* pH less than 7.35, $Paco_2$ greater than 42 mm Hg, HCO_3 greater than 26 mEq/L. *Chronic:* pH less than 7.35, $Paco_2$ greater than 42 mm Hg, HCO_3 normal or slight increase
- Serum HCO_3: Reflects acid–base balance; initial values normal unless mixed disorder is present.
- Serum electrolytes: Usually not altered
- Chest radiography: Determines the presence of underlying pulmonary disease.
- Drug screen: Determines the quantity of drug if patient is suspected of taking an overdose.

Treatment and Management

Respiratory acidosis is treated by carrying out the following:

1. Improve ventilation.
2. Administer bronchodilators or antibiotics for respiratory infections as indicated.
3. Administer oxygen as indicated.
4. Administer adequate fluids (2 to 3 L/day) to keep mucous membranes moist and help remove secretions.

Nursing Points-of-Care: Respiratory Acidosis

Nursing assessment includes:

1. Obtain history of pneumonia, chronic obstructive pulmonary disease (COPD), narcotic use, or emphysema.
2. Obtain baseline vital signs.
3. Assess for signs and symptoms of respiratory acidosis.
4. Obtain baseline values for laboratory tests, especially $Paco_2$.

Key nursing interventions include:

1. Providing safety precautions when a patient is confused
2. Monitoring laboratory results for changes, especially pH and $Paco_2$
3. Monitoring for changes in vital signs
4. Monitoring oxygen and mechanical ventilator when in use
5. Elevating the head of the patient's bed
6. Encouraging the patient to perform deep-breathing exercise
7. Performing chest percussions to break up mucus when appropriate

Respiratory Alkalosis: Carbonic Acid Deficit

Respiratory alkalosis is usually caused by hyperventilation, which causes "blowing off" of carbon dioxide and a decrease in H_2CO_3 content. Respiratory alkalosis can be acute or chronic.

Pathophysiology and Etiology

Acute respiratory alkalosis results from pulmonary disorders that produce hypoxemia or stimulation of the respiratory centers. Underlying causes of hypoxemia include high fever, pneumonia, congestive heart failure, pulmonary emboli, hypotension, asthma, and inhalation of irritants. Causes of stimulation of respiratory centers include anxiety (most common), excessive mechanical ventilation, CNS lesions involving the respiratory center, and salicylate overdose (an early sign).

Signs and Symptoms

Respiratory alkalosis causes light-headedness, the inability to concentrate, numbness and tingling of the extremities (circumoral paresthesia), tinnitus, palpitations, epigastric pain, blurred vision, precordial pain (tightness), sweating, dry mouth, tremulousness, seizures, and loss of consciousness.

Diagnostic Tests

- ABG values: pH greater than 7.45, $Paco_2$ less than 38 mm Hg, HCO_3 less than 22 mEq/L
- Serum electrolytes: Presence of metabolic acid–base disorders
- Serum phosphate: May fall to less than 0.5 mg/dL.
- ECG: Determines cardiac dysrhythmias

Treatment and Management

Treatment of patients with respiratory alkalosis consists of the following:

1. Treating the source of anxiety (instruct patient to breathe slowly into a paper bag)
2. Administering a sedative as indicated
3. Treating the underlying cause (Metheny, 2000)

Table 4–6 presents a summary of acute acid–base imbalances.

Nursing Points-of-Care: Respiratory Alkalosis

Nursing assessment includes:

1. Obtain a patient history of hysteria, fever, or severe infection.
2. Check for signs and symptoms of respiratory alkalosis.
3. Obtain baseline vital signs.
4. Obtain ABG values.

Key nursing interventions include:

1. Encouraging the patient who is hyperventilating to breathe slowly
2. Having the patient rebreathe expired air by breathing into a paper bag
3. Administering a sedative as directed
4. Listening to the patient who is in emotional distress

> Table 4–6 **SUMMARY OF ACUTE ACID-BASE IMBALANCES**

The Body's Reaction to Acid-Base Imbalance

Condition	pH	$Paco_2$	HCO_3	How the Body Compensates
Respiratory acidosis	↓	↑ or normal	↑	Kidneys conserve HCO_3 and eliminate H*, to increase pH
With compensation	Slightly ↓ or normal	↑	↑	
Respiratory alkalosis	↑	↓ or normal	↓	Kidneys eliminate HCO_3 and conserve H*, to decrease pH
With compensation	Slightly ↓ or normal	↓	↓	
Metabolic acidosis	↓	↓	↓ or normal	Hyperventilation to blow off excess CO_2 and conserve HCO_3
With compensation	Slightly ↓ or normal	↓	↓	
Metabolic alkalosis	↑	↑	↑ or normal	Hypoventilation to ↑ CO_2; kidneys keep H* and excrete HCO_3
With compensation	Slightly ↓ or normal	↑	↑	

Common Causes of Acid-Base Imbalance

Respiratory acidosis	Asphyxis, respiratory depression, CNS depression
Respiratory alkalosis	Hyperventilation, anxiety, PE (causing hyperventilation)
Metabolic acidosis	Diarrhea, renal failure, salicylate overdose such as ASA (aspirin)
Metabolic alkalosis	Hypercalcemia, overdose on an alkaline substance such as antacid

**Compensatory response.*

NURSING PLAN OF CARE

ELECTROLYTE IMBALANCE

Focus Assessment

Subjective

- History of precipitating illness or disorder
- Complaints of weakness, lethargy, and fatigue
- Use of drugs that may cause problem

Objective

- Serum laboratory values consistent with specific electrolyte imbalance
- Urine specific gravity, pH, and osmolarity consistent with specific electrolyte imbalance

(Continued on following page)

- Neuromuscular, cardiovascular, and neurologic assessment findings consistent with specific electrolyte imbalance

Patient Outcome/Evaluation Criteria

Patient will:

- Maintain vital signs within normal limits.
- Be mobile without evidence of weakness, pain, or fractures.
- Have an adequate cardiac output, blood pressure with normal range, absence of clinical signs of heart failure and cardiac dysrhythmias.
- Exhibit voiding pattern and urine characteristics with normal range.
- Have no injury caused by neuromuscular or sensory alterations.
- Have an effective breathing pattern with normal depth and rate.

Nursing Diagnoses

- Sensory perceptual alterations secondary to hyponatremia
- Altered health maintenance related to poor dietary habits or perceptual or cognitive impairment
- Constipation related to weakened peristalsis
- Fluid volume deficit related to failure of the regulatory mechanism
- Impaired physical mobility related to activity intolerance, decreased strength and endurance, pain, discomfort, neuromuscular impairment, or musculoskeletal impairment related to electrolyte imbalance
- Ineffective breathing pattern related to biochemical imbalances
- Altered comfort related to injuring agent (e.g., stones associated with excessive calcium)
- Risk for injury related to confusion, altered thought processes resulting from: (1) electrolyte imbalance, tetany, and seizures; (2) severe hypocalcemia or sensory changes; (3) hypercalcemia; or (4) severe hypokalemia, hypocalcemia, or hypophosphatemia
- Impaired gas exchange related to altered oxygen resulting from laryngeal spasm in patients with severe hypokalemia, hyperkalemia, hypocalcemia, or hypophosphatemia
- Altered urinary elimination pattern related to changes in renal function resulting from hypercalcemia
- Risk for impaired verbal communication related to confusion, lethargy, or electrolyte imbalance

Nursing Management

1. Identify patient populations at risk for electrolyte imbalances.
2. Consult with physician if the signs and symptoms of fluid or electrolyte imbalance persist or clinically worsen.
3. Monitor pertinent client assessment data for potential effects related to electrolyte imbalances:
   a. abnormalities in serum electrolytes as indicated.
   b. vital signs for trending.

(Continued on following page)

NURSING PLAN OF CARE

ELECTROLYTE IMBALANCE *(Continued)*

- c. ECG for dysrhythmias.
- d. patient response to electrolyte replacement therapy.
- e. loss of electrolyte-rich body fluids, such as nasogastric suctioning, ileostomy drainage, diarrhea, wound drainage, or diaphoresis.
- f. side effects of prescribed electrolyte supplements.
- g. intake and output and possibly daily weights.
- h. signs of tetany
- i. signs of CNS depression

4. Administer supplemental electrolytes as indicated.
5. Closely monitor serum potassium levels in patients taking diuretics with digoxin.
6. Medicate for pain as needed.
7. Obtain ordered specimens for laboratory analysis of serum and urine electrolytes and ABGs as indicated.
8. Maintain I.V. solution containing electrolytes at a constant flow rate.
9. Provide a safe environment for patients with neurologic and neuromuscular manifestations of electrolyte imbalances.
10. Use an infusion pump when administering parenteral potassium and magnesium.
11. Incorporate seizure precautions into nursing care when indicated.
12. Encourage compliance with therapeutic regimen.
13. Maintain patent I.V. line.

***Sources:** Sparks & Taylor (1998), Hogan & Wane (2003).*

Patient Education

Provide written material and verbal instructions regarding any medications.

Provide information on predisposing factors associated with specific electrolyte imbalances.

Review indicators of digitalis toxicity, if appropriate.

Provide information on dietary sources of electrolytes in deficit situations when appropriate.

Educate regarding salt substitutes, potassium-sparing diuretics, and other predisposing drugs.

Provide information on over-the-counter medications (e.g., magnesium and aluminum hydroxide, antacids and phosphorus-binding antacids, laxatives, multivitamin and mineral supplements) when appropriate.

Educate the patient with cancer about symptoms of hypercalcemia.

(Continued on following page)

Educate the patient about appropriate use of laxatives if deficit is caused by abuse.

Educate the patient on the high phosphorus content of processed foods, carbonated beverages, and over-the-counter medications when appropriate.

Home Care Issues

Patients' disease states that might require home electrolyte replacement therapy include:

- Cardiopulmonary disorders: potassium replacement.
- Gastrointestinal disorder: intractable diarrhea, hyperemesis gravidarum
- Patients receiving chemotherapy
- Electrolyte replacement therapies usually last from 1 to 7 days. The electrolytes are provided through a peripheral indwelling venous access device unless a long-term access device is available.
- Assess patients taking oral electrolyte supplements for compliance.

Key Points

- The seven major electrolytes and their symbols are:
  - *Cations:*
  - Sodium: Na^+
  - Potassium: K^+
  - Calcium: Ca^{2+}
  - Magnesium: Mg^{2+}
  - *Anions:*
  - Chloride: Cl^-
  - Phosphate: HPO_4^-
  - Bicarbonate: HCO_3^-
- The prefix hypo: Deficit in an electrolyte
- The prefix hyper: Excess in an electrolyte
- Key nursing interventions for electrolyte imbalances:
  - Monitor laboratory values
  - Frequent assessments of neurologic, cardiovascular respiratory, GI, integumentary status; special senses; body weight; and vital signs
  - Monitor ECG.
  - Monitor for phlebitis.
  - Monitor for symptoms of fluid overload.
  - Accurate intake and output

- Safety precautions when the patient is confused
- Patients taking digitalis need to be monitored carefully for digoxin toxicity.
- Monitor arterial blood gases when appropriate.

- Key laboratory values that the nurse must recognize:
  - Potassium K^+ 3.5 to 5.5 mEq/L
  - Calcium: Na^+ 135 to 145 mEq/L
  - Magnesium (Mg^{2+}) 1.5 to 2.5 mEq/L
  - Phosphate (HPO_4^-) 3.0 to 4.5 mg/dL
  - Chloride (Cl^-) 95 to 108 mEq/L
- Critical guidelines for infusion potassium include:
  - Never give potassium I.V. push.
  - Concentrations of potassium greater than 60 mEq should not be given in a peripheral vein.
  - Concentrations greater than 8 mEq/100 mL can cause pain and irritation of peripheral veins, leading to phlebitis.
  - Do not add potassium to a hanging container.
  - Administer potassium at a rate not exceeding 10 mEq/h through peripheral veins.
- Calcium and phosphate have a reciprocal relationship: When one is elevated, the other is decreased.
- Patients with calcium imbalances may need seizure precautions.
- Monitor for calcemia in patients receiving massive transfusions of citrated blood.
- Trousseau's sign and Chvostek's sign are specific for calcium deficit.
- Patients with calcium excess (i.e., hypercalcemia) need to be treated with saline diuresis and may need hemodialysis.
- The most dangerous symptom of hypocalcemia is laryngospasm.
- The four major acid–base imbalances in the body are respiratory acidosis (carbonic acid excess), respiratory alkalosis (carbonic acid deficit), metabolic acidosis (base bicarbonate deficit), and metabolic alkalosis (bicarbonate excess).
- Acid–base balance is maintained through three major reaction-specific buffer systems that regulate hydrogen ion concentration: the carbonic acid–bicarbonate system, the phosphate buffer system, and the protein buffer system.

Critical Thinking: Case Study

A 65-year-old man presented to the emergency room with complaints of chronic tiredness and increased skin pigmentation. On examination his blood pressure was low: 98/60 mm Hg. Blood test revealed a plasma potassium level of 6.8 mEq/L and a plasma sodium level of 132 mEq/L. The BUN was 20 mg/dL and the serum creatinine was 1.2 mg/dL

What is the electrolyte imbalance? What is the underlying cause? What nursing diagnoses would apply to this patient? What would be the treatment options for this patient?

Media Link: Use the enclosed CD–ROM for more critical thinking activities and the answers to this case study.

Post-Test

In questions 1 through 8, match the signs and symptoms in Column I to the clinical manifestation in Column II.

Column I	Column II
1. CNS depression, drowsiness, lethargy	**a.** Hypomagnesemia
2. Hyperirritability, tremors, increased tendon reflexes	**b.** Hypermagnesemia
3. Carpopedal spasm, laryngeal spasm, convulsions	**c.** Hypocalcemia
4. Bone tumors, prolonged immobilization, increased PTH secretion	**d.** Hypercalcemia
5. Fatigue, headache, apprehension, serum Na^+ 115	**e.** Hypernatremia
6. Serum Na^+ 150, urine Na^+ less than 40 mEq/L, urine specific gravity greater than 1.125	**f.** Hyponatremia
7. ECG with flat or inverted T wave, depressed ST segment	**g.** Hypokalemia
8. ECG with peaked, narrow T wave, shortened QT interval, prolonged PR interval followed by disappearance of P wave	**h.** Hyperkalemia

9. Treatment for a patient with metabolic alkalosis includes:

a. Removal of underlying cause

b. I.V. fluid administration with NaCl

c. Replacement of potassium deficit

d. All of the above

10. To correct metabolic acidosis, the parenteral fluid of choice is:

a. $NaHCO_3$

b. NaCl

   c. Albumin
   d. 5 Percent dextrose in water

11. The pH range of arterial blood is:
    a. 7.25 to 7.35
    b. 7.35 to 7.45
    c. 7.45 to 7.55
    d. 7.56 to 8.05

12. A nursing diagnosis that would be appropriate for the patient with calcium deficit would be:
    a. Ineffective breathing pattern related to biochemical imbalances
    b. Altered comfort related to injuring agent
    c. Risk for injury related to electrolyte imbalance, tetany, and seizures
    d. Altered urinary elimination pattern related to changes in renal function

Media Link: Use the enclosed CD–ROM with this text for more practice test questions and answers along with rationales.

References

Hogan, M.A., & Wane, D. (2003). *Fluids, Electrolytes and Acid Base Balance.* Upper Saddle River, NJ: Prentice–Hall.

Horne, C., & Derrico, D. (1999). Mastering ABGs. *American Journal of Nursing,* 99(8), 26–33.

Lee, C.A., Barrett, C.A., & Ignatavicius, D. (1996). *Fluids and Electrolytes* (4th ed.). Philadelphia: F.A. Davis.

Metheny, N.M. (2000). Fluids and Electrolyte Balance. In Metheny N.M. (ed.). *Nursing Considerations* (4th ed.). Philadelphia: Lippincott-Williams & Wilkins, pp. 59–181.

National Student Nurses' Association (1997). Specific Electrolyte Imbalances. In McEntee, M.A., & Gil, G.M. (eds.). *Fluids and Electrolytes.* Albany, NY: Delmar, pp. 36–70.

Narins, R. (1994). *Clinical Disorders of Fluid and Electrolyte Metabolism* (5th ed.). New York: McGraw–Hill, p. 282

Phillips, L.D., & Kuhn, M. (1999). *Manual of IV Medications* (2nd ed.). Philadelphia: Lippincott.

Sparks, S.M., & Taylor, C.M. (1998). *Nursing Diagnosis Reference Manual* (4th ed.). Springhouse, PA: Springhouse Corporation.

Weldy, N.J. (1996). *Body Fluids and Electrolytes. A Programmed Presentation* (7th ed.). St. Louis: Mosby, pp. 83–119, 127.

Answers to Chapter 4 Post-Test

1. **b**
2. **a**
3. **c**
4. **d**
5. **f**
6. **e**
7. **g**
8. **h**
9. **d**
10. **a**
11. **b**
12. **c**

Unit 2

Basic Infusion Practice

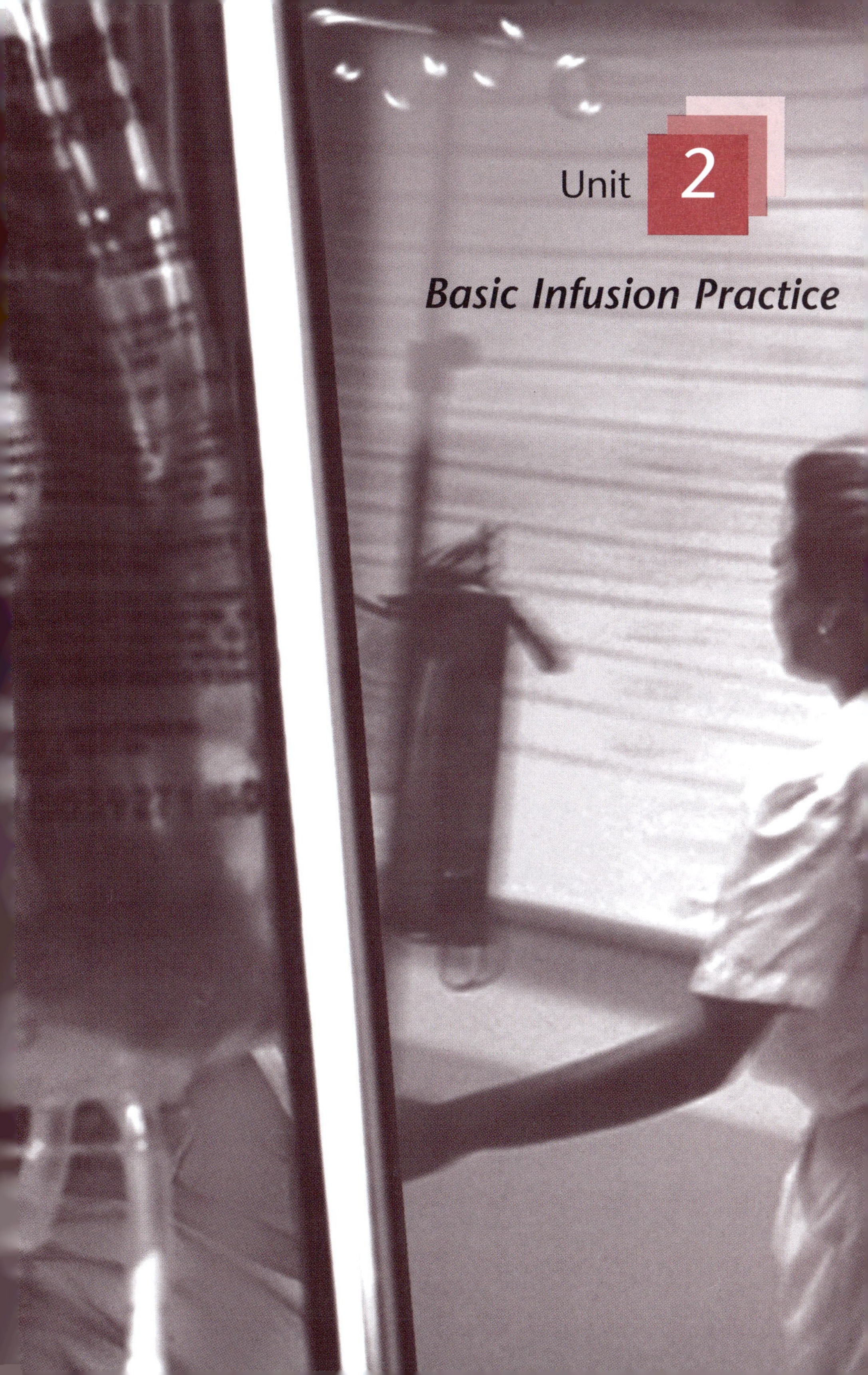

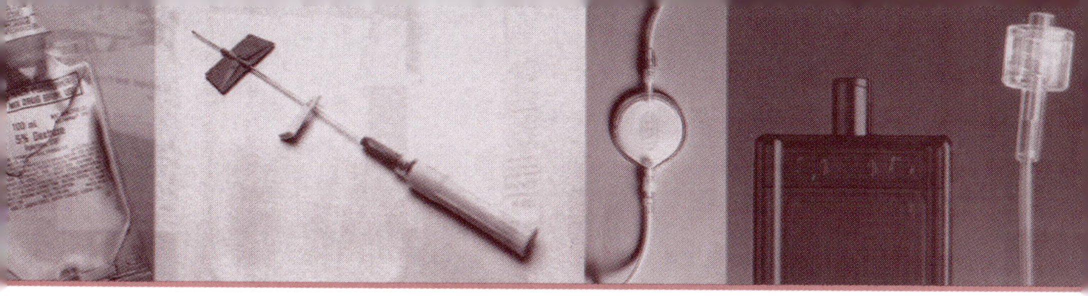

Chapter 5
Parenteral Solutions

Let the patient's taste decide. You will say that, in cases of great thirst, the patient's craving decides that it will drink a great deal of tea, and that you cannot help it. But in these cases be sure that the patient requires diluents for quite other purposes than quenching the thirst; he wants a great deal of some drink, not only of tea, and the doctor will order what he is to have, barley water or lemonade, or soda water and milk, as the case may be.

—Florence Nightingale, 1859

Chapter Contents

LEARNING OBJECTIVES

Upon completion of this chapter, the reader will be able to:

1. Define terminology related to parenteral solutions.
2. Identify the three objectives of parenteral therapy.
3. List the key elements in intravenous (I.V.) solutions.
4. List the uses of maintenance fluids.
5. List the four functions of glucose as a necessary nutrient when administered parenterally.
6. Explain the roles of vitamin C and vitamin B complex in maintenance therapy.
7. Describe the uses of hypotonic, isotonic, and hypertonic fluids.
8. Identify the major groupings of I.V. solutions.
9. Compare the advantages and disadvantages of dextrose, sodium chloride, hydrating fluids, and multiple electrolyte fluids.
10. Identify the main role of hydrating fluids.
11. Compare the properties of a crystalloid with those of a colloid solution.
12. Identify the use of alkalinizing and acidifying fluids.
13. State the most commonly used hypotonic multiple electrolyte solution.
14. State the most commonly used isotonic multiple electrolyte fluid.
15. State the use of albumin, hetastarch, and dextran.

GLOSSARY

Balanced solution Parenteral solution that contains electrolytes in proportions similar to those in plasma; also contains bicarbonate or acetate ion

Catabolism The breakdown of chemical compounds by the body; an energy-producing metabolic process

Colloid A substance (e.g., blood, plasma, albumin, dextran) that does not dissolve into a true solution and is not capable of passing through a semipermeable membrane

Crystalloid A substance that forms a true solution and is capable of passing through a semipermeable membrane (e.g., lactated Ringer's solution, isotonic saline)

Dehydration A deficit of body water; can involve one fluid compartment or all three

Hydrating fluid A solution of water, carbohydrate, sodium, and chloride used to determine adequacy of renal function
Hypertonic solution A solution with an osmolarity higher than that of plasma
Hypotonic solution A solution with an osmolarity lower than that of plasma
Isotonic solution A solution with the same osmolarity as plasma
Maintenance therapy Fluids that provide all nutrients necessary to meet daily patient requirements
Normal saline Solution of salt (0.9 percent sodium chloride)
Plasma substitute A solution of a synthetic substance, such as dextran, used as a substitute for plasma
Replacement therapy Replenishment of losses when maintenance cannot be met and when patient is in a deficit state
Restoration therapy Reconstruction of fluid and electrolyte needs on a continuing basis until homeostasis returns

Rationales and Objectives of Parenteral Therapy

The complex subject of fluids and electrolytes is the foundation for understanding parenteral fluid administration. Chapters 3 and 4 provide the requisite background knowledge for this chapter on parenteral therapy.

To understand the use of parenteral solutions the nurse must understand two important concepts: (1) the rationale for the physician's order of I.V. therapy and (2) the type of solution ordered, together with the composition and clinical use of that solution. Objectives or rationales for administration of I.V. therapy fall into three broad categories:

1. Maintenance therapy for daily body fluid requirements
2. Replacement therapy for present losses
3. Restoration therapy for concurrent or continuing losses.

These three objectives differ with regard to the time necessary to complete the therapy, the purpose of the I.V. fluid, and the type of patient who is to receive the I.V. solution. Factors affecting the choice of objective in prescribing parenteral fluid and the rate of administration by the physician are the patient's renal function, daily maintenance requirements, existing fluid and electrolyte imbalance, clinical status, and disturbances in homeostasis as a result of parenteral therapy (Metheny, 2000).

Maintenance Therapy

Water has the priority in maintenance therapy. The body needs water to replace insensible loss, which can occur as perspiration from the skin and moisture from respirations. The average adult loses 500 to 1000 mL of water over 24 hours through insensible loss. Water is also an important dilutor for waste products excreted by the kidneys. Approximately 30 mL of fluid is needed per kilogram of body weight (i.e., 15 mL/kg) for maintenance needs (Metheny, 2000). In addition, an individual's fluid requirements are based on age, height, weight, and amount of body fat.

Maintenance therapy provides nutrients that meet the daily needs of a patient for water, electrolytes, and dextrose. Water has priority. The typical patient profile for maintenance therapy is an individual who is allowed nothing by mouth (NPO) or whose oral intake is restricted for any reason. Remember that insensible loss is approximately 500 to 1000 mL every 24 hours. Maintenance therapy should be 1500 mL per square meter (m^2) of body surface over 24 hours (Metheny, 2000). For example, a man weighing 85 kg (187 lb) has a body surface area of 2 (m^2); 1500 times 2 equal 3000; therefore, he needs 3000 mL of fluids for maintenance therapy.

Balanced solutions for maintenance therapy include water, daily needs of sodium and potassium, and glucose. Glucose, a necessary component in maintenance therapy, is converted to glycogen by the liver. It has four main uses in parenteral therapy:

1. Improves hepatic function.
2. Supplies necessary calories for energy.
3. Spares body protein.
4. Minimizes ketosis.

NURSING FAST FACT!

The basic caloric requirement for an adult is 1600 calories/day for a 70-kg adult at rest. Approximately 100 to 150 g of carbohydrates are needed daily to minimize protein catabolism and prevent starvation. One liter of 5 percent dextrose in water contains 50 g of dextrose (Metheny, 2000).

Hospitalized patients receiving additional saline or glucose infusions are prone to developing potassium deficiency. In addition, hospitalized patients are usually under physiologic stress. Excretion of potassium in their urine can increase to 60 to 120 mEq/day even with limited intake. Tissue injury significantly increases the loss of potassium. Normal dietary intake of potassium is 80 to 200 mEq/day.

Vitamins are necessary for utilization of other nutrients. Vitamin C and vitamin B complex are used frequently in parenteral therapy, especially for postoperative patients. Vitamin C promotes wound healing, and vitamin B complex has a role in metabolism of carbohydrates and maintenance of gastrointestinal (GI) function (Weinstein, 1997).

Replacement Therapy

Replacement therapy is necessary to take care of the fluid, electrolyte, or blood product deficits of patients in acute distress; this type of therapy is supplied over a 48-hour period. Examples of conditions of patients needing replacement infusion therapy (and their replacement requirements) are:

- Hemorrhage (for replacement of cells and plasma)
- Low platelet count (for replacement of clotting factors)
- Vomiting and diarrhea (for replacement of losses of electrolytes and water)
- Starvation (for replacement of losses of water and electrolytes)

When the maintenance of body requirements cannot be met, the physician should institute replacement therapy. The physician must figure the losses and calculate replacement over a 48-hour period. Kidney function is the first thing that should be checked before replacement therapy is begun. Patients requiring replacement therapy, except those in shock, require potassium. Patients under stress from tissue injury, wound infection, or gastric or bowel surgery also require potassium. Adequate replacement is achieved using 20 mEq/L of potassium (Metheny, 2000).

NURSING FAST FACT!

Never give more than 120 mEq of potassium in a 24–hour period unless cardiac status is monitored continuously, because it can create a life-threatening situation.

Carefully monitor balanced solutions with potassium for the following patients:

1. Those with dysfunction of the:
   - Renal system
   - Cardiovascular system
   - Adrenal glands
   - Pituitary gland
   - Parathyroid gland
2. Those with deficits of:
   - Sodium
   - Calcium
   - Base bicarbonate
   - Blood volume (hypovolemic)
3. Those with excess of:
   - Base bicarbonate
   - Extracellular potassium
   - Extracellular calcium

NURSING FAST FACT!

Key nursing assessment: Check kidney function before administering potassium in replacement therapy.

Restoration Therapy

Restoration therapy for concurrent losses is achieved on an ongoing daily basis. Critical evaluation of concurrent losses of fluid and electrolyte therapy is done at least every 24 hours. Accurate documentation of intake and output is extremely important in this type of management of fluid and electrolyte therapy. Restoration of homeostasis depends on the nursing assessment of intake of I.V. fluids as well as on the documentation of all body fluid losses. The types of clinical patients who require 24-hour evaluation are those with draining fistulas, abscesses, nasogastric tubes, burns, and abdominal wounds.

The fluid and electrolyte management of these patients cannot be completed in 48 hours. Therefore, maintenance therapy and replacement therapy do not meet these patients' needs. A day-by-day restoration of vital fluids and electrolytes is necessary. With these types of patients, you will see frequent changes in the types of solutions ordered, in the amounts of electrolytes ordered based on laboratory values ordered, and in the rate of infusion.

The type of restoration fluid ordered depends on the type of fluid that is being lost. For example, excessive loss of gastric fluid must be replaced by solutions resembling that fluid; with nasogastric suctioning, chloride, potassium, and sodium are lost continually. Restoration of electrolyte imbalance is imperative for proper homeostatic management therapy. Rather than waiting to make daily rounds to evaluate the 24-hour totals and change infusion orders, physicians are ordering multiple electrolyte solutions to be used as a replacement solution through the main infusion system on an ongoing basis. This replacement need is reevaluated every 1 to 8 hours. Table 5–1 presents an example of how restoration fluids are ordered and administered. Restoration of fluids and electrolytes is challenging for nurses. One must be on time and accurate so as not to overload.

Key Elements in Parenteral Solutions

The key elements that make up parenteral fluids include water, carbohydrates (glucose), protein, vitamins, electrolytes, and pH.

> Table 5–1 **ADMINISTRATION OF RESTORATION FLUIDS**

The physician orders 1000 mL of 5% dextrose/0.45% sodium chloride every 8 hours as a primary solution. A multiple electrolyte solution, such as lactated Ringer's solution, is ordered in addition to the primary solution to replace nasogastric output milliliter for milliliter over 4 hours. The primary I.V. solution is continuously infused at 125 mL/h. If the nasogastric suction container is emptied of 400 mL of gastric secretions, the nurse will need to infuse 400 mL of lactated Ringer's solution over the next 4 hours, or 100 mL/h. (See sample schedule below.) The primary solution (5% dextrose/0.5% sodium chloride) will infuse at 125 mL, and the lactated Ringer's solution will infuse at 100 mL/h for a total of 225 mL/h. The nurse will then empty the nasogastric suction container 4 hours later and recalculate the replacement solution.

Time	8 AM	9 AM	10 AM	11 AM	12 noon	1 PM
Gastric suction, mL	400				300	
Primary fluids, mL	125	125	125	125	125	125
Restoration fluids (lactated Ringer's solution), mL	100	100	100	100	75	75
Total, mL	225	225	225	250	200	200

Water

Normal daily maintenance requirements for water in an adult are roughly 1000 mL/day. These water needs are increased in patients with sensible water losses such as respiratory rate above 20, fever, and diaphoresis, as well as in low–humidity environments; in patients with decreased renal concentration ability; and in elderly people. The average adult loses 500 to 1000 mL in the form of insensible water every 24 hours. Water must be provided for adequate kidney function.

NURSING FAST FACT!

High humidity, such as that in an incubator, minimizes insensible water loss (Metheny, 2000).

Carbohydrates (Glucose)

Glucose, a nutrient included in maintenance, restoration, and replacement therapies, is converted into glycogen by the liver, which improves hepatic function. By supplying calories for energy, it spares body protein. Sources of carbohydrates include dextrose (glucose) and fructose. When glucose is supplied by infusion, all the parenteral glucose is bioavailable.

The addition of 100 g of glucose per day minimizes starvation. Every 2 L of 5 percent dextrose in water contains 100 g of glucose.

Amino Acids

Amino acids (protein) are the body-building nutrients whose major functions are contributing to tissue growth and repair, replacing body cells, healing wounds, and synthesizing vitamins and enzymes. Amino acids are the basic units of protein. The parenteral proteins currently used are elemental, provided as synthetic crystalline amino acids. These proteins are available in concentrations of 3.5 to 15 percent and are used in total parenteral nutrition (TPN) centrally or peripherally. When administered by infusion, protein bypasses the GI and portal circulation (Metheny, 2000).

The usual daily requirement is 1 g of protein/kg of body weight. For example, a 54-kg woman needs 54 g of protein per day.

Vitamins

Vitamins are added to restorative and replacement therapies. Certain vitamins (i.e., the fat-soluble A, D, E, and K and water-soluble B and C vitamins) are necessary for growth and act as catalysts for metabolic processes. Some disease conditions alter vitamin requirements (Metheny, 2000). Vitamins B and C are the most frequently used in parenteral therapy. Vitamin B complex is important in the metabolism of carbohydrates and the maintenance of GI function, which is especially important in postoperative patients. Vitamin C promotes wound healing.

Electrolytes

Electrolytes are the major additives to replacement and restorative therapies. Correction of electrolyte imbalances is important in the prevention of serious complications associated with excess or deficit of electrolytes. There are seven major electrolytes in normal body fluids and the same seven major elements are supplied in manufactured I.V. solutions. (Chapter 4 reviews these electrolyte functions.) The electrolytes of major importance in parenteral therapy are potassium, sodium, chloride, magnesium, phosphorus, calcium, and bicarbonate or acetate ion (important for acid–base balance).

pH

The pH reflects the degree of acidity or alkalinity of a solution. Blood pH is not a significant problem for routine parenteral therapy. Normal kidneys can achieve an acid–base balance as long as enough water is supplied. The USP standards require that solution pH must be slightly acidic (a pH of between 3.5 and 6.2). Many solutions have a pH of 5. The acidity of solutions allows them to have a longer shelf life.

NURSING FAST FACT!

As the acidity of a solution increases, the solution's ability to irritate vein walls increases.

Osmolarity of Parenteral Solutions

The tonicity (osmolarity) of intravenous solutions refers to the effect of the concentration or osmotic pressure of dissolved particles in the solution. The concentration of dissolved particles directly determines the direction of the fluid shift between the extracellular and intracellular compartments. Administration of intravenous fluids is guided by the tonicity of the solution and falls into three categories: isotonic or isosmolar, hypotonic, and hypertonic (Kraft, 2000). The effect of I.V. fluid on the body fluid compartments depends on how its osmolarity compares with the patient's serum osmolarity. Intravenous fluids can change the fluid compartment in one of three ways:

1. Expand the intravascular compartment
2. Expand the intravascular compartment and deplete the intracellular and interstitial compartments
3. Expand the intracellular compartment and deplete the intravascular compartment

NOTE > Review Chapter 3 for further information on osmolarity and diagrams of fluid shifts.

Isotonic or Isomolar Fluids

Isotonic solutions have an osmolarity of 250 to 375 mOsm/L. Blood and normal body fluids have an osmolarity of 285 to 295 mOsm/kg. These fluids are used to expand the extracellular fluid (ECF) compartment. No net fluid shifts occur between isotonic solutions because the osmotic pressure gradient is the same inside and outside the cells. Many isotonic solutions are available. Examples include 0.9 percent sodium chloride, 5 percent dextrose in water, and lactated Ringer's solution.

Isotonic solutions are commonly used to treat fluid loss, dehydration, and hypernatremia (sodium excess). Five percent dextrose solution is used for dehydration because it replaces fluid volume without disrupting the interstitial and intracellular environment. However, this solution becomes hypotonic when dextrose is metabolized; the solution should be used cautiously in patients with renal and cardiac disease because of the increased risk of fluid overload (Kraft, 2000). This solution also does not provide enough daily calories and can lead to protein breakdown if used for extended periods of time.

Hypotonic Fluids

Hypotonic fluids have an osmolarity lower than 250 mOsm/L. By lowering serum osmolarity, the body fluids shift out of blood vessels into cells and interstitial spaces. The resulting osmotic pressure gradient draws water into the cells from the ECF, causing the cells to swell. Hypotonic solutions are used for patients who have hypertonic dehydration, water replacement, and diabetic ketoacidosis after initial sodium chloride replacement (Kraft, 2000). Examples of hypotonic solutions include 0.45 percent sodium chloride (half-strength saline), 0.33 percent sodium chloride, and 2.5 percent dextrose in water.

Hypotonic solutions hydrate cells and can deplete the circulatory system. Water moves from the vascular space to the intracellular space when hypotonic fluids are infused.

Hypertonic Fluids

Hypertonic fluids have an osmolarity of 375 mOsm/L or higher. The resulting osmotic pressure gradient draws water from the intracellular space increasing extracellular volume and causing cells to shrink. Examples of hypertonic fluids include 5 percent dextrose in 0.45 percent sodium chloride, 5 percent dextrose in 0.9 percent sodium chloride, 5 percent dextrose in lactated Ringer's, 10 percent dextrose in water, and colloids (albumin 25 percent, plasma protein fraction, dextran, and hetastarch).

These fluids are used to replace electrolytes, to treat hypotonic dehydration, and in temporary treatment of circulatory insufficiency and shock. When hypertonic dextrose solutions are used alone, they also are used to shift ECF from the interstitial fluid to the plasma.

NURSING FAST FACTS!

Caution: *The danger with the use of isotonic solutions is circulatory overload. These solutions do not cause fluid shifts into other compartments. The problem with overexpanding the vascular compartment is that the fluid dilutes the concentration of hemoglobin and lowers hematocrit levels.*

Caution: *Hypertonic solutions are irritating to vein walls and may cause hypertonic circulatory overload. Some hypertonic solutions are contraindicated in patients with cardiac or renal disease because of the increased risk of congestive heart failure and pulmonary edema.*

Do not give hypotonic solutions to patients with low blood pressure because it will further a hypotensive state.

Give hypertonic solutions slowly to prevent circulatory overload.

Types of Parenteral Solutions

Crystalloid Solutions

Crystalloids are materials capable of crystallization (i.e., have the ability to form crystals). Crystalloids are solutes that, when placed in a solution, mix with and dissolve into a solution and cannot be distinguished from the resultant solution. Because of this, crystalloid solutions are considered true solutions that are capable of diffusing through membranes. The vascular fluid is 25 percent of the ECF, and 25 percent of any crystalloid administered remains in the vascular space. Crystalloids must be given in three to four times the volume to expand the vascular space to a degree equal to that brought about by a **colloid** solution. Types of crystalloid solutions include dextrose solutions, sodium chloride solutions, multiple electrolyte solutions, and alkalizing and acidifying solutions.

Dextrose Solutions

Carbohydrates can be administered by the parenteral route as dextrose, fructose, or invert sugar. Dextrose is the most commonly administered carbohydrate. The percentage solutions express the number of grams of solute per 100 g of solvent. Thus a 5 percent dextrose in water (D5W) infusion contains 5 g of dextrose in 100 mL of water.

NURSING FAST FACTS!

One milliliter of water weighs 1 g, and 1 mL is 1 percent of 100 mL. Milliliters, grams, and percentages can be used interchangeably when calculating solution strength. Thus, 5 percent dextrose in water equals 5 g of dextrose in 100 mL, and 1 L of 5 percent dextrose in water contains 50 g of dextrose. (Example: 250 mL of 20 percent dextrose in water solution contains 50 g of dextrose.)

Hypotonic dextrose solutions hydrate the intracellular compartment more than they hydrate the intravascular space.

An adult at bed rest needs approximately 1600 calories daily; this is a basal figure and does not allow for fever or other causes of increased metabolism (Metheny, 2000). When carbohydrate needs are inadequate, the body will use its own fat to supply calories. Dextrose fluids are used to provide calories for energy, reduce catabolism of protein, and reduce protein breakdown of glucose to help prevent a negative nitrogen balance.

The monohydrate form of dextrose used in parenteral solutions provides 3.4 kcal/g. It is difficult to administer enough calories by I.V. infusion, especially with 5 percent dextrose in water, which provides only

170 calories per liter. One would have to administer 9 L to meet calorie requirements, and most patients cannot tolerate 9000 mL of fluid in 24 hours. Concentrated solutions of carbohydrates in 20 to 70 percent dextrose are useful for supplying calories. These solutions containing high percentages of dextrose must be administered slowly for adequate absorption and utilization by the cells (Metheny, 2000).

Dextrose is a nonelectrolyte, and the total number of particles in a dextrose solution does not depend on ionization. Dextrose is thought to be the closest to the ideal carbohydrate available because it is well metabolized by all tissues. The tonicity of dextrose solutions depends on the particles of sugar in the solution. Dextrose 5 percent is rapidly metabolized and has no osmotically active particles after it is in the plasma. The osmolarity of a dextrose solution is determined differently from that of an electrolyte solution. Dextrose is distributed inside and outside the cells, with 8 percent remaining in the circulation to increase blood volume. The USP pH requirements for dextrose are 3.5 to 6.5 (Metheny, 2000).

Dextrose in water is available in various concentrations including 2.5, 5, 10, 20, 30, 40, 50, and 70 percent. Dextrose is also available in combination with other types of solutions. The 5 percent and 10 percent concentrations can be given peripherally. Concentrations higher than 10 percent are given through central veins. A general exception is the administration of limited amounts of 50 percent dextrose given slowly through a peripheral vein for emergency treatment of hypoglycemia (usually 3 mL/min) (Deglin & Vallerand, 2002).

The other two types of carbohydrates used for infusions, fructose and invert sugar, have their own specific uses. Fructose is similar to glucose but is less irritating to veins. The important point about fructose is that it can be metabolized by adipose tissue independent of insulin. However, fructose cannot be used if the patient is in acidosis. Invert sugar contains the same equimolar quantities of glucose and fructose, but less invert sugar is lost in the urine (Metheny, 2000).

ADVANTAGES

- Acts as a vehicle for administration of medications.
- Provides nutrition.
- Can be used as treatment for hyperkalemia (using high concentrations of dextrose).
- Can be used in treatment of patients with dehydration.
- Provides free water.

DISADVANTAGES

The main disadvantage of dextrose solutions intravenously is vein irritation, which is caused by the slightly acidic pH of the solution. Vein irritation, vein damage, and thrombosis may result when hypertonic dextrose solutions are administered in a peripheral vein (Hankin & Hedrick, 2001).

If solutions of 20 to 70 percent dextrose are infused rapidly, they act as an osmotic diuretic and pull interstitial fluid into plasma, causing severe cellular **dehydration.** Any solution of dextrose infused rapidly can place the patient at risk for dehydration. To prevent this adverse reaction, infuse the dextrose solution at the prescribed rate.

If 20 to 70 percent dextrose is infused too rapidly, it can irritate the vein wall. Rapid infusion of 20 to 70 percent dextrose can also lead to transient hyperinsulin reaction, in which the pancreas secretes extra insulin to metabolize the infused dextrose. Sudden discontinuation of any hypertonic dextrose solution may leave a temporary excess of insulin.

To prevent hyperinsulinism, infuse an isotonic dextrose solution (5 to 10 percent) to wean the patient off hypertonic dextrose. The infusion rate should be gradually decreased over 48 hours. When administering dextrose solutions, remember that they do not provide any electrolytes. Dextrose solutions cannot replace or correct electrolyte deficits, and continuous infusion of 5 percent dextrose in water places patients at risk for deficits in sodium, potassium, and chloride. In addition, dextrose cannot be mixed with blood components because it causes hemolysis (i.e., agglomeration) of the cells.

Before any medication is added to a dextrose solution, compatibility information should be checked. Dextrose may also affect the stability of admixtures (e.g., ampicillin sodium) (Hankins & Hedrick, 2001).

NURSING FAST FACTS!

Do not play "catch up" if the solution infusion is behind schedule. Make sure the I.V. solution does not "run away" and that it does not infuse rapidly into the patient.

All dextrose solutions are acidic (pH 3.5 to 5.0) and may cause thrombophlebitis. Assess the I.V. site frequently.

Table 5–2 presents the types and contents of available dextrose solutions.

Sodium Chloride Solutions

Sodium chloride solutions are available in 0.25, 0.45, 0.9, 3, and 5 percent concentrations. Sodium chloride 0.9 percent solution, often referred to as normal saline, has 154 mEq of both sodium and chloride, or about 9 percent higher than normal plasma levels of sodium and chloride ions without other plasma electrolytes. The term *normal saline* is therefore misleading.

There are many clinical uses of sodium chloride solutions, including treatment of shock, hyponatremia, use with blood transfusions, resuscitation in trauma situations, fluid challenges, metabolic alkalosis hypercalcemia, and fluid replacement in diabetic ketoacidosis, to list a few.

> Table 5–2 **CONTENTS OF AVAILABLE INTRAVENOUS FLUIDS**

Solution	Osmolarity	Dex-trose, g/100 mL	pH	Cal/ 100 mL	Na	Cl	K	Ca	Mg	Acetate	Lactate
				Dextrose in Water (D/W)							
2.5% D/W	Hypotonic	2.5	4.5	8							
5% D/W	Isotonic	5	4.8	17							
10% D/W	Hypertonic	10	4.7	34							
20% D/W	Hypertonic	20	4.8	68							
50% D/W	Hypertonic	50	4.6	170							
70% D/W	Hypertonic	70	4.6	237							
				Sodium Chloride (NaCl)							
0.2% NaCl (1/4 strength)	Hypotonic		4.5		34	34					
0.45% NaCl (1/2 strength)	Hypotonic		5.6		77	77					
0.9% NaCl (full strength)	Isotonic		6.0		154	154					
3% NaCl	Hypertonic		6.0		513	513					
5% NaCl	Hypertonic		6.0		855	855					
				Dextrose and Sodium Chloride (D/NaCl)							
0.2% D and 0.9% NaCl	Isotonic	2.5	4.5	8	154	154					
5% D and 0.2% NaCl	Isotonic	5	4.6	17	34	34					
5% D and 0.45 NaCl	Hypertonic	5	4.6	17	77	77					
5% D and 0.9% NaCl	Hypertonic	5	4.4	17	154	154					
				Multiple Electrolyte Solutions							
Lactated Ringer's solution	Isotonic	6.5			130	109	4	3			28
Ringer's injection	Isotonic	5.5			147	156	4	4			
Normosol-R	Isotonic	6.4		18	140	98	5		3	27	
Plasmalyte-A	Isotonic	5.5			140	98	5		3	27	
Isolyte E	Isotonic	6.0			140	103	10		3	49	
				Speciality Solutions							
1/6 *M* sodium lactate	Isotonic (335)	6.5			167						167
10% Mannitol	Hypertonic	5.7									
20% Mannitol	Hypertonic	5.7									

(Continued on following page)

Solution	Osmolarity	Dextrose, g/100 mL	pH	Cal/100 mL	Na	Cl	K	Ca	Mg	Acetate	Lactate
$NaHCO_3$	Isotonic (333)	8.0			595						595
6% Dextran and 0.9% NaCl	Isotonic	5.0			154	154					
10% Dextran and 0.9% NaCl	Isotonic	5.0			154	154					

Ca = Calcium; Cal = calories; Cl = chloride; K = potassium; Mg = magnesium; Na = sodium.

Sodium chloride solutions should be used cautiously in patients with congestive heart failure, edema, or hypernatremia because it replaces ECF and can lead to fluid overload.

Table 5–2 presents the types and content of available sodium chloride solutions.

ADVANTAGES

- Provides ECF replacement when chloride loss is greater than or equal to sodium losses (e.g., a patient undergoing nasogastric suctioning).
- Treats patients with metabolic alkalosis in the presence of fluid loss (the 154 mEq of chloride helps compensate for the increase in bicarbonate ions).
- Treats patients with sodium depletion.
- Initiates or terminates a blood transfusion (the saline solutions are the only solutions to be used with any blood product).

DISADVANTAGES

- Provides more sodium and chloride than patients need, causing hypernatremia. The adult dietary sodium requirements are 90 to 250 mEq daily. Three liters of sodium chloride (0.9 percent) provides a patient with 462 mEq of sodium, a level that exceeds normal tolerance. To prevent this overload of electrolytes, assess for signs and symptoms of sodium retention.
- Can cause acidosis in patients receiving continuous infusions of 0.9 percent sodium chloride because sodium chloride provides one third more chloride than is present in ECF. The excess chloride leads to loss of bicarbonate ions, leading to an imbalance of acid.
- May cause low potassium levels (i.e., hypokalemia) because of the lack of the other important electrolytes over a period of time.
- Can lead to circulatory overload. Isotonic fluids expand the ECF compartment, which can lead to overload of the cardiovascular compartments.

NURSING FAST FACT!

During stress, the body retains sodium, adding to hypernatremia.

Hypotonic saline (0.45 percent) can be used to supply normal daily salt and water requirements safely. Hypertonic saline solution (3 to 5 percent) is used only to correct severe sodium depletion and water overload.

Hyperosmolar saline (3 or 5 percent NaCl) can be dangerous when administered incorrectly.

Nurses should follow these steps to ensure safe administration of hyperosmolar saline:

- Check serum sodium level before and during administration.
- Administer only in intensive care settings.
- Monitor aggressively for signs of pulmonary edema.
- Only small volumes of hyperosmolar fluids are usually administered.
- Use a volume-controlled device or electronic infusion pump (NSNA, 1997).

AGE-RELATED CONSIDERATIONS 5–1

Be aware of the increased dangers of administering saline solutions to elderly patients, patients with severe dehydration, and patients with chronic glomerulonephritis.

Dextrose Combined with Sodium Chloride

When sodium chloride is infused, the addition of 100 g dextrose prevents formation of ketone bodies. Dextrose prevents **catabolism,** which is the breakdown of chemical compounds by the body. Consequently, there is a loss of potassium and intracellular water.

Carbohydrates and sodium chloride fluid combinations are best used when there has been an excessive loss of fluid through sweating, vomiting, or gastric suctioning (Kuhn, 1999). See Table 5–2 for types of available dextrose and sodium chloride solutions.

ADVANTAGES

- Temporarily treats patients with circulatory insufficiency and shock caused by hypovolemia in the immediate absence of a plasma expander.
- Provides early treatment of burns, along with plasma or albumin.
- Replaces nutrients and electrolytes.
- Acts as a **hydrating solution** to assist in checking kidney function before replacement of potassium.

DISADVANTAGE

- Same as for sodium chloride solutions (see earlier section): hypernatremia, acidosis, and circulatory overload.

Hydrating Solutions (Combinations of Dextrose and Hypotonic Sodium Chloride)

Solutions that contain dextrose and hypotonic saline provide more water than is required for excretion of salt and are useful as hydrating fluids. Hydrating fluids are used to assess the status of the kidneys. The administration of a hydrating solution at a rate of 8 mL/m^2 of body surface per minute for 45 minutes is called a fluid challenge. When urinary flow is established, it indicates that the kidneys have begun to function; the hydrating solution may then be replaced with a specific electrolyte solution. If the urinary flow is not restored after 45 minutes, the rate of infusion should be reduced and monitoring of the patient should continue without administration of electrolyte additives, especially potassium (Metheny, 2000). Carbohydrates in hydrating solutions reduce the depletion of nitrogen and liver glycogen and are also useful in rehydrating cells.

Hydrating solutions are potassium free. Potassium is essential to the body but can be toxic if the kidneys are not functioning effectively and are therefore unable to excrete the extra potassium (Kuhn, 1999). See Table 5–2 for types of hydrating fluids.

ADVANTAGES

- Help assess the status of the kidneys before replacement therapy is started.
- Hydrate patients in dehydrated states.
- Promote diuresis in dehydrated patients.

DISADVANTAGE

- Require cautious administration in edematous patients (e.g., patients with cardiac, renal, or liver disease).

NURSING FAST FACT!

Do not give potassium to any patient unless kidney function has been established. Use hydrating fluid to check kidney function.

Multiple Electrolyte Fluids

A variety of balanced electrolyte fluids are available commercially. Balanced fluids are available as hypotonic or isotonic maintenance and replacement solutions. Maintenance fluids approximate normal body electrolyte needs; replacement fluids contain one or more electrolytes in amounts higher than those found in normal body fluids. Balanced fluids also may contain lactate or acetate (yielding bicarbonate), which helps to combat acidosis and provide a truly "balanced solution." See Table 5–2 for types of multiple electrolyte solution.

NURSING FAST FACTS!

Multiple electrolyte fluids are recommended for use in patients with trauma, alimentary tract fluid losses, dehydration, sodium depletion, acidosis, and burns.

Do not use gastric replacement fluid in patients with hepatic insufficiency or renal failure.

Many types of multiple electrolyte replacement fluids are available. Special fluids are available from each manufacturer for gastric replacement, which provide the typical electrolytes lost by vomiting or gastric suction. These isotonic fluids usually contain ammonium ions, which are metabolized in the liver to hydrogen ions and urea, replacing hydrogen ions lost in gastric juices. Lactated Ringer's injection is considered an isotonic multiple electrolyte solution.

Hypertonic multiple electrolyte solutions are also used as replacement fluids. Usually 5 percent dextrose has been added to them, which raises the osmolarity of the solution.

Ringer's Solution and Lactated Ringer's

The Ringer's solutions (i.e., Ringer's injection and lactated Ringer's injection) are classified as balanced or isotonic solutions because their fluid and electrolyte contents are similar to those of plasma. They are used to replace electrolytes at physiologic levels in the ECF compartment.

RINGER'S SOLUTION (INJECTION)

Ringer's injection is a fluid and electrolyte replenisher, which is used rather than 0.9 percent sodium chloride for treating patients with dehydration after reduced water intake or water loss. Ringer's solution (injection) is similar to **normal saline** (i.e., 0.9 percent sodium chloride) with the substitution of potassium and calcium for some of the sodium ions in concentrations equal to those in the plasma. Ringer's injection, however, is superior to 0.9 percent sodium chloride as a fluid and electrolyte replenisher and it is preferred to normal saline for treating patients with dehydration after drastically reduced water intake or water loss (e.g., with vomiting, diarrhea, or fistula drainage). This solution has some incompatibilities with medications, so it is necessary to check drug compatibility literature for guidelines.

NURSING FAST FACT!

Ringer's injection does not contain enough potassium or calcium to be used as a maintenance fluid or to correct a deficit of these electrolytes.

Ringer's injection is used for the following:

- Treatment of any type of dehydration
- Restoration of fluid balance before and after surgery
- Replacement of fluids resulting from dehydration, GI losses, and fistula drainage

Use this solution instead of lactated Ringer's when the patient has liver disease and is unable to metabolize lactate.

ADVANTAGES

- Tolerated well in patients who have liver disease.
- May be used as blood replacement for a short period of time.

DISADVANTAGES

- Provides no calories.
- May exacerbate sodium retention, congestive heart failure, and renal insufficiency.
- Contraindicated in renal failure.

LACTATED RINGER'S SOLUTION

This solution is also called Hartmann's solution. Lactated Ringer's is the most commonly prescribed solution, with an electrolyte concentration closely resembling that of the ECF compartment. This solution is commonly used to replace fluid loss resulting from burns, bile, and diarrhea.

Lactated Ringer's is used for the following:

- Rehydration in all types of dehydration
- Restoration of fluid volume deficits
- Replacement of fluid lost as a result of burns
- Treatment of mild metabolic acidosis
- Treatment of salicylate overdose

NURSING FAST FACT!

Lactated Ringer's solution has some incompatibilities with medications, so it is necessary to check drug compatibility literature for guidelines.

ADVANTAGES

- Contains the bicarbonate precursor to assist in acidosis.
- Most similar to body's extracellular electrolyte content.

DISADVANTAGES

- Three liters of lactated Ringer's solution contains about 390 mEq of sodium, which can quickly elevate the sodium level in a patient who does not have a sodium deficit.
- Lactated Ringer's solution should not be used in patients with impaired lactate metabolism, such as those with liver disease, Addison's disease, severe metabolic acidosis or alkalosis, profound hypovolemia, or profound shock or cardiac failure.
- In the above conditions, serum lactate levels may already be elevated.

Resuscitation of Trauma Patients by Using Crystalloid Solutions

The controversy over the type and method of fluid to be used in resuscitation of the acutely injured patient is well documented. Both crystalloid and colloid fluids are capable of restoring circulating volume (Jordan, 2000).

Crystalloid fluids used for trauma resuscitation include lactated Ringer's solution and 0.9 percent sodium chloride. Crystalloid fluids fill both the interstitial and intravascular spaces. Advantages of crystalloid fluid include cost effectiveness, nonallergenic properties, and reduced viscosity, leading to improved microcirculation (American College of Surgeons Committee, 1998).

NURSING FAST FACT!

At present isotonic sodium chloride is recommended as the first line fluid in resuscitation of hypovolemic trauma patients (Revell, Porter, & Greaves, 2002).

Alkalizing and Acidifying Infusion Fluids

ALKALIZING FLUIDS

Metabolic acidosis can occur in clinical situations in which dehydration, shock, liver disease, starvation, or diabetes causes retention of chlorides, ketone bodies, or organic salts or when too large an amount of bicarbonate is lost. Treatment consists of infusion of an alkalizing fluid. Two I.V. fluids are available when there are excessive bicarbonate losses and metabolic acidosis occurs: 1/6 molar isotonic sodium lactate and 5 percent sodium bicarbonate injection. The lactate ion must be oxidized in the body to carbon dioxide before it can affect the acid–base balance. Sodium lactate to bicarbonate requires 1 to 2 hours. Oxygen is needed to increase bicarbonate concentrations. The isotonic solution sodium bicarbonate injection provides bicarbonate ions in clinical situations in which there are excessive bicarbonate losses.

Alkalizing fluids are used in treating vomiting, starvation, uncontrolled diabetes mellitus, acute infections, renal failure, and severe acidosis with severe hyperpnea (sodium bicarbonate injection).

The 1/6 molar sodium lactate solution is useful whenever acidosis has resulted from sodium deficiency; however, it is contraindicated in patients suffering from lack of oxygen and in those with liver disease. Patients receiving this fluid should be watched for signs of hypocalcemic tetany.

NURSING FAST FACT!

Sodium bicarbonate injection is used to relieve dyspnea and hyperpnea; the bicarbonate ion is released in the form of carbon dioxide through the lungs, leaving behind an excess of sodium.

Acidifying Fluids

Metabolic alkalosis is a condition associated with an excess of bicarbonate and deficit of chloride. Isotonic sodium chloride (0.9 percent) provides conservative treatment of metabolic alkalosis. Ammonium chloride is the solution used to treat metabolic alkalosis. Acidifying fluids are used for severe metabolic alkalosis caused by a loss of gastric secretions or pyloric stenosis.

An advantage is that the ammonium ion is converted by the liver to hydrogen ion and to ammonia, which is excreted as urea. However, a disadvantage is that ammonium chloride must be infused at a slow rate to enable the liver to metabolize the ammonium ion. In fact, rapid infusion can result in toxicity, causing irregular breathing and bradycardia.

NURSING FAST FACT!

Ammonium chloride must be used with caution in patients with severe hepatic disease or renal failure and is contraindicated in any condition in which a high ammonium level is present.

Potassium Chloride Solutions

Several premixed solutions of potassium chloride (KCl) are available from the manufacturer. Potassium 20 or 40 mEq is added to 5 percent dextrose in water or 5 percent dextrose and 0.45 percent sodium chloride. Follow special nursing considerations in administration of I.V. potassium chloride. Chapter 4 provides more information about potassium chloride, including the critical guidelines for the administration of potassium chloride fluids.

NURSING FAST FACT!

As packaged from the manufacturer, potassium has a clear red label to distinguish it from I.V. solutions without additives.

Colloid Solutions

Patients with fluid and electrolyte disturbances occasionally require treatment with colloids. Colloid solutions contain protein or starch molecules that remain distributed in the extracellular space and do not form a "true" solution. When colloid molecules are administered, they remain in the vascular space for several days in patients with normal capillary endothelia. These fluids increase the osmotic pressure within the plasma space, drawing fluid to increase intravascular volume.

Colloid solutions do not dissolve and do not flow freely between fluid compartments. Infusion of a colloid solution increases intravascular colloid osmotic pressure (pressure of plasma proteins).

Dextran

Dextran fluids are polysaccharides that behave as colloids. They are available as low molecular weight dextran (dextran 40) and high molecular weight dextran (dextran 70). Dextran 70 is more effective than dextran 40 as a substitute for plasma expansion. It is important to monitor the patient's pulse, blood pressure, and urine output every 5 to 15 minutes for the first hour of administration of dextran and then every hour after that. Dextran should be administered at a rate of 20 mL/kg of body weight over 24 hours to prevent hypersensitivity reactions and decrease the risk of bleeding (Phillips & Kuhn, 1999).

Dextran fluids are used for **plasma substitution** or expansion. An advantage of dextran use is that the intravascular space is expanded in excess of the volume infused. Disadvantages are the possibility of hypersensitivity reactions (i.e., anaphylaxis) and an increased risk of bleeding.

NURSING FAST FACT!

Dextran is contraindicated in patients with severe bleeding disorders, congestive heart failure, and renal failure. It is important to draw blood for typing and cross-matching before administering dextran.

Albumin

Albumin is a natural plasma protein prepared from donor plasma. This colloid is available as a 5 or a 25 percent solution. Five percent albumin is osmotically and oncotically equivalent to plasma. The 25 percent solution is equivalent to 500 mL of plasma or two units of whole blood (Phillips & Kuhn, 1999).

Albumin is used for maintenance of blood volume, emergency treatment of shock caused by acute blood loss, hypovolemic shock caused by plasma rather than whole blood loss, hypoproteinemic conditions, and treatment of erythroblastosis fetalis (25 percent solution).

- These products are subject to an extended heating period during preparation and therefore do not transmit viral disease.

DISADVANTAGES

- May precipitate allergic reactions (e.g., urticaria, flushing, chills, fever, or headache).
- May cause circulatory overload (greatest risk with 25 percent albumin).
- May cause pulmonary edema.
- May alter laboratory findings.

Mannitol

Mannitol is a sugar alcohol substance that is available in concentrations from 5 to 25 percent. It is used to promote diuresis in patients with oliguric acute renal failure, to promote excretion of toxic substances in the body, to reduce excess cerebrospinal fluid (CSF), to reduce intraocular pressure, and to treat intracranial pressure and cerebral edema.

ADVANTAGE

- May reduce excess CSF within 15 minutes.

DISADVANTAGES

- May cause fluid and electrolyte imbalances.
- May cause cell dehydration or fluid overload by drawing fluid from cells into the vascular system.
- Requires cautious use for patients with impaired cardiac or renal system (Hankins & Hedrick, 2001).

Hetastarch

Hetastarch (hydroxyethyl glucose) is a synthetic colloid made from starch. It is available under the name Hespan as a 6 or 10 percent solution, diluted in isotonic sodium chloride in a 500-mL container. These starches are not derived from donor plasma and are therefore less toxic and less expensive. Hetastarch is equal in plasma volume expansion properties to 5 percent human albumin.

ADVANTAGE

- Hetastarch does not interfere with blood typing and crossmatching, as do other colloidal solutions.

DISADVANTAGE

- Possibility of allergic reaction

Hetastarch may alter the coagulation mechanism (i.e., with transient prolongation of the prothrombin, partial thromboplastin, and clotting times). Thus, this solution is contraindicated in patients with severe bleeding disorders, severe congestive heart failure, and anuric renal failure (Terry & Hedrick, 1995).

NURSING FAST FACT!

Use hetastarch cautiously in patients whose conditions predispose them to fluid retention.

Table 5–3 presents a summary of common I.V. fluids.

> Table 5–3 **QUICK-GLANCE CHART OF COMMON I.V. FLUIDS**

Solutions	Indications	Precautions
	Dextrose Solutions	
5% Dextrose 10% Dextrose 20% Dextrose 50% Dextrose 70% Dextrose	Spares body protein. Provides nutrition. Provides calories. Provides free water. Acts as a diluent for I.V. drugs. Treats dehydration. Treats hyperkalemia.	Possible compromise of glucose tolerance by stress, sepsis, hepatic and renal failure, corticosteroids, and diuretics Does not provide any electrolytes. May cause vein irritation, water intoxication, and possible agglomeration. Use cautiously in the early postoperative period to prevent water intoxication; ADH secretions as a stress response to surgery Hypertonic fluids may cause hyperglycemia, osmotic diuresis, hyperosmolar coma, or hyperinsulinism.
	Sodium Chloride (NaCl) Solutions	
0.2% NaCl 0.45% NaCl 0.9% NaCl 3% NaCl 5% NaCl	Replaces ECF and electrolytes. Replaces sodium and chloride. Treats hyperosmolar diabetes. Acts as diluent for I.V. drug administration. Used for initiation and discontinuation of blood products. Replaces severe sodium and chloride deficit. Helps to correct water overload. Acts as an irrigant for intravascular devices.	Hyponatremia (excessive use of 0.25% or 0.45% NaCl); calorie depletion; hypernatremia or hyperchloremia; circulatory overload; deficit of other electrolytes Can induce hyperchloremic acidosis because of a loss of bicarbonate ions. Does not provide free water or calories. Use with caution in older adults.

(Continued on following page)

Solutions	Indications	Precautions
	Combination Dextrose and Sodium Chloride Solutions	
5% Dextrose/ 0.2% NaCl (hydration solution) 5% Dextrose/ 0.45% NaCl (hydration solution) 5% Dextrose/ 0.9% NaCl	Assesses kidney function. Hydrates cells. Promotes diuresis. For temporary treatment of circulatory insufficiency hydrating fluids. Replaces nutrients and electrolytes. Supplies some calories. Reduces nitrogen depletion. Used in place of plasma expanders.	Use with caution in patients with edema and those with cardiac, renal, or liver disease. Do not use in patients in diabetic coma. Do not use in patients who are allergic to corn.
	Multiple Electrolyte Solutions	
A. Maintenance solutions	Provide free water, calories, and electrolytes.	
Plasma-Lyte M (Baxter) (an electrolyte solution and 5% dextrose)	Provides routine maintenance Relieves physiologic stress leading to inappropriate release or ADH.	Water intoxication May cause increased potassium levels.
B. Replacement solutions	Provide calories and electrolytes.	
Plasma-Lyte R (Baxter) injection Plasma-Lyte 148 and 5% dextrose	Provides fluid and electrolyte replacement.	Hypernatremia Fluid overload
5% Dextrose in Ringer's injection	Provides calories. Spares protein. Replaces ECF losses and electrolytes.	Contraindicated in patients with renal failure Use with caution in patients with congestive heart failure Composition similar to plasma Tolerated well in patients with liver disease
5% Dextrose and lactated Ringer's solutions	Treats mild metabolic acidosis. Replaces fluid losses from burns and trauma. Replaces fluid losses from alimentary tract. Rehydrates in all types of dehydration.	Contraindicated in patients with lactic acidosis Circulatory overload May cause metabolic acidosis. Ionic composition similar to plasma Contains bicarbonate precursor
	Specialty Fluids	
A. Alkalizing	Treats metabolic acidosis. Relieves dyspnea and hyperpnea.	
Sodium bicarbonate 1/6 Molar sodium lactate	Corrects metabolic acidosis. Reduces severe hyperkalemia. Treats uncontrolled diabetes mellitus, acute infections, and renal failure.	1/6 Molar contraindicated in patients suffering from the lack of oxygen or in those with liver disease, hypocalcemia (tetany), or hypernatremia

(Continued on following page)

> Table 5–3 **QUICK-GLANCE CHART OF COMMON I.V. FLUIDS** *(Continued)*

Solutions	Indications	Precautions
B. Plasma expanders		
Dextran 70 (6%) and 0.9% NaCl Dextran 40 (10%) and 0.9% NaCl	Provides plasma expansion. Treats perioperative shock. Counteracts shock or anticipated shock related to trauma, surgery, burns, or hemorrhage. Prevents venous thrombosis and pulmonary embolism during surgery.	Hypersensitivity reactions Increased risk of bleeding Preexisting hypervolemic conditions should be considered (e.g., renal or cardiac disease) Do not add any medications to dextran solutions.
10% Mannitol 20% Mannitol	Reduces intraocular pressure. Decreases intracranial pressure, reducing cerebral edema. Promotes diuresis and excretion of toxic substances. Increases granulocyte yield during leukapheresis.	Hypervolemia Extravasation Skin irritation Tissue necrosis Interferes with laboratory testing Preexisting conditions should be considered with caution owing to possible crystal formation.
5% Albumin 25% Albumin	Restores circulatory dynamics. Counteracts shock or impending shock caused by hypovolemia. Provides protein (for hypoproteinemia). Treats hyperbilirubinemia and erythroblastosis fetalis.	Allergic reactions Circulatory overload Alteration of laboratory tests Extensive heating period during preparation prevents transmission of viral disease.
6% Hetastarch in 0.9% NaCl 10% Hetastarch in 0.9% NaCl	Provides fluid replacement. Restores circulatory dynamics. Provides volume expansion.	May alter coagulation mechanism. Allergic reactions Hypervolemia Do not use with severe bleeding disorder. Does not interfere with blood typing and cross-matching.

NURSING PLAN OF CARE

ADMINISTRATION OF PARENTERAL FLUIDS

Focus Assessment

Subjective

- History of present illness of fluid loss

Objective

- Observe ability to ingest and retain fluids.
- Vital signs

(Continued on following page)

- Weight
- Assess symptoms of fluid disturbance.
- Assess for complications associated with infusion therapy (phlebitis, erratic flow rates, infiltration).

Patient Outcome/Evaluation Criteria

Patient will:

- Demonstrate improved fluid balance as evidenced by urine output of 30 mL/h with normal specific gravity, stable vital signs, moist mucous membranes, good skin turgor, and capillary refill of less than 3 seconds.
- Verbalize understanding of condition and treatment.
- Report to the nurse any complications related to the parenteral infusion (i.e., redness, swelling, or pain at the infusion site; sharp pains running up the arm at the I.V. site; dizziness or headache).

Nursing Diagnoses

- Anxiety (mild, moderate, severe) related to threat to or change in health status; misconceptions regarding therapy
- Altered nutrition less than body requirements related to inability to ingest or digest food or absorb nutrients; inadequate nutrient replacement
- Decreased cardiac output related to reaction to parenteral solution, contamination
- Fluid volume excess related to infusion of I.V. fluid
- Knowledge deficit related to new procedure and maintaining I.V. therapy
- Fluid volume deficit related to deviations affecting intake and absorption of fluids; factors influencing fluid needs (e.g., hypermetabolism state)
- Impaired tissue integrity related to irritating fluids
- Risk for infection related to broken skin or traumatized tissue
- Risk for altered tissue perfusion: cerebral–renal related to fluid volume imbalance.
- Risk for sleep pattern disturbance related to external sensory stimuli (e.g., I.V. fluid and tubing)

Nursing Management

1. Administer I.V. fluids at room temperature.
2. Administer I.V. medications at prescribed rate and monitor for results.
3. Use open containers immediately.
4. Monitor I.V. site during infusion.
5. Monitor for
   a. signs and symptoms of fluid overload
   b. urine output and specific gravity
   c. trending of pertinent laboratory values (electrolytes, PT, PTT, serum amylase)

(Continued on following page)

NURSING PLAN OF CARE

ADMINISTRATION OF PARENTERAL FLUIDS *(Continued)*

6. Monitor for I.V. patency before administering I.V. medications.
7. Replace I.V. cannula and apparatus every 48 to 72 hours.
8. Replace fluid containers at least every 24 hours.
9. Flush I.V. lines between administration of incompatible solutions with sodium chloride
10. Record intake and output.
11. Provide information outlining current I.V. therapy.
12. Maintain standard precautions.

Patient Education

Instruct on reason for therapy (e.g., replacement fluid, vitamins, nutrition, volume replacement).

Instruct to report signs and symptoms of complications (e.g., burning at infusion site, redness, any discomfort).

Explain need for increased oral intake if appropriate.

Teach patient how to follow sodium and fluid restriction if appropriate.

Teach patient to weigh self daily.

Review signs and symptoms of dehydration and overhydration with patient.

Teach patient to change positions slowly if any dizziness or lightheadedness occurs.

Teach to report to the nurse any pain, swelling, leaking, redness, or harness at the I.V. site.

Most infusion therapies in the home are used for delivery of specific treatment such as antibiotics, chemotherapy, total parenteral nutrition, growth hormones, blood products, and hydration therapy.

Home Care Issues

Home care for hydration therapy is used for dehydration and fluid and electrolyte imbalance resulting from:

- Cardiopulmonary disorders
- Fistulas
- Hyperemesis gravidarum
- Intractable diarrhea

(Continued on following page)

- Chemotherapy (before and after)
- Radiation enteritis
- Short bowel syndrome
- Short-term therapy lasts from 1 to 7 days and is usually administered via a peripheral lock or long-term access device.
- Educate patients about the need for therapy, aseptic technique, setup and administration of specific solution, and possible complications.

Key Points

Parenteral Solutions

- Three main objectives of I.V. therapy are to:
  - Maintain daily requirements
  - Replace previous losses
  - Restore concurrent losses
- Solutions have an osmolarity of hypotonic, isotonic, or hypertonic:
  - Hypotonic is 250 mOsm/L or below.
  - Isotonic ranges from 250 to 375 mOsm/L.
  - Hypertonic is above 375 mOsm/L.
- Give hypertonic solutions slowly to prevent circulatory overload.
- As the acidity of the solution increases, irritation to the vein wall increases.
- Do not play "catch-up" with I.V. solutions that are behind schedule; recalculate the infusion.
- Always check compatibility before adding medication to dextrose solutions.
- Do not give potassium solutions to any patient unless kidney function has been established.
- Infusates are categorized as:
  - Crystalloids: Solutions that are considered true solutions and whose solutes, when placed in a solvent, mix, dissolve, and cannot be distinguished from the resultant solutions. Crystalloids are able to move through membranes. Examples are dextrose and sodium chloride solutions and lactated Ringer's solution.
  - Colloids: Substances whose particles, when submerged in a solvent, cannot form a true solution because their molecules cannot dissolve, but remain suspended and distributed in the fluid. Examples are dextran, albumin, mannitol, blood products, and hetastarch.

Critical Thinking: Case Study

Over a 16-hour period of time, a 6-year-old child was inadvertently given 800 mL of 3 percent sodium chloride solution instead of the prescribed 0.45

percent sodium chloride. She developed lethargy, convulsions, and coma before the error was discovered. Despite resuscitative efforts the child died.

Identify the mEq of each electrolyte in the I.V. solutions.

Identify the tonicity of each of the electrolyte solutions.

Refer to Chapter 1 on legal aspects for factors involved in malpractice.

What types of safeguards should be in place for the pediatric patient receiving I.V. fluids?

Media Link: The answers to this case study, along with more critical thinking scenarios, are on the enclosed CD–ROM

Post-Test

1. Match the term in column I with the definition in column II.

Column I	Column II
_____Crystalloid	**a.** Substance that does not dissolve and does not pass through a semi-permeable membrane
_____Hydrating solution	**b.** Ability to restore equilibrium
_____Homeostasis	**c.** Solution of water, carbohydrate, and sodium chloride used to check kidney function
_____Colloid	**d.** Breakdown of chemical compounds by the body's energy, producing metabolic process
_____Catabolism	**e.** A substance that forms a true solution

2. The three objectives of I.V. therapy are:
   - **a.** Maintenance, peristaltic, and replacement therapy
   - **b.** Replacement, expansion, and restoration therapy
   - **c.** Maintenance, replacement, and restoration therapy
   - **d.** Restoration, hydration, and dehydration therapy
3. The functions of glucose in parenteral therapy include all of the following **EXCEPT:**
   - **a.** Provides calories for energy.
   - **b.** Helps to prevent negative nitrogen balance.
   - **c.** Reduces catabolism of protein.
   - **d.** Serves as vehicle for blood transfusions.
4. Maintenance solutions are used for patients who are:
   - **a.** Ingesting nothing by mouth for a short period of time
   - **b.** Experiencing hemorrhage

c. Dehydrated from GI losses

d. Experiencing draining fistulas

5. What is the most commonly used multiple electrolyte solution?

   a. 5 Percent dextrose in water

   b. 0.9 Percent sodium chloride

   c. Lactated Ringer's solution

   d. 5 Percent dextrose and sodium chloride

6. What is the most common complication of dextran administration?

   a. Fluid overload

   b. Hypersensitivity reactions

   c. Hyponatremia

   d. Hyperkalemia

7. What is the purpose of a colloid solution?

   a. To expand the interstitial compartment

   b. To replace electrolytes

   c. To expand the intravascular compartment

   d. To correct acidosis

8. Dextrose and hypotonic sodium chloride solutions are considered hydrating fluids because:

   a. They provide more water than is required for excretion of sodium.

   b. The water they provide equals that needed for excretion of sodium.

   c. They maximize retention of potassium in the cell.

   d. They maximize the retention of sodium.

9. The expected outcome of administering a hypertonic solution is to:

   a. Shift ECF from intracellular space to plasma

   b. Hydrate cells

   c. Supply free water to vascular space

10. Which of the following solutions are used to prime the administration set when blood is to be administered?

    a. 5 Percent dextrose in water

    b. Lactated Ringer's

    c. 0.9 Percent sodium chloride

    d. 5 Percent dextrose and 0.45 percent sodium chloride

Media Link: Additional practice questions are located on the enclosed CD–ROM.

References

American College of Surgeons (1998). *Committee on Trauma: Advanced Trauma Life Support.* Chicago: American College of Surgeons.

Deglin, J.H., & Vallerand, A.H. (2005). *Davis's Drug Guide for Nurses* (9th ed.). Philadelphia: F.A. Davis.

Hankins, J., & Hedrick, C. (2001). Parenteral fluids. In Hankins, J., Lonsway, R.A., Hedrick, C., & Perdue, M. (eds.). *Intravenous Therapy: Clinical Principles and Practices* (2nd ed.). Philadelphia: W.B. Saunders, pp. 141–164.

Jordan, K.S. (2000). Fluid resuscitation in acutely injured patients. *Journal of Intravenous Nursing*, 23(2), 81–87.

Kee, J.L., & Paulanka, B.J. (2000). *Fluids and Electrolytes with Clinical Applications: A Programmed Approach* (6th ed.). Albany NY: Delmar.

Kraft, P.A. (2000). The osmotic shift. *Journal of Intravenous Nursing*, 23(4), 220–224.

Kuhn, M. (1999). *Pharmacotherapeutics: A Nursing Process Approach* (4th ed.). Philadelphia: F.A. Davis, pp. 173–193.

Metheny, N.M. (2000). Fluid and electrolyte balance. In Metheny, N.M. (ed.). *Nursing Considerations* (4th ed.). Philadelphia: Lippincott-Williams & Wilkins, pp. 169–171.

National Student Nurses Association (1997). Specific electrolyte imbalances. In McEntee, M.A. & Gill, G.M. (eds.). *Fluids and Electrolytes.* Albany, NY: Delmar, pp. 36–70.

Phillips, L.D., & Kuhn, M. (1999). *Manual of I.V. Drugs* (2nd ed.). Philadelphia: J.B. Lippincott.

Revell, M., Porter, K., & Greaves, I. (2002). Fluid resuscitation in prehospital trauma care: A consensus view. *Emergency Medicine Journal*, 19(6), 494–499.

Answers to Chapter 5 Post-Test

1. **e, c, b, a, d**
2. **c**
3. **d**
4. **a**
5. **c**
6. **a**
7. **c**
8. **b**
9. **a**
10. **c**

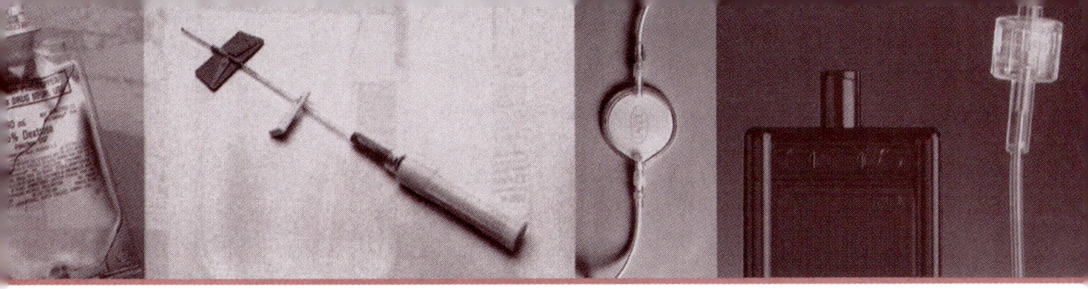

Chapter 6
Equipment

All rituals and ceremonials which our modern worship of efficiency may devise, and all our elaborate scientific equipment will not save us if the intellectual and spiritual elements in our art are subordinated to the mechanical, and if the means come to be regarded as more important than ends.

—Isabel M. Stewart, 1929

Chapter Contents

LEARNING OBJECTIVES

Upon completion of this chapter, the reader will be able to:

1. Define the terminology related to I.V. equipment.
2. Identify the types and characteristics of three infusate containers.
3. Identify the use of vented and nonvented administration sets with the appropriate solution containers.
4. Identify the types and characteristics of peripheral and central infusion devices.
5. State the major advantages and disadvantages associated with over-the-needle catheters and scalp vein needles.
6. Identify the characteristics and uses of electronic infusion devices.
7. Describe the use of filters in the infusion of solutions and blood products.
8. Describe the use of miscellaneous adjuncts to aid in the administration of safe infusions.
9. Identify the Infusion Nurses Society (INS) and the Centers for Disease Control and Prevention (CDC) recommendations for standards of practice related to equipment safety and use.

GLOSSARY

Cannula A tube or sheath used for infusing fluids

Check valve A device that functions to prevent retrograde solution flow; also called a backcheck valve

Coring Visible, as well as microscopic, particles of rubber bung displaced by the spike during piercing of the glass container or needle during access of implanted vascular access devices

Drip chamber Area of the I.V. tubing usually found under the spike where the solution drips and collects before running through the I.V. tubing

Drop factor The number of drops needed to deliver 1 mL of fluid

Filter A special porous device used to prevent the passage of undesired substances

Gauge Size of cannula opening

Hub Female connection point of an I.V. cannula where the tubing or other equipment attaches

Implanted port A catheter surgically placed into a vessel or body cavity and attached to a reservoir; the reservoir is placed under the skin

Infusate I.V. solution

Lumen The space within an artery, vein, or catheter

Macrodrip Drop factor of 10 to 20 drops equivalent to 1 mL based on manufacturer's specifications

Microaggregate Microscopic collection of particles, such as platelets, leukocytes, and fibrin that can exist in stored blood

Microdrip Drop factor of 60 drops/mL

Midclavicular catheter Long (20 to 24 in) I.V. access device made of a soft flexible material inserted into one of the superficial veins of the peripheral vascular system and advanced to proximal axillary or subclavian veins

Midline Peripherally inserted catheter with the tip terminating in the proximal portion of the extremity, usually 6 inches in length

Patient-controlled analgesia (PCA) A drug administration system that allows the patient to self-administer and regulate delivery of medication for pain control on an as-needed basis

Peripherally inserted central catheter (PICC) Long (20 to 24 in) I.V. access device made of a soft flexible material inserted into one of the superficial veins of the peripheral vascular system and advanced to the superior vena cava

Port Point of entry

PRN (pro re na'ta) According to circumstances. Used to describe devices used for intermittent infusions

Psi Pounds per square inch; a measurement of pressure: 1 psi equals 50 mm Hg or 68 cm H_2O

Radiopaque Material used in I.V. catheter that can be identified by radiographic examination

Rubber bung Stopper of glass container composed of numerous substances including rubber, chemical particles, and cellulose fibers

Stylet Needle or guide that is found inside a catheter used for vein penetration

Tunneled catheter A catheter designed to have a portion lie within a subcutaneous passage before exiting the body

Infusion Therapy Equipment

The nurse's role in infusion therapy equipment use includes the decision-making process of equipment acquisition; knowledge of operation of equipment to ensure safe, effective delivery of infusion therapy; and financial accountability. There is a relationship between the industry that manufacturers the equipment, health care providers, and the patient that is collaborative and mutually dependent (Perucca, 2001).

The public holds industry, medical institutions, and professionals accountable for the safe and effective delivery of health care. Medical products and equipment are the collaborative responsibility of industry and medical professionals.

Infusion Delivery Systems

Two infusion systems are available for delivery of I.V. fluids: the glass system and the plastic system (Fig. 6–1). Sterile evacuated glass containers became available in 1929. The rigid glass containers are composed of a

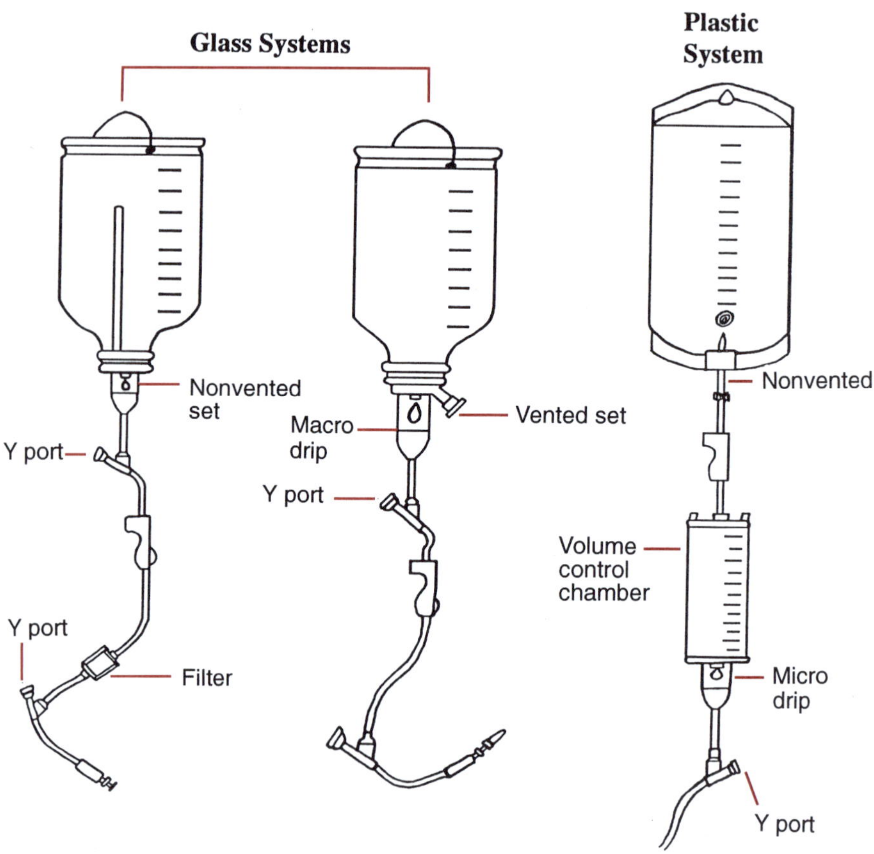

Figure 6–1 ■ Comparison of glass and plastic infusion delivery systems. (Drawings by Timothy D. Mitas.)

standard mix of materials, glass, metal, and rubber. The combination of materials is a disadvantage because of incompatibilities with fluids and additives and the breakdown of the materials during heat sterilization. In 1950, plastic containers became accessible for the storage and delivery of blood products. Today, the plastic system is used 90 to 95 percent of the time for administering solutions and blood products.

The Glass System

Two types of glass systems are available: one is the closed glass system and another is the open glass system. Both glass systems have partial vacuum and require air vents. In the open-glass system, air enters through a plastic tube in the container and collects in the air space in the bottle, allowing for displacement of the solution. In the closed-glass system, air is filtered into the container via vented tubing. The closed-glass system must use vented tubing to allow air into the container. Although plastic containers are used in most situations, the glass system remains the container of choice for infusates that cannot adapt to plastic bags because of incompatibilities with the chemical or properties of plastic.

NURSING FAST FACT!

In the open-glass system, the straw must extend above the fluid level to prevent bubbling of the air through the solution. Bubbling increases the risk of contamination.

The closed glass system has a stopper, also called the **rubber bung.** During insertion of the administration set, **coring** can occur, which results in the introduction of fragments of the rubber core into the solution. Twisting the spike through the rubber bung can displace visible and microscopic particles of the rubber bung. Because of the combination of materials in the glass system, some disadvantages have been experienced when using this system during heat sterilization procedures.

Checking the Glass System for Clarity

To ensure safety in the administration of solutions, the nurse must check the solution's clarity and expiration date before connecting it to the administration set. To check the glass system, hold the glass bottle up to the light and check for flashes of light, floating particles, or discoloration. The glass system should be crystal clear; if it is not, mark the container as contaminated and return it to the central supply station. Check the expiration date on the label.

ADVANTAGES

- Crystal clear; allows good visualization of contents
- Graduations on glass easy to read.
- Inert; has no plasticizers

DISADVANTAGES

- Breakage and shattering of glass
- Storage problems
- Coring (because of the rubber bung)
- Cumbersome disposal
- Rigidity
- Container constructed of mixed materials

The Plastic System

Most I.V. fluids are packaged in plastic containers that are flexible or semirigid (Fig. 6–2). The flexible plastic container has several unique features. The entire structure that comes in contact with the fluid, including the closure, is made of the same material; it is all polyvinyl chloride (PVC) or other suitable material. There is no combination of metal, rubber, or glass as in the rigid glass system. The plastic system is a truly closed system.

Plastic containers are commonly made of PVC, which is a polymeric material. The plasticizer diethylhexylphthalate (DEHP) is added to plas-

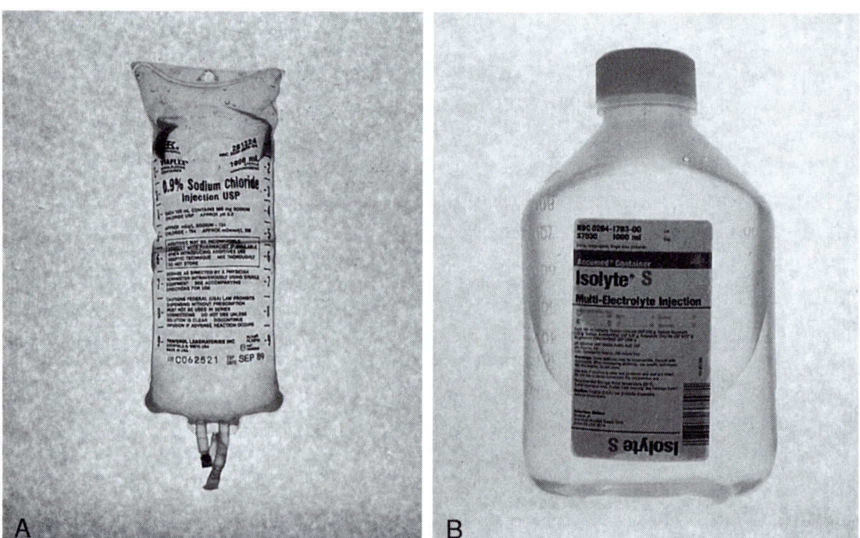

Figure 6–2 ■ Plastic infusion system. I.V. solutions are available in both *(A)* a flexible plastic container and *(B)* a more rigid type of container. (Courtesy of D. Anderson, Chico, CA.)

tic to make it pliable, but it is not chemically bonded to the vinyl and can leach out into the solution (Kaplan, 1999). The introduction of PVC plastic solution containers has been accompanied by concerns of compatibility, specifically with the DEHP. Many manufacturers are providing non-DEHP PVC fluid containers. Refer to Table 6–1 for more information on DEHP and to Table 6–2 for a list of manufacturers of non-DEHP solution containers.

The plastic system does not contain a vacuum; therefore, the containers must be flexible and collapsible. The plastic system does not need air to replace fluid flowing from the container. Either a vented or a nonvented administration set is acceptable for delivery of the infusate. A membrane seals both the medication and the administration ports of the container, and entry of air into this system is prevented. Because there is no rubber bung on the plastic system, spiking the system can be accomplished by means of a simple twisting motion (Fig. 6–3). Because the plastic can be easily perforated during use, careful attention should be paid to the integrity of this container during preparation and infusion delivery.

> Table 6–1 **CONCERNS OVER PVC AND DEHP**

Polyvinyl chloride (PVC) is a commonly used plastic found in many consumer, industrial, and medical products. A phthalate (DEHP) is a plasticizer that is added to PVC that allows PVC to become flexible. In 1972, potential hazards of transfusing blood that contained DEHP derived from blood bags and tubing were identified. In 1986, California Proposition 65 listed DEHP as a chemical that is known to cause cancer. In 1988, the Environmental Protection Agency (EPA) identified DEHP as a probable human carcinogen.

When incinerated, PVC releases hydrogen chloride gas (identified as a toxic air pollutant and cause of acid rain) and possible dioxin. When PVC products are incinerated, they produce HCl, a corrosive gas that has been identified as a toxic air pollutant. PVC materials are also not biodegradable, and DEHP may leach into the soil.

There are two reasons why the use of PVC I.V. containers is contraindicated in many I.V. therapies:

1. Absorption
2. Leaching

DEHP is not chemically bound to the polymer and can leach out during use. This extraction occurs either by DEHP's directly leaching out of the PVC product or when an extracting material (blood or I.V. fluids) diffuses into the PVC matrix, dissolves the plasticizer, and then the two diffuse out together. The most important factors in DEHP's leaching from medical devices are temperature, concentration of the phthalate, agitation, storage time, and surrounding media. DEHP is leached from PVC blood bags, I.V. bags, and tubing into blood, blood products, and medical solutions (HealthCare Without Harm, 1999). Certain drugs (e.g., Taxol, cyclosporine, diazepam, miconazole, nitroglycerine, warfarin, sodium carmustin), fat emulsions, and blood products enhance the leaching of DEHP (B. Braun, 1999).

HealthCare Without Harm (*www.noharm.org/DEHP*) initiated a collaborative international campaign advocating environmentally responsible health care. In the 1980s, I.V. solutions were provided by B. Braun in non-PVC bags. (Health Care without Harm, 1999).

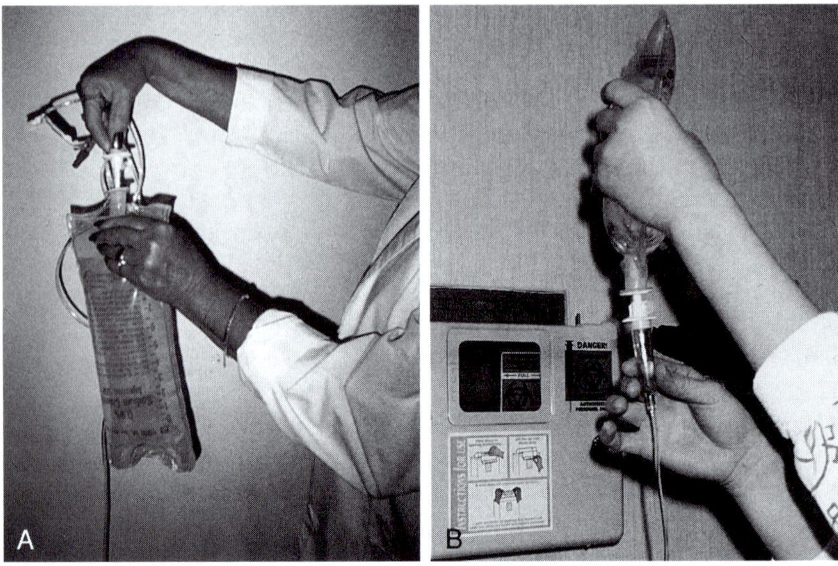

Figure 6–3 ■ Spiking the plastic container. *(A)* To spike the plastic container, insert the piercing pin of the I.V. tubing into the outlet port of the infusion bag using a twisting motion to ensure that the seal is pierced completely open. *(B)* Invert the container and squeeze the drip chamber to fill.

Never write directly on a flexible plastic bag with a ballpoint or indelible marker; the pen may puncture the bag and the marker ink may absorb into the plastic.

The advantages of the semirigid, hard plastic unit are that it is made of polyolefin, contains no plasticizers, and the fluid level marks are easier to read. This system is also impermeable to moisture. Semirigid containers must be vented to add air to the infusion system.

The flexible and semirigid plastic systems, when used in a series with other similar containers, may promote movement of residual air into the I.V. line.

ADVANTAGES

- Closed system
- Flexible
- Lightweight
- Container composed of one substance
- Better storage

DISADVANTAGES

- Punctures easily
- Fluid level difficult to determine
- Composed of plasticizers
- Not completely inert (potential for leaching)
- Environmentally unsafe

Checking the Plastic System for Clarity

The plastic container should be held up to the light and checked for clarity. If the plastic system is not crystal clear, any discoloration or floating particles in the solution should be identified and labeled as contaminants. The plastic system must be squeezed to check for pinholes. Check the expiration date on the label to ensure patient safety and be sure the outer wrap of the plastic system is free of pooled solution.

Use-Activated Containers

Use-activated containers (Fig. 6–4) are compartmentalized with premeasured ingredients that form an admixture when mixed. The containers are

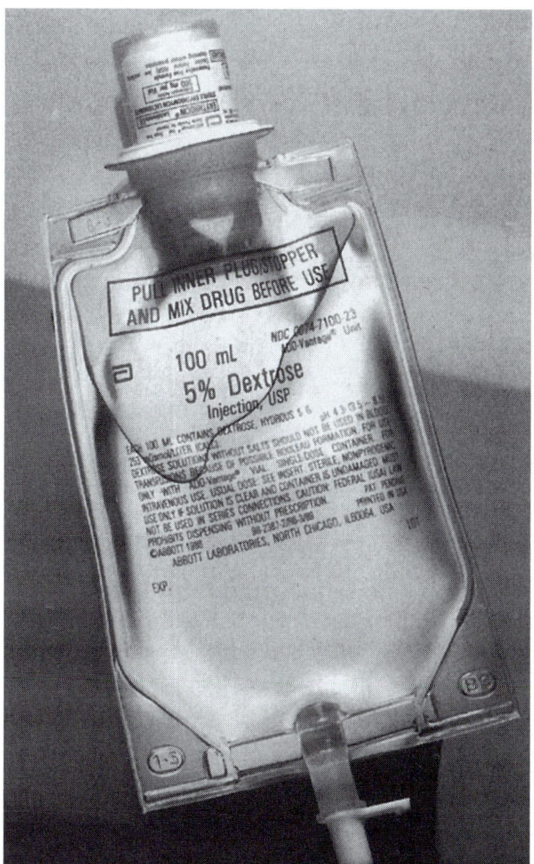

Figure 6–4 ■ Use-activated system. This Abbott ADD-Vantage system allows drugs to be reconstituted quickly and safely in an appropriate amount of diluent immediately before use. (Courtesy of Abbott Laboratories, North Chicago, IL. Used with permission.)

useful for high-use infusions that have a short shelf life after admixture. These systems are useful in the emergency department because they enable ease of use in acute situations (such as in an ambulance), in field use, and during transport. The ambulatory and home care settings also benefit from use-activated systems. These systems are more expensive, however.

To activate the container, the nurse deliberately ruptures the container's seal or diaphragm by compressing opposing parts or applying pressure to rupture the internal reservoir. The primary disadvantage of the system occurs when this step is not completed appropriately.

NURSING FAST FACT!

A concern with use-activated containers is the belated rupture of the medication reservoir with a potentially harmful concentration of drug being administered (Peucca, 2001).

Administration Sets

The most frequently used administration sets include:

- Single-line sets, which include primary (standard) sets, secondary sets (also called "piggyback" sets), and volume-controlled (also called metered-volume) sets
- Primary Y sets
- Administration sets, which vary among manufacturers and drop factor, all have the basic components (Fig. 6–5).

Basic Components of Administration Sets

The basic components of administration sets include:

1. *Spike/piercing pin:* The spike/piercing pin is a sharply tipped plastic tube designed to be inserted into the infusate container. It is connected to the flange, drop orifice, and drip chamber.
2. *Flange:* The flange is a plastic guard that helps prevent touch contamination during insertion of the spike.
3. *Drop orifice:* The drop orifice is an opening that determines the size and shape of the fluid drop. The size of this drop orifice determines the **drop factor.**
4. *Drip chamber:* The drip chamber is a pliable, enlarged clear plastic tube that contains the drop orifice. It is connected to the tubing.
5. *Tubing:* The plastic tubing connects to the drip chamber. Depending on the manufacturer, the tubing may have a variety of clamps, ports, connectors, or filters built into the system. The

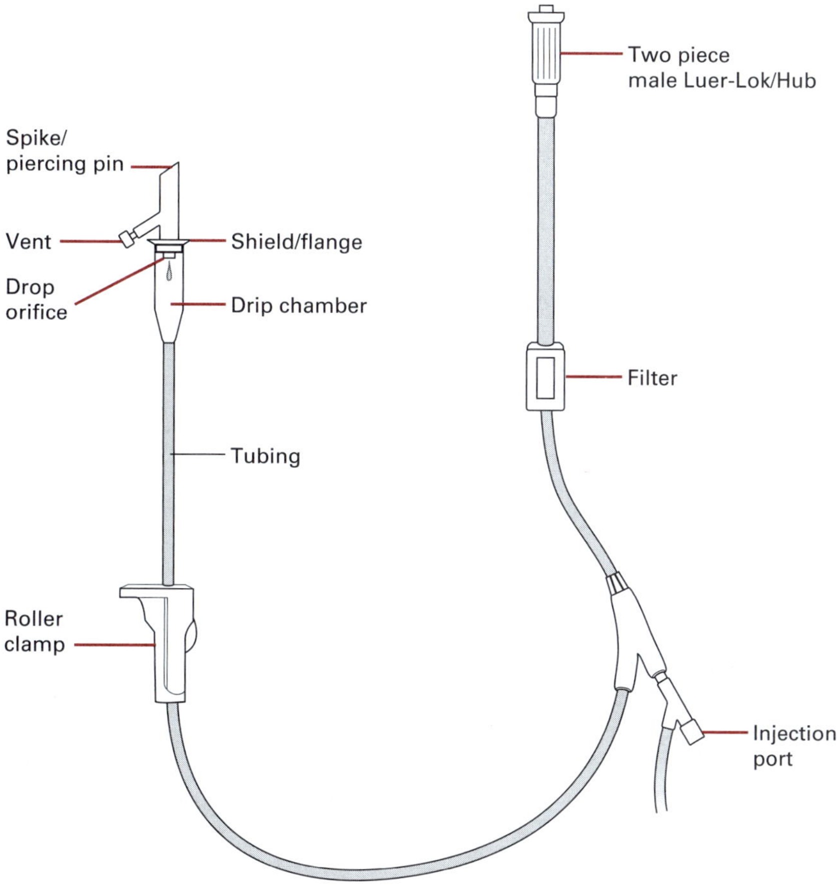

Figure 6–5 ■ Basic administration system.

average length of primary tubing is 66 to 100 inches. The length of secondary administration sets averages from 32 to 42 inches.

6. *Clamp:* The flow clamp control device operates on the principle of compression of the tubing wall. Each manufacturer supplies a clamp (roller, screw, or slide), and all operate on the principle of compression. The roller and screw clamps are equally reliable. The slide clamp is viewed as less reliable in controlling flow.
7. *Injection ports:* Injection ports serve as an access into the tubing and are located at various points along the administration set. Usually the ports are used for administration of medication. Small (21- to 25-gauge) needles should be used to access these ports to ensure resealing.
8. *Backcheck valve:* The valve allows the primary solution to resume after the piggyback is completed.

9. *Hub:* The adaptor to connect the administration set to the I.V. catheter or a needleless system is also called the male Luer-Lok.
10. *Final filter:* The final filter removes foreign particles from the infusate. It can be purchased as part of the administration set tubing, or filters can be added on.

Single-Line Administration Sets

Single-line sets have only one spike that extends proximally from the drip chamber. Only one main bag of infusate is used with this system. The tubing distal to the **drip chamber** terminates in one male-adapter end that connects to the **hub** of a vascular access device.

Primary Sets

Primary sets are referred to as standard sets and are available as vented or nonvented. Vented sets have an air filter attached to the spike pin that allows air to enter the container. Vented sets must be used on the closed-glass system. Nonvented sets have a straight spike pin without an air vent device. Nonvented sets can be used on any open-glass or plastic system. Primary sets are available in **macrodrip** form (10 to 20 drops/mL) or in **microdrip** form (60 drops/mL). Primary sets can have one, two, or three access ports, and often have inline filters with backcheck valves (Schiff, 2001). The calibration is clearly specified on the box of each administration set, as well as in the accompanying literature. The microdrip set, also called a minidrip or pediatric set, is used when small amounts of fluid are required (Fig. 6–6).

A **check valve** (also called backcheck valve) is a device that functions to prevent retrograde flow of the solution. Check valves are inline components of many primary administration sets. The check valve is an important feature when secondary I.V. lines are in place for intermittent infusions. The check valve inhibits the backflow of secondary **infusate** into the primary infusate.

Check valves function when the:

- Primary infusate is infusing at the prescribed rate by gravity.
- Secondary infusate, of a lesser volume, is piggybacked into the primary line.
- Level of the secondary infusate is higher than the primary container.
- Clamp on the tubing of the secondary container is opened, activating the backcheck valve because of the pressure exerted by the piggyback solution.
- Secondary infusate container empties and its fluid descends into its tubing; the decreased pressure in the line causes the backcheck valve to release, thus activating flow in the primary line (Fig. 6–7).

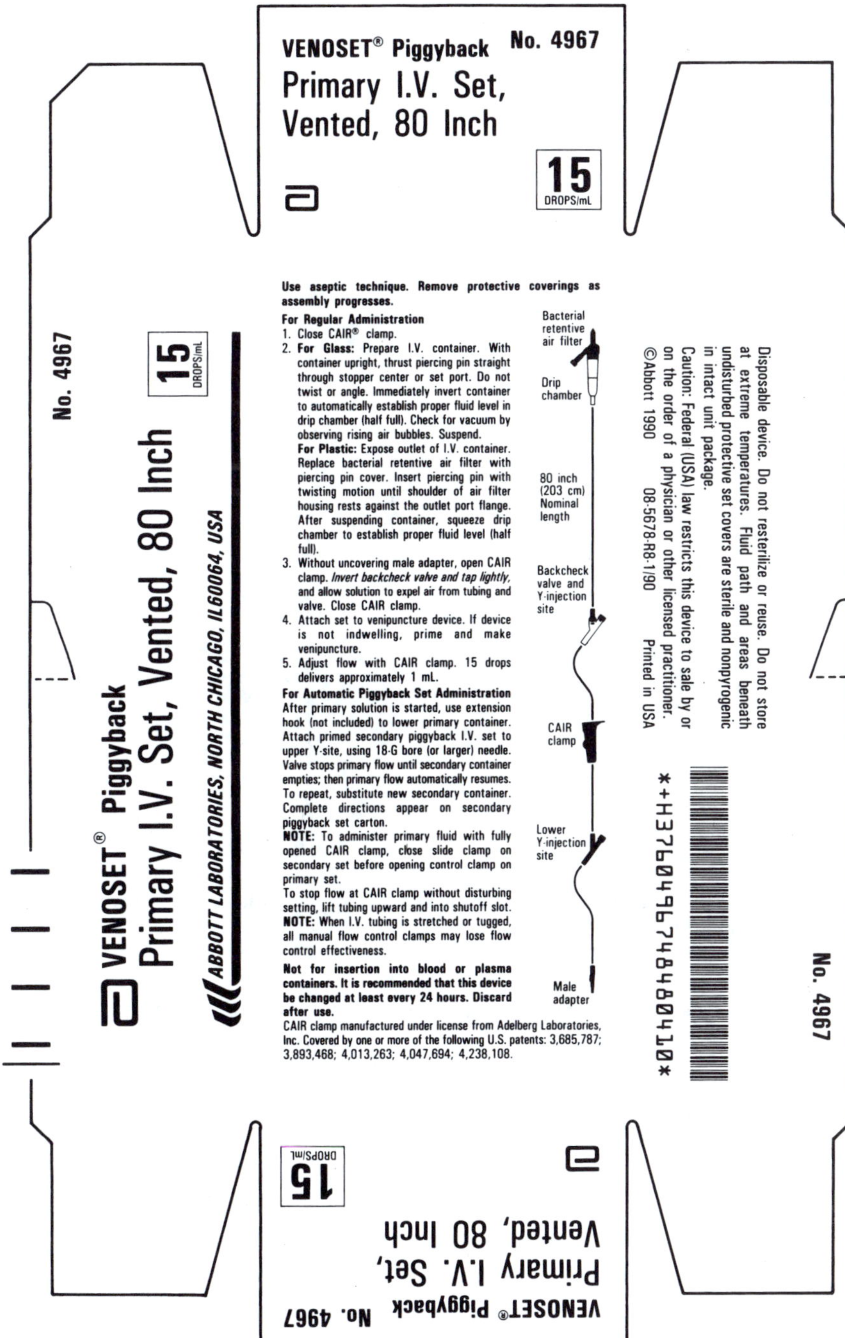

Figure 6–6 ■ Primary administration set package. (Courtesy of Abbott Laboratories, Hospital Products Division, North Chicago, IL.)

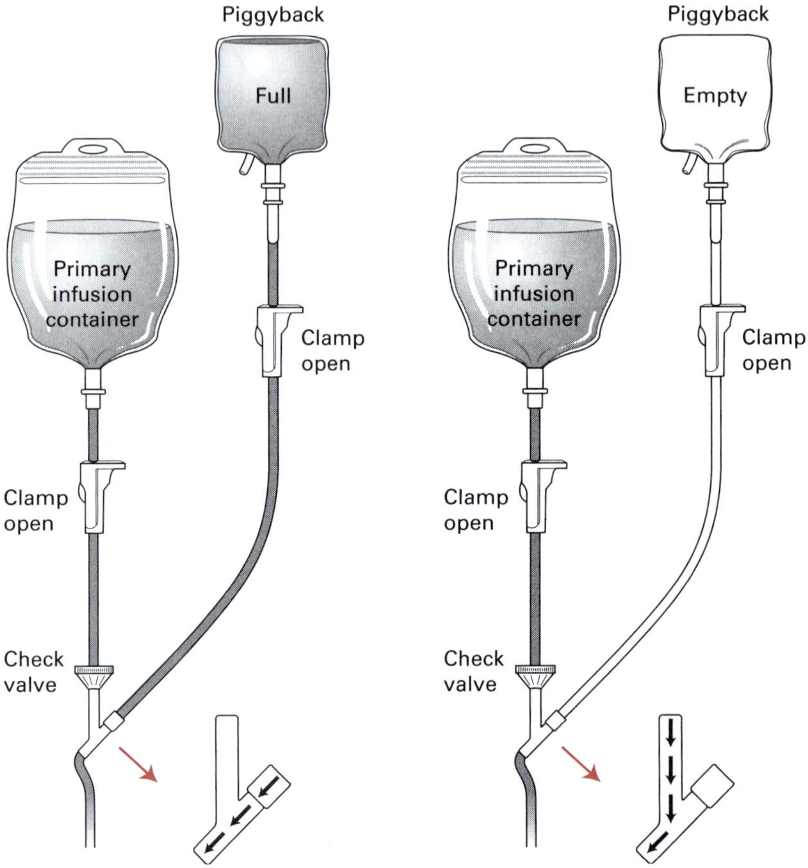

Figure 6–7 ■ Check valve (also called backcheck valve) acts to prevent retrograde solution flow.

INS Standard. Primary and secondary continuous administration sets shall be changed every 72 hours and immediately on suspected contamination or when the integrity of the product or system has been compromised. (INS, 2000, 54)

An organization that exhibits an increased rate of catheter-related bloodstream infection with the practice of 72-hour administration set changes should return to a 48-hour administration set change. (INS, 2000, 24)

Secondary Administration Sets

Two types of secondary administration sets are available: the piggyback set and the volume-controlled set.

PIGGYBACK SET

The piggyback set has short tubing (30 to 36 inches) with a standard drop factor of 10 to 20 drops/mL. It is used to deliver 50 to 100 mL of infusate. These sets are widely used because of the administration of multiple drug therapies to patients. They are connected with a needleless adapter into an **injection port** immediately distal to the backcheck valve of the primary tubing (Josephson, 1999). In setting up the piggyback set, the primary infusion container is positioned lower than the secondary container, using the extension hook provided in the secondary line box.

VOLUME-CONTROLLED SET

The volume-controlled set, also called a metered-volume chamber set, is designed for intermittent administration of measured volumes of fluid with a calibrated chamber. These sets are calibrated in much smaller increments than other infusion devices, thus limiting the amount of solution available to the patient (usually for reasons of safety). Most chambers hold 100 to 150 mL of solution, but neonatal chambers may hold only 10 to 50 mL. The volume-controlled set is most frequently used for pediatric patients and critically ill patients when small, well-controlled delivery of medication or solution is needed (Fig. 6–8).

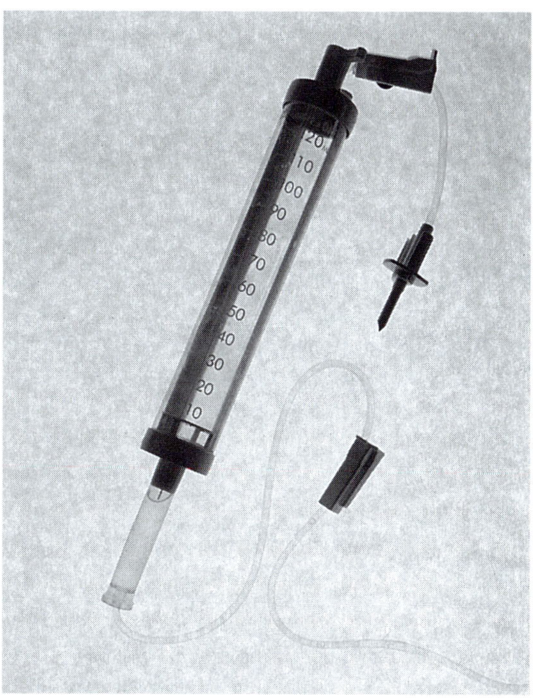

Figure 6–8 ■ Volume chamber control set for intermittent infusion. (Courtesy of D. Anderson, Chico, CA.)

INS Standard. Primary intermittent administration sets shall be changed every 24 hours and immediately upon suspected contamination or when the integrity of the product or system has been compromised. (INS, 2000, 54)

Primary Y Administration Sets

The primary Y administration set is used for rapid infusion or for administration of more than one solution at a time. Each leg of the Y set is capable of being the primary set. The Y set has two separate spikes with a separate drip chamber and short length of tubing with individual clamps. Primary Y sets are made up of large-bore tubing because this tubing is meant to infuse large amounts of fluid in acute situations. Blood components can be administered through primary Y sets. A Y set allows for priming of the administration set before the blood is administered. Most blood administration Y sets contain inline filters with a pore size of 170 microns and have a drop factor of 10 to allow for the safe infusion of blood cells (AABB, 2002).

Primary Y sets are not provided as vented sets, so caution is needed when using bottles with venting straws or a venting apparatus added to the bottle. Collapsible containers should be used with Y sets. Any air emboli associated with tubing of this inner lumen size are considered significant (Perucca, 2001).

INS Standard. Administration sets that are used to accommodate blood or blood components shall be changed after each unit of blood or at the end of 4 hours. (INS, 2000, S4)

Pump-Specific Administration Sets

Pump-specific administration sets are made specifically for use with electronic infusion devices (EIDs). These sets also come in a number of configurations, with each set specific for respective electronic delivery systems. For specifics on each pump administration set, see the literature that accompanies each EID.

Lipid Administration Sets

Lipids or fat emulsions are supplied in glass containers and require special vented tubing that is supplied by the manufacturer. Lipid-containing infusates have been known to leach phthalates from bags and tubing made of PVC. Fat emulsions are supplied in glass containers with non-PVC infusion sets.

Nitroglycerin Administration Sets

Nitroglycerin tubing is available in certain infusion pump sets. Safe care can be accomplished with or without a nitroglycerin-specific administration set, as long as the potential risks are understood. Nitroglycerin is incompatible with standard PVC tubing. Studies have shown that nitroglycerin adheres to the plastic in the tubing and fluid bag. Nitroglycerin sets can be made with non-PVC sets. Nitroglycerin-specific sets are more expensive; however, when used with the glass system they offer a system that does not create an adhering surface for nitroglycerin. The use of specialty sets remains controversial and much debated (Trissel, 2000).

Accessory Devices for Administration Sets

Accessory, or add-on, devices for administration sets include:

- Filters
- Extension tubings
- Adapters and connectors
- Stopcocks
- Injection access ports
- Needleless systems

When an add-on device is used, it should be of a Luer-Lok configuration. Aseptic technique and infection control measures must be followed for all add-on device changes. Adding accessories to an existing administration set is referred to as breaching the infusion line. Whenever an infusion line is breached, the possibility for the introduction of contaminates exists.

> **INS Standard.** When add-on devices are used, they should be changed with each catheter or administration set replacement, or whenever the integrity of either product is compromised. (INS, 2000, 35)

Filters

Inline I.V. Solution Filters

Inline, or "final," **filters** are used in the delivery of I.V. therapy to filter out microorganisms, which, if alive, will multiply in the bloodstream or, if dead, will enter the tissue and cause a sterile abscess. The use of inline filtration in intravenous infusions guards against inadvertent infusion of particulate matter; air and lipid emboli; endotoxins; and microorganisms such as bacteria, protozoa, and fungi (Dunleavy & Sevick, 2001). There are two groups of particulate matter: (1) nonviable contaminants such as particles of metal, lint, asbestos, rubber, cotton, dust, and glass and (2) viable contaminants, consisting of bacteria and fungi. Inline filters remove undissolved drug powders or crystals and precipitates from incompatible admixtures.

The U.S. Centers for Disease Control and Prevention (CDC) does not recommend the use of inline filters as a routine infection-control measure. This is based on the belief that these filters are not cost effective in preventing infrequently occurring infusion-related infections because they may also increase personnel time and the incidence of infections (CDC, 2002).

The Infusion Nurses Society standards (2000) favor the inline filters for removal of bacteria, fungi, particulate matter, air, and some endotoxins from I.V.-delivered fluids. This position is also supported by a recommendation published in 1994 by the U.S. Food and Drug Administration (FDA). The National Coordinating Committee on Large Volume Parenteral has established priorities for the use of filters and recommends the use of filters with tissue plasminogen activator (TPN) admixtures; for immunodeficient or immunocompromised patients; and for I.V. infusions containing additives, especially those that are heavily precipitated

Inline filters are available in a variety of forms, sizes, and materials:

- Filters measuring 170 microns remove most debris from blood.
- Filters measuring 0.5 to 1.2 microns remove most particulate matter but do not remove fungi or bacteria.
- Filters measuring 0.45 micron remove fungi or bacteria.
- Filters measuring 0.22 micron remove all fungi and bacteria but can reduce flow rates.

The smallest human capillary is slightly larger than a red blood cell (approximately 6 microns). Well mixed infusate solutions may contain microprecipitates in the range of 1 to 50 microns. The use of inline filters ensures removal of particles that can pass rigorous visual inspection (Dunleavy & Sevick, 2001). Infusion-related phlebitis, a common complication occurring in up to 70 percent of patients receiving I.V. therapy, can be attributed to physical (microprecipitates and particulate matter) and chemical (irritating pharmaceuticals and additives) causes, as well as increased manipulation of I.V. sets and materials (Maki & Mermel, 1998).

> **INS Standard.** A 0.22-micron filter is considered a bacterial/particulate retentive, air-eliminating filter and is recommended for use to decrease the potential of air emboli, reduce the risk of phlebitis, and prevent bacteria contamination. To achieve final filtration, the filter should be located as close to the **cannula** site as possible. The filter should be an integral part of the administration set. (INS, 2000, 38)

Two commonly used inline filters are the depth filter and the membrane filter.

DEPTH FILTERS

The depth filter is composed of fibers or fragmented material that has been pressed or bonded to form a maze; the pore size is nonuniform. Fluid flows through a random path that absorbs and traps the particles. These filters can clog when large amounts of particles are retained. Depth filters prime easily and are capable of air elimination.

MEMBRANE FILTERS

Membrane filters are screen filters with uniformly sized pores. Filters range in size from 170 microns (largest) to 0.22 micron (smallest). They allow liquids but not particles to pass through them. The finer the membrane, the more fully it will filter the liquid. A 5-micron screen will retain on the flat portion of the membrane all particles larger than 5 microns. Filters of 0.2 microns are for bacteria, fungus, and air retention. The 0.22-micron air-venting filters automatically vent air through a nonwettable (hydrophobic) membrane and permit uniform high-gravity flow through large wettable (hydrophilic) membrane.

To be effective, an infusion membrane filter must have the ability to:

- Maintain high flow rates
- Automatically vent air
- Retain bacteria, fungi, particulate matter, and endotoxins
- Tolerate pressures generated by infusion pumps
- Act in a nonbinding fashion to drugs

Membrane filters are used when:

1. An additive has been combined with the solution.
2. The injection port on the tubing is used.
3. The patient is susceptible to infusion phlebitis.
4. The infusion is given centrally.
5. The solution is a three-in-one TPN solution.

Prescribed therapies in which a 0.2-micron filter is contraindicated include administration of blood or blood components, lipid emulsions, and low-dose (less than 5 micron/mL) solutions. Other contraindications include the administration of low-volume medications (total amount less than 5 mg over 24 hours), I.V. push medications, medications in which pharmacologic properties are altered by the filter membrane, and medications that adhere to the filter membrane.

All filters have a certain pressure value at which they will allow the passage of air from one side of a wetted hydrophilic membrane to the other. This pressure valve is called the bubble point.

Filters are also rated according to the pounds per square inch (**psi**) of pressure they can withstand. The filter should withstand the psi exerted by the infusion pump or rupture may occur. If the psi rating of the housing is less than that of the membrane, excess force will break the housing.

When using a positive-pressure EID, consideration should be given to the psi rating of a filter. The psi exerted by the device should never exceed the psi capacity of the filter (INS, 2000, 38).

Filters for Parenteral Therapy

An air-eliminating 0.2-micron filter set designed for 96-hour bacteria and endotoxin retention is indicated for use with I.V. administration sets for the removal of inadvertent particulate debris, microbial contaminates and their associated endotoxin, and entrained air that may be found in solutions intended for I.V. administration (Pall, 2000) (Fig. 6–9A, B).

A filter set for total nutritional admixture administration has a 1.2-micron air-eliminating filter. This filter set is indicated for use with any

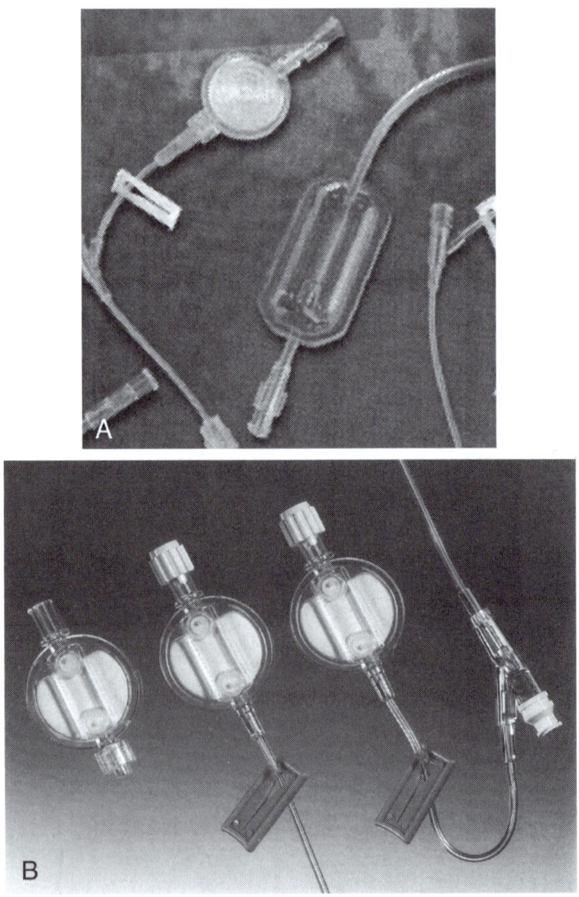

Figure 6–9 ■ *(A)* Inline 0.22-micron filter: Filterflow. (Courtesy of B. Braun Medical Inc., Bethlehem, PA.) *(B)* The Supor AEF 0.2-micron filter set for removal of inadvertent particulate debris and bacterial contamination with minimal drug binding. (Courtesy of Pall Corporation, Port Washington, NY.)

nutritional I.V. administration containing lipids for the removal of inadvertent particulate debris, fungal contaminants, and entrained air (Pall, 2000; Fig. 6–10).

When lipid emulsions are administered, a 0.45-micron filter is available for the removal of inadvertent particulate debris; air; and microbial contaminates such as *Candida albicans, Moraxella osloensis, Staphylococcus aureus,* and *Klebsiella pneumoniae* (Fig. 6–11).

Blood Filters

The American Association of Blood Banks states that blood must be transfused through a sterile, pyrogen-free transfusion set that has a filter capable of retaining particles that are potentially harmful to the recipient (ABB, 2002). Commercially available filters include the standard clot filter, the microaggregate filter, and the leukocyte depletion filter. For further details on blood filters, see Chapter 13.

> **INS Standard.** Blood filters are used to remove particulate matter from blood and its components. Nurses should be knowledgeable regarding filters and filter requirements of various blood components. (INS, 2000, 38)

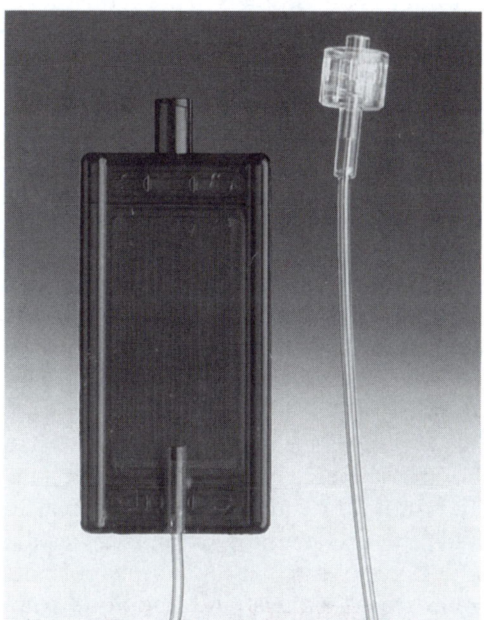

Figure 6–10 ▪ Air-eliminating filter set designed for total nutrient admixture solutions. This filter has a 1.2-micron nylon membrane that provides an effective barrier for the patient from inadvertent particulate contamination, uncontrollable precipitate contamination, and entrained air. (Courtesy of Pall Corporation, Port Washington, NY.)

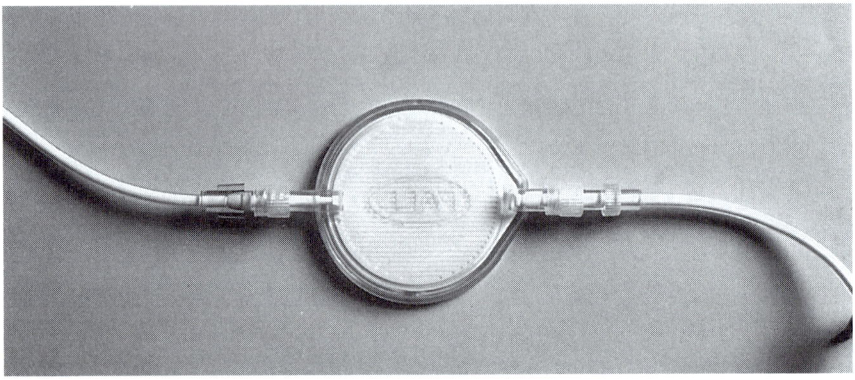

Figure 6–11 ■ Lipipor emulsive filter contains a 0.45-micron filter used for removal of inadvertent particulate debris, entrained air, and microbial contamination of drug lipid emulsions. (Courtesy of Pall Corporation, Port Washington, NY.)

STANDARD CLOT FILTERS

Blood administration sets have a standard clot filter of 170 to 260 microns. They are intended to remove coagulated products, microclots, and debris resulting from collection and storage. These filters allow passage of smaller particles called microaggregates, which are composed of nonviable leukocytes, primarily granulocytes, platelets, and fibrin strands. The microaggregates can cause pulmonary dysfunction (adult respiratory distress syndrome) when large quantities of stored bank blood are infused (Menitove, 1999).

MICROAGGREGATE FILTERS

A supplementary filter (transfusion filter) can be added to an in-use administration set, permitting infusion of blood, easy replacement of the filter (if clogging occurs), and multiple infusions of blood units. The 20- to 40-micron **microaggregate** blood filters remove most debris from the transfusion product but can slow the administration of blood to an undesirable rate. The 40-micron filter allows blood to be transfused easily in the specified period of time; however, filtration is less refined. The 80-micron filter is the filter of choice in many institutions because of its safe level of filtration and high flow rate potential (Perucca, 2001). A microaggregate filter is a free-flow, low priming volume device that provides a 40-micron rated screen filter medium for the removal of potentially harmful blood components, microaggregates, and nonblood component particulate matter (Pall, 2000) (Fig. 6–12).

LEUKOCYTE DEPLETION FILTERS

Leukocyte depletion filters are used to remove leukocytes (including leukocyte-mediated viruses) from red blood cells and platelets.

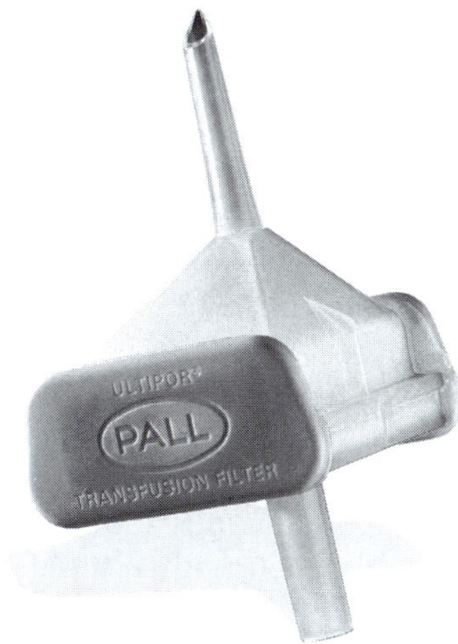

Figure 6–12 ■ Microaggregate blood transfusion filter. (Courtesy of Pall Corporation, Port Washington, NY.)

Leukocyte-poor filters are classified according to efficiency level, not micron size (Pall Biomedical Corporation, 2000). These filters can be used to remove 99.9 percent of leukocytes from red blood cells, platelets, and plasma (Pall, 2000).

Websites

Pall Medical Filter information: *www.pall.com/medical*

Extension Tubings

Extension tubings are add-on sets used to add I.V. line length. Commonly used with active patients, these sets, which come in various lengths, aid in tubing changes without the need for site manipulation. Extension tubing is also frequently used as primary tubing for syringe pumps and ambulatory pumps. Disadvantages are an added cost and an additional site for bacteria to enter the system.

Adapters and Connectors (Loops)

J-, U-, or T-shaped adapters and connectors may be used at the injection site. The T port is a common add-on device that is usually about 4 to 6 inches long and is made of standard or microbore tubing with a hard plastic T-shaped connector on one end. One leg of the T connector attaches to the I.V. device with the other a resealable latex port.

The J loop or U connector has the same purpose as the T connector. Their rigid shape is maintained when connected to an I.V. site.

Disadvantages of I.V. adapter and connector loops are increased cost and increased potential for infection because of the increased opportunity for manipulation and risk of separation. Their use should be limited (Fig. 6–13).

INS Standard. All add-on devices should be of Luer-Lok design. Tape should not be used as a means of junction securement. (INS, 2000, 35)

Stopcocks

A stopcock is a device that controls the direction of flow of an infusate through manual manipulation of a direction-regulating valve (Fig. 6–14). A stopcock is usually a three- or four-way device. A three-way stopcock connects two lines of fluid to a patient and provides a mechanism for either one to run to the patient (similar to a faucet). With a four-way stopcock, the valve can be manipulated so that one or both lines can run to the patient, alone, or in combination.

The general use of stopcocks is strongly discouraged because of the issue of contamination. When the stopcock portals are uncapped they are vulnerable to touch contamination. The stopcock itself is small and requires handling in such a way that sterility can easily be compromised. Syringes are frequently attached to I.V. push administration, and the portal is poorly protected after use (Perucca, 2001).

NURSING FAST FACT!

Caution should be exercised when using a stopcock because of the risk of contamination of the I.V. system or accidental disconnection if a Luer-Lok connection is not used or if the stopcock is accidentally turned. Also, the infusion might be interrupted or administered incorrectly.

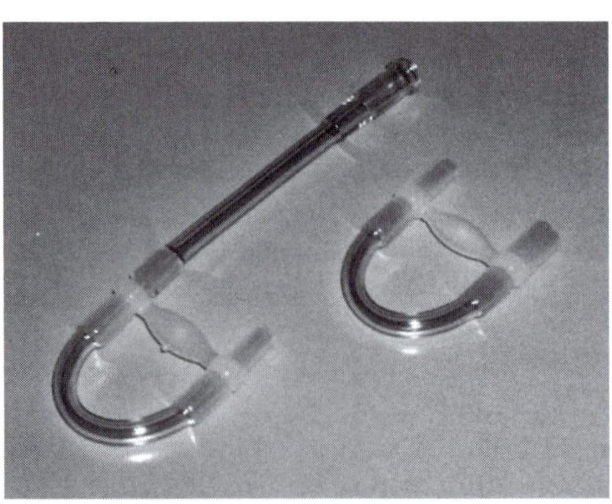

Figure 6–13 ■ J- and U-shaped add-on devices. (Courtesy of Becton Dickinson, Franklin Lakes, NJ.)

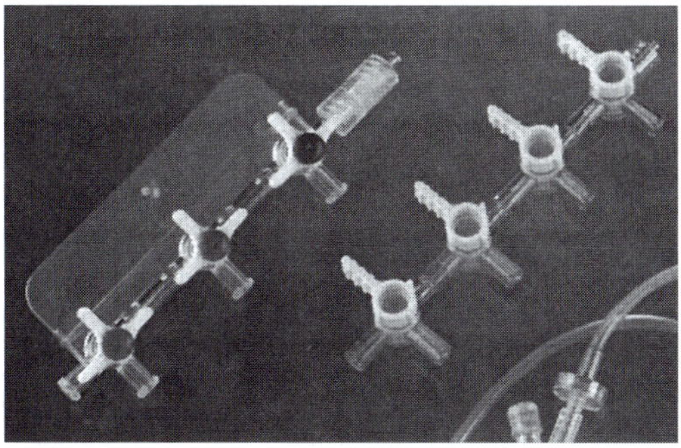

Figure 6–14 ■ Stopcocks. (Courtesy of B. Braun Medical Inc., Bethlehem, PA.)

Injection Access Ports

Injection access ports or caps are locking devices also known as resealable **PRN** devices. A **locking device** is a capped resealable diaphragm that may have a Luer-Lok or Luer slip connection. The diaphragms may be made of latex, but many manufacturers are now making latex-free diaphragms because of increased sensitivities to latex. This type of device can convert continuous I.V. infusion to an intermittent device when a resealable plug is inserted into the cannula hub. The resealable lock is used for saline or heparin flush (Fig. 6–15).

A disadvantage of the resealable lock is that it can separate at the hub or plug junction, allowing bacteria to enter the system because of inadequate flushing of blood cells from under the latex rubber. In addition, an occlusion or blood clot can occur within the locking device.

> **INS Standard.** Injection access ports should be aseptically cleansed with an approved antimicrobial solution immediately before use. (INS, 2000, 41)

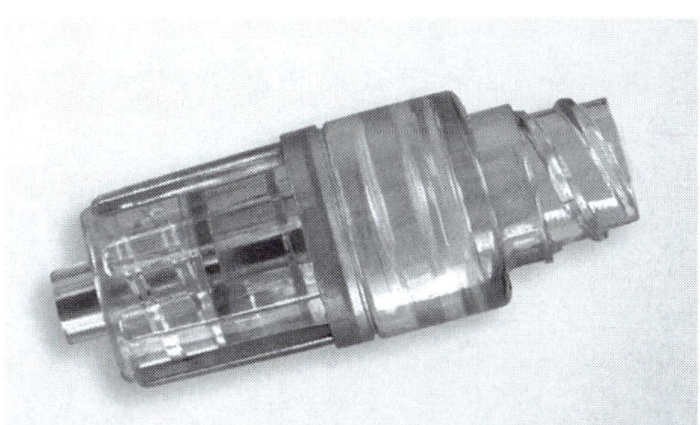

Figure 6–15 ■ PRN valve with needleless technology: Clearlink Access System. (Courtesy of Baxter International Inc., Round Lake, IL.)

NURSING FAST FACT!

Large-bore needles or frequent needle punctures may remove a plug of rubber from the port, resulting in coring. The risk of coring is difficult to predict; therefore, injection caps should be routinely changed according to institutional protocol.

Needleless Systems

The Needlestick Safety and Prevention Act, which took effect in April of 2001, reinforces the need to use safe needles to reduce injuries. Needleless systems and needle safety systems are the state-of-the-art technology of needle systems and are used to connect I.V. devices, administer infusates and medications, and sample blood.

Estimates indicate that 600,000 to 800,000 needlestick and other percutaneous injuries occur annually in the United States (EPINet, 2000). The current cost for a single percutaneous injury is estimated at between $500 and $1000, with more than $500 million being spent annually for needlestick injuries.

The use of protected needles or needleless equipment significantly decreases the risk of needlestick injuries (NIOSH, 2000). An increasing number and variety of needle devices with safety features are now available. Examples of safety device designs include:

- Needleless connectors
- Protected needle connectors
- Needles that retract into a syringe or vacuum tube holder
- Hinged or sliding shields attached to phlebotomy needles, winged steel needles
- Protective encasements to receive an I.V. stylet
- Sliding needle shields attached to disposable syringes and vacuum tube holders
- Self-blunting phlebotomy and winged steel needles
- Retractable finger/heel-stick lancets

Figure 6–16 is an example of a needlefree system, and Figure 6–17 shows examples of a protected needle.

The shielded needle design provides FDA guidelines that require that the device be designed to require the worker's hands to remain behind the needle as it is covered (FDA, 1995). The shielded needle provides protection for the practitioner after the stylet is withdrawn from the catheter during insertion into a vein. The needle is usually locked within a needle guard (Fig. 6–17).

To purchase a report on needlestick prevention devices, contact the Emergency Care Research Institute (ECRI) which is an independent, nonprofit agency evaluating medical devices:

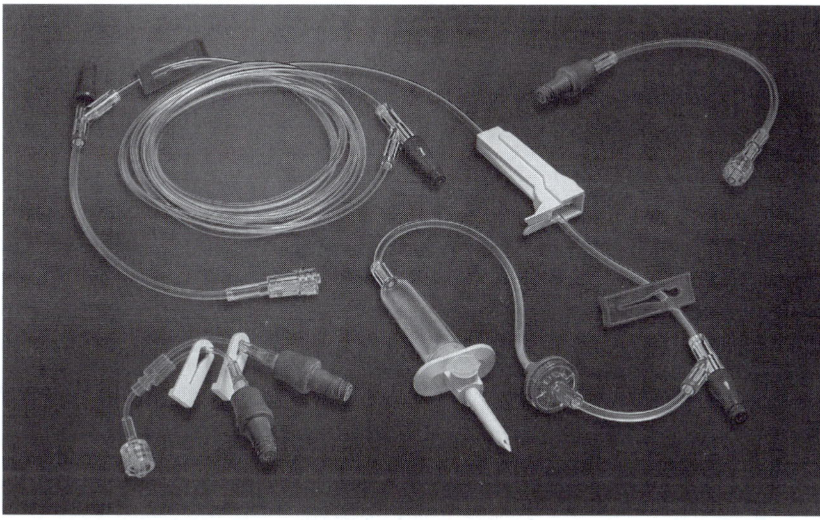

Figure 6–16 ■ Life Shield Clave needleless system. (Courtesy of Abbott Laboratories, North Chicago, IL.)

ECRI
5200 Butler Pike
Plymouth Meeting, PA 19462
610-825-6000 ext. 5888

Websites

Emergency Care Research Institute (ECRI): *www.ECRI.com*
Centers for Disease Control and Prevention (CDC): *www.cdc.gov/niosh/2000*
Service Employees International Union (SEIU): *www.serv.org/new*
International Health Care Worker Safety Center: *hsc.virginia.edw/epinet*

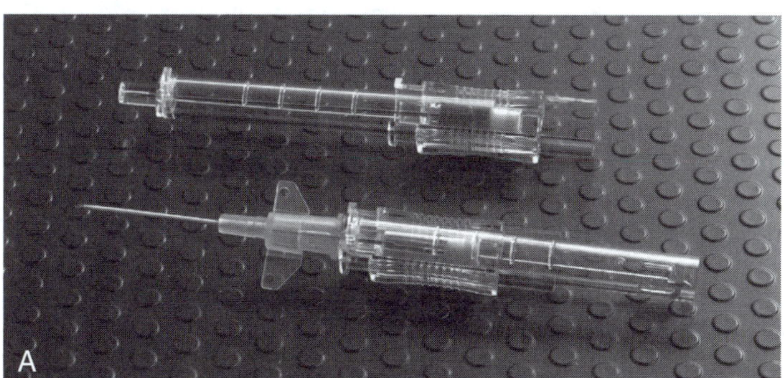

Figure 6–17 ■ *(A)* Protectiv I.V. catheter needle protection system. (Courtesy of Medex, Inc., Carlsbad, CA.)

(Continued on following page)

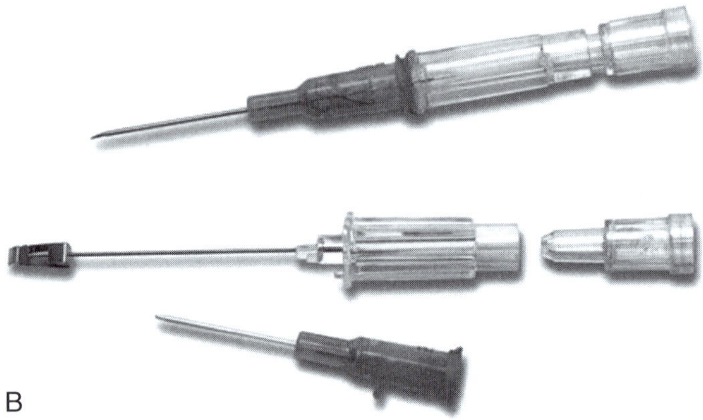

B

Figure 6–17 *(Continued)* ■ *(B)* Introcan safety I.V. catheter with passive safety. (Courtesy of B. Braun Medical Inc., Bethlehem, PA.)

NOTE > See Chapter 1 for further information on risks of needlestick injuries. Table 6–2 presents a list of *I.V. safety products and devices.*

Peripheral Infusion Devices

Several types of peripheral infusion devices are commercially available: scalp vein needles, over-the-needle catheters, through-the-needle catheters, midline catheters, and dual-**lumen** catheters. The catheter-type devices usually have **radiopaque** material or stripping added to ensure radiographic visibility. Radiopacity aids in the identification of a catheter embolus, a rare complication. The hub of a cannula is plastic and color coded to indicate the length and **gauge.**

Catheters are made of various biocompatible materials such as polytetrafluoroethylene (Teflon) and Vialon (Becton Dickinson). Teflon is less thrombogenic and less inflammatory than polyurethane or PVC, and Vialon is a newer material that is nonhemolytic and free of plasticizers. Teflon, a polyurethane material, has been shown to provide low cost, low rates of infiltration, and comparatively low rates of phlebitis. Vialon is slick when wetted and softens after insertion, minimizing venous trauma and clot induction. For a comparison of the types of peripheral infusion devices, see Table 6–3.

INS Standard. The cannula selected shall be of the smallest gauge and the shortest length possible to accommodate the prescribed therapy. Catheters shall be radiopaque. A short peripheral catheter is defined as one that is smaller than 3 inches in length. The term "cannula" refers to a stainless steel needle or the catheter. (INS, 2000, 44)

> Table 6–2 **SAFETY PRODUCTS AND DEVICES**

Alternatives to Poylvinyl Chloride (PVC) and DEHP	
Blood bags:	Baxter Healthcare
Central line catheters and PICC lines:	B. Braun, Becton Dickinson, Horizon Medical Products, Klein-Baker Medical, Utah Medical Products, Inc. and Vygon
I.V. Bags:	B. Braun, Biometrix, Budget Medical Products, Curlin Medical, Cryovac, Kawasumi, Horizon Medical Products, MPS Acacia, Medex, Inc., Natvar, Pactiv, and Cryovac
Needleless and Needle Protector Systems	
I.V. Medication Delivery Systems:	Used to administer medication or fluids through an I.V. catheter port or I.V. connector site.
Needleless I.V. Access-Blunted Cannulas	Life Shield System, Abbott Laboratories Interlink® IV Access System, Baxter/Becton Dickinson Ultrasite® Needle-free IV system, B. Braun Medical POSIFLOW valve, Becton Dickinson SmartSite Needle-Free System, Alaris Medical Systems Safsite System, B. Braun Medical Clave™ connector, ICU Medical AVI Checkvalve, 3M Health Care
Recessed/Protected Needles	LifeShield Connector, Abbott Laboratories NeedleLock Device, Baxter Healthcare Corp. Versa-Lok and Pro-Lok, Beech Medical Click Lock and Piggy Lock, ICU Medical Centurion Uni-Guard Piggy Back Connector, Tri-State Hospital Supply Corp.
I.V. Insertion Equipment:	Used to access the bloodstream for I.V. administration.
Shielded or Retracting Peripheral I.V. Catheters	Introcan® Safety IV catheter, B.Braun Medical Insyte™ Auto Guard™ shielded IV catheter, Becton Dickinson IV Safe™ M.C. Johnson Co., Inc. Saf-T-Intima™ IV catheter safety system, Becton Dickinson Protectiv and Protective Plus IV Catheter safety system, Johnson & Johnson Medical, Inc. Protectiv® Acuvance® I.V. Safety Catheter, Ethicon EndoSurgery, Inc. Secure peripheral venous catheter, Vadus, Inc.
Shielded Midline I.V. Catheters	Biovue ™ PICC/Midline catheter with Protective Safety Introducer, Johnson & Johnson Medical, Inc.

Sources: *CDC/EPINET/products. www.med.Virginia.EDU/medcntr/centers/epinet/products.html#1*
HealthCare Without Harm

> Table 6–3 COMPARISON OF PERIPHERAL INFUSION DEVICES

Cannula	Advantages	Disadvantages	Uses
Scalp-vein needle	Excellent for one-time I.V. medication, blood withdrawal, in patients allergic to nylon or Teflon Wings allow ease of insertions and secure taping Attached extension permits easy tubing change	Needle increases the risk of infiltration Not recommended for use in flexor areas Needle not flexible Repuncture by contaminated needle possible	Infants and children Elderly and other adults with small veins Adults receiving short-term therapy
Over-the-needle	Easy to insert Stays patent longer Catheter tip tapered to prevent peelback Radiopaque feature makes radiographic detection easy Infiltration rare	Depending on the hub, sometimes difficult to secure with tape Long inflexible stylet increases the risk of accidental puncture; pressure marks from hub	Long-term therapy Delivery of viscous liquids: blood and total parenteral nutrition
	Winged cannula easy to tape Stable; allows for greater patient mobility	Some catheters drag through the skin on insertion Increased risk of phlebitis	Arterial monitoring
Through-the-needle	Permits insertion of catheter into the SVC Less likely to damage veins Stable	Needle remains secured outside the skin; risk of catheter embolus Plastic catheter may support infection or trigger phlebitis in central veins	Long-term therapy Delivery of viscous liquid Delivery of drugs Central venous pressure monitoring

Scalp-Vein Steel Needles

The wing-tipped or butterfly needles are types of scalp-vein steel needles. Scalp-vein needles are made of stainless steel with odd-numbered gauges (i.e., 17-, 19-, 21-, 23-, 25-) and lengths of 0.5 to 1.0 inch. The wings attached to the shaft are made of rubber or plastic, and the flexible tubing extending behind the wings varies from 3 to 12 inches long (Fig. 6–18).

These needles are most frequently used for short-term therapy, usually in patients with expected indwelling catheter times of less than 24 hours, such as with single-dose therapy, I.V. push medications, or blood sample retrieval (Perucca, 2001). Steel needles are biocompatible, and low rates of inflammation or phlebitis have been documented. Steel cannulas do not flex or yield with resistance; therefore, the steel tip can easily puncture the vasculature after placement, increasing the risk of infiltration.

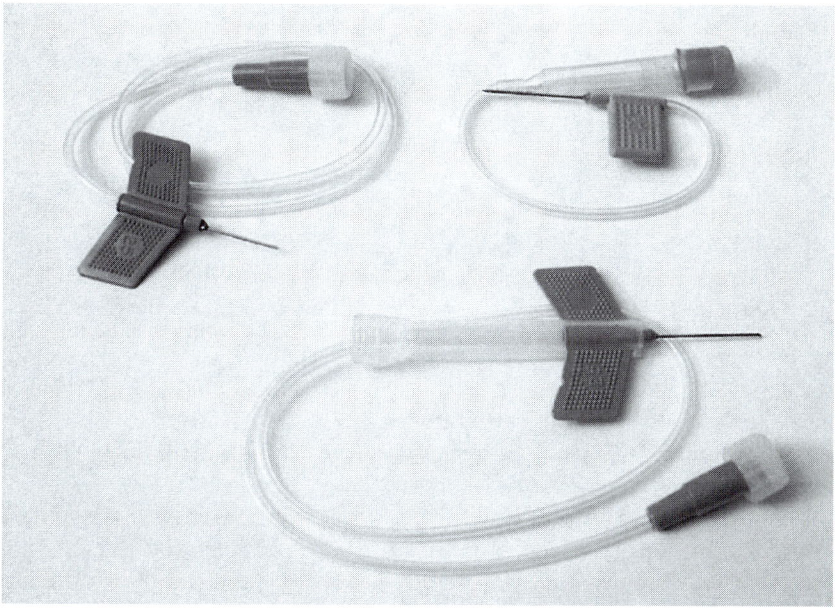

Figure 6–18 ■ Types of scalp vein needles. (Courtesy of Becton Dickinson, Franklin Lakes, NJ.)

INS Standard. Because stainless steel needles tend to dislodge and infiltrate more frequently than catheters, their use should be limited to short-term or single-dose administration. (INS, 2000, 44)

Over-the-Needle Catheters

The most widely used infusion device is the over-the-needle catheter (ONC), which consists of a needle with a catheter sheath (Fig. 6–19). The point of the needle extends beyond the tip of the catheter. After venipuncture, the needle (**stylet**) is withdrawn and discarded, leaving a flexible catheter within the vein. The cannula consists of a catheter with a length of 0.5 to 2.0 inches and gauges of even numbers ranging from 12 to 24. Use the following as a guide regarding when to use the different gauge catheters:

- 14- to 16-gauge: multiple trauma, heart surgery, transplantation procedures
- 18-gauge: major trauma or surgery, blood administration
- 20-gauge: minor trauma or surgery, blood administration
- 22-gauge: pediatric use, person with small veins, administration of platelets or plasma. (Avoid using 22-gauge catheters when administering packed red blood cells, whole blood, and antibiotic therapy.)

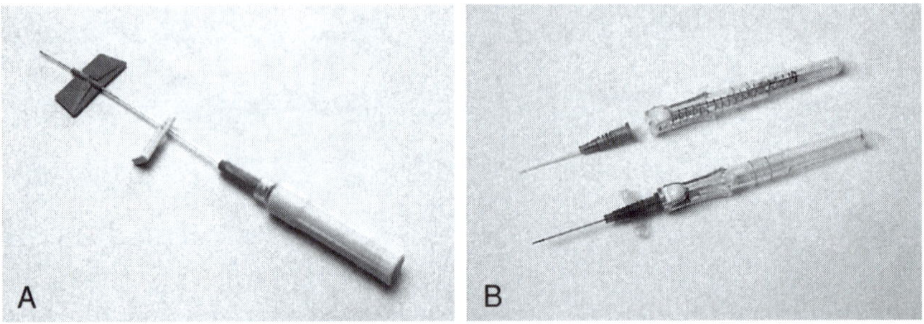

Figure 6–19 ■ Over-the-needle catheters. *(A)* Integrated I.V. catheter with safety shield SAF-T-INTIMA. *(B)* Insyte with safety shield. (Courtesy of Becton Dickinson, Franklin Lakes, NJ.)

Teflon over-the-needle catheters tend to increase the risk of infusion-related phlebitis with small peripheral venous catheters (Maki & Mermel, 1998).

Vialon, an elastomer of polyurethane, is a high-strength material that provides a smooth-surfaced catheter for easy insertion. After it is inside a vein, Vialon becomes soft and pliable, permitting the catheter to float in the vein rather than against the intima of the vein wall. Vialon is also designed to minimize local reactions under conditions of extended use.

INS Standard. Radiopaque over-the-needle catheters are recommended for routine infusion therapy. (INS, 2000, 44)

NURSING FAST FACT!

With any catheter, use the shortest length and the smallest gauge to deliver the ordered therapy. Also, use a vein large enough to sustain sufficient blood flow because this will decrease irritation to the vein wall.

Catheter Designs

THIN WALL

The thin-walled over-the-needle catheter is constructed of plastic and its thinner wall provides higher flow rates because of its larger internal lumen. Thin-walled catheters are smoother on insertion because they have a more tapered fit to the inner stylet. The thin-walled construction also causes the catheter to become less able to hold its shape once it is inserted and warmed to body temperature. This soft, "flimsy" catheter is easier on the intima of the vein but collapses with negative pressure.

FLASHBACK CHAMBERS

The flashback chamber is a small space at the hub of the stylet. When the stylet punctures the vein during catheter insertion, the increased pressure in the vein is immediately relieved into the catheter stylet with a flow of blood in the flashback chamber. This allows the nurse to see that the blood return is continuing as the catheter is advanced and secured. The safest catheters use a flashback chamber that allows the rapid return of blood but prohibits any blood spillage.

ADDITION OF WINGS

Adding wings to the design of I.V. catheters and scalp-vein needles is intended to improve insertion technique and catheter maintenance. The wings are usually flexible plastic protrusions from the hub of the device. Winged catheters provide more control when the after is manipulated, thereby preventing contamination.

COLOR CODING

The peripheral catheter hubs incorporate international color-coding standards. Universal color-coding standards allow visual recognition of the catheter gauge size. This standard has not been applied to gauge sizes of midline or central infusion catheters. The color codes are:

- Yellow: 22-gauge
- Pink: 20-gauge
- Green: 18-gauge
- Gray: 16-gauge

NURSING FAST FACT!

Looking at color-coding should never substitute for reading the package label.

Dual-Lumen Peripheral Catheters

The dual-lumen peripheral catheter is available in a range of catheter gauges with corresponding lumen sizes. Two totally separate infusion channels exist, making it possible to infuse two solutions simultaneously. They are available as 16-gauge catheters with 18- and 20-gauge lumens or as 18-gauge catheters with 20- and 22-gauge lumens. Dual-lumen catheters are also available as midlines.

NURSING FAST FACT!

Controversy still exists regarding simultaneous infusions of known incompatible solutions or medications through a dual-lumen peripheral catheter because of the limited hemodilution achievable in any peripheral vessel.

Through-the-Needle Catheters

A through-the-needle catheter (TNC) consists of a catheter between 14 and 19 gauges in diameter lying inside a needle. The needle may be from 1 to 2 inches long, and the catheter may be 8 to 36 inches long. The newer type of through-the-needle catheters, seen mainly in peripherally inserted central venous access devices, have a steel or plastic encasement that can be removed after the catheter is advanced into the vein. After the catheter is placed, the needle is withdrawn and secured outside the skin. Because the catheter is radiopaque, confirmation by radiographic examination can be done before administration of viscous solutions.

Midline Catheters

Any catheter placed between the antecubital area and the head of the clavicle is called a midline catheter. **Midline catheters** are designed for intermediate-term therapies of up to 28 days of isotonic or near-isotonic therapy. The catheters are 6 inches long and are made of elastomeric hydrogel. Approximately 2 hours after insertion, this type of catheter becomes 50 times softer, allowing it to increase 2 gauges in size and 2.5 cm in length. It is placed midline in the antecubital region in the basilic, cephalic, or median antecubital site and is then advanced into the larger vessels of the upper arm for greater hemodilution (Fig. 6–20).

Radiologic confirmation of the tip location is recommended in the following clinical situations:

- Difficulty with catheter advancement
- Pain or discomfort after catheter advancement
- Inability to obtain free-flowing blood return
- Inability to flush the catheter easily
- A guidewire that is difficult to remove or is bent after removal

INS Standard. The choice of catheter and appropriate nursing care for midline catheters should be established in organizational policy and procedure. (INS, 2000, 44)

NOTE > Guidelines for PICC and midline catheters are presented in Chapter 12.

Central Infusion Devices

Long-term I.V. therapy may require venous access over weeks, months, or even years. Special central venous catheters have been designed specifi-

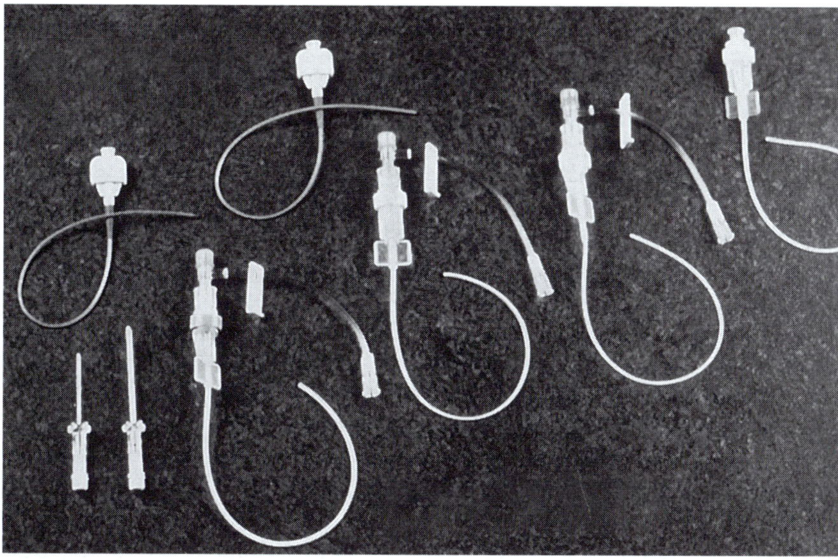

Figure 6–20 ■ Examples of midline catheters. (Courtesy of BARD Access Systems, Salt Lake City, UT.)

cally for long-term access, patient comfort, and decreased complications associated with multiple therapies. There are three general types of placement of central venous lines: centrally placed percutaneous catheters, central venous tunneled catheters, and implanted ports, all of which must be inserted by a physician, and peripherally inserted central catheters (PICCs), which can be inserted by a nurse specifically trained in their insertions.

Central catheters are made of soft, medical grade silicone elastomers, thermoplastic polyurethane, or PVC and are commercially available in many designs. Polyurethane catheters are the most commonly used catheters because of the material's versatility, malleability (tensile strength and elongation characteristics), and biocompatibility (Perucca, 2001).

NOTE > Additional information on central venous catheters is given in Chapter 12.

Central lines include:

- Percutaneous catheters
- Central venous tunneled catheters
- Implantable venous access ports
- PICCs

NOTE > Various types of central line catheters in use today are discussed in detail in Chapter 12.

Percutaneous Catheters

In 1961, the first I.V. catheter for accessing the central circulation was introduced (Stewart & Sanislow, 1961). The percutaneously inserted catheter may consist of polyurethane, a stiffer material, which makes the catheter easy to advance, allowing catheter insertion outside the operating room. The percutaneous catheter is placed by an infraclavicular approach through the subclavian vein (or the jugular or femoral vein) and secured by suturing. The final tip location should be in the superior vena cava (SVC). The catheter may remain in place for a few days to several weeks. This type of catheter provides access to larger venous circulation for the delivery of hypertonic solutions. These catheters can have single, double, triple, or quadruple lumena.

Central Venous Tunneled Catheters

Central venous **tunneled catheters** (CVTCs) are made of soft, medical grade silicone elastomers. CVTs have a Dacron cuff near the subcutaneous exit site of the catheter that anchors it in place, acts as a securing device, and serves as an antimicrobial barrier. CVTCs are surgically inserted through percutaneous cutdown under local or general anesthesia. The distal catheter tip is advanced into the vessel and is placed in the SVC. The proximal end is subcutaneously tunneled to an incisional exit site on the anterior or posterior trunk of the body. The usual exit sites for CVTCs are the mid- to lower thoracic or upper abdominal regions. Types of tunneled catheters include Broviac, Hickman, Raaf, and Groshong. These catheters are 20 to 30 inches long and have a 17- to 22-gauge internal lumen diameter. The thickness of the silicone wall varies by manufacturer. Silicone catheters can be single, dual, triple, or quadruple lumen (Fig. 6–21).

Implantable Venous Access Ports

The implantable venous access port is a completely closed system consisting of an implanted device with a drug reservoir, or port, with a self-sealing system connected to an outlet catheter. The device is surgically implanted into a convenient body site in a subcutaneous pocket. The self-sealing septum can withstand up to 2000 needle punctures. This device provides venous access for blood withdrawal, I.V. solution infusion, blood transfusion, and chemotherapy. The **implanted port** must be

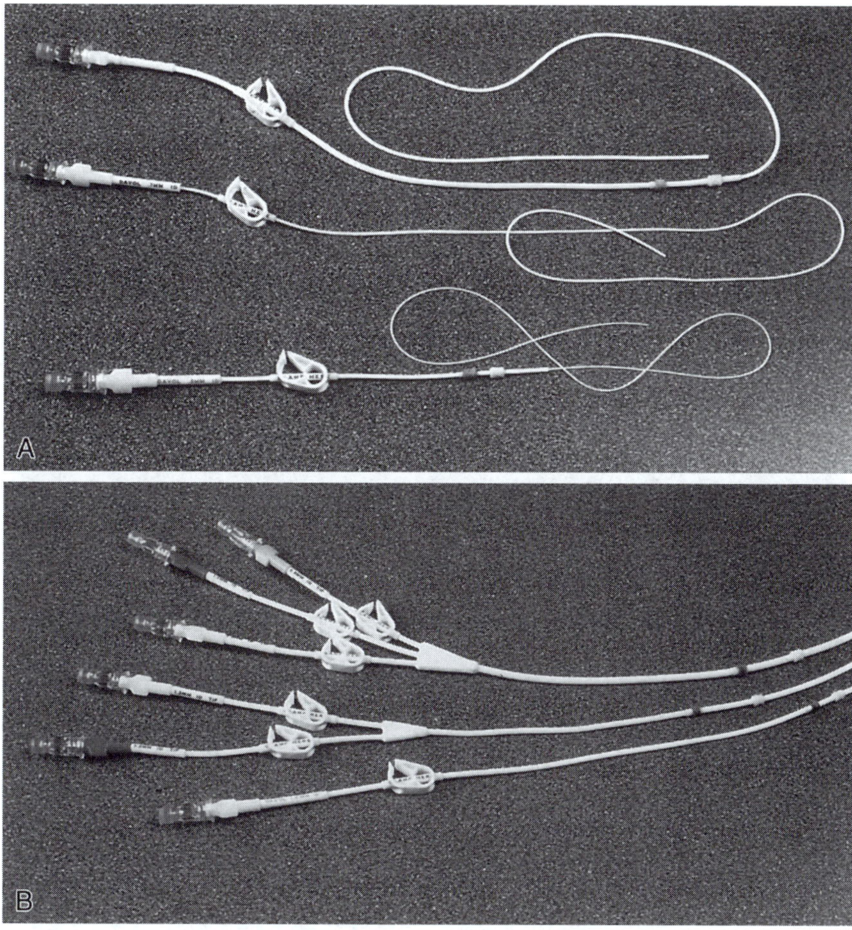

Figure 6–21 ■ *(A)* Hickman *(top)* and Broviac *(bottom two)* catheters. *(B)* Triple-lumen *(top)*, double-lumen *(middle)*, and single-lumen *(bottom)* central venous tunneled catheters.

accessed with a Huber needle (noncoring) for safe and proper penetration of the septum of the port. Because these are noncoring needles, they contribute to the long lifetime of the port. The needles are sized from 19 to 24 gauge and range from 1 to 2 inches in length. The needles are available in 90-degree or straight-needle designs (Fig. 6–22).

Peripherally Inserted Central Venous Catheters

A PICC is placed with tip location in the SVC. This catheter usually ranges from 16 to 26 gauges and from 20 to 24 inches in length. The peripheral

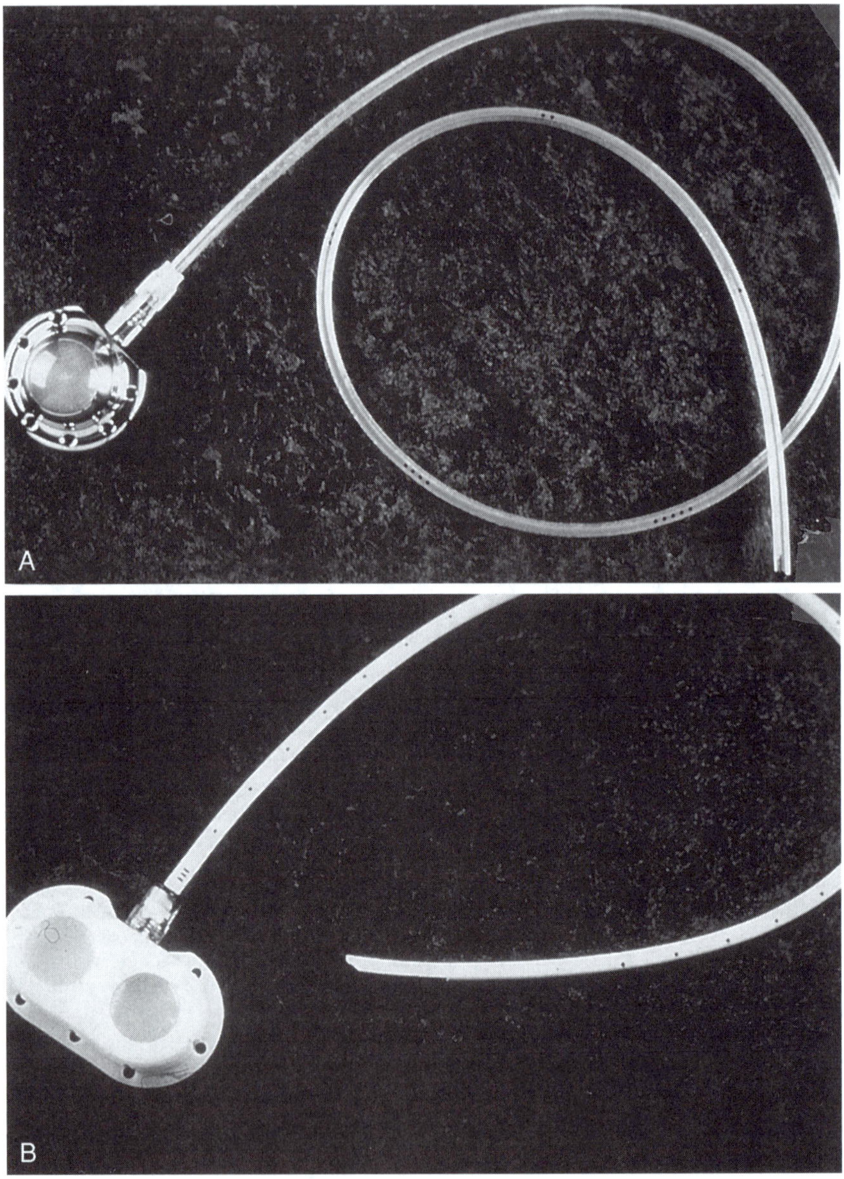

Figure 6–22 ■ *(A)* Dome port with Groshong valve. *(B)* MRI dual port. (Courtesy of BARD Access Systems, Salt Lake City, UT.)

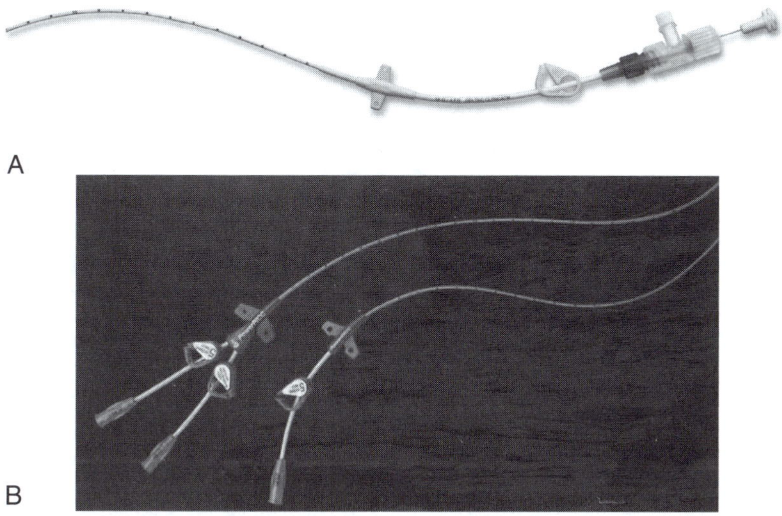

Figure 6–23 ■ Peripherally inserted central catheters (PICC). *(A)* CliniCath, single lumen. *(B)* PowerPicc.™

catheter is inserted into a peripheral site and advanced into the SVC. To reach the SVC in the average adult, a catheter at least 20 inches long is required. The catheter is made of silicone, which has proven reliability and biocompatibility over the years in central venous catheter application as well as a variety of implant uses. Silicone elastomer is soft, flexible, nonthrombogenic, and biocompatible (Fig. 6–23A). A new product is the PowerPicc™, which combines efficacy of PICC and maximum injection rates with a new bifurcation design, and easy to read labeling (Fig. 6–23B).

A PICC may be used to deliver all types of therapy. It is the appropriate choice for parenteral nutrition with dextrose content greater than 10 percent, continuous infusion of vesicant medications or medications with the ability to cause necrosis if they infiltrate, therapies with extreme variations in tonicity of pH, or anticipated extended I.V. therapy.

> **INS Standard.** The catheter selected for a PICC shall be a radiopaque catheter designed for central placement by peripheral access. The length of the catheter should be such that the tip resides in the SVC. (INS, 2000, 44)

Infusion Regulation Devices

Historically, infusion systems were regulated with a roller clamp, which the nurse adjusted manually with the roller or screw clamp on the admin-

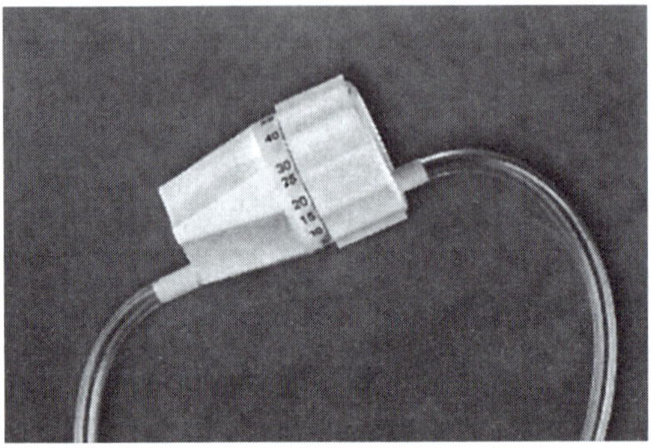

Figure 6–24 ■ Mechanical controller: Rate flow regulator. (Courtesy of B. Braun Medical Inc., Bethlehem, PA.)

istration set. Today numerous mechanical and electronic devices are available to assist nurses in maintaining an accurate infusion rate.

> **INS Standard.** A flow-control device is used to assist in regulating a prescribed administration rate. (INS, 2000, 39)

Mechanical Gravity Devices

Flow-regulating mechanisms that attach to the primary infusion administration sets are called mechanical gravity control devices (or mechanical controllers). They are manually set to deliver specified volumes of fluid per hour. They are available as dials, with clocklike faces, or a barrel-shaped device with cylindrical controls. Flow markings on the dials help to approximate the drops per minute, based on the set drop factor, but should be verified by counting the drops (Fig. 6–24).

> **INS Standard.** Manual flow-control devices should achieve accurate delivery of prescribed therapy with minimal deviation and are an adjunct to nursing care and are not intended to alleviate the nurse's responsibility for monitoring the flow rate of the therapy. (INS, 2000, 39)

Electronic Infusion Devices

The use of electronic infusion devices (EIDs) or flow-control devices should be guided by the patient's age and condition, setting, and prescribed therapy. These devices provide an accurate flow rate, are easy to use, and have alarms that signal problems with the infusion. However, hourly assessment, responsibility, and accountability for safe infusion still lie with the professional nurse. To use these devices effectively, the nurse should know: (1) indications for their use, (2) their mechanical operation, (3) how to troubleshoot, (4) their psi rating, and (5) safe usage guidelines.

Infusion control devices have come a long way since their introduction in 1958. The very early models had serious accuracy and safety problems: air embolisms, fluid containers that ran dry, and clogged catheters were common. The pumps were large, hard to troubleshoot, and limited in their reliability and usability.

IVAC Corporation introduced the concept of the rate controller in 1972; today there are many models and types on the market, including:

- Controllers
- Positive-pressure infusion pumps
- Volumetric pumps
- Peristaltic pumps
- Syringe pumps
- Patient-controlled analgesia (PCA) systems
- Multichannel and dual channel
- Ambulatory pumps
- Disposable pumps (elastomeric balloon pumps)

NURSING FAST FACT!

Because of the many controllers and volumetric and peristaltic pumps on the market, refer to the manufacturer's recommendations for troubleshooting guidelines for set up and of each EID.

INS Standard. EIDs shall be used when warranted by the patient's age, condition, setting, and prescribed therapy. The nurse is responsible and accountable for the use of the EID. (INS, 2000, 39)

Controllers

Controllers operate strictly on gravity flow and do not exert positive pressure greater than the head height of the infusion bag, which is usually 2 psi. Some controllers can reach a psi of 5, but this pressure is uncommon. The maximum flow rate is affected by how high the I.V. container is hung above the I.V. site. Controllers cannot detect infiltrations. After the I.V. catheter leaves the vein and infiltrates into the tissues, the pressure drops. Because the infusion device is "looking" for pressure to signal an infiltration, it may be a long time with significant fluid accumulation before the infuser actually detects infiltration. It is always best to recommend that the nurse monitor the infusion visually and not rely on the infusion device to detect infiltrations.

NURSING FAST FACT!

One psi and 50 mm Hg exert the same amount of pressure.

A drop sensor and electric feedback mechanism regulate the gravity flow of the fluid. Controllers reduce the potential for rapid infusion of large amounts of solution (runaways) and empty bottles. Controllers assist the nurse in detecting infiltrations and maintaining accurate flow rates. It is estimated that 80 percent of I.V. fluid and drug administration can safely be regulated by the use of a controller.

The I.V. bag is usually hung 36 inches above a patient's head for adequate gravity pressure. When there is resistance to the flow, the controller's alarm will sound, signaling that it cannot maintain the preset rate. Resistance can occur when the patient is restless and frequently changing positions, if the catheter tip is at a flexion point, or if the patient lies on the tubing. Many of the newer controllers can deliver blood components safely.

Positive-Pressure Infusion Pumps

Positive-pressure infusion pumps average 10 psi, with up to 15 psi considered to be safe, although newer technology has the psi set as low as 0.1 psi. Older pumps still in use may pump at dangerous pressures of 16 to 22 psi. Pressures greater than 15 to 20 psi should be used with extreme caution.

Positive-pressure infusion pumps are used for delivering high volumes and complex therapies in high-acuity situations. The pumps are more precise than controllers; accurately deliver the fluid as programmed; and have many features, such as the ability to keep track of fluid amounts and to sound alarms for various malfunctions. These pumps totally control the flow rate (Fig. 6–25).

NURSING FAST FACT!

All positive pressure pumps should have an "anti–free-flow" alarm to prevent inadvertent free-flowing solution.

Volumetric Pumps

Volumetric pumps calculate the volume delivered by measuring the volume displaced in a reservoir that is part of the disposable administration set. The pump calculates every fill and empty cycle of the reservoir. The reservoir is manipulated internally by a specific action of the pump. The industry standard for the accuracy of electronic volumetric infusion pumps is plus or minus 5 percent (Perucca, 2001).

Pressure terminology includes the terms "fixed" and "variable." With fixed infusion pressure, the pump is set internally to infuse up to a certain psi but not more (occlusion limit). Variable-pressure pumps allow individual judgment about the psi needed to safely deliver therapy. Nurses can adjust a variable-pressure pump through programming. Variable-

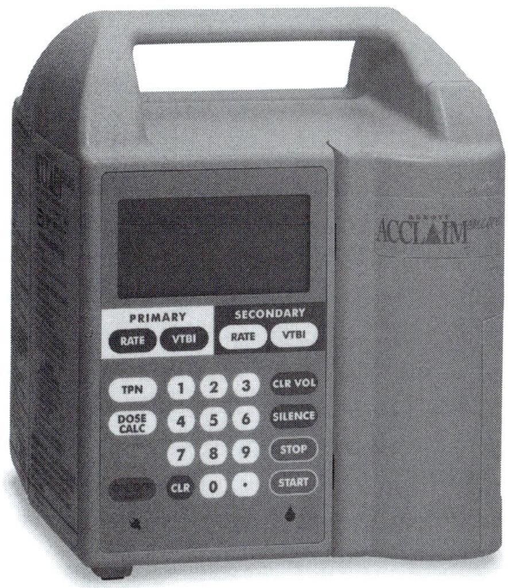

Figure 6–25 ■ Infusion pump: ACCLAIM Encore pump. (Courtesy of Abbott Laboratories, North Chicago, IL.)

pressure devices have a conservative upper limit (usually 10 psi) and a lower limit of 2 psi similar to that of a controller. A psi setting of 4 to 8 is common.

Volumetric pumps have proved invaluable in neonatal, pediatric, and adult intensive care units, where critical infusions of small volumes of fluid or doses of high-potency drugs are indicated. A cartridge pumps the solution to be delivered; therefore, blood and red blood cells can be administered without damage to the blood cells.

Many pumps use microprocessor technology for a more compact unit and for easier troubleshooting. All volumetric pumps require special tubing.

NURSING FAST FACT!

To ensure safe, efficient operation, review the literature that accompanies the pump to become familiar with the operation of the pump. Observe all precautions.

Peristaltic Pumps

Peristaltic refers to the controlling mechanisms: a peristaltic device moves fluid by intermittently squeezing the I.V. tubing. The device may be rotary or linear. In a rotary peristaltic pump, a rotating disk or series of rollers compresses the tubing along a curved or semicircular chamber, propelling the fluid when pressure is released. In a linear device, one or more projections intermittently press the I.V. tubing. Peristaltic pumps are used primarily for the infusion of enteral feedings.

Syringe Pumps

Syringe pumps are piston-driven infusion pumps that provide precise infusion by controlling the rate by drive speed and syringe size, thus eliminating the variables of the drop rate. Syringe pumps are valuable for critical infusions of small doses of high-potency drugs. A lead, screw motor-driven system pushes the plunger to deliver fluid or medication at a rate of 0.01 to 99.9 mL/h. It is a precisely accurate delivery system that can be used to administer very small volumes. Some models have program modes capable of administration in mg/kg per minute, mcg/min, and mL/h. The syringe is usually filled in the pharmacy and stored until used.

These pumps are used most frequently for delivery of antibiotics and small-volume parenteral therapy. Syringe pump technology was applied to PCA infusion devices. Syringe pumps are used frequently in the areas of anesthesia, oncology, and obstetrics.

The volume of the syringe pump is limited to the size of the syringe; a 60-mL syringe is usually used. However, the syringe can be as small as 5 mL. The tubing usually is a single, uninterrupted length of kink-resistant tubing with a notable lack of Y injection ports. Syringe pumps can use primary or secondary sets, depending on the intended use (Perucca, 2001) (Fig. 6–26A, B).

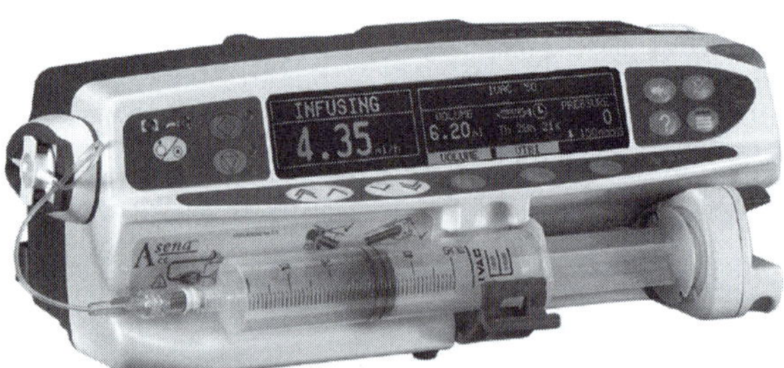

A

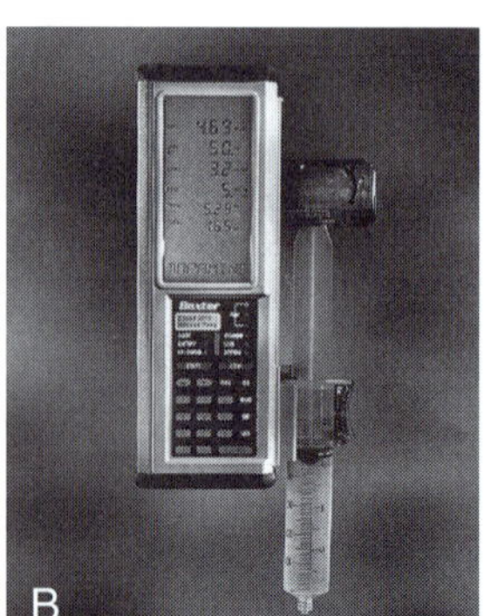

B

Figure 6–26 ■ Syringe pumps. *(A)* The ASENA CC syringe pump. (Courtesy of Alaris Medical Systems, San Diego, CA.) *(B)* Autosyringe AS50 infusion pump. (Courtesy of Baxter International Inc., Round Lake, IL.)

Patient-Controlled Analgesia Pumps

Patient-controlled analgesia pumps have been developed to assist patients in controlling their pain at home or in the hospital. PCA pumps can be used to deliver medication through I.V., epidural, or subcutaneous routes. These pumps are different from other infusion devices in that they have a remote bolus control in which the patient or nurse can deliver a bolus of medication at set intervals. PCA pumps are available in ambulatory or pole-mounted models.

There are three types of PCA pumps: basal, continuous, and demand. All three afford some type of pain control with varying degrees of patient interaction.

- The basal mode is designed to achieve pain relief with minimal medication with intermittent dosing, thus allowing the patient to remain alert and active without sedation.
- The continuous mode of therapy is designed for patients who need maximum pain relief; it usually does not fluctuate from hour to hour and should completely relieve pain or achieve a constant effect.
- The demand mode dose is delivered by intermittent infusion when a button attached to the pump is pushed. The demand dose can be used alone or with the basal type of infusion.

NURSING FAST FACT!

Patient-controlled analgesia pumps must be programmed with parameters to prevent overmedication. These pumps are designed with a special key or locking device for security of the medications.

INS Standard. Nurses should be knowledgeable about the preparation and use of the PCA devices, including programming the device to deliver prescribed therapy, administration and maintenance procedures, and the use of lock-out devices. In addition, nurses should have knowledge of the pharmacologic implications of the medication, monitor the patient for therapeutic response, recognize untoward responses, implement nursing interventions as required, and document in the medical record. (INS, 2000, 72)

Multichannel and Dual-Channel Pumps

Multiple-drug delivery systems are computer generated, and many use computer-generated technology. Multichannel and dual-channel pumps can deliver several medications and fluids simultaneously or intermittently from bags, bottles, or syringes. Multichannel pumps (usually with three or four channels) require manifold-type sets to set up all channels,

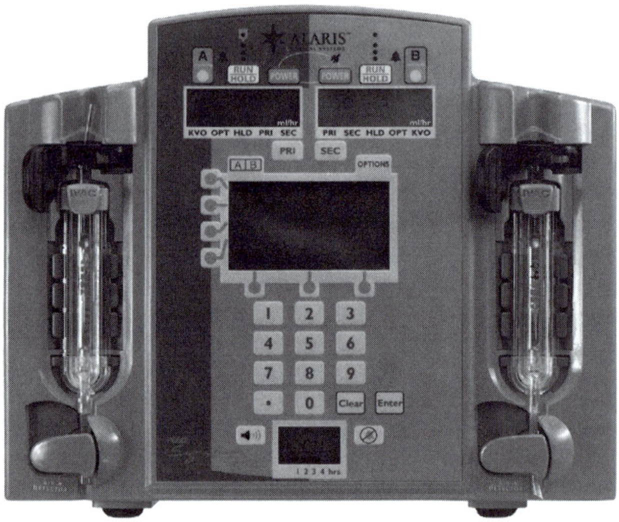

Figure 6–27 ■ Dual channel infusion system. (Courtesy of Alaris Medical Systems, San Diego, CA.)

whether or not they are in use; each channel must be programmed independently. Programming a multichannel pump can be challenging (Fig. 6–27).

Dual-channel pumps offer a two-pump mechanism assembly, with a common control and programming panel. This type of pump uses one administration set for each channel.

Ambulatory Pumps

Ambulatory pumps are lightweight, compact infusion pumps. These have made a significant breakthrough in long-term care. This device allows the patient freedom to resume a normal life. Ambulatory pumps range in size and weight; most weigh less than 6 lb and are capable of delivering most infusion therapies. Features include medication delivery, delivery of several different dose sizes at different intervals, memory of programs, and safety alarms. The main disadvantage of ambulatory pumps is limited power supply; they function on a battery system that requires frequent recharging (Fig. 6–28).

New Technology

Medication Safety Systems

Newer pumps are available with modular point-of-care platforms that integrate infusion, patient monitoring, and clinical best practice guidelines for optimal outcomes (Fig. 6–29).

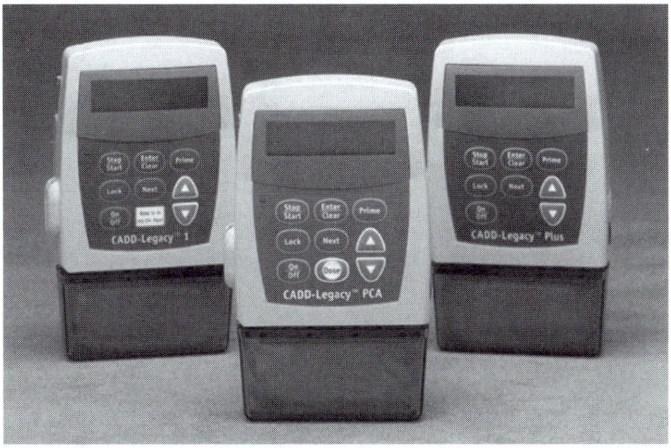

Figure 6–28 ■ Ambulatory pumps. CADD Legacy system. (Courtesy of Deltec, Inc., St. Paul, MN.)

Website

Alaris Medical Systems: *www.alarismed.com*

Medication safety systems in modular form are available to prevent medication errors (Figs. 6–30 and 6–31).

Fluid Removal System

The System 100 Fluid Removal System (CHF Solutions) is a mechanical pump and ultrafiltration system engineered to remove excess fluid from patients with fluid-overload via peripheral access. This pump can remove 2 to 3 L of excess fluid from the blood stream in 4 to 8 hours.

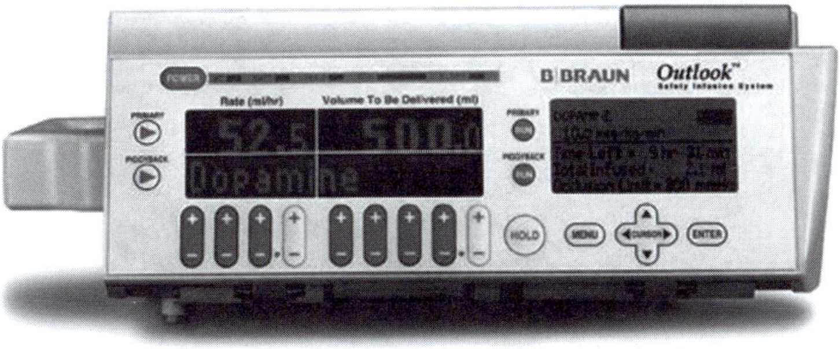

Figure 6–29 ■ Infusion pump with I.V. safety systems: Dose Scan and Dose Guard barcoding. Horizon Outlook. (Courtesy of B. Braun Medical Inc., Bethlehem, PA.)

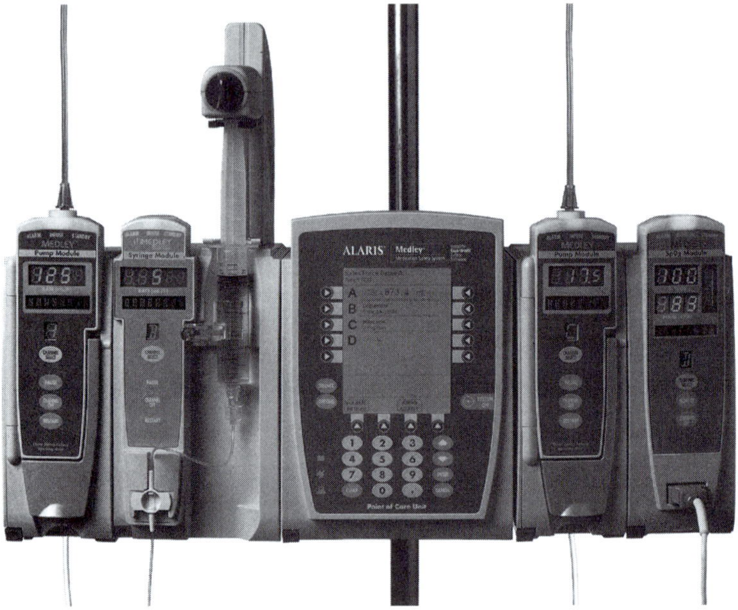

Figure 6–30 ■ Medication safety system: Modular point-of-care computer. Medley medication safety system. (Courtesy of Alaris Medical Systems, San Diego, CA.)

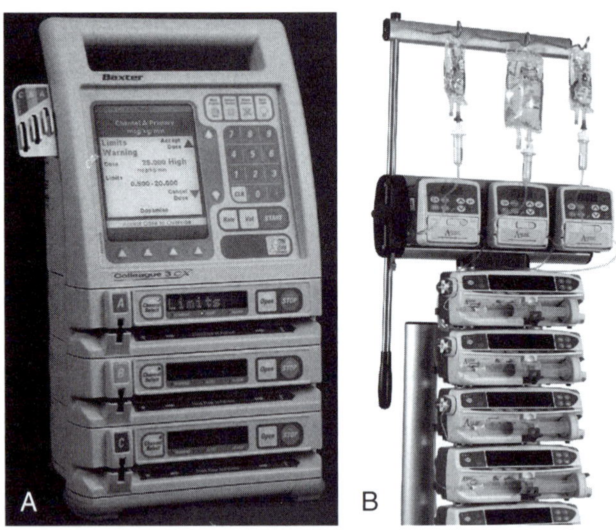

Figure 6–31 ■ Multichannel pumps. *(A)* Colleague CX volumetric infusion pump. (Courtesy of Baxter International Inc., Round Lake, IL.) *(B)* The ASENA infusion system with docking station. Volumetric pump and choice of syringe pumps. (Courtesy of Alaris Medical Systems, San Diego, CA.)

Website

CHF Solutions: *www.chfsolutions.com*

Disposable Pumps

The elastomeric balloon pump system is a portable device with an elastomeric reservoir, or balloon, that works on flow restrictions. The balloon, which is made of a soft rubberized material capable of being inflated to a predetermined volume, is safely encapsulated inside a rigid, transparent container. When the reservoir is filled, the balloon exerts positive pressure to administer the medication with an integrated flow restrictor that controls the flow rate. This system requires no batteries or electronic programming and is not reusable (Fig. 6–32).

Elastomeric balloon devices are used primarily for the delivery of antibiotics. The typical volume for these devices is 50 to 100 mL, but these balloons are available in sizes up to 250 mL.

Programming Electronic Infusion Devices

To be able to program any type EID, one needs to be familiar with the terminology for delivering infusion and the device enhancements, including alarms.

Infusion Terminology

- *Rate:* Amount of time over which a specific volume of fluid is delivered. Infusion pumps deliver in increments of milliliters per hour. The most common rate parameters for regular infusion pumps are 1 to 999 mL/h. Many newer pumps are capable of setting rates that offer parameters of 0.1 mL in increments of 0.1 to 99.9 mL, then in 1-mL increments up to 999 mL. Many newer pumps are capable of setting rates that satisfy both regular infusion and microinfusion needs. Better-quality pumps that offer combination rates do not allow the rate to be set above 99.9 without a deliberate act to enter the adult values.
- *Volume infused:* Measurement that tells how much of a given solution has been infused. This measurement is used to monitor the amount of fluid infused in a shift. It can also be used in home health to monitor the infusion periodically during the day or over several days. The "counter" must be returned to 0 at the beginning of each shift.
- *Volume to be infused:* Usually the amount of solution hanging in the solution container. A pump is designed to sound an alarm when the volume to be infused is reached.
- *Tapering or ramping:* These are terms that are used to describe the progressive increase or decrease of the infusion rate. Pumps that will increase or taper infusion rates are gaining popularity. The

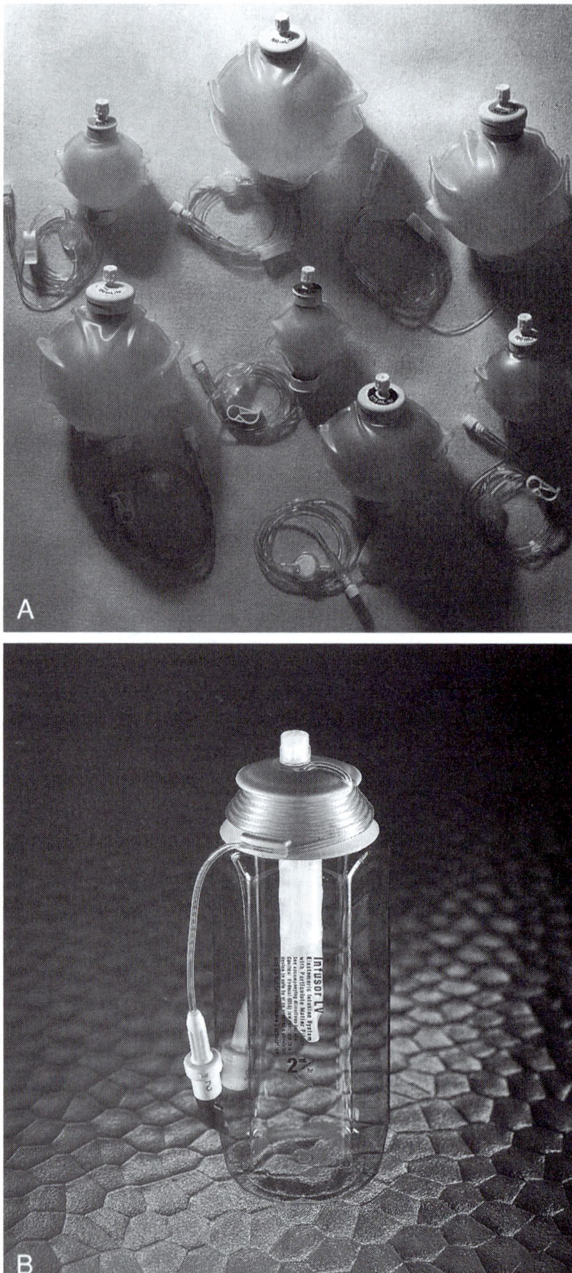

Figure 6–32 ■ Small-volume infusion pumps. *(A)* Eclipse elastomeric pumps come in a variety of sizes ranging in volume from 50 to 500 mL. (Courtesy of B. Braun Medical Inc., Bethlehem, PA.) *(B)* Infusor LV system. (Courtesy of Baxter Interantional Inc., Round Lake, IL.)

pump can use its own program to mathematically calculate the ramping rate once the duration of infusion and total volume to be infused is given.

- *Timed infusion:* This refers to an infusion governed by a 24-hour clock within the device. With times infusion, the device must have a sufficient internal back-up battery to maintain the clock accurately at all times. Timed-infusions are used for ramping and tapering, automatic piggybacking, and intermittent doing.

Enhancement Terminology

- *Drop sensors:* Used with a controller to confirm the presence or absence of flow. The drop sensor is attached to the drop chamber of the administration set or can be located internally on the controller as the flow passes through a chamber.

NURSING FAST FACT!

The drop chamber must remain still to ensure that the counter senses or detects each drop as it falls. Splashing or multiple drops result in sudden rate changes.

Alarm Terminology

- *Air-in-line:* Designed to detect only visible bubbles or microscopic bubbles. This alarm is necessary for all positive-pressure pumps and infusion controllers. Volumetric pumps are usually equipped with air-in-line detectors.
- *Occlusion:* Standard alarm for infusion devices. Controllers may be able to indicate only "no flow." With an occlusion alarm, controllers are able to indicate upstream (between pump and container) or downstream (between patient and pump) occlusion by absence of flow. Many newer pumps are able to differentiate between upstream (or proximal) and downstream (or distal) occlusions. This is often detected by changes in pressure.

NURSING FAST FACT!

In a number of EIDs, the pressure is "user" selectable from 0.10 to 10 psi. Occlusion alarms at low psi settings are common because the pumps are sensitive to even slight changes in pressure and very small I.V. catheter or patient movement. Many of the current EIDs infuse fluids using very low infusion pressures, often lower than the pressure of a gravity delivery. These devices are not, however, designed to detect infiltrations. When an infiltration occurs, the inline pressure may actually drop; therefore, the EID will not detect the infiltration. Visual monitoring of the I.V. site by a professional nurse is mandatory for patients with EIDs.

- *Infusion complete:* Alarm triggered by a preset volume limit ("infusion complete"). These alarms are helpful in preventing the fluid container from running dry because they can be set to sound before the entire solution container is infused.
- *Low battery or low power:* Gives the user ample warning of the pump's impending inability to function. A low-battery alarm means that the batteries need to be replaced or external power source needs to be connected. As a protective measure, when low-battery and low-power alarms are continued over a preset number of minutes, the pumps usually convert to a keep-vein-open (KVO) rate. The preset KVO rate is usually between 0.1 and 5 mL.
- *Nonfunctional or malfunctional:* Alarm that means the pump is operating outside parameters and the problem cannot be resolved. When this alarm sounds, the pump should be disconnected from the patient and returned to biomedical engineering or to the manufacturer for evaluation. The alert signifying a nonfunctional alarm may be worded in many ways, depending on the manufacturer.
- *Not infusing:* Indicates that all of the pump infusion parameters are not set. This feature prevents tampering or setting changes from happening accidentally. The pump must be programmed or changed and then told to "start."
- *Parameters or timed-out:* Reminds the programmer that all settings have not been completed.
- *Tubing:* Used generally with controllers. Ensures that the correct tubing has been loaded into the pump. If tubing is incorrectly loaded, this alarm will also sound.
- *Door:* Indicates that the door that secures the tubing is not closed. Cassette pumps may give a "cassette" alarm if the cassette is unable to infuse within device operating parameters.
- *Free flow:* Detects the rapid infusion of fluid, which can occur when the set is removed from the pump. Disengaging the tubing from the pump requires a deliberate act. Most newer devices have free-flow protection, meaning that when the door is opened accidentally, there should be no fluid flow to the patient without nurse intervention.

Additional Electronic Infusion Device Enhancements

Many other functions have been added to newer pumps. These include:

- Preprogrammed drug compatibility
- Retrievable patient history data
- Infiltration or thrombus detection alarm
- Central venous pressure monitor
- Positive pressure fill stroke
- Modular self-diagnosing capability
- Printer read-out
- Nurse call system

- Remote site programming
- Syringe use for secondary infusion
- Adjustable occlusion pressures
- Opaque infusions (for blood, fat emulsions, iron dextran)
- Secondary rate settings
- Lock level for security
- Barcoding

NOTE > See Appendix A for a Summary of Recommendations from the CDC (2002) on Procedures for Maintenance of Intravascular Catheters, Administration Sets, and Parenteral Fluids.

NURSING PLAN OF CARE

PATIENTS RECEIVING PERIPHERAL I.V. THERAPY

Focus Assessment

Subjective

- Knowledge of therapies and equipment used to deliver therapy

Objective

- Suitable vascular access device for length and type of therapy
- Adequate level of consciousness and compliance

Patient Outcome/Evaluation Criteria

Patient will:

- Demonstrate appropriate technique or procedures for self care.
- Be free of injury and complications associated with I.V. therapy.

Nursing Diagnoses

- Risk for injury related to environmental conditions, lack of knowledge regarding equipment
- Knowledge deficit related to new procedure and maintaining I.V. therapy
- Impaired physical mobility related to placement and maintenance of I.V. cannula
- Anxiety (mild, moderate, or severe) related to new equipment technology
- Ineffective management of therapeutic regimen individual related to noncompliance (cost)

(Continued on following page)

NURSING PLAN OF CARE

PATIENTS RECEIVING PERIPHERAL I.V. THERAPY *(Continued)*

Nursing Management

1. Monitor to patient for:
   a. breaks in the integrity of the infusion equipment
   b. patient's knowledge of equipment
2. Help the patient and/or family identify potential areas of conflict; cultural mores, or cost
3. Follow the manufacturer's guidelines on the setup and maintenance of specific EIDs.
4. Select and prepare infusion pumps as indicated.
5. Correct any malfunctioning equipment.
6. Plug equipment into electrical outlets connected to an emergency power source.
7. Have equipment periodically checked by bioengineers as appropriate.
8. Set alarm limits on equipment as appropriate.
9. Respond to equipment alarms appropriately.
10. Consult with other healthcare team members and recommend equipment and devices for patient use.
11. Compare machine-derived data with nurse's perception of patient's condition.
12. Explain potential risks and benefits of using equipment technology.
13. Follow INS Standards of Practice in rotation of I.V. sites, fluid container, administration set, and dressing changes.
14. Maintain integrity of the infusion site, and equipment at all times.
15. Use filters when appropriate.
16. Use appropriate administration set (vented or nonvented) with the appropriate fluid container.
17. Inspect fluid containers, administration sets, and cannulas for integrity before use.

Patient Education

- Instruct the patient by demonstrating the preparation and administration of therapy.
- Teach the patient and family how to operate equipment, as appropriate.
- Advise the patient regarding pump alarms and advise him or her to contact the nurse if the alarm is triggered.
- Instruct the patient and family on the use of PCA pumps for pain control.

(Continued on following page)

- Teach the patient and family the expected patient outcomes and side effects associated with using the equipment.
- Document the patient's and family's understanding of the education provided to them.

Home Care Issues

Reimbursement is a challenge in the home care setting. Before any equipment is acquired, the reimbursement status of the clientele served and the anticipated need should be thoroughly explored (Perucca, 2001).

Home care infusion devices are designed to allow the patient maximum portability and freedom of movement. The aim is for small, quiet, lightweight infusion pumps with pouches to enclose the infusion container. Equipment used at home must offer safety features because the caregiver in most situations is the patient or family.

Equipment used frequently in home care management includes:

- Medical teaching dolls (Legacy Products): Facilitate visual, hands-on approach to educate patients of all ages and families about vascular access site, equipment, and procedures
- Vascular access devices: Easy to administer medication by home healthcare professional, patient, or family
- Tubing, connectors, and filters: Include needleless systems for use in home to prevent needlestick injuries
- EIDs: Syringe pumps, elastomeric infusers, ambulatory pumps
- Premixed medications
- Transport storage pouch

Key Points

- Types of infusion delivery systems include glass and plastic (rigid and flexible).
- Check all solutions for clarity and expiration date. Squeeze to check for leaks, floating particles, and clarity.
- Concerns over PVC and DEHP: The plasticizer phthalate (DEHP) is added to many I.V. products for flexibility. EPA warns that PVC leaches into I.V. solutions and toxic absorption can occur. Many new products on market without DEHP.
- Administration sets
  - Single-line sets: Most frequently used; follow INS standards for frequency of set changes. Available in vented and nonvented sets.
  - Primary (standard) set, volume-controlled sets
  - Primary Y sets: Most often used with blood components
  - Pump-specific sets: Used with EIDs

- Lipid administration sets: Used with fat emulsion, which are supplied in glass containers with special vented tubing
- Nitroglycerin administration sets

- Filters
  - Inline I.V. solution filters
  - Depth: Filters in which pore size is not uniform
  - Membrane (screen): Air-venting, bacteria-retentive, 0.22-micron filter
  - Blood filters
  - Standard clot: 170 to 220 microns; used on blood administration sets to remove coagulated products, microclots, and debris
  - Microaggregate: 20, 40, and 80 microns; can be added to an in-use blood administration set, permitting infusion of blood, and easy replacement of the filter for delivery of multiple units
  - Leukocyte depletion: Used to remove 95 to 99.9 percent of leukocytes from red blood cells
- Adaptors and connectors
  - J-, U-, or T-shaped ports that are used at the injection site. Add-on devices add length for manipulation. Add-on devices are used only when an integral system is not available to deliver the prescribed therapy.
- Stopcocks
  - Control the direction of flow of an infusate through manual manipulation of a direction regulation valve
- Resealable locks (PRN device)
  - Attach to hub of catheter and convert the cannula into an intermittent device
- Needleless systems
  - State-of-the-art technology to replace needles to connect I.V. devices and administer infusates
- Peripheral infusion devices
  - Scalp vein needles: For short-term therapy; odd-numbered gauges
  - Over-the-needle catheters: For peripheral therapy, made from Teflon, Vialon; even-numbered gauges
  - Through-the-needle catheters: Example is a PICC
  - Midline catheters: 6 inches long; indwelling time, 28 days
- Central infusion devices
  - Percutaneous catheters
  - Central venous tunneled catheters (CVTCs)
  - Implantable ports: Closed system composed of implanted device with reservoir, port, and self-sealing system; require the use of a noncoring needle to access port
  - Peripherally inserted central catheters (PICCs): Inserted peripherally and threaded to the SVC; can be placed by physicians, nurses, or nurse practitioners
- Infusion regulation devices
  - EIDs

- Controller: Used in 80 percent of situations requiring rate control device; gravity-dependent; many are nonvolumetric; some volumetric controllers available with peristaltic action
- Pumps
  - Volumetric: Calibrated in milliliters per hour; require special cassette or cartridge to be used with the machine, very accurate, and used in delivery of high-potency drugs or when accuracy is imperative
  - Peristaltic: Calibrated in milliliters per hour; used primarily for delivery of enteral feedings; have a rotary disk or rollers to compress tubing
  - Syringe: Piston-driven pump that controls rate of infusion by drive speed and syringe size
  - Patient-controlled analgesia (PCA): Can be used at home or in hospital to deliver pain medication
  - Ambulatory infusion: Lightweight, compact infusion pumps
  - Elastomeric balloons: Portable device designed with an elastomeric reservoir for delivery of medication

Critical Thinking: Case Study

A pediatric client is admitted to the unit with pneumonia. A peripheral I.V. is ordered. What equipment would you choose for this infusion and why? What safety factors would you consider? What education would you provide the parents?

Media Link: The answers to this case study and other critical thinking activities are on the enclosed CD–ROM.

Post-Test

In **1** through **5**, match the term in Column I with the definition in Column II.

Column I	**Column II**
1. Cannula	**a.** A female connection point of an I.V. cannula where the tubing or other equipment attaches
2. Drip chamber	**b.** Point of entry
3. Lumen	**c.** Area of the I.V. tubing usually found under the spike where the solution drips and collects
4. Hub	**d.** Space within an artery, vein, or catheter
5. Port	**e.** A tube or sheath used for infusing fluids

6. When using a flexible plastic system, what type of administration set could you choose?
   a. Vented
   b. Nonvented
   c. Vented or nonvented; both work with this system
7. A 0.22-micron filter should be used when:
   a. An additive has been combined with the solution
   b. The patient is susceptible to infusion phlebitis
   c. The infusion is delivered by the central route
   d. All of the above
8. The standard blood administration set has a clot filter of how many microns?
   a. 170
   b. 40
   c. 20
   d. 10
9. Microaggregate filters are used for:
   a. Administration of protein solutions
   b. Administration of whole blood and packed cells stored more than 5 days
   c. Removal of bacteria for infusion
   d. Filtering air from the set
10. A disadvantage of the glass system is that it:
    a. Is breakable and difficult to store
    b. Reacts with some solutions and medications
    c. May be difficult to read fluid levels
    d. May develop leaks

Media Link: Use the CD–ROM enclosed with this text for more practice test questions and answers along with rationales.

References

American Association of Blood Banks (2002). *Technical Manual* (14th ed.). Bethesda, MD: AABB.

B. Braun Medical Inc. (1999). Is the IV container as important as the solution being infused? Intravenous Nurses Society Annual Conference. Charlotte, NC, May 3–5.

HealthCare Without Harm (1999). Citizen petition for a food and drug administration regulation or guideline to label medical devices that leach phthalate plasticizers and to establish a program to promote alternative. *www.noharm.org* (available June 14, 1999).

Intravenous Nursing Society (1997). Position paper: Midline and midclavicular catheters. *Journal of Intravenous Nursing,* 20(4), 175–178.

Intravenous Nursing Society (2000). Intravenous Nursing Standards of Practice. *Journal of Intravenous Nursing,* 21, S35–44, 72.

Kaplan, L.K. (1999). Vinyl debate heats up. *Infusion* (Newsline), 5(8), 6, 10.

Maki D.G., & Mermel L.A. (1998). Infection due to infusion therapy. In Bennett, J.V., & Brachman, P.S. (eds.). *Hospital Infections* (4th ed.). Philadelphia: Lippincott-Raven, p 690.

Menitove J. (ed.) (1999). *Standards for Blood Banks and Transfusion Services* (19th ed.). Arlington, VA: American Association of Blood Banks.

Pall Biomedial Corporation (2000). New York, NY: Pall Biomedical Products Corporation.

NIOSH (2000). *NIOSH Alert: Preventing Needlestick Injuries in Health Care Settings.* Publication No. 2000–108. Washington, DC: Centers for Disease Control and Prevention.

Perucca, R. (2001). Intravenous therapy equipment. In Hankins, J., Lonsway, R.A., Hedrick, C., & Perdue, M. (eds.). *Intravenous Therapy: Clinical Principles and Practice* (2nd ed.). Philadelphia: W.B. Saunders, pp. 300–334.

Schiff, L. (2001). IV administration sets. *RN* 11(64), 61.

Trissel, L.A. (2000). *Handbook on Injectable Drugs* (11th ed.). Bethesda, MD: American Society of Health-System Pharmacists.

U.S. Centers for Disease Control and Prevention (2002). Guideline for prevention of intravascular catheter related infections. *MMWR Morbidity and Mortality Weekly Report,* 51, RR-10.

U.S. Food and Drug Administration (1995). Supplement guidance on the content of premarket notification submissions for medical devices with sharps injury prevention features. Rockville, MD: U.S. Food and Drug Administration.

Answers to Chapter 6 Post-Test

1. **e**
2. **c**
3. **d**
4. **a**
5. **b**
6. **c**
7. **d**
8. **a**
9. **b**
10. **a**

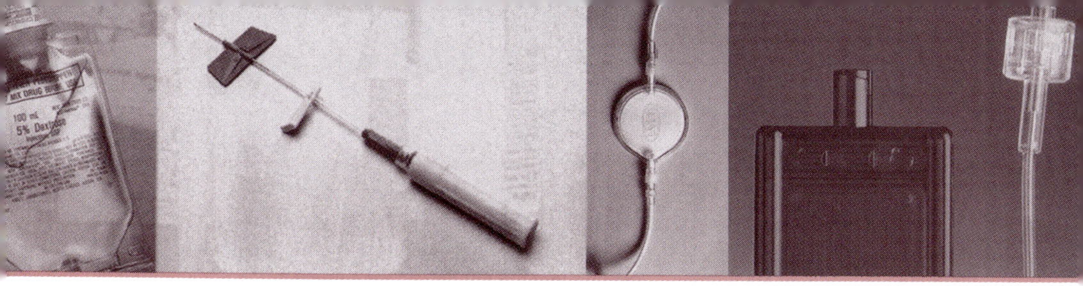

Chapter 7
Techniques for Peripheral Intravenous Therapy

Challenges make you discover things about yourself that you really never knew. They're what make the instrument stretch—what make you go beyond the norm.

—Cicely Tyson, American Actress

Chapter Contents

LEARNING OBJECTIVES

Upon completion of this chapter, the reader will be able to:

1. Define the terminology related to venous access.
2. Recall the anatomy and physiology related to the venous system.
3. Identify the five tissue structures that the infusion nurse must penetrate for a successful venipuncture.
4. Identify the peripheral veins appropriate for venipuncture.
5. List the factors affecting site selection.
6. Demonstrate Phillips' 15-step approach for initiating I.V. therapy.
7. List the sites appropriate for labeling.
8. Identify the key components of the documentation process for peripheral I.V. therapy.
9. State the Infusion Nursing Standards of Practice for peripheral infusions.
10. Recall the steps in performing a saline lock flush.
11. Describe the advantages and disadvantages of resealable locking devices.
12. Identify the uses of lidocaine and topical creams for initiating I.V. therapy.
13. Calculate drops per minute using varied drop-factor tubing.
14. Apply the nursing process to care of individuals receiving I.V. therapy.

GLOSSARY

Antimicrobial An agent that destroys or prevents the development of microorganisms

Bevel Slanted edge on opening of a needle or cannula device

Cannula Hollow plastic tube used for accessing the vascular system

Dermis The corium layer of the skin composed of connective tissue, blood vessels, nerves, muscles, lymphatics, hair follicles, and sebaceous and sudoriferous glands

Distal Farther from the heart; farthest from point of attachment (below the previous site of cannulation)

Drop factor The number of drops needed to deliver 1 mL of fluid

Endothelial lining A thin layer of cells lining the blood vessels and heart

Epidermis The outermost layer of skin covering the body, which is composed of epithelial cells and is devoid of blood vessels

Gauge Size of a cannula (catheter) opening; gradual measurements of the outside diameter of a cannula

Macrodrip Drop factor of 10 to 20 drops equivalent to 1 mL based on manufacturer

Microabrasion Superficial break in skin integrity that may predispose the patient to infection

Microdrip Drop factor of 60 drops/mL

Palpation Examination by touch

Prime To fill the administration set with infusate for the first time

Proximal Nearest to the heart; closest point to attachment (above the previous site of cannulation)

Anatomy and Physiology Related to I.V. Practice

To perform I.V. therapy accurately, nurses must know the anatomy and physiology of the skin and venous system and be familiar with the physiologic response of veins to heat, cold, and stress. It is also important to become familiar with the skin thickness and consistency at various sites.

Skin

The skin consists of two main layers, the **epidermis** and the **dermis,** which overlie the superficial fascia. The epidermis, composed of squamous cells that are less sensitive than underlying structures, is the first line of defense against infections. The epidermis is thickest on the palms of the hands and soles of the feet and is thinnest on the inner surfaces of the extremities. Thickness varies with age and exposure to the elements, such as wind and sun.

The dermis, a much thicker layer, is located directly below the epidermis. The dermis consists of blood vessels, hair follicles, sweat glands, sebaceous glands, small muscles, and nerves. As with the epidermis, the thickness of the dermis varies with age and physical condition. The skin is a special-sense touch organ, and the dermis reacts quickly to painful stimuli, temperature changes, and pressure sensation. This is the most painful layer during venipuncture because of the large amount of blood vessels and the many nerves contained in this sheath.

The hypodermis, or fascia, lies below the epidermis and dermis and provides a covering for the blood vessels. This connective tissue layer varies in thickness and is found over the entire body surface. Because any infection in the fascia, called superficial cellulitis, spreads easily throughout the body, it is essential to use strict aseptic technique when inserting infusion devices. This superficial tissue layer connects with deeper fascia (Fig. 7–1).

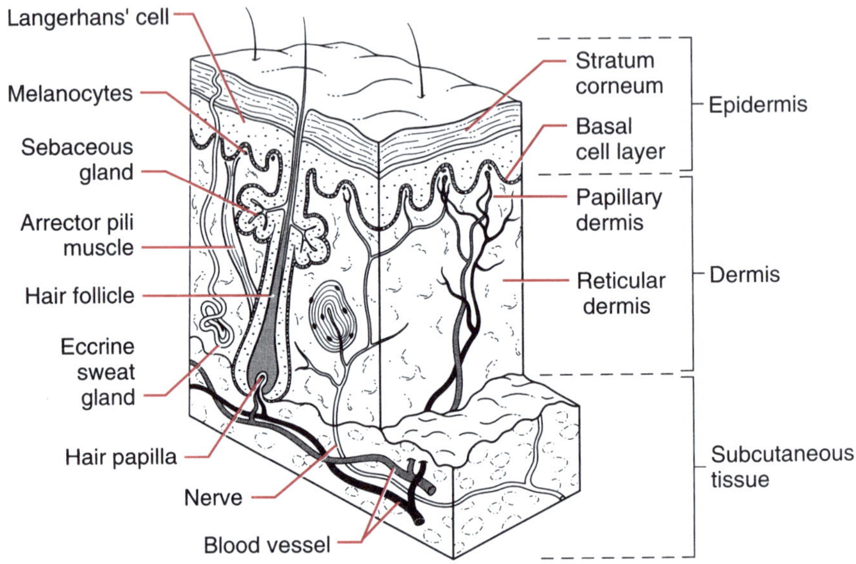

Figure 7–1 ■ Anatomy of skin.

Sensory Receptors

There are five types of sensory receptors, four of which affect parenteral therapy. The sensory receptors transmit along afferent fibers. Many types of stimulation, such as heat, light, cold, pressure, and sound, are processed along the sensory receptors (Guyton & Hall, 2000). Sensory receptors related to parenteral therapy include:

1. Mechanoreceptors, which process skin tactile sensations and deep tissue sensation (**palpation** of veins)
2. Thermoreceptors, which process cold, warmth, and pain (application of heat or cold)
3. Nociceptors, which process pain (puncture of vein for insertion of the **cannula**)
4. Chemoreceptors, which process osmotic changes in blood and decreased arterial pressure (decreased circulating blood volume)

NURSING FAST FACT!

To decrease the patient's pain during venipuncture, keep the skin taut by applying traction to it and move quickly through the skin layers and past the pain receptors.

> Table 7–1 COMPARISON OF ARTERY AND VEIN

Artery*	Vein*
Thick-walled	Thin-walled
25% of arterial wall	10% of vein wall
Lacks valves	Greater distensibility
Pulsates	Valves present approximately every 3 in

Has three tissue layers.

Venous System

The body transport mechanism, the circulatory system, has two main subdivisions—the cardiopulmonary and the systemic systems. The systemic circulation, particularly the peripheral veins, is used in I.V. therapy. Veins function similarly to arteries but are thinner and less muscular (Table 7–1).

The wall of a vein is only 10 percent of the total diameter of the vessel, compared with 25 percent in the artery. Because the vein is thin and less muscular, it can distend easily, allowing for storage of large volumes of blood under low pressure. Approximately 75 percent of the total blood volume is contained in the veins.

Some veins have valves, particularly those that transport blood against gravity, as in the lower extremities. Valves, made up of endothelial leaflets, help prevent the **distal** reflux of blood. Valves occur at points of branching, producing a noticeable bulge in the vessel (Smeltzer & Bare, 2003). Arteries and veins have three layers of tissue that form the wall: the tunica intima, tunica adventitia, and tunica media (Fig. 7–2).

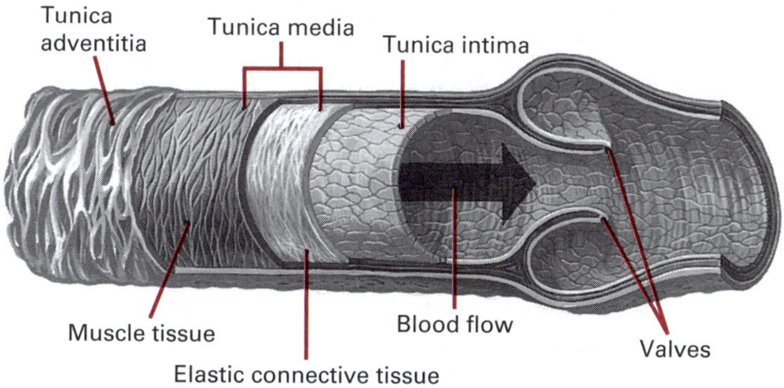

Figure 7–2 ■ Anatomy of a vein. (Source: Medical Economics Publishing, Montvale, NJ, with permission.)

Venous blood flows slower in the periphery and increases in turbulence in the larger veins of the thorax. This increased flow rate is an important aspect in administering hypertonic fluids in larger vasculatures (Fabian, 1998).

The following lists the amount of blood flow in certain veins:

- Cephalic and basilic veins: 45 to 95 mL/min
- Subclavian vein: 150 to 300 mL/min
- Superior vena cava: 2000 mL/min

Tunica Adventitia

The outermost layer, called the tunica adventitia, consists of connective tissue that surrounds and supports a vessel. The blood supply of this layer, called the vasa vasorum, nourishes both the adventitia and media layers. Sometimes during venipuncture, you can feel a "pop" as you enter the tunica adventitia.

Tunica Media

The middle layer, called the tunica media, is composed of muscular and elastic tissue with nerve fibers for vasoconstriction and vasodilation. The tunica media in a vein is not as strong and rigid as it is in an artery, so it tends to collapse or distend as pressure decreases or increases. Stimulation by change in temperature or mechanical or chemical irritation can produce a response in this layer. For instance, cold blood or infusates can produce spasms that impede blood flow and cause pain. Application of heat promotes dilatation, which can relieve a spasm or improve blood flow.

NURSING FAST FACT!

During venipuncture, if the tip of the catheter has nicked the tunica adventitia or is placed in the tunica media layer, a small amount of blood will appear in the catheter; however, the catheter will not thread because it is trapped between layers. If you cannot get a steady backflow of blood, the needle might be in this layer, so advance the stylet of the cannula slightly before advancing the catheter.

Tunica Intima

The innermost layer, called the tunica intima, has one thin layer of cells, referred to as the **endothelial lining.** The surface is smooth, allowing blood to flow through vessels easily. Any roughening of this bed of cells during venipuncture while the catheter is in place, or on discontinuing the system, fosters the process of thrombosis formation and discomfort. (See Chapter 9 for complications.)

Veins of the Hands and Arms

Several veins can be used to infuse I.V. fluids, but the veins of the hands or arms are most commonly used (Figs. 7–3 and 7–4). When selecting the best site, many factors must be considered, such as ease of insertion and access, type of needle or catheter that can be used, and comfort and safety for the patient. Table 7–2 provides information on identifying and selecting the most effective I.V. site for the clinical situation of the patient.

Approaches to Venipuncture

Performing a successful venipuncture requires mastery and knowledge of infusion therapy as well as psychomotor clinical skill. Many aseptic approaches to venipuncture techniques provide safe parenteral therapy. The Phillips 15-step venipuncture method, outlined in Table 7–3 and explained in detail in this chapter, is an easy-to-remember step approach for beginning practitioners.

The Infusion Nurses Society (INS) has developed the Infusion Nursing Standards of Practice to protect patients and nurses who administer infusion therapy. Guidelines supporting quality client care have been published by the Occupational Safety and Health Administration (OSHA) and the Centers for Disease Control and Prevention (CDC). As a nurse ini-

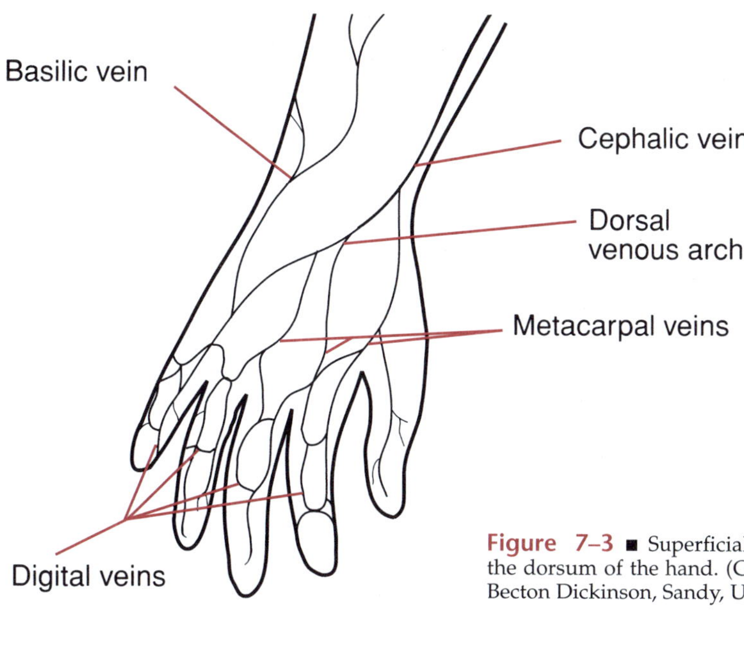

Figure 7–3 ■ Superficial veins of the dorsum of the hand. (Courtesy of Becton Dickinson, Sandy, UT.)

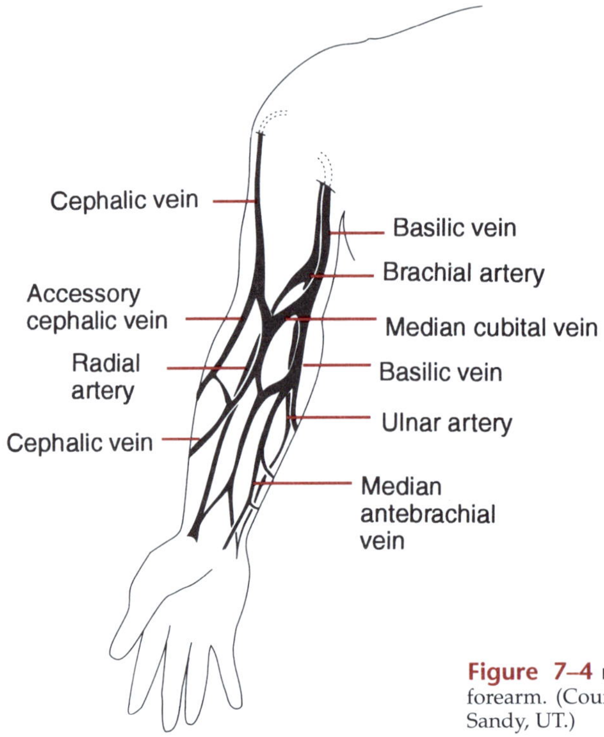

Figure 7–4 ■ Superficial veins of the forearm. (Courtesy of Becton Dickinson, Sandy, UT.)

> Table 7–2 **SELECTING AN INSERTION SITE FOR THE SUPERFICIAL VEINS OF THE DORSUM OF THE HAND AND THE ARM**

Vein and Location	Insertion Device	Considerations
Digital Lateral and dorsal portions of the fingers	Small-gauge cannula 20- to 22-gauge catheter 21- to 25-gauge steel needle	Use a padded tongue blade to splint the cannula. Use only solutions that are isotonic without additives because of the risk of infiltration.
Metacarpal Dorsum of the hand formed by union of digital veins between the knuckles	20- to 22-gauge to $^{3}/_{4}$–1 inch in length over the needle catheter 21- to 25-gauge steel needle (short-term)	Good site to begin therapy Usually easily visualized Avoid if infusing antibiotics, potassium chloride, or chemotherapeutic agents.
Cephalic Radial portion of the lower arm along the radial bone of the forearm	18- to 22-gauge cannulas, usually over-the-needle catheter	Large vein, easy to access First use most distal section and work upward for long-term therapy Useful for infusing blood and chemically irritating medications

(Continued on following page)

Vein and Location	Insertion Device	Considerations
Basilic Ulnar aspect of the lower arm and runs up the ulnar bone	18- to 22-gauge, usually over-the-needle catheter	Difficult area to access Large vein, easily palpated, but moves easily; stabilize with traction during venipuncture. Often available after other sites have been exhausted.
Accessory cephalic Branches off the cephalic vein along the radial bone	18- to 22-gauge, usually over-the-needle catheter	Medium to large size and easy to stabilize May be difficult to palpate in persons with large amounts of adipose tissue Valves at cephalic junction may prohibit cannula advancement Short length may prohibit cannula use
Upper cephalic Radial aspect of upper arm above the elbow	16- to 20-gauge, usually over-the-needle catheter	Difficult to visualize Excellent site for confused patients (who tend to pull at their I.V. line)
Median antebrachial Extends up the front of the forearm from the median antecubital veins	18- to 22-gauge, usually over-the-needle catheter	Area has many nerve endings and should be avoided Infiltration occurs easily.
Median basilic Ulnar portion of the forearm	18- to 22-gauge, usually over-the-needle catheter	Good site for I.V. therapy
Median cubital Radial side of forearm; crosses in front of the brachial artery at the antecubital space	16- to 22-gauge, usually over-the-needle catheter	Good site for I.V. therapy
Antecubital In the bend of the elbow	All sizes especially 16- to 18-gauge; used for midline catheters and peripherally inserted central catheters and blood collection	Should be reserved for blood draws for laboratory analysis only, unless in an emergency Uncomfortable placement site, owing to the arm extending in an unnatural position Area difficult to splint with armboard If used in an emergency situation, change site within 24 hours

tiating infusion therapy, be aware of these standards, as well as those of your own institution (Elkin, Perry, & Potter, 2003).

INS standards have been integrated throughout the 15 steps.

Precannulation

Before initiating cannulation, you must follow steps 1 through 5: checking the physician's order, handwashing, preparing the equipment,

> Table 7–3 **PHILLIPS 15-STEP VENIPUNCTURE METHOD**

Precannulation

1. Checking physician's order
2. Hand hygiene
3. Equipment preparation
4. Patient assessment and psychological preparation
5. Site selection and vein dilation

Cannulation

6. Needle selection
7. Gloving
8. Site preparation
9. Vein entry, direct versus indirect
10. Catheter stabilization and dressing management

Postcannulation

11. Labeling
12. Equipment disposal
13. Patient education
14. Rate calculations
15. Documentation

assessing and preparing the patient, and selecting the vein and the site of insertion.

Step 1: Checking the Physician's Order

A physician's order, other authorized individual, or standing order, is necessary to initiate I.V. therapy. The order should be clear, concise, legible, and complete. All I.V. solutions should be checked against the physician's order. The order should include:

- Date and time of the day
- Infusate name
- Route of administration
- Dosage of administration
- Volume to be infused
- Rate of infusion
- Duration of infusion
- Physician's signature

INS Standard. Verbal orders written by a nurse in the medical record in a hospital setting should be signed by the prescriber within an appropriate time frame.

Verbal orders taken in a home setting must be sent to the prescriber for signature. (INS, 2000, 10)

A written order is required for cannula placement in the arm of a patient who has undergone a mastectomy or axillary node removal. (INS, 2000)

Step 2: Hand Hygiene

Hand hygiene has been shown to significantly decrease the risk of contamination and cross-contamination. Touch contamination is a common cause of transfer of pathogens. Soap and water are adequate for handwashing before the insertion of a cannula; however, an antiseptic solution such as chlorhexidine may be used. Wash hands for 15 to 20 seconds before equipment preparation and before insertion of a catheter. Do not apply hand lotion after handwashing (CDC, 2002). The agent that you use for washing has an effect on effectiveness. Bar, powdered, leaflet, or liquid soaps that do not contain an antibacterial agent are unacceptable for surgical scrubs.

The CDC (2002) recommends the following for hand hygiene:

- Decontaminate hands after removing gloves.
- Before eating and after using a restroom, wash hands with a non-antimicrobial soap and water or with antimicrobial soap and water.
- Antimicrobial-impregnated wipes may be considered as an alternative to washing hands with non-antimicrobial soap and water.
- When using an alcohol-based hand gel, apply product to palm of one hand and rub hands together, covering all surfaces of hands and fingers until hands are dry.

Numerous studies have been published in the last decade that focus on fingernails and infection control. The majority echoes the message—that healthcare workers who wear artificial nails are more likely to harbor pathogens than those who do not (Barber, 2003).

Do not wear artificial fingernails or extenders when having direct contact with patients at high risk (those in intensive care units or operating rooms). Keep natural tips $^1/_4$ inch long (CDC 2002).

INS Standard. Hand washing shall be performed before and immediately after all clinical procedures and after removal of gloves. (INS, 2000, S25)

Several studies have demonstrated that skin underneath rings is more heavily colonized than comparable areas of skin on fingers without rings. Consideration should be give to limiting jewelry when delivering of health care to patients who are immunocompromised or at high risk for infection (CDC, 2002).

Websites

Web-Based Hygiene Resources
CDC, Atlanta, Georgia: *www.cdc.gov/ncidod/hip*

Step 3: Equipment Preparation

Inspect the infusate container at the nurses' station, in the clean utility, or in the medication room. In modern practice, two systems are available—glass system (open or closed) and plastic system (rigid or soft).

To check the glass system, hold the container up to the light to inspect for cracks as evidenced by flashes of light. Glass systems are crystal clear. Rotate the container and look for particulate contamination and cloudiness. Inspect the seal and check the expiration date.

To check a plastic system, squeeze the soft plastic infusate container to check for breaks in the integrity of the plastic; squeeze the system to detect pinholes. Observe for any particulate contamination and check the expiration date. The plastic systems are not crystal clear. The outer wrap of the soft plastic systems should be dry.

Select either a vented or nonvented primary tubing set or a secondary set, depending on the rationale for infusion. It is wise to "**spike**" the solution container and "prime" the administration set at the nurses' station to detect defective equipment. Choose the correct tubing to match the solution container. For closed glass, use vented only; for plastic, use either vented or nonvented. (See Chapter 6 for more detailed information on I.V. equipment.)

Step 4: Patient Assessment and Psychological Preparation

Selection of the vascular access device and insertion site requires integration of data obtained from the patient care issues, patient assessment, and the specific infusion therapy prescribed. Selection of the vascular access device requires collaboration efforts with input from physician, nurse, patient, and caregiver (Otto, 2003). It is important to use step 4 to gather the necessary information needed to perform a successful venipuncture and infusion therapy.

First, provide privacy for the patient. Explain the procedure to minimize his or her anxiety. Instruct the patient regarding the purpose of the I.V. therapy, the procedure, what the physician has ordered in the infusate and why, the mobility limitations, and signs and symptoms of potential complications.

Evaluate the patient's psychological preparedness for the I.V. procedure by talking with him or her before assessing the vein. The nurse should consider aspects such as autonomy, handedness, and independence, along with invasion of personal space when I.V. placement is necessary. Often the patient has a fear of pain associated with venipuncture because of the lack of understanding or the memory of a previously negative encounter related to necessity of the therapy.

Questions to ask the patient:

- What is your primary medical diagnosis?
- Do you have a chronic disease that places you at risk of complications?
- Do you have epilepsy?
- Do you have a history of vasovagal reactions during venipuncture or when you see blood?
- Do you have fragile peripheral veins, and do they roll?
- Have you had previous vascular access devices?
- Will you be in one setting for the course of therapy or will you be transferred to another setting?
- If you will be going home with the access device, are you (or a caregiver) willing to learn how to manage the device at home (Hadaway, 1999)?

Step 5: Site Selection and Vein Dilatation

Site selection is based on INS standards.

> **INS Standard.** Vein selection shall include assessment of the patient's condition, age, and diagnosis; vein condition size and location; and type and duration of therapy. The vein shall accommodate the gauge and length of the cannula required by the prescribed therapy. (INS, 2000 S49)

VEIN DILATATION

Several factors should be considered before a venipuncture is attempted. These factors help nurses make competent choices of location for the infusion.

1. *Type of solution:* Fluids that are hypertonic (i.e., more than 375 mOsm), such as antibiotics and potassium chloride, are irritating to vein walls. Select a large vein in the forearm to initiate this therapy. Start at the best, lowest vein.
2. *Condition of vein:* A soft, straight vein is the ideal choice for venipuncture. Palpate the vein by moving the tips of the fingers down the vein to observe how it refills. The dorsal metacarpal veins in elderly patients are a poor choice because blood extravasation (i.e., hematoma) occurs more readily in small, thin veins. When a patient is hypovolemic, peripheral veins collapse more quickly than larger veins.

Avoid:

- Bruised veins
- Red, swollen veins
- Veins near previously infected areas
- Sites near a previously discontinued site

CULTURAL AND ETHNIC CONSIDERATIONS: PERFORMING I.V. THERAPY 7–1

Transcultural nursing is becoming a specialty field; however, every nurse must use transcultural knowledge to facilitate culturally appropriate care. Practitioners performing I.V. therapy must make every effort to deliver culturally sensitive care that is free of inherent biases based on gender, race, and religion.

Culturally diverse nursing care must take into account six cultural phenomena that vary with application and use, yet are evident in all cultural groups: (1) communication, (2) space, (3) social organization, (4) time, (5) environmental control, and (6) biologic variations.

In preparing to perform I.V. therapy–related procedures on patients from different cultures, it is important to remember some key guidelines:

- Plan care based on the communicated needs and cultural background.
- Learn as much as possible about the patient's cultural customs and beliefs.
- Encourage the patient to share cultural interpretations of health, illness, and health care.
- Be sensitive to the uniqueness of the patient.
- Identify sources of discrepancy between the patient's and your own concepts of health and illness.
- Communicate at the patient's personal level of functioning.
- Modify communication approaches to meet cultural educational needs.
- Understand that respect for the patient and his or her communication needs is central to the therapeutic relationship.
- Communicate in a nonthreatening manner.
- Follow acceptable social and cultural amenities.
- Adopt special approaches when the patient speaks a different language (e.g., translators or AT&T).
- Use a caring tone of voice and facial expression.
- Speak slowly and distinctly but not loudly.
- Use gestures, pictures, and play acting to help the patient understand.
- Repeat the message in a different way.
- Be alert to words the patient seems to understand and use them frequently.
- Keep messages simple and repeat them.
- Avoid using technical medical terms and abbreviations.
- If available, use an appropriate language dictionary.
- Use interpreters to improve communication (Giger & Davidhizar, 1999).

3. *Duration of therapy:* Choose a vein that supports I.V. therapy for at least 72 hours. Start at the best, lowest vein. Use the hand only if a nonirritating solution is being infused. Long courses of infusion therapy make preservation of veins essential. Perform venipuncture distally with each subsequent puncture **proximal** to previous puncture and alternate arms.

Avoid:

- A joint flexion
- A vein too small for cannula size

4. *Cannula size:* Hemodilution is important. The **gauge** of the cannula should be as small as possible. When performing transfusion therapy, an 18-gauge catheter is preferred so the cellular portion of blood will not be damaged during infusion.
5. *Patient age:* Infants do not have the accessible sites that older children and adults have owing to infants' increased body fat. Veins in the hands, feet, and antecubital region may be the only accessible sites. Veins in elderly persons are usually fragile; approach venipuncture gently and evaluate the need for a tourniquet (Fabian, 1995).

NURSING FAST FACT!

Fragile veins can be penetrated with less extravasation of blood if a tourniquet is not used and an indirect (two-step) method is used.

6. *Patient preference:* Consider the patient's personal feelings when determining the catheter placement site. Evaluate the extremities, taking into account the dominant hand.
7. *Patient activity:* Ambulatory patients using crutches or a walker will need cannula placement above the wrist so the hand can still be used.
8. *Presence of disease or previous surgery:* Patients with vascular disease or dehydration may have limited venous access. Avoid phlebitis-infiltrated sites or a site of infection. If a patient has a condition with poor vascular venous return, the affected side **must be avoided**. Examples are cerebrovascular accident, mastectomy, amputation, orthopedic surgery of the hand or arm, and plastic surgery of the hand or arm.
9. *Presence of shunt or graft:* Do not use a patient's arm or hand that has a patent graft or shunt for dialysis.
10. *Patients receiving anticoagulation therapy:* Patients receiving anticoagulant therapy have a propensity to bleed. Local ecchymoses and major hemorrhagic complications can be avoided if the nurse is aware that the patient is taking anticoagulant therapy. Precautions can be taken when initiating I.V. therapy. Venous distention can be accomplished with minimal tourniquet pressure. Use the smallest cannula that will accommodate the vein and deliver the ordered infusate. The dressing must be removed gently using alcohol or adhesive remover.

11. *Patient with allergies:* Determine whether a patient has allergies. Allergies to iodine need to be identified because iodine is contained in products used to prep the skin before venipuncture. Question the patient regarding allergies to shellfish. If there is a doubt, use 70 percent isopropyl alcohol to prep the skin and cleanse the ports. Other allergies of concern to delivery of safe patient care include allergies to medications, foods, animals, and environmental substances.

Websites

Allergy, Asthma, & Immunology Online: *www.allergy.mcg.edu*

Other sites:

NURSING FAST FACTS!

Always question the patient regarding allergies before administering medications, especially those given parenterally. Question patients on latex allergy specifically.

Cannulation of the lower extremities in adults should be avoided, because this increases the risk of thrombophlebitis and embolism (INS, 2000, 43).

There are many ways to increase the flow of blood in the upper extremities. Factors affecting the capacity for dilatation are blood pressure, presence of valves, sclerotic veins, and multiple previous I.V. sites.

The following list provides ways to dilate veins.

1. *Gravity:* Position the extremity lower than the heart for several minutes.
2. *Fist clenching:* Instruct the patient to open and close his or her fist. Squeezing a rubber ball or rolled washcloth works well.
3. *Tapping:* Using thumb and the second finger, flick the vein; this releases histamines beneath the skin and causes dilatation.
4. *Warm compresses:* Apply warm towels to the extremity for 10 minutes. A new technology available is a warming mitt warmed to 52 degrees; alternatively, a passive warming mitt, which is not heated, can be used for 15 minutes prior to venipuncture and during the venipuncture procedure. In a recent study Walling and Lenhardt (2003) found that the success rate for cannula insertion was 94 percent with active warming. Do not use a microwave oven to heat towels; the temperature can become too hot and cause a burn.

5. *Blood pressure cuff:* This is an excellent choice for vein dilatation. Pump the cuff up slightly (e.g., about 30 mm Hg). This method prevents constriction of the arterial system.

NURSING FAST FACT!

Care must be exercised when using a blood pressure cuff not to start the I.V. too close to the cuff, which causes excessive back pressure.

6. *Tourniquet:* Apply the tourniquet 6 to 8 inches above the venipuncture site if the blood pressure is within normal range. If the patient is hypertensive, the tourniquet should be placed high on the extremity; occasionally, the tourniquet is not needed in the case of severely hypertensive patients. With hypotensive patients, move the tourniquet as close as possible to the venipuncture site without contamination of the prepped area. (See Chapter 10 for multiple tourniquet techniques.)

NURSING FAST FACT!

Use the tourniquet only once. Using the same tourniquet on more than one patient can result in cross-contamination. Tourniquets may be sources of latex exposure (INS, 2000, 42).

Use a nonlatex tourniquet (Becton Dickinson [1-800-237–2762] or Baumgarten's Plastiband [1-800-247–5547]) or place clothing or a stockinette over the latex tourniquet.

INS Standard. Site selection should be routinely initiated in the distal areas of the upper extremities, and subsequent cannulation should be made proximal to the previously cannulated site. Avoid using veins at areas of flexion unless the area is immobilized. Veins in the antecubital fossa should be reserved for peripheral central line and midline access and for drawing blood samples. (INS, 2000, 43)

7. *Multiple tourniquets:* Applying additional tourniquets to increase the oncotic pressure and bring deep veins into view is discussed in detail in Chapter 10.
8. *Transillumination:* Use of a penlight or Venoscope to illuminate veins in patients with dark skin is discussed in detail in Chapter 9.
9. Ultrasonography can be used to place peripheral I.V. catheters for short-term therapy when traditional landmark methods for placement fail (LaRue, 2000).

Cannulation

Cannulation involves steps 6 through 10: selecting the needle, gloving, preparing the site, direct or indirect entry into the vein, and stabilizing the catheter and managing the dressing.

Nursing goals for choosing an appropriate site include the following:

- The site must tolerate the rate of flow.
- The site must be capable of delivering the medications ordered.
- The site must tolerate the gauge of cannula needed.
- The patient must be comfortable with the site chosen.
- The site must not impede the patient's activities of daily living (Fabian, 1998).

Table 7–4 presents tips for selecting veins.

Step 6: Needle Selection

Infusions may be delivered with a plastic or steel cannula. (See Chapter 6 for needle choice and sizes.) The choice of catheter depends on the purpose of the infusion and the condition and availability of the veins. Steel needles are generally avoided, except for bolus injections or infusions lasting only a few hours. Inflexible steel needles greatly increase the risk of vein injury and infiltration.

Catheters made of radiopaque material are the best quality. Most hospitals, clinics, and home care agencies have policies and procedures for the selection of catheters. Recommended gauges are:

- 18- to 20-gauge for infusion of hypertonic or isotonic solutions with additives
- 18- to 20-gauge for blood administration
- 22- to 24-gauge for pediatric patients
- 22-gauge for fragile veins in elderly persons if unable to place a 20-gauge catheter

> Table 7–4 **TIPS FOR SELECTING VEINS**

- A suitable vein should feel relatively smooth, pliable with valves well spaced.
- Veins will be difficult to stabilize in a patient who has recently lost weight.
- Debilitated patients and those taking corticosteroids have fragile veins that bruise easily.
- Sclerotic veins are common among narcotics addicts.
- Sclerotic veins are common among the elderly population.
- Dialysis patients usually know which veins are good for venipuncture.
- Start with distal veins and work proximally.
- Veins that feel bumpy, like running your finger over a cat's tail, are usually thrombosed or extremely valvular.

The tip of the catheter should be inspected for integrity before venipuncture to note the presence of burrs on the needle, peeling of catheter material, or other abnormalities.

NURSING FAST FACT!

Only two attempts at venipuncture are recommended because multiple unsuccessful attempts cause unnecessary trauma to the patient and limit vascular access. When aseptic technique is compromised (i.e., in an emergency situation), the cannula is also considered compromised and a new catheter should be placed within 24 hours.

INS Standard. The cannula selected shall be the smallest gauge and shortest length to accommodate the prescribed therapy. Catheters shall be radiopaque. (INS, 2000, 44)

INS Standard. A peripheral short catheter shall be removed every 72 hours and immediately on suspected contamination, complication, or therapy discontinuation. An organization that fails to maintain an ongoing phlebitis rate of 5 percent or less with the practice of 72-hour catheter site rotation should return to a 48-hour site rotation interval. (INS, 2000, 55)

Step 7: Gloving

The CDC (2002) recommends following standard precautions whenever exposure to blood or body fluids is likely. Latex and vinyl gloves protect wearers from contact with blood and body fluids. However, latex, a natural material, is more flexible than vinyl and molds to the wearer's hand, allowing freedom of movement. Its lattice-type structure allows tiny punctures to reseal automatically.

NURSING FAST FACT!

Latex and the powder used in the gloves are associated with potentially severe allergic reactions in susceptible persons. Avoid using this material if you have experienced any reactions to their use. (For more information on latex allergy, see Chapter 1.)

Gloves made of polyvinyl chloride, the synthetic rubber known as vinyl, do not reseal, are less flexible and less durable, and are of limited usefulness in high-risk, heavy-usage situations.

ANESTHETIC AGENTS

Although not all patients require anesthetics, the infusion nurse should make an individualized determination for each patient. Factors to consider include depth of insertion location of the vein, gauge of the needle, composure of the patient, presence of allergies, patient preference, payment sources, and time available for adequate response (Moureau & Zonderman, 2000).

NOTE > At this step, after donning gloves, the nurse would use a topical transdermal cream, iontophoresis, or intradermal lidocaine 1 percent injectable to produce anesthesia prior to skin preparation. Refer to the section in this chapter on controversial practices for a description of steps in use of these products.

Step 8: Site Preparation

Hair should be removed only with scissors or clippers. Shaving is not recommended because of the potential for **microabrasions**, which increase the risk of infection. The use of depilatories is not recommended because of the potential for allergic reactions. Electric hair removal devices are not used unless they are effective and meet the criteria for preservation of skin integrity (INS, 2000, 45).

Cleansing the insertion site reduces the potential for infection. The following **antimicrobial** solutions may be used to prepare the cannula site:

- Iodophor (povidone-iodine)
- 70 Percent isopropyl alcohol
- Chlorhexidine (ChloraPrep®; Med-Flex Hospital Products, Inc.)
- Tincture of iodine, 2 percent

A recent study (Hibbard, Mulberry & Brady, 2002) concluded that a 2 percent ChloraPrep® (combination of 2 percent chlorhexidine gluconate and 70 percent isopropyl alcohol) significantly reduced microbial counts over a 24-hour period of time and was not associated with skin irritation. This study suggested that ChloraPrep® is an appropriate solution for use in preparing a venipuncture site to help reduce the risk of nosocomial infection.

Aqueous benzalkonium-like compounds and hexachlorophene should not be used as preparatory solutions before venipuncture (INS, 2000, 54).

In preparing the site, use a vigorous circular motion, working from the center outward to a diameter of 2 to 3 inches for 20 seconds. The solutions should be allowed to air dry. Use 70 percent alcohol as a defatting agent before application of the povidone-iodine. If the patient is allergic to iodine, use 70 percent alcohol with friction for at least 30 seconds.

INS Standard. Do not apply 70 percent isopropyl alcohol after a povidone-iodine prep because alcohol negates the effect of the povidone-iodine. (INS, 2000, 47)

Step 9: Vein Entry

Gloves should be in place before venipuncture and kept on until after the cannula is stabilized. Gloves should be removed only after the risk of exposure to body fluids has been eliminated. Venipuncture can be performed using a direct (one-step) or indirect (two-step) method. The direct method is appropriate for small-gauge needles, fragile hand veins or rolling veins and carries an increased risk of causing a hematoma. The indirect method can be used for all venipunctures. Procedures Display 7–1: Venipuncture describes the steps to use.

PROCEDURES DISPLAY 7–1

VENIPUNCTURE

Step 1: Pull skin below puncture site to stabilize the skin and prevent the rolling of the vein.

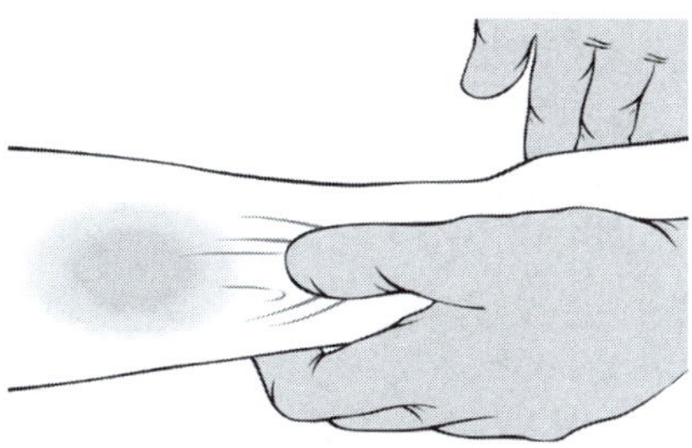

Step 2: Grasp the flashback chamber.
Step 3: Insert the needle of choice **bevel** up at a 30- to 45-degree angle, depending on the vein location and catheter, while applying traction on the vein to keep skin taut.

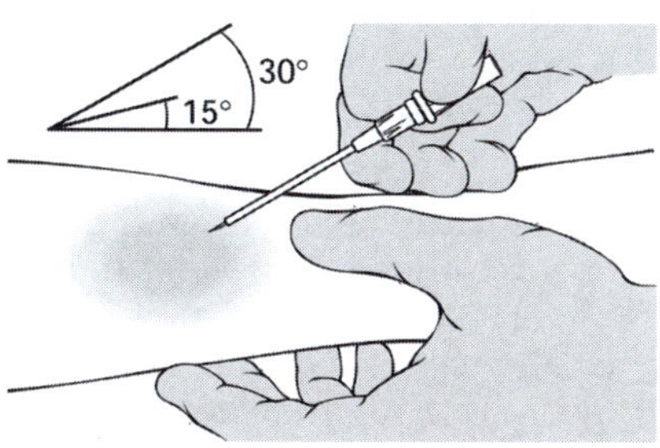

(Continued on following page)

PROCEDURES DISPLAY 7–1

VENIPUNCTURE *(Continued)*

Step 4: Insert the catheter by direct or indirect method with a steady motion.

For the Direct (One-Step) Method:

A. Insert the cannula directly over the vein at a 30- to 45-degree angle.

B. Penetrate all layers of the vein with one motion.

For the Indirect (Two-Step Method):

A. Insert the cannula at a 30- to 45-degree angle to the skin alongside the vein; gently insert the cannula distal to the point at which the needle will enter the vein.

B. Maintain parallel alignment and advance through the subcutaneous tissue.

C. Relocate the vein and decrease the angle as the cannula enters the vein.

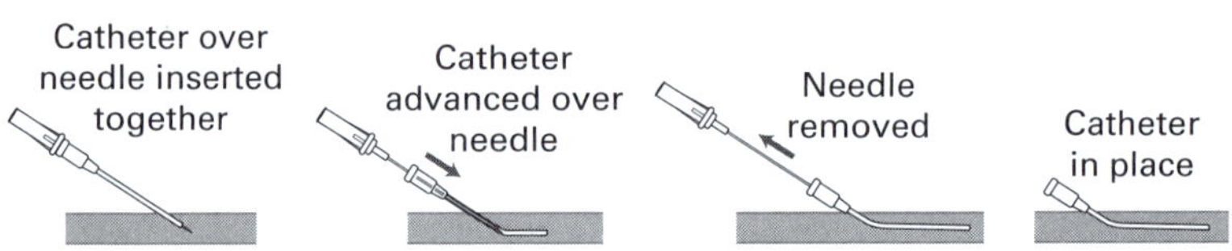

Jabbing, stabbing, or quick thrusting should be avoided because such actions may cause rupture of delicate veins. For performing a venipuncture on difficult veins, follow these guidelines:

- For paper-thin transparent skin or delicate veins: Use the smallest catheter possible (preferably 22-gauge); use direct entry; consider not using a tourniquet; decrease angle of entry to 15 degrees; apply minimal tourniquet pressure.
- For an obese patient or if you are unable to palpate or see veins: Create a visual image of venous anatomy and select a longer catheter [preferably 2 inch].
- If the veins roll when venipuncture is attempted: Apply traction to the vein with thumb during venipuncture, keeping skin taut; leave tourniquet on to promote venous distention; use a blood pressure cuff for better filling of the vein; use 16- or 18-gauge catheter.

Step 5: After the bevel enters the vein and blood flashback occurs, lower the angle of the catheter and stylet (needle) as one unit and advance into the vein. After the catheter tip and bevel are in the vein, advance the catheter forward off the stylet and into the vein. A steady backflow of blood indicates a successful entry. If the

(Continued on following page)

catheter is shorter than the needle, backflow may occur before the catheter tip is fully in the vein.

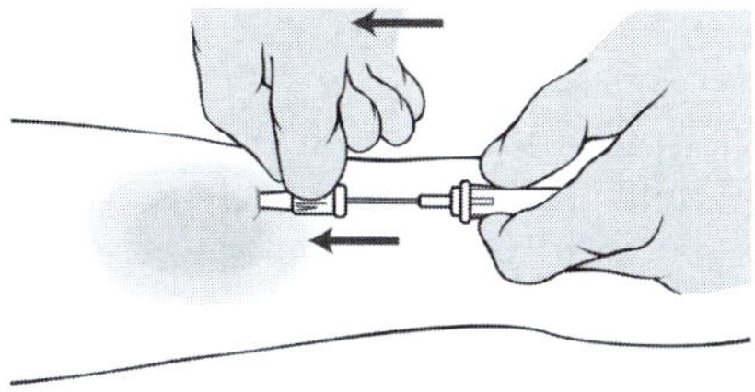

Step 6: After the vein is entered, cautiously advance the cannula into the vein lumen. Hold the catheter hub with your thumb and middle finger and use your index finger to advance the catheter, maintaining skin traction. A one-handed technique is recommended to advance the catheter off the stylet so that the opposite hand can maintain proper traction on the skin and maintain vein alignment. [A two-handed technique can be used, but this increases the risk of vessel rupture during threading of a rigid cannula in a nonstabilized vein.]

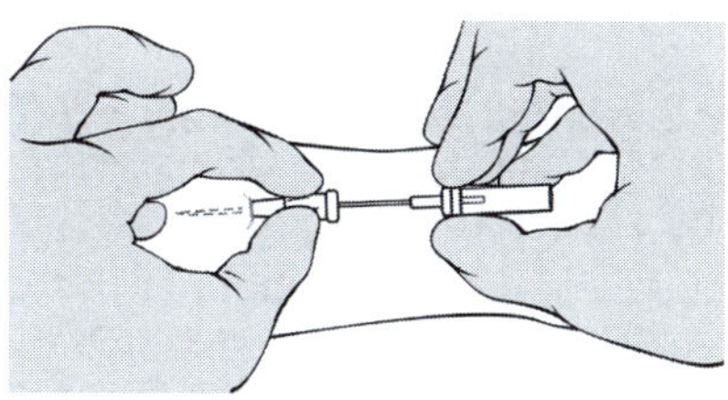

Step 7: While the stylet is still partially inside the catheter, release the tourniquet.
Step 8: Remove the stylet.
Step 9: Connect the adaptor on the administration set to the hub of the catheter.
[Figures Courtesy of Critikon, a Johnson & Johnson Company.]

NURSING FAST FACT!

Blood may ooze from the catheter, depending on the brand of needle used. If there is no blood, the catheter may not be placed correctly or may have penetrated the vein wall. If this is the case, remove the catheter and restart with a sterile cannula.

If the vein has sustained a through-and-through puncture and a hematoma develops, immediately remove the catheter and apply direct pressure to the site. Do not reapply a tourniquet to an extremity immediately after a venipuncture because a hematoma will form.

TROUBLESHOOTING TIPS

Common reasons for failure of venipuncture include:

- Failure to release the tourniquet promptly when the vein is sufficiently cannulated. Intravascular oncotic pressure may cause bleeding outside the vein.
- Using a "stop and start" technique that beginners who lack confidence use. This tentative approach can injure the vein, causing bruising.
- Inadequate vein stabilization. Not using traction to hold the vein causes the stylet to push the vein aside.
- Failure to recognize that the cannula has gone through the opposite vein wall.
- Stopping too soon after insertion so only the stylet, not the cannula, enters the lumen (intima) of the vein. Blood return disappears when the stylet is removed because the cannula is not in the lumen.
- Inserting the cannula too deeply, below the vein. This is evident when the cannula won't move freely because it is imbedded in fascia or muscle. The patient also complains of severe discomfort.
- Failure to penetrate the vein wall because of improper insertion angle (too steep or not steep enough), causing the cannula to ride on top of or below the vein (Millam & Hadaway, 2000).

Step 10: Catheter Stabilization and Dressing Management

CATHETER STABILIZATION

The catheter should be stabilized in a manner that does not interfere with visualization and evaluation of the site. Stabilization reduces the risk of complications related to I.V. therapy such as phlebitis, infiltration, sepsis, and cannula migration.

There are three methods appropriate for stabilization of the catheter hub: the U method, the H method, and the chevron method (Table 7–5).

When tape is used, it should be applied only to the cannula hub or wings and should not be applied directly to the skin–cannula junction site (INS, 2000, 49).

Using an armboard to stabilize the catheter site is not usually necessary with over-the-needle catheters. If it is necessary because of an erratic flow rate caused by the patient's frequent change of position, use a disposable lightweight armboard. To absorb perspiration, cover the armboard with a washcloth or a paper cover (usually provided with armboards). Secure the armboard with two or three pieces of double-backed tape to protect the patient's skin. Do not tape over the site but do leave the patient's fingers free for movement.

> **INS Standard.** Cannulas need to be stabilized in a manner that does not interfere with assessment and monitoring of the infusion site or impede delivery of the prescribed therapy. (INS, 2000, 49)

> Table 7–5 **STABILIZING THE CATHETER***

U Method	**H Method**	**Chevron Method**
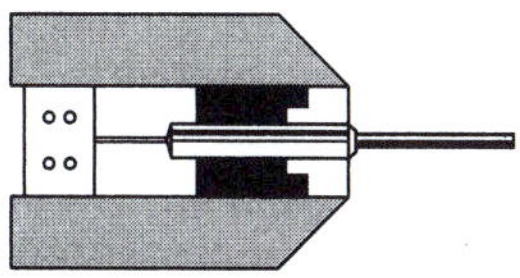	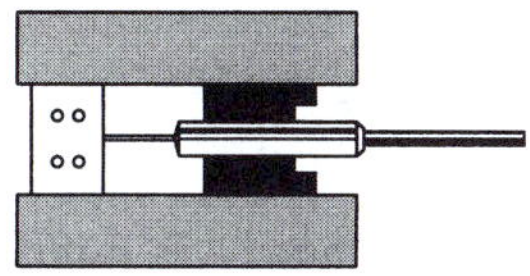	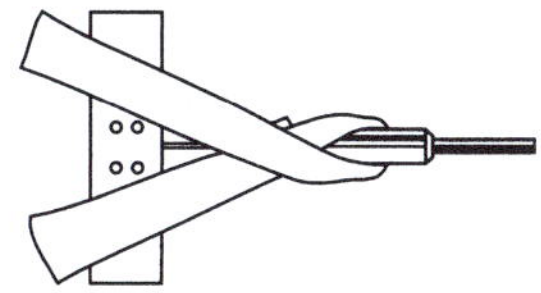
Use for Winged Set	**Use for Winged Set**	**Use for Winged Set**
1. Cut three strips of $^{1}/_{2}$-inch tape. With sticky side up, place one strip under tubing. **2.** Bring each side of the tape up, folding it over the wings of the needle. Press it down, parallel with the tubing. **3.** Loop the tubing and secure it with a piece of 1-inch tape.	**1.** Cut three strips of 1-inch tape. **2.** Place one strip of tape over each wing, keeping the tape parallel with the needle. **3.** Place another strip of tape perpendicular to the first two. Place over the wings to stabilize wings and hub.	**1.** Cover the venipuncture with transparent dressing or 2 × 2 gauze dressing. **2.** Cut a long 5- to 6-inch strip of $^{1}/_{2}$-inch tape. Place one strip of tape, sticky side under hub, parallel with the dressing. **3.** Cross the end of the tape over the opposite side of the needle so that the tape sticks to the patient's skin. **4.** Apply a piece of 1-inch tape across the wings of the chevron. Loop the tubing and secure it with another piece of 1-inch tape.

**For all methods, include on the last piece of tape the date, time of insertion, size of gauge, length of needle or catheter, and your initials.*

A new method of catheter securement became available in the 1990s as an alternative to the traditional tape and/or suture securement. This new method is an adhesive pad with an integrated posted retainer designed to hold the catheter in place more securely than allowed by tape. Statlock (Venetec International, San Diego, CA) is one manufacturer of this sort of adhesive anchor/built-in retainer (Moureau & Lannucci, 2003). In addition, a very new device is the I.V. House UltraDressing with flexible fabric to wrap around a patient's hand after the I.V. is started. See Figures 7–5 and 7–6.

JUNCTION SECUREMENT

The use of junction securement minimizes the risk of complications related to infusion therapy. A method of securement should always be used at junction points of I.V. tubing and add-on devices. Examples of junction securement are Luer locks, clasping devices, and threaded devices. The use of tape is not recommended because of the potential

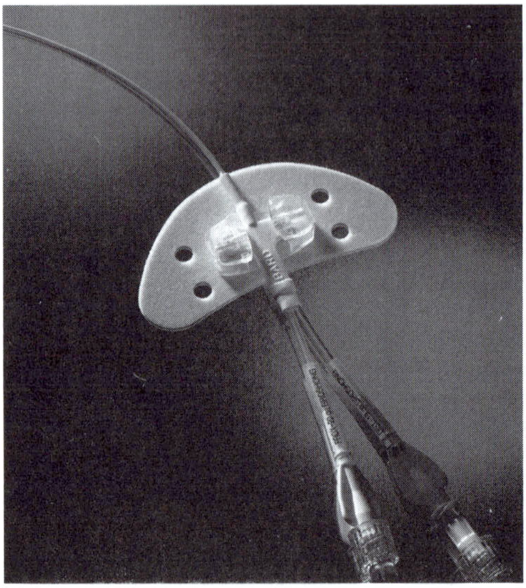

Figure 7–5 ■ Statlock IV/PICC catheter securement device. (Courtesy of Venetec International, Mission Viejo, CA.)

risks of air embolism and hemorrhage that may lead to a life-threatening situation caused by separation of the I.V. system and risk of infection (INS, 2000, 57).

DRESSING MANAGEMENT

There are two methods for dressing management: (1) a gauze dressing secured with tape and (2) a transparent semipermeable membrane dress-

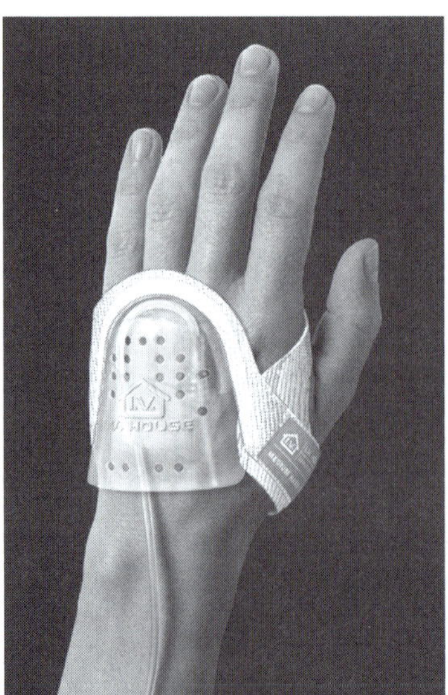

Figure 7–6 ■ I.V. House UltraDressing that consists of flexible fabric with thumb holes and a polyethylene dome that wraps around a patient's hand after an I.V. is started. This prevents accidental snagging of the loop or catheter hub. (Courtesy of I.V. House, Inc. Hazelwood, MO.)

ing (TSM). A sterile gauze dressing can be applied aseptically with edges secured with tape.

INS Standard. Gauze dressings should be changed every 48 hours on peripheral sites or when the integrity of the dressing is compromised. (INS, 2000, 50)

To apply the gauze dressing:

1. Cleanse the area of excess moisture after venipuncture.
2. Secure the cannula hub.
3. Apply the dressing.

INS Standard. The use of a nonocclusive type adhesive bandage strip in place of a gauze dressing is not recommended. (INS, 2000, 50)

Transparent semipermeable membrane dressings should be applied aseptically and changed every 48 to 72 hours, depending on the standard of practice within the institution. The dressing and catheter should be replaced together, unless the integrity of the dressing is impaired; then removal of the dressing with replacement of a new sterile TSM is required. Do not use ointment of any kind under a TSM dressing. Adhesive-coated semipermeable film is available from many manufacturers. The TSM dressing should be applied only to the cannula hub and wings.

To apply a TSM:

1. Cleanse the area of excess moisture after venipuncture.
2. Center the transparent dressing over cannula site and partially over the hub.
3. Press down on the dressing, sealing the catheter site.
4. Apply tape to secure administration set. (See Procedures Display 7–2: Applying a Dressing.)

INS Standard. TSM dressings should be changed on peripheral short catheters at the time of site rotation or sooner if the integrity has been compromised. (INS, 2000, 50)

NURSING FAST FACTS!

- *Do not put tape over the transparent film because it is difficult to remove the transparent film when the dressing needs to be changed.*
- *Polyurethane dressings are semipermeable. That is, they are impervious to extrinsic microbial contaminates and liquid-phase moisture and variably permeable to oxygen, carbon dioxide, and water vapor. Other studies in healthy volunteers have shown little effect of these dressing on the cutaneous flora.*

PROCEDURES DISPLAY 7–2
APPLYING A DRESSING

Step 1: Cover the insertion site and catheter hub with the transparent dressing.

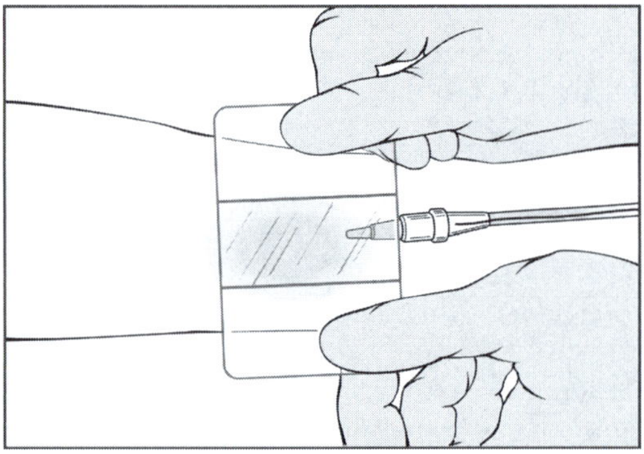

Step 2: Pinch the transparent dressing around the catheter hub to secure the hub.

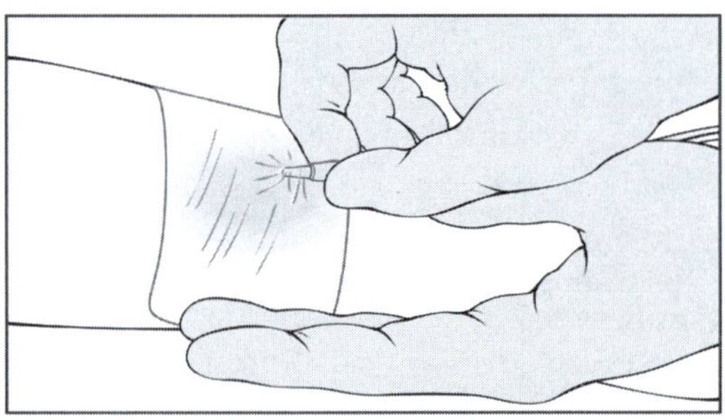

Step 3: Label the insertion site, noting the catheter gauge, date and time of insertion, and initials of the person who performed the venipuncture.

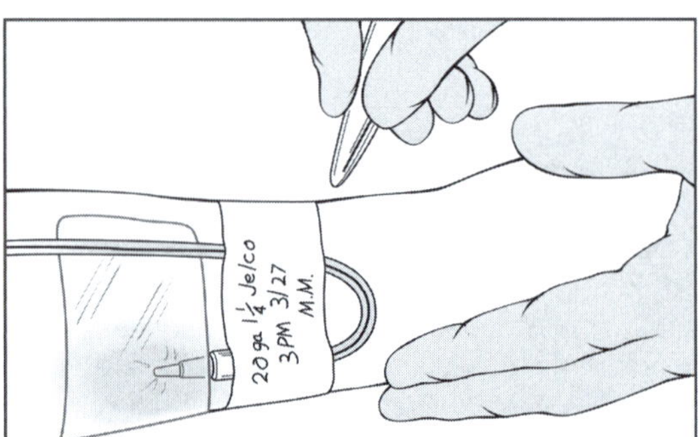

[Figures Courtesy of Critikon, a Johnson & Johnson Company.]

Advantages of TSM dressings include that they allow continuous inspection of the site, are more comfortable than gauze and tape, and permit patients to bathe and shower without saturating the dressing (Maki & Mermel, 1998). A disadvantage of TSM dressings is that they are more costly than gauze and tape (Maki & Mermel, 1998).

Ongoing clinical trials based on the knowledge that cutaneous occlusive dressings with tape or impervious plastic films result in an explosive increase in cutaneous microflora, with overgrowth of gram-negative bacilli and yeast.

Step 11: Labeling

The I.V. setup should be labeled in three spots: the insertion site, the tubing, and the solution container, which should be time stripped.

> **INS Standard.** Distinctive legible labeling shall provide pertinent and easily identified information relative to the cannula, dressing, solution, medication, and administration set. (INS, 2000, 17)

1. The venipuncture site should be labeled on the side of the transparent dressing or across the hub. Do not place the label over the site because this obstructs visualization of the site. Include on the label:
   - Date and time
   - The type and length of the catheter (e.g., 20-gauge, 1-inch)
   - The nurse's initials
2. Label the tubing according to agency policy and procedure so that practitioners on subsequent shifts will be aware of when the tubing must be changed.
3. Place a time strip on all parenteral solutions with the name of the solution and additives, initials of the nurse, and the time the solution was started.

NURSING FAST FACT!

Time strips are helpful for assessing whether the solution is on schedule.

Step 12: Equipment Disposal

Recapping needles increases the risk of needlestick injuries to the practitioner. Needles and stylets should be disposed of in nonpermeable tamper-proof containers. In accordance with the Occupational Safety and Health Administration (OSHA) and the Joint Commission on Accreditation of Healthcare Organizations, needles and stylets should not be recapped, broken, or bent (JCAHO, 2000; CDC, 2001). After venipuncture is complete, dispose of all paper and plastic equipment in a container suitable for burning.

INS Standard. Needles and stylets (sharps) shall be disposed of in nonpermeable, tamper-proof containers. (INS, 2000, 31)

Step 13: Patient Education

Patients have the right to receive information on all aspects of their care in a manner they can understand, as well as the right to accept or refuse treatment (INS, 2000, 12).

After the catheter is stabilized, the dressing applied, and the labeling complete:

- Inform the patient of any limitations on movement or mobility.
- Explain all alarms if an electronic control device is used.
- Instruct the patient to call for assistance if the venipuncture site becomes tender or sore or if redness or swelling develops.
- Advise the patient that the venipuncture site will be checked by the nurse.

INS Standard. When a patient requires continued care in his or her home, the nurse shall provide comprehensive education to the patient and caregiver that includes the behavioral domains of cognitive, affective, and psychomotor, along with a written set of instructions on all pertinent aspects of treatment. (INS, 2000, 12)

Step 14: Rate Calculations

Many clinical environments require delivery of I.V. medications, unusual infusion rates, and administration of primary and secondary infusions, so I.V. therapists must be capable of accurate calculations. Calculating the proper I.V. rate for medication and solution delivery can be time intensive. All I.V. infusions should be monitored frequently for accurate flow rates and complications associated with infusion therapy.

NOTE > Refer to the section on math calculations (pp. 295–300) for further guidance on rate calculations.

Step 15: Monitoring and Documentation

Monitoring of the patient should include cannula, exit site, and surrounding area; flow rate; clinical data; patient response; and compliance to the prescribed therapy. The frequency of monitoring provides for patient protection and is an integral part of quality and risk management. Information that is obtained by monitoring should be communicated to other healthcare professionals responsible for the patient's care by documentation (INS, 2000, S23).

Documentation of I.V. therapy procedure generally includes:

- Date and time of insertion
- Manufacturer's brand name and style of device (in some settings lot number)
- The gauge and length of the device
- Specific name and location of the accessed vein
- The infused solution and rate of flow
- Infusing by gravity or pump
- The number attempts for a successful I.V. start
- Condition of extremity prior to access
- The patient's specific comments related to the procedure
- Patient response, excessive anxiety, patient movement, or an untoward response
- Signature (Dugger, 2001)

Documentation should be legible, accessible to healthcare professionals, and readily retrievable.

INS Standard. Documentation in the patient's medical record should contain sufficient information to identify infusion procedures, prescribed treatments, complications, nursing interventions, and patient outcomes. (INS, 2000, 17)

Observation of the patient and the delivery of infusion therapy provide data for nursing interventions. Documentation of observations and nursing interventions include the following:

- Tenderness
- Temperatures at and around the site
- Discoloration
- Swelling
- Draining
- Actions taken by the nurse

Documentation of infusion device removal is crucial. Documentation of a peripheral I.V. device removal should include the site condition, integrity and length of catheter, any complications incurred, date, time, and initials of the person removing the device (Dugger, 2001).

Patient education is lacking in most audits of charts; therefore, documentation of patient response to the procedure needs to be included in the charting format. This needs to be addressed in narrative charting or in a check-off format, which includes the status of the patient, the reason for restart, the procedure used, and comments.

Table 7–6 summarizes the steps of starting a peripheral infusion.

NOTE > Refer to Appendix A for CDC (2001) recommendations for the use of peripheral venous catheters.

> Table 7–6 **SUMMARY OF STEPS IN INITIATING I.V. THERAPY**

Precannula Insertion

1. Check physician order; confirm all parts of the order for accuracy.
2. Wash hands for 15 to 20 seconds using antiseptic solution or antimicrobial wipes. Prepare equipment: Check for breaks in integrity and check expiration date; spike and prime the infusion system.
3. Provide privacy. Explain procedure to the patient. Evaluate the patient's psychological preparation for I.V. therapy.
4. Make assessment of site and vein dilatation.
5. Assess both arms keeping the factors for vein selection in mind. Make a choice whether to use blood pressure cuff or tourniquet for dilatation. Use other methods for venous distension, such as warm packs, gravity, or tapping, if necessary.

Cannula Insertion

6. Choose the appropriate catheter for duration of infusion and type of infusate based on facility policy and procedure. Rewash hands.
7. Use gloves, following universal precautions for exposure to blood or body fluids.
8. Prepare site by using 70% alcohol to cleanse the site followed by a 20-second scrub with povidone-iodine or chlorhexidine. Let the povidone-iodine or chlorhexidine air dry. Do not remove. If the patient is allergic to iodine, use alcohol for a 30-second vigorous scrub as a substitute. Do not retouch. Put on gloves before venipuncture.
9. Insert the over-the-needle catheter with the direct or indirect method. Thread the catheter while removing the stylet needle. Connect the catheter hub to I.V. tubing or insert a locking device (PRN device).
10. Stabilize the catheter hub with the chevron taping method or use transparent dressing directly over the hub and site. There are two methods of dressing management: (1) 2-inch × 2-inch gauze with all edges taped; change every 48 hours or (2) transparent film (TSM) applied with aseptic technique and changed every 48 to 72 hours or if the integrity of the dressing is compromised.

Postcannula Insertion

11. Label the insertion site with cannula size, date, time, and initials; label the tubing with the date and time; strip the solution.
12. To facilitate equipment disposal, use OSHA and JCAHO standards for disposal of the needle.
13. Explain to the patient the limitations, provide information on the equipment being used, and give instructions for observation of the site.
14. Remember when doing rate calculations that if a roller clamp or electronic controller is used, the drops per minute should be calculated based on the drop factor.
15. Monitor the patient for response to prescribed therapies. Document the procedure performed, how the patient tolerated the venipuncture, and what instructions were given to the patient.

Discontinuation of the I.V. Cannula

I.V. therapy should be discontinued if the integrity of the cannula is compromised or the physician orders the discontinuation of therapy. To discontinue the I.V. cannula:

1. Put on gloves.
2. Obtain a dry 2-inch by 2-inch gauze pad. Avoid one with alcohol because it causes stinging and promotes bleeding.

3. Loosen the tape and apply the gauze pad loosely over the site.
4. Remove the cannula and transparent dressing as one unit, without pressure over the site.
5. After the catheter is removed, apply direct pressure with the sterile gauze pad over the site.
6. An adhesive bandage may be applied to the venipuncture site after bleeding is controlled.
7. Document the site appearance, how the patient tolerated the procedure, and the intactness of the cannula.

Intermittent Infusion Devices

Intermittent infusion devices or resealable locks, also called PRN (as needed) devices, intermittent I.V. lock devices, and saline or heparin locks have been a standard of practice in most care settings for more than a decade. Flushing is performed to ensure and maintain patency of the catheter and prevent mixing of medications and solutions that are incompatible. Routine flushing shall be performed with the following:

- Administration of blood and blood components
- Blood sampling
- Administration of incompatible medications or solutions
- Administration of medication
- Intermittent therapy
- When converting from continuous to intermittent therapies.

Intermittent infusion devices have both advantages and disadvantages.

ADVANTAGES

- Provide access to the vascular system, allowing for more flexibility than hanging I.V. fluids.
- Allow for reduced volume of fluid administered, which can be important for cardiac patients.
- Can be used to collect blood samples for glucose tolerance tests, eliminating multiple puncture sites.
- Provide access for delivery of emergency medications.

DISADVANTAGES

- Occlusion or blood clotting within the lock
- Possibility of speed shock and damage from drug being rapidly introduced into the circulation

Intermittent Infusion Maintenance

The CDC (2001) recommends that heparin be used only when intermittent infusion devices are used for blood sampling. This is a change based on studies that suggest that 0.9 percent sodium chloride is just as effective as heparin in maintaining catheter patency and reducing phlebitis. How devices are kept patent is determined by institution policy.

Currently, the INS recommends using sodium chloride injection for flushing peripheral I.V. cannulas.

> **INS Standard.** Flushing with 0.9 percent sodium chloride injection solution to ensure and maintain patency of an intermittent peripheral I.V. cannula should be performed at intervals. (INS, 2000, 56)

Sodium Chloride Lock Flush

Cost-effectiveness is a driving factor influencing the choices of clinical practice in today's healthcare delivery. Use of 0.9 percent sodium chloride rather than heparin to maintain heparin locks has been investigated as a way of reducing cost.

ADVANTAGES

- Fewer steps
- Lower cost

DISADVANTAGES

- Loss of patency
- Risk of phlebitis

Heparin Lock Flush

Heparin inhibits reactions that lead to blood coagulation and the formation of fibrin clots in vitro and in vivo. The anticoagulant effect of heparin is almost immediate. Heparin acts indirectly by means of a plasma cofactor, thereby neutralizing several activated clotting factors. Because of these properties, it can be used therapeutically as a flushing agent.

Heparinized saline has been used successfully for many years and is a recognized standard of practice in the medical community. It is recommended that the lowest possible concentration of heparin (10 to 100 U) be used.

ADVANTAGES

- Reduced risk of phlebitis
- Low incidence of side effects when properly used
- Low risk of tort liability with heparin flushing practices
- One dose of heparin solution will maintain anticoagulation within the lumen of the device for up to 4 hours.

Despite pressures to reduce costs by eliminating the flush, legally and ethically hospitals can support only policies that benefit or at least have no adverse effect on the patient.

DISADVANTAGES

- Must be used with caution in patients with known hypersensitivity to pork and beef.
- Local and systemic allergic-type reactions with the use of multidose vial preparations are thought to be associated with a preservative hypersensitivity.
- Has one extra step.
- Increased cost to patients
- Complications, including hypersensitivity reactions, transient increases in activated partial thromboplastin time, and delayed fibrinolysis with platelet aggregation and thrombocytopenia
- Bioincompatibilities

NURSING FAST FACT!

Do not use the heparin sequence in flushing a peripheral I.V. unless backed by institutional policy or specifically ordered by a physician.

When flushing the device, positive pressure within the lumen of the catheter must be maintained during and after administration of the flush solution to prevent reflux of blood into the cannula lumen.

INS Standard. The amount of heparin and the frequency of the flush should be such that the patient's clotting factors are not altered. (INS, 2000, 56)

Table 7–7 presents a comparison of the heparin and saline lock flush procedures.

Controversial Practices

Controversy exists regarding the administration of anesthetics either on or in the skin before venipuncture. These include the use of lidocaine (1 percent Xylocaine hydrochloride), intradermal injection as well as transdermal application of Xylocaine creams and iontophoresis. Table 7–8 presents types of anesthetic agents.

Lidocaine

Lidocaine has been used in clinical practice since 1948 and is one of the safest anesthetics. Lidocaine is an amide that works by stopping impulses at the neural membrane. The anesthetized site is numb to pain, but the patient perceives touch and pressure and has control of his or her muscles. The anesthetic becomes effective within 15 to 30 seconds and lasts 30 to 45 minutes. The nurse must have knowledge of the actions and side

> Table 7–7 **COMPARISON OF HEPARIN LOCK FLUSH AND SODIUM CHLORIDE (SALINE) LOCK FLUSH**

Preservative-Free 0.9% Sodium Chloride Flush	Heparin Lock Flush (10–100 U/mL)
Wash hands. Don gloves. Use aseptic technique/observe standard precautions. **1.** Swab port with appropriate antiseptic. **2.** Connect saline-filled syringe to catheter via insertion into prepared injection/access port. **3.** Slowly aspirate until positive blood return is obtained to confirm patency. **4.** Slowly inject saline maintaining positive pressure **5.** Disconnect syringe from port.	Wash hands. Don gloves. Use aseptic technique/observe standard precautions. **Heparin Flush Only** **1.** Swab port with appropriate antiseptic. **2.** Connect heparin-filed syringe to catheter via insertion port. **3.** Slowly aspirate until positive blood return to confirm catheter patency. **4.** Slowly inject flush maintaining positive pressure **5.** Disconnect syringe from injection port. Use SASH (Saline-Administration-Saline-Heparin) method **1.** Swab port with 70 percent isopropyl alcohol or Betadine. **2.** Connect saline-filled syringe to injection/access port. **3.** Slowly aspirate until positive blood return to confirm catheter patency. **4.** Flush with saline. **5.** Cleanse port with appropriate antiseptic solution. **6.** Connect medication to injection port. **7.** Administer medication. **8.** Disconnect medication from port. **9.** Cleanse port. **10.** Connect second saline-filled syringe to injection port. **11.** Flush with saline. **12.** Cleanse port. **13.** Connect heparin-filled syringe to port, slowly aspirate to reconfirm positive blood aspirate. **14.** Slowly inject heparin flush, maintaining positive pressure. **15.** Disconnect syringe from port.

Source: *INS, 2002 Policies and Procedures.*

effects associated with lidocaine. A history of previous allergies precludes the administration of lidocaine.

The use of lidocaine is a simple process:

1. Check for patient allergy and lidocaine sensitivity.
2. Select the appropriate arm, apply the tourniquet, and select a suitable vein.
3. Draw up 0.1 mL of 1 percent lidocaine (plain) in a TB syringe. More than 0.1 mL increases the risk of vasospasm.
4. Put on gloves.

> Table 7–8 **TYPES OF ANESTHETIC AGENTS**

Transdermal applications
- ELA-Max cream (Ferndale Laboratories, Ferndale, CA)
- EMLA cream (Astra Pharmaceuticals, Wayne, PA)
- LaerCaine Compound (Dr. L. H. Dixon, Unit Dose Packaging, Phoenix, AZ)
- Tetracaine 4 percent cream (amethocaine 4 percent)
- Hydrogel mixtures (compounded individually by pharmacists)
- Ethyl chloride spray (Chloroethane) (Gebauer Company, Cleveland, OH)
- TAC (tetracaine, adrenaline, epinephrine, and cocaine)
- LET (tetracaine, epinephrine, and lidocaine)

Injectables
- Lidocaine 1 percent
- Iontophoretic agent
- NumbyStuff (Iontocaine) (IOMED Clinical Systems, Salt Lake City, UT)
- Bacteriostatic normal saline

5. Prep site with alcohol for 30 seconds and allow it to dry.
6. Reapply the tourniquet. The vein should be fully dilated, pulled taut by stretching, and stabilized while the local anesthetic is administered.
7. Insert the needle at a 15- to 25-degree angle. Inject the lidocaine intradermally into the side of the vein next to the desired insertion site. Do not nick the vein.
8. Withdraw the needle. Allow 5 to 10 seconds for the anesthetic to take effect.
9. Continue with the steps in starting the I.V. (e.g., prep skin with Betadine).

INS Standard. Local anesthesia, including lidocaine, shall not be routinely used for the insertion of a cannula. (INS, 2000, 46)

NURSING FAST FACTS!

Local anesthetics should not be injected into a vein because of the possibility of an undesirable systemic effect. The local anesthetic will not "freeze" the venipuncture site if it is injected into the vein (Fig. 7–7).

Some clinicians believe administration of lidocaine before catheter insertion increases patient comfort and decreases anxiety. However, lidocaine may expose a patient to complications that include (but are not limited to) allergic reaction, anaphylaxis, inadvertent injection of the drug into the vascular system, and obliteration of the vein.

Transdermal Analgesia

ELA-Max (Ferndale Laboratories) and EMLA (Astra) creams are examples of transdermal analgesic topical creams. ELA-Max contains 4 percent lidocaine. ELA-Max contains microscopic, phospholipid spheres called

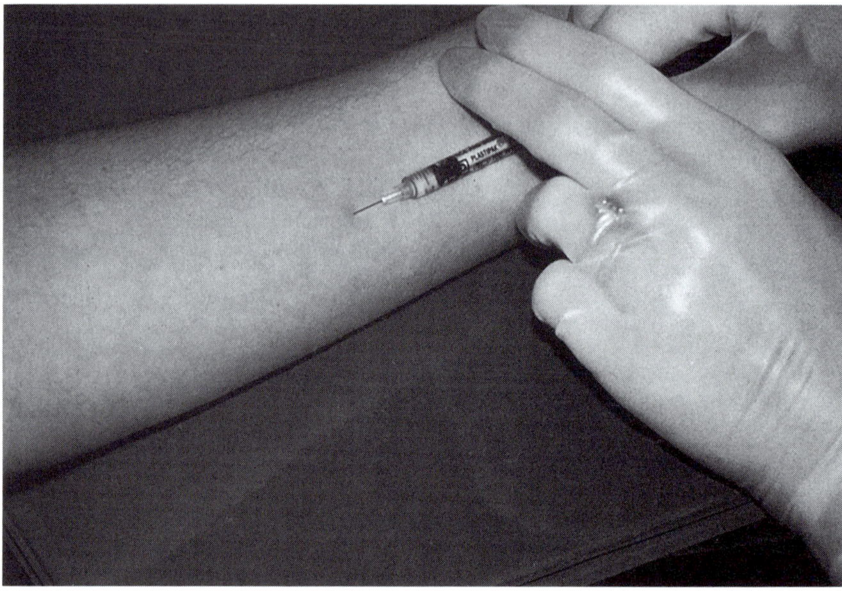

Figure 7–7 ■ Intradermal lidocaine administered before venipuncture using 0.1 to 0.2 mL of 1 percent lidocaine and a tuberculin syringe entering the skin at a 15- to 25-degree angle.

Accusomes^{Tm}. Accusomes^{Tm} act as microscopic vessels that help deliver the drug through the skin. It is not necessary to cover the area after application, but it is recommended when using on young children to prevent accidental ingestion or removal of the cream. This transdermal analgesic takes effect in 30 minutes.

Follow these steps when applying ELA-Max cream:

1. Wear gloves and use clean technique.
2. Prepare the affected area by washing with mild soap and water. Do not use alcohol or acetone.
3. Apply a small amount of cream and gently massage it into the skin. Next, squeeze enough cream to completely cover the affected area so that no skin is visible beneath the cream
4. The cream should remain undisturbed for 30 to 60 minutes.
5. Remove the occlusive dressing, if one is used; remove the cream by wiping with a clean gauze or tissue. Additional skin preparation or cleaning may now be performed (Ferndale Laboratories, 2003).

Figure 7–8 shows application of a transdermal analgesic agent. With ELA-Max cream an occlusive dressing does not have to be used.

Iontophoresis

Iontophoresis is a drug delivery method that uses a small external electric current to deliver water-soluble, charged drugs into the skin. Lidocaine

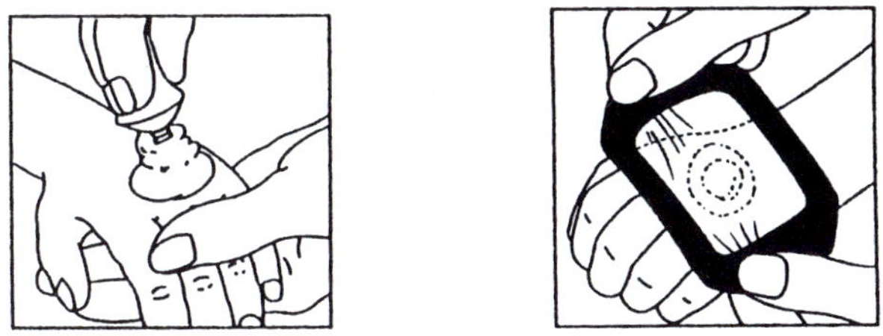

A B

Figure 7–8 ■ *(A)* Application of EMLA cream to the intended venipuncture site. *(B)* Placement of an occlusive dressing over the cream. (Courtesy of Astra Pharmaceutical Products, Inc., Westborough, MA.)

HCl and epinephrine are both positively charged in the pH 4.5 Iontocaine solution, and both drugs are delivered simultaneously by the Phoresor System from the positive electrode to provide dermal anesthesia. Iontocaine is actively pushed into the skin by a low-level direct current. The area of skin under the electrode is anesthetized within 7 to 10 minutes and has a penetration depth of 10 mm. Iontophoresis of Iontocaine causes a transient, local blanching. Iontocaine is indicated for production of local dermal analgesia. Iontocaine is contraindicated in patients with a known history of hypersensitivity to local anesthetics of the amide type (Iomed, 1997).

Bacteriostatic Normal Saline

Bacteriostatic normal saline provides anesthetic action with reduced risk because of inclusion of the preservative benzyl alcohol. Instillation is either intradermal or subcutaneous, forming a wheal just below or to the side of the vein. The anesthetic action is immediate. The benzyl alcohol acts on the nerve endings to produce a short period of local anesthesia. Advantages of using bacteriostatic normal saline over the injectable anesthetic agents include availability, biocompatibility without risk of allergic reactions, and no vasoconstriction. Preservatives in normal saline are not approved for use in neonates or with intrathecal devices (McNelis, 1998; Moureau & Zonderman, 2000).

Calculating the I.V. Rate

Primary I.V. Rate Calculations

The ability to calculate I.V. rates is essential in many clinical environments. Intravenous practitioners must be able to calculate accurately. For proper I.V. rate calculations for medication and solution delivery, two key components must be understood:

1. The drip rate of the I.V. administration set to be used (called the **drop factor**)
2. The amount of solution to be infused over 1 hour.

Macrodrip Sets

To calculate the drip rate correctly, note the drop factor of the administration set. This is usually located on the side, front, or back of the administration package. Drop factors provided by the administration set for **macrodrip** tubing are as follows:

Primary (macrodrip) sets:

- 10 drops = 1 mL
- 15 drops = 1 mL
- 20 drops = 1 mL

Use macrodrip sets whenever (1) a large amount of fluid is ordered to be infused over a short period of time or (2) the microdrips per minute are too many, making counting too difficult (Buchholz, 2003).

Microdrip Sets

Special administration sets such as pediatric (**microdrip**) sets and transfusion administration sets are also available. All manufacturers of microdrip sets are consistent in having 60 drops equaling 1 mL.

Pediatric (microdrip) sets:

- 60 drops = 1 mL

Use microdrip sets whenever (1) the I.V. is to be administered over a long period of time, (2) a small amount of fluid is to be administered, or (3) the macrodrops per minute are too few (Buchholz, 2003).

NURSING FAST FACT!

Blood flow through veins exerts a pressure: if the I.V. is too slow, blood pressure may force blood into the administration set, where it clots. The I.V. will stop.

Blood Administration Sets

Transfusion administration needs a larger drop orifice, so all manufacturers of administration sets specific for blood use 10-drop orifices.

Blood administration sets:

- 10 drops = 1 mL

Table 7–9 presents a drop factor conversion chart.

> Table 7–9 **CONVERSION CHART: RATE CALCULATION**

	Drop Factors			
Order: mL/h	**10 Drops/mL**	**15 Drops/mL**	**20 Drops/mL**	**60 Drops/mL**
10	2	3	3	10
15	3	4	5	15
20	3	5	7	20
30	5	8	10	30
50	8	13	17	50
75	13	19	25	N/A
80	13	20	27	N/A
100	17	25	33	N/A
120	20	30	40	N/A
125	21	31	42	N/A
150	25	38	50	N/A
166	27	42	55	N/A
175	29	44	58	N/A
200	33	50	67	N/A
250	42	63	83	N/A
300	50	75	100	N/A

Microdrip tubing is not appropriate for rates over 50 mL/h.

Determining the Amount of Solution to Be Infused

The physician orders the amount of solution to be infused. Orders are written in one of two ways: (1) in the total amount over a specified length of time, such as 1000 mL over 8 hours; or (2) in the amount to be delivered per hour (e.g., 125 mL/h).

Formula for I.V. Flow Rates Using Drops per Minute

After the drop factor of the tubing and the amount of solution to be infused are known, the following formula can be used to calculate the drop rate per minute:

mL per hour × drops per mL (drop factor [DF]) ÷ 60 (minutes in an hour) = drops per minute

$$\text{Formula: } \frac{\text{mL/h} \times \text{DF}}{\text{minutes}} = \text{drop (gtt)/min}$$

Formula for I.V. Flow Rates Using an Electronic Rate Control Device

Calculations are particularly important when an electronic rate control device is not being used or when an electronic controller is used that does not have a mechanism to dial in milliliters per hour.

NOTE > Rule: Problems in I.V. calculations are solved in two steps. Step 1 is used to solve problems requiring an infusion pump and to simplify the math needed for microdrip and macrodrip. Step 2 will solve micro- and macrodrip problems (Buchholz, 2003).

MACRODRIP INFUSION

Example: Physician orders are for 125 mL/h and the primary tubing selected has a drop factor of 15. Two steps are needed.

$$\text{Formula: } \frac{\text{mL/h} \times \text{DF}}{\text{minutes}} = \text{gtt/min}$$

$$\text{Step 1: } \frac{125 \times 15}{60} = \text{gtt/min}$$

$$\text{Step 2: } = 31 \text{ gtt/min}$$

MICRODRIP INFUSION

When using a microdrip (pediatric tubing) that is 60 drops/mL, the drops per minute equal the milliliters per hour, so only one step is needed.

Example: The physician orders 35 mL of solution per hour for a 2-year-old girl. You would set up your rate calculation as follows, using only one step.

$$\text{Formula: } \frac{\text{mL/h} \times \text{DF}}{\text{minutes}} = \text{gtt/min}$$

$$\text{Step 1: } \frac{35 \times 60}{60} = \text{gtt/min} = 35 \text{ gtt/min}$$

NOTE > Do the practice problems in Math Calculations Worksheet 7-2 at the end of this chapter to test your comprehension of rate calculation.

The conversion chart in Table 7–9 can be cut and laminated for use in your clinical practice to assist in rate calculation.

Formula for I.V. Flow Rates Using Milliliters per Hour

When using an electronic infusion device that has a setting for milliliters per hour, the amount of solution to be infused in 1 hour is programmed into the infusion pump.

Example: The physician orders the I.V. solution at 125 mL/h. Only one step is required. The rate for the pump would be dialed in for 125 mL/h.

Adjusting the Flow Rate

It is the responsibility of the nurse to maintain the rate of flow of I.V. fluid, especially those with additives. Many factors can interfere with the flow: kinking of the tube, movement of the client, the effect of gravity, or placement of the catheter. It is not at the discretion of the nurse to arbitrarily speed up or slow down the flow rate.

NURSING FAST FACT!

Recalculation of flow rates must be included in hospital policy and must not vary from the original rate by more than 25 percent.

A recalculation of the flow rate is indicated when, during routine observation, the flow rate of the I.V. has either increased or decreased. Recalculate the flow rate to administer the total milliliters remaining over the number of hours remaining of the original order.

Example: The order reads 1000 mL of 5 percent dextrose in water over 8 hours. The drop factor is 15 gtt/mL and the I.V. is correctly set at 31 gtt/min. You would expect that after 4 hours, 50 percent of the total or 500 mL of the solution would be infused. However, in checking the I.V. bag the fourth hour after starting the I.V., you find 600 mL remaining. You would compute a new flow rate for the 600 mL to run for the remaining 4 hours.

Step 1: Hourly volume to be infused:

$$\frac{600}{4\text{ hours}} = 150\text{ mL/h}$$

Step 2: Know the drop factor of the tubing: 15

Calculation of example:

$$\frac{15 \times 150}{60} = 37.5 = 38\text{ gtt/min}$$

(It is standard practice to round up if the fraction is above 0.5.)

Secondary Infusion: Solutions to Be Infused in Less Than 1 Hour

A physician may order that a medication be dissolved in a small amount of I.V. fluid (usually 50 to 100 mL) and run "piggyback" to the regular I.V. fluid (Picker, 1999).

To set the rate of the secondary infusion the formula must be changed to adjust for the time change.

Formula:

$$\frac{\text{mL per hour} \times \text{drops per mL (drop factor)}}{\text{Hourly volume (varies)}} = \text{drops per minute}$$

Example: Kefzol 0.5 g in 100 mL of dextrose in water to run intravenous piggyback (IVPB) over 30 minutes. Administration set is 20 drop factor.

$$\frac{20 \times 100 \text{ mL}}{30 \text{ minutes}} = 2000$$

$$= 67 \text{ gtt/min}$$

NOTE > Do the practice problems in Math Calculations Worksheet 7-3 at the end of this chapter to test your comprehension of recalculations and secondary infusions.

NURSING PLAN OF CARE

INITIATION OF VENIPUNCTURE

Focus Assessment

Subjective

- Interview the patient regarding previous experiences with venipunctures.
- Review the purpose of I.V. and patient diagnosis.
- Question regarding previous experience with I.V. therapy.

Objective

- Assess arms for access.
- Assess condition of skin and substructures.
- Review medical chart of history (i.e., shunts, previous surgeries, stroke) and current medical diagnosis.
- Assess presence of tattoos.
- Assess presence of edema.
- Review trends in vital signs.

Patient Outcome/Evaluation Criteria

Patient will:

- Remain free of complications associated with the presence of the catheter, including absence of pain, swelling, or redness.
- Verbalize comfort and minimal restrictions to activities of daily living immediately after catheter insertion.
- Demonstrate improved fluid balance.

(Continued on following page)

- Verbalize understanding of need for I.V. access and consent to procedure.

Nursing Diagnoses

- Anxiety (mild, moderate, or severe) related to threat to or change in health status; misconceptions regarding therapy
- Fear related to insertion of cannula
- Knowledge deficit related to new procedure and maintaining I.V. therapy
- Impaired physical mobility related to pain or discomfort resulting from placement and maintenance of I.V. cannula
- Impaired skin integrity related to I.V. cannula or I.V. solution
- Pain related to physical trauma (e.g., cannula insertion)
- Risk of infection related to broken skin or traumatized tissue

Nursing Management

1. Verify the physician's order for I.V. therapy.
2. Educate the patient about procedure.
3. Maintain standard precautions.
4. Adhere to hand hygiene guidelines
5. Use strict aseptic technique during insertion and maintenance of the cannula.
6. Examine the solution for type, amount, expiration date, character of solution, and integrity of container.
7. Determine compatibility of all I.V. fluids and additive consulting appropriate literature.
8. Select and prepare an I.V. infusion pump as indicated.
9. Administer I.V. fluids at room temperature.
10. Monitor for I.V. therapy complications (e.g., phlebitis, infiltration, site infection).
11. Replace I.V. cannula and administration sets according to INS Standards of Practice
12. Maintain integrity of occlusive dressing.
13. On discontinuing of I.V. cannula observe I.V. site for signs and symptoms of infection, infiltration, or phlebitis; assess that the catheter removed is intact; and educate the patient on post infusion complications.

Source: *Elkin, Perry, & Potter (2003).*

Patient Education

Instruct on purpose of I.V. therapy.

Educate regarding limitations of movement.

Instruct to notify the nurse if pump alarms.

Instruct to report discomfort at the infusion site.

Documentation should include the responses of the patient family and caregiver to teaching. All infusion therapy modalities should be explained to all those involved in patient care.

Websites

Patient education: www.patient-education.com

Other sites:

Home Care Issues

Home care issues for the initiation and maintenance of I.V. therapy revolve around technical procedures, as well as the monitoring of therapy. The technical procedures that the patient is expected to learn and perform depend on his or her cognitive ability, willingness to learn, and the specific technique being taught. Another home care issue is the number of visits that will be required to maintain the line and the proximity of the patient's home to a healthcare facility.

In alternative care settings, such as the home, the nurse may have to adapt to poor lighting, not having an adjustable bed, and lack of privacy (Perucca, 2001).

Many common household items contain latex. Home-bound patients who perform self-catheterization or undergo intermittent catheterization are at risk for latex-related allergic reactions. Synthetic rubber, polyethylene, silicon, or vinyl can be used effectively in the home care setting.

Territoriality (i.e., the need for space) serves four functions: security, privacy, autonomy, and self-identification. People tend to generally feel safer in their own territory because it is arranged and equipped in a familiar manner. Most people believe there is a degree of predictability associated with being in one's own personal space and that this degree of predictability is hard to achieve elsewhere (Giger & Davidhizar, 2004).

Patients or their caregivers are often expected to:

- Administer solutions or medications, and add mix medications
- Change dressings.
- Change administration sets.
- Set up or monitor pump equipment.

The patient and his or her family must be taught universal precautions and aseptic technique in the home care setting.

NURSING FAST FACTS!

- *The home care nursing staff is responsible for the routine restarts of peripheral I.V. or blood draws.*
- *Requirements for clinical documentation in the home are generally the same as those for acute care except for environmental issues. The principle diagnosis is critical for medical reimbursement, and the record must reflect total patient care, including the assessment, care plan, evaluations, implementation of care, and outcomes (Dugger, 2001). Joint Commission on Accreditation of Healthcare Organizations (JCAHO) standards for home care require that an agency document the use of clinical practice guidelines, critical pathways, and standards of practice in the decision-making process (JCAHO, 2000).*

Key Points

- The first step is an understanding of the anatomy and physiology of the venous system. The five layers in the approach to successful venipuncture are the epidermis, dermis, tunica adventitia, tunica media, and tunica intima.
- A working knowledge of the veins in the hand and forearm is vital so the practitioner can successfully locate an acceptable vein for venipuncture and cannula placement. Keep in mind the type of solution, condition of vein, duration of therapy, patient age, patient preference, patient activity, presence of disease, previous surgery, presence of shunts or grafts, allergies, and medication history.
- The steps in performing the placement of a catheter that can support I.V. therapy for 48 to 72 hours are as follows:

  Precannulation
  - Step 1: Check physician's order.
  - Step 2: Wash hands.
  - Step 3: Prepare equipment.
  - Step 4: Assess the patient and his or her psychological preparedness.
  - Step 5: Select site and dilate vein.

  Cannula Placement
  - Step 6: Needle selection
  - Step 7: Gloving
  - Step 8: Site preparation
  - Step 9: Vein entry
  - Step 10: Catheter stabilization and dressing management

  Postcannulation
  - Step 11: Labeling
  - Step 12: Equipment disposal

- Step 13: Patient instructions
- Step 14: Rate calculation
- Step 15: Documentation

- The choice of using heparin or saline to maintain latex injection ports (locks) is determined by the agency's policies and procedures and the physician's order. Check these before using the steps in heparin or saline lock flush.
- Locks must be flushed every 8 hours if not being used for medication administration.
- Use of Xylocaine hydrochloride before venipuncture. Use 0.1 to 0.2 mL of 1 percent xylocaine injected intradermal. Wait 5 to 10 seconds before continuing the steps of the venipuncture.
- Use of topical transdermal analgesia cream, such as a combination of lidocaine 2.5 percent and prilocaine 2.5 percent. Apply in thick layer and cover with occlusive dressing for 1 hour.
- Rate calculations: To calculate drop rates of gravity infusions, I.V. nurses must know (1) the drop factor of the administration set and (2) the amount of solution ordered.

  Macrodrip sets:
  - 10 gtt = 1 mL
  - 15 gtt = 1 mL
  - 20 gtt = 1 mL

  Microdrip sets:
  - 60 gtt = 1 mL
  - Transfusion administration sets: usually 10 gtt = 1 mL

Critical Thinking: Case Study

An order is received to convert a patient's continuous I.V. infusion to a saline lock. The patient is complaining of pain and has a new order for Demerol 25 mg I.V. What equipment must be gathered?

What are the priorities of nursing care? What nursing interventions must be implemented?

Media Link: Answers to this critical thinking exercise and additional exercises are on the CD–ROM.

Worksheet 7–1

Superficial Veins of the Upper Extremities

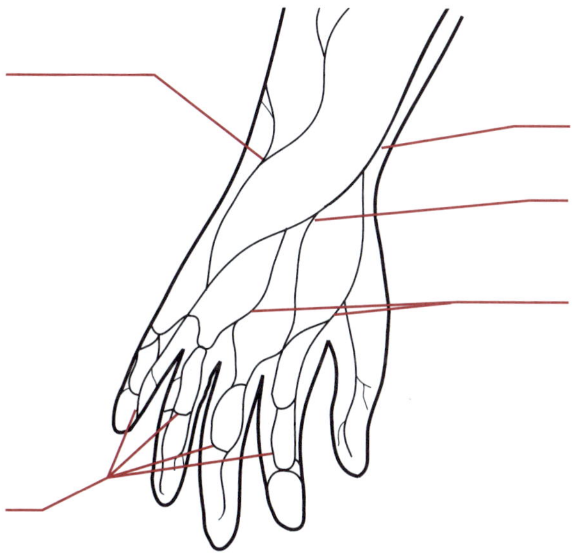

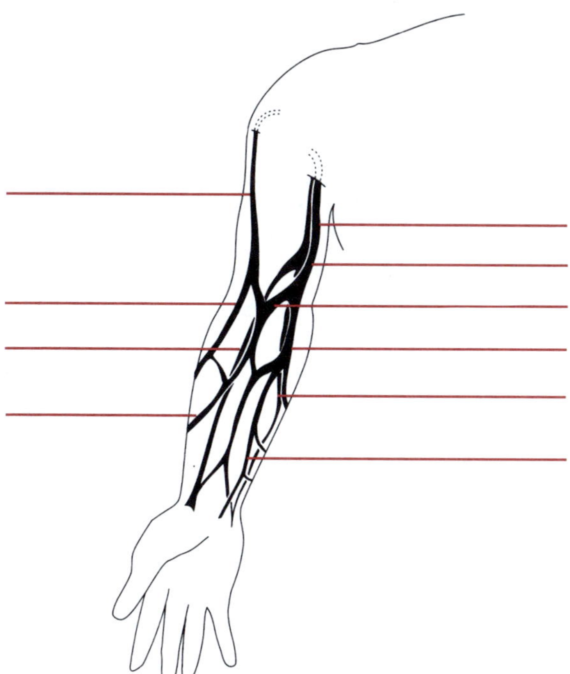

Worksheet Answers 7–1

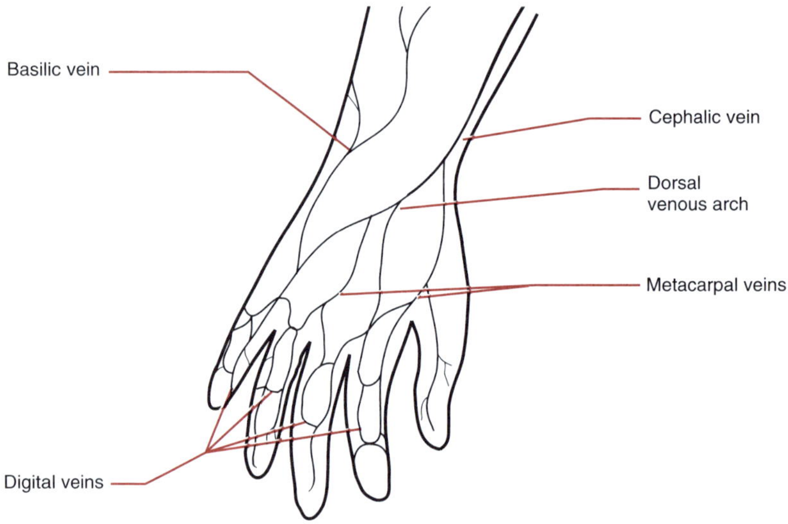

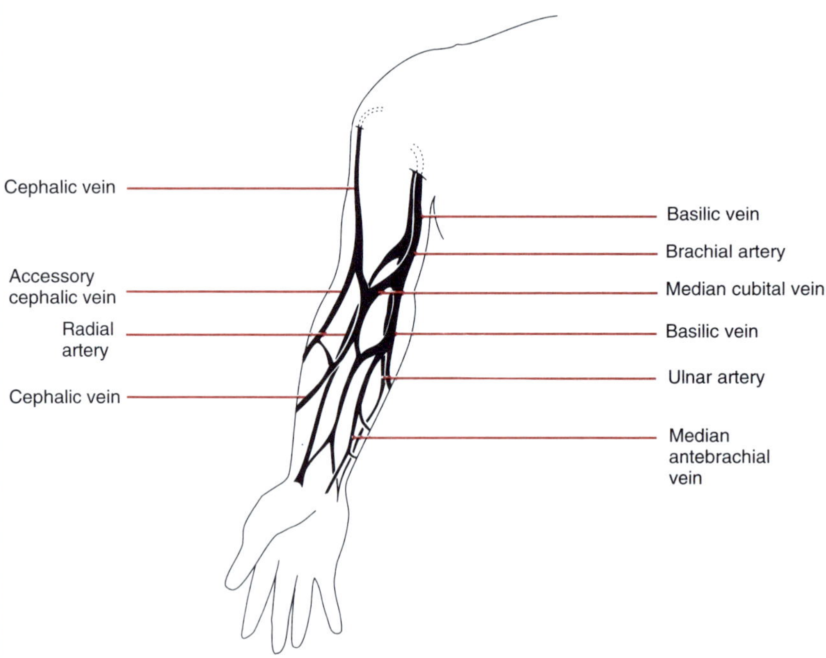

Worksheet 7–2

Basic Calculation of Primary Infusions

1. The order reads 1000 mL of 5 percent dextrose in water at 125 mL/h. You have available 20 drop factor tubing. Calculate the drops per minute.

2. The order is for 1000 mL of 5 percent dextrose and 0.45 percent sodium chloride at 150 mL/h. You have available 15 drop factor tubing. Calculate the drops per minute.

3. The order is for 250 mL (1 U) of packed cells over 2 hours. Remember, blood tubing is always 10 drop factor. Calculate the drops per minute.

(Continued on following page)

Worksheet 7–2 *(Continued)*

4. The order is for 45 mL/h of 5 percent dextrose and sodium chloride solution on an 8-month-old baby. Calculate the drops per minute if you have to use a controller that is drops per minute. (Remember, use microdrip tubing.)

5. The order reads 3000 mL of a multiple electrolyte fluid over 24 hours. You have available 20 drop factor tubing. Calculate the drops per minute.

6. The order is for 250 mL of 5 percent dextrose in water to run at 25 mL/h. You will be infusing it using an infusion pump.

(Continued on following page)

Worksheet 7–2

7. The order is for 500 mL of lactated Ringer's solution to be administered at 75 mL/h. You have available 15 drop factor tubing. Calculate the drops per minute

8. Calculate problem 7 using 20 drop factor tubing.

9. The order reads 50 mL/h of 5 percent dextrose in water to rehydrate an 85-year-old woman. You assess the patient and find her cardiovascular status compromised. What tubing do you choose, microdrip or macrodrip? Why? Calculate the drops per minute using 15 drop factor tubing and 60 drop factor tubing.

(Continued on following page)

10. The order is for aminophylline 500 mg in 250 mL of 5 percent dextrose in water to be infused at 50 mL/h. You will be infusing it via an infusion pump.

Worksheet 7–2 Answers

1. Formula: $\dfrac{\text{mL/h} \times \text{DF}}{\text{minutes}} = \text{gtt/min}$

Step 1: $\dfrac{125 \times 20}{60} = \text{gtt/min}$

Step 2: $\dfrac{125}{3} = 42 \text{ gtt/min}$

2. Formula: $\dfrac{\text{mL/h} \times \text{DF}}{\text{minutes}} = \text{gtt/min}$

Step 1: $\dfrac{150 \times 15}{60} = \text{gtt/min}$

Step 2: $\dfrac{150}{4} = 38 \text{ gtt/min}$

3. Formula: $\dfrac{\text{mL}}{\text{hours}} = \text{mL/h}$

Step 1: $250 \div 2 = 125 \text{ mL/h}$

Formula: $\dfrac{\text{mL/h} \times \text{DF}}{\text{minutes}} = \text{gtt/min}$

Step 2: $\dfrac{125 \times 10}{60} = \text{gtt/min}$

Step 3: $\dfrac{125}{6} = 21 \text{ gtt/min}$

4. Formula: $\dfrac{\text{mL/h} \times \text{DF}}{\text{minutes}} = \text{gtt/min}$

Step 1: $\dfrac{45 \times 60}{60} = 45 \text{ gtt/min}$

Only one step needed for microdrop infusions.
When using 60 gtt tubing the gtt/min = the amount of the hourly infusion volume.

(Continued on following page)

Worksheet 7–2 Answers *(Continued)*

5. Formula: $\frac{\text{mL}}{\text{hours}} = \text{mL/h}$

Step 1: $\frac{3000}{24} = \underline{125\ \text{mL/h}}$

Formula: $\frac{\text{mL/h} \times \text{DF}}{\text{minutes}} = \text{gtt/min}$

Step 2: $\frac{125 \times 20}{60} = \text{gtt/min}$

Step 3: $\frac{125}{3} = 42\ \text{gtt/min}$

6. Formula: $\frac{\text{mL/h} \times \text{DF}}{\text{minutes}} = \text{gtt/min}$

Step 1: $\frac{25 \times 60}{60} = 25\ \text{gtt/min}$

Only one step needed for infusion pumps (microdrip sets).

7. Formula: $\frac{\text{mL/h} \times \text{DF}}{\text{minutes}} = \text{gtt/min}$

Step 1: $\frac{75 \times 15}{60} = \text{gtt/min}$

Step 2: $\frac{75}{4} = 19\ \text{gtt/min}$

8. Formula: $\frac{\text{mL/h} \times \text{DF}}{\text{minutes}} = \text{gtt/min}$

Step 1: $\frac{75 \times 20}{60} = \text{gtt/min}$

Step 2: $\frac{75}{3} = 25\ \text{gtt/min}$

(Continued on following page)

Worksheet 7–2 Answers

9. Formula: $\frac{\text{mL/h} \times \text{DF}}{\text{minutes}} = \text{gtt/min}$

Microdrip:

Step 1: $\frac{50 \times 60}{60} = 50 \text{ gtt/min}$

Macrodrip:

Step 1: $\frac{50 \times 15}{60} = \text{gtt/min}$

Step 2: $\frac{50}{4} = 13 \text{ gtt/min}$

Microdrip would be a better choice because of the difficulty regulating a 13-gtt drip rate. Also, with a compromised patient, there is more flexibility if needed to adjust the rate lower with a microdrip set.

10. Formula: $\frac{\text{mL/h} \times \text{DF}}{\text{minutes}} = \text{gtt/min}$

Step 1: $\frac{50 \times 60}{60} = 50 \text{ gtt/min}$

Only one step needed for infusion pump.

Worksheet 7–3

Recalculations and Secondary Infusions

1. The physician orders a fluid challenge of 250 mL of sodium chloride over 45 minutes. You have 20 drop factor tubing available. Calculate the drops per minute in order to accurately deliver the 250 mL over 45 minutes.

2. Administer vinblastine sulfate 50 mg diluted in 50 mL of 0.9 percent sodium chloride over 15 minutes. You have available macrodrip 15.

3. Administer 500 mg of acyclovir in 100 mL of 5 percent dextrose in water over 1 hour. You have available macrodrip 20 gtt.

(Continued on following page)

Worksheet 7–3

4. Administer trimethoprim–sulfamethoxazole 400 mg in 125 mL of dextrose in water over 90 minutes. You have available a microdrip set and macrodrip 15 gtt.

5. At 12 noon you discover that an infusion set to deliver 100 mL per hour from 7 AM to 5 PM has 400 mL left in the infusion bag. Recalculate the infusion using a macrodrip 10 gtt.

6. Recalculate the flow rate in drops per minute for an infusion that is scheduled for 12 hours of 1000 mL of lactated Ringer's solution. At the sixth hour, there is 850 mL remaining. It is infusing using a macrodrip 20 gtt.

(Continued on following page)

Worksheet 7–3 *(Continued)*

7. Recalculate the flow rate in drops per minute for an infusion that is scheduled for 6 hours of 1000 mL of 5 percent dextrose in water. At the end of hour 4, there is 360 mL remaining. It is infusing using a macrodrip 15 gtt.

8. Recalculate the flow rate for an infusion of 100 mL of 0.9 percent sodium chloride solution to run for 4 hours. At the end of the second hour, there is 90 mL remaining. You have available a microdrip and macrodrip 15 gtt.

9. The order is for carbenicillin disodium 2 g of IVPB diluted in 50 mL of 5 percent dextrose in water to infuse in 15 minutes. You have available macrodrip 20 gtt. Calculate the drip rate.

10. The order is written for vancomycin 500 mg in 100 mL of 5 percent dextrose in water over 30 minutes. You will be infusing it with an infusion pump.

Worksheet 7–3 Answers

1. Formula: $\frac{\text{mL/h} \times \text{DF}}{\text{minutes}} = \text{gtt/min}$

   Step 1: $\frac{250 \times 20}{45} = \text{gtt/min}$

   Step 2: $\frac{250 \times 4}{9} = \frac{1000}{9} = \underline{111 \text{ gtt/min}}$

2. Formula: $\frac{\text{mL/h} \times \text{DF}}{\text{minutes}} = \text{gtt/min}$

   Step 1: $\frac{50 \times 15}{15} = \underline{50 \text{ gtt/min}}$

3. Formula: $\frac{\text{mL/h} \times \text{DF}}{\text{minutes}} = \text{gtt/min}$

   Step 1: $\frac{100 \times 20}{60} = \text{gtt/min}$

   Step 2: $\frac{100}{3} = 33 \text{ gtt/min}$

4. Formula: $\frac{\text{mL/h} \times \text{DF}}{\text{minutes}} = \text{gtt/min}$

   Step 1: $\frac{125 \times 15}{90} = \text{gtt/min}$

   Step 2: $\frac{125}{6} = 21 \text{ gtt/min}$

5. Formula: $\frac{\text{mL}}{\text{hours}} = \text{mL/h}$

   Step 1: $\frac{400}{5} = 80 \text{ mL/h}$

   Formula: $\frac{\text{mL/h} \times \text{DF}}{\text{minutes}} = \text{gtt/min}$

(Continued on following page)

Worksheet 7–3 Answers *(Continued)*

Step 2: $\frac{80 \times 10}{60} = \text{gtt/min}$

Step 3: $\frac{80}{6} = 13 \text{ gtt/min}$

6. Formula: $\frac{\text{mL}}{\text{hours}} = \text{mL/h}$

Step 1: $\frac{850}{6} = 142 \text{ mL/h}$

Formula: $\frac{\text{mL/h} \times \text{DF}}{\text{minutes}} = \text{gtt/min}$

Step 2: $\frac{142 \times 20}{60} = \text{gtt/min}$

Step 3: $\frac{142}{3} = 47 \text{ gtt/min}$

7. Formula: $\frac{\text{mL}}{\text{hours}} = \text{mL/h}$

Step 1: $\frac{360}{2} = 180 \text{ mL/h}$

Formula: $\frac{\text{mL/h} \times \text{DF}}{\text{minutes}} = \text{gtt/min}$

Step 2: $\frac{180 \times 15}{60} = \text{gtt/min}$

Step 3: $\frac{180}{4} = 45 \text{ gtt/min}$

8. Formula: $\frac{\text{mL}}{\text{hours}} = \text{mL/h}$

Step 1: $\frac{90}{2} = 45 \text{ mL/h}$

(Continued on following page)

Worksheet 7–3 Answers

Formula: $\frac{\text{mL/h} \times \text{DF}}{\text{minutes}} = \text{gtt/min}$

Step 2: $\frac{45 \times 15}{60} = \text{gtt/min}$

Step 3: $\frac{45}{4} = 11 \text{ gtt/min}$

9. Formula: $\frac{\text{mL/h} \times \text{DF}}{\text{minutes}} = \text{gtt/min}$

Step 1: $\frac{50 \times 20}{15} = \text{gtt/min}$

Step 2: $\frac{50 \times 4}{3} = \text{gtt/min}$

Step 3: $\frac{200}{3} = 67 \text{ gtt/min}$

10. Formula: $\frac{\text{mL/h} \times \text{DF}}{\text{minutes}} = \text{gtt/min}$

Step 1: $\frac{100 \times 60}{30} = \text{gtt/min}$

Step 2: $\frac{100}{2} = 50 \text{ gtt/min}$

Post-Test

In **1** through **5**, match the definition in Column II to the term in Column I:

Column I	Column II
1. Antimicrobial	**a.** Peripheral vascular access device made of polyurethane
2. Cannula	**b.** Slanted portion of cannula device or needle
3. Bevel	**c.** To fill the administration set with infusate for the first time
4. Prime	**d.** To insert the administration set into the infusate container
5. Spike	**e.** An agent that destroys or prevents the development of microorganisms

6. List the four steps in maintaining patency of a saline locking device when giving a medication.

1.

2.

3.

4.

7. Before equipment setup and venipuncture, how many seconds of hand hygiene procedure with an antimicrobial soap are recommended?

a. 10 to 30

b. 15 to 20

c. 30 to 60

d. 45 to 60

8. I.V. therapy labels should be on which areas?

a. Catheter site, tubing, and solution container

b. Tubing, solution container, and chart

c. Solution container, catheter site, and patient's armband

9. The order reads 1000 mL of 5 percent dextrose and lactated Ringer's solution at 125 mL/h. Calculate the drip rate using 20 gtt factor tubing.

____________gtt/min

10. What is the recommended frequency in which a patient receiving infusion therapy should be monitored?

a. Systematic, ongoing and documented

b. Every 4 hours and documented

c. Every shift or every 8 to 12 hours and documented

d. Every 24 hours and documented

References

Barber, P. (2003). Scratch that. *Nurseweek,* June 2.

Buchholz, S. (2003). Henle's *Med-Math* (4th ed.). Philadelphia: Lippincott Williams & Wilkins, pp. 188–204.

Dugger, B. (2001). Documentation. In Hankins, J., Lonsway, R.A., Hedrick, C., & Perdue, M.B. (eds.). *Intravenous Therapy: Clinical Principles and Practice* (2nd ed.). Philadelphia: W.B. Saunders, pp. 459–468.

Elkin, M.K., Perry, A., & Potter, P.A. (2003). *Nursing Interventions and Clinical Skills* (3rd ed.). St. Louis: Mosby.

Fabian, B. (1998). Basic I.V. skills: Adult and pediatric. National Academy presentation: November 1998, Phoenix, AZ.

Ferndale Laboratories (2003). ELA-MAX package insert. Ferndale, CA: Ferndale Laboratories.

Giger, J.N., & Davidhizar, R.E. (2004). *Transcultural Nursing: Assessment and Intervention.* St. Louis: Mosby.

Guyton, A.C., & Hall, J.E. (2001). *Textbook of Medical Physiology* (10th ed.). Philadelphia: W.B. Saunders.

Hadaway, L. (1999). Choosing the right vascular access device, part I. *Nursing 99,* 99(2), 18.

Hibbard, J.S., Mulberry, G.K., & Brady, A. (2002). A clinical study comparing the skin antisepsis and safety of chloraprep, 70 isopropyl alcohol and aqueous chlorhexidine. *Journal of Infusion Nursing,* 25(4), 244–249.

Infusion Nursing Society (2000). Revised intravenous nursing standards of practice. *Journal of Intravenous Nursing,* 21 (Suppl), 65.

Iomed Clinical Systems. (1997). Iontoaine (product literature). Salt Lake City: Iomed, Inc,

Joint Commission on Accreditation of Healthcare Organizations (1999–2000). Comprehensive accreditation manual for health care. Oakbrook Terrace: IL. Joint Commission on Accreditation of Healthcare Organizations.

LaRue, G.D. (2000). Efficacy of ultrasonography in peripheral venous cannulation, *Journal of Intravenous Nursing,* 23(1) 29–34.

Maki, D.G., & Mermel, L.A. (1998). Infection due to infusion therapy. In Bennett, J., & Brachman, P. (eds.). *Hospital Infections* (4th ed.). Philadelphia: Lippincott-Raven, pp. 689–716.

McNelis, K.A. (1998). Intradermal bacteriostaic 0.9% sodium chloride containing the preservative benzyl alcohol compared with intradermal lidocaine hydrochloride 1% for alleviation of intravenous cannulation pain. *AANA Journal*, 66, 585–590.

Millam, D.A., & Hadaway, L. (2000). On the road to successful I.V. starts. *Nursing 2000*, 4, 34–42.

Moureau, N., & Lannucci, A.L. (2003). Catheter securement: Trends in performance and complications associated with the use of either traditional methods or an adhesive device. *Journal of Vascular Access Devices* 8(1), 29–33.

Moureau, N., & Zonderman, A. (2000). Does it always have to hurt? *Journal of Intravenous Therapy*, 23(4), 213–218.

Otto, S.E. (2003). Understanding the immune system: Overview for infusion assessment. *Journal of Infusion Nursing*, 26(2), 79–85.

Perucca, R. (2001). Obtaining vascular access. In Hankins, J., Lonsway, R.A., Hedrick, C., & Perdue, M.B. (eds.). *Intravenous Therapy: Clinical Principles and Practice* (2nd ed.) Philadelphia: W.B. Saunders, pp. 370–399.

Smeltzer, S.C., & Bare, B.G. (2003). *Brunner and Suddarth's Textbook of Medical-Surgical Nursing* (9th ed.). Philadelphia: J.B. Lippincott, Williams & Wilkins.

U.S. Centers for Disease Control and Prevention. (2001). Centers for Disease Control and Prevention intravascular device-related infections prevention; Guideline availability; notice. Atlanta: US Department of Health and Human Services.

U.S. Centers for Disease Control and Prevention. (2002). Guideline for hand hygiene in health-care settings. Atlanta: US Department of Health and Human Services. 51 (RR16) 1–44.

Venetec. (2000). Statlock virtually eliminates catheter restarts in new clinical trial. San Diego: Venetec International. Press Release.

Walling A.D, & Lenhardt, R. (2003). Local warming and insertion of peripheral venous cannulas: Single blinded prospective randomized controlled trail and single blinded randomized crossover trial. *American Family Physician*, 67(2), 401.

Answers to Chapter 7 Post-Test

1. **e**
2. **a**
3. **b**
4. **c**
5. **d**
6. Check patency; flush with 1 mL of sodium chloride; administer medication; flush with 1 mL of sodium chloride using positive pressure.
7. **b**
8. **a**
9. 42 gtt/min
10. **a**

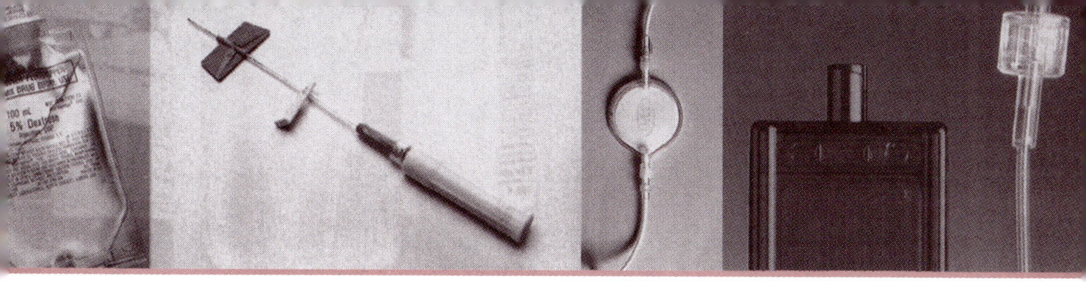

Chapter 8
Phlebotomy Techniques

Medicine is not only a science, but also the art of letting our own individuality interact with the individuality of the patient.
—Albert Schweitzer

Chapter Contents

LEARNING OBJECTIVES

Upon completion of this chapter, the reader will be able to:

1. List the various types of anticoagulants used in blood collection.
2. Identify the tube color codes for vacuum collection.

LEARNING OBJECTIVES *continued*

3. Describe phlebotomy safety supplies and equipment.
4. Identify the various supplies that should be carried on a specimen collection tray.
5. Identify the types of equipment needed to collect blood by venipuncture.
6. Describe the patient identification process.
7. List essential information for test requisitions.
8. Identify the most common sites for venipuncture for blood collection.
9. Describe the venipuncture procedure and steps for evacuated tube method and syringe method.
10. State the order of draw for collection tubes.

GLOSSARY

Acid–citrate–dextrose (ACD) An additive commonly used in specimen collection for blood donations to prevent clotting. Ensures that the RBC maintains their oxygen-carrying capacity.

Anticoagulant Substance introduced into the blood or a blood specimen to keep it from clotting

Assay Determination of the purity of a substance or the amount of any particular constituent of a mixture

Citrate–phosphate–dextrose (CPD) Anticoagulant typically used for blood donations.

Ethylenediaminetetraacetic acid (EDTA) Anticoagulant additive used to prevent the blood clotting sequence by removing calcium and forming calcium slats. EDTA prevents platelet aggregation and is useful for platelet counts and platelet function tests.

Hemoconcentration Increased localized blood concentration of large molecules such as proteins, cells, and coagulation factors

Hemolysis Rupture or lysis of the blood cells

Multiple-sample needle Used with the evacuated tube method of blood collection, these needles are attached to a holder/adapter and allow for multiple specimen tube fills and changes without blood leakage.

National Committee for Clinical Laboratory Standards (NCCLS) Nonprofit organization that recommends quality standard and guidelines for clinical laboratory procedures

National Phlebotomy Association (NPA) Professional organization for phlebotomists that offers continuing education activities and certification examination for phlebotomists

Oxalates Anticoagulants that prevent blood-clotting sequence by removing calcium and forming calcium salts

Phlebotomist Individual who practices phlebotomy
Phlebotomy Incision of a vein for blood collection
Single-sample needle Used for collecting a blood sample from a syringe.
Syringe method Method of venipuncture whereby a syringe is used to collect blood that is then transferred to collection tubes
Vacuum (evacuated) tube system Color-coded specimen collection tube that contains a vacuum so as to aspirate blood when a needle enters a patient's vein. The tubes are part of a blood collection method that also requires a double-pointed needle and special plastic holder (adapter).

Introduction to Phlebotomy

Purpose of Phlebotomy

Blood and other specimen collections are important to the entire health assessment of the client. Laboratory analysis of a variety of specimens is used for three important purposes:

1. Diagnostic testing, which is used to contribute to the client's diagnosis
2. Therapeutic assessments, which are used to develop the appropriate therapy or treatment of the medical condition
3. Monitoring of a patient's health status, which is used to make sure the therapy or treatment is working to alleviate the medical condition

Professional Competencies

The role of the nurse may include **phlebotomy**, along with the responsibility of preserving veins for infusion therapy. The nurse has the unique position of using a single venipuncture to permit both the withdrawal for blood and the initiation of an infusion, thereby preserving veins.

Usually a **phlebotomist** or blood collector must complete a phlebotomy program. Nurses are usually trained on the job or in an infusion course. There are professional organizations that recognize phlebotomists independently. All sponsor certification examinations for healthcare workers.

NURSING FAST FACT!

If specimens are incorrectly acquired, labeled, or transported by the healthcare practitioner, the laboratory tests can be useless or can even be harmful to the client.

NOTE > Review Chapter 1: Risk Management for further information on competencies and quality improvement standards.

Websites

The following is a list of organizations and their Websites:
American Society of Clinical Pathologists (ASCP): *www.ascp.org*
The National Phlebotomy Association (NPA): *www.scpt.com*
The American Society for Clinical Laboratory Science (ASCLS): *www.nca-info.org*
American Medical Technologists (AMT): *www.amt1.com*
American Society of Phlebotomy Technicians (ASPT): *www.aspt.org*

The nurse performing phlebotomy procedures or the phlebotomist must have the following knowledge base to perform blood withdrawal procedures safely (American Society of Clinical Pathologists, 1999):

Demonstrates knowledge of:

- Basic anatomy and physiology
- Medical terminology
- Potential sources of error
- Safety measures and infection control practices
- Standard operating procedures
- Fundamental biology

Selects appropriate:

- Courses of action
- Quality control procedures
- Equipment/methods and reagents
- Site for blood collection

Prepares Patient and Equipment
Evaluates

- Specimen and patient situations
- Possible sources of error and inconsistencies

Steps in Collection of Blood Specimens

Healthcare Worker Preparation

All healthcare workers must be familiar with current recommendations and hospital policies for handling blood and body fluids. All specimens should be treated as if they are hazardous and infectious.

NOTE > Review Chapter 1: Risk Management for further information on competencies and quality improvement standards. Refer to Chapter 2 for guidelines on standard precautions.

Prior to performing any type of specimen collection, the nurse or phlebotomist should have gathered the necessary protective equipment, phlebotomy supplies, test requisitions, writing pens, and appropriate patient information. Refer to Table 8–1 for a list of supplies that should be included in a blood collection tray.

Blood Collection

Blood collection includes obtaining serum, plasma, or whole blood from the patient. Serum consists of plasma minus fibrinogen and is obtained by drawing blood in a dry tube and allowing it to coagulate. A majority of the diagnostic tests require serum. Plasma consists of stable components of blood minus cells. Anticoagulant tubes are used to prevent blood from clotting. Whole blood is required in many tests such as complete blood count and bleeding times.

In preparing for blood collection the healthcare worker carries out essential steps to ensure a successful blood specimen collection. **The National Committee for Clinical Laboratory Standards** (1998b) has recommendations for safe blood collection. These steps may vary in individual facilities based on the characteristics of their patient populations. Some steps may be carried out simultaneously. The recommended steps include:

1. Preparation of the healthcare worker
2. Assessing the patient's physical disposition

> Table 8–1 **BLOOD COLLECTION TRAY CONTENTS**

Marking pen or pencil
Vacuum tubes containing the anticoagulants
Safety holders for vacuum tubes (single-use disposable)
Needles for vacuum tubes and syringes
Tourniquets (latex and non-latex)
Gloves (non-sterile-exam)
70% Isopropyl alcohol and iodine prep pads or ChloraPrep pads (chlorhexidine)
Sterile gauze pads

Tape
Band Aids
Biohazardous waste container
Safety lancets
Microcollection blood serum separator tubes
Antimicrobial hand gel – if bacteriocidal soap not available

3. Identifying the patient
4. Approaching the patient
5. Selecting a puncture site
6. Selecting and preparing equipment and supplies
7. Preparing the puncture site
8. Choosing a venipuncture method
9. Collecting the samples in the appropriate tubes and in the correct order.
10. Labeling the samples
11. Assessing the patient after withdrawal of the blood specimen
12. Considering any special circumstances that occurred during the phlebotomy procedure
13. Assessing criteria for sample recollection or rejection
14. Prioritizing patients and sample tubes.

Accessing, Identifying, and Approaching the Patient

The nurse or phlebotomist must be aware of the physical or emotional disposition of the patient, which can have an impact on the blood collection process. Cues that can help in the phlebotomy process include the following (Garza & Becan-McBride, 2002, 235):

- *Diet:* It is important to note whether the patient has been fasting or not.
- *Stress:* A patient who is excessively anxious or emotional may need extra time.
- *Age:* The elderly may have more difficult or frail veins from which to choose for the venipuncture site. Pediatric patients often need additional support for venipuncture.
- *Weight:* Obese patient may require special equipment, such as a large blood pressure cuff for the tourniquet or a longer needle to penetrate the vein.

NOTE > Chapter 10 covers special problems in venipuncture.

Patient Identification Process

Prior to any specimen collection procedure, the patient must be correctly identified by using a two-step process:

- The patient should be asked to state his or her first and last names.
- Confirm a match between patient's response, the test requisition, and some form of identification, such as hospital identification bracelet, driver's license, or another identification card.

A hospitalized patient should always wear an identification bracelet indicating his or her first and last names and a designated hospital number.

Patients in outpatient clinics usually have the same procedures as inpatient clients, with use of identification bracelet or predistributed identification cards before any specimens are collected.

NURSING FAST FACT!

Technology has advanced such that many hospitals have one- and two-dimensional barcode technologies to enable more information to be encoded. Barcodes tend to be very accurate and cost-effective for larger organizations.

Blood specimen collection for blood banking, such as typing and crossmatching, may require additional patient identification procedures and armband application.

Care must be taken in identification of emergency room patients. Often when patients come to the emergency room, they are unconscious and/or unidentified. Each hospital has policies and procedures for dealing with these cases, which usually includes assigning the patient an identification tag with a hospital or medical record number.

Test Requisitions

Laboratory tests must be ordered by a qualified healthcare practitioner. The documented requests are usually transmitted in the form of paper-based requisition or by computer. The requisition should contain the following information (Garza & Becan-McBride, 2002, 239):

- Patient's full name
- Patient's identification or medical record number
- Patient's date of birth
- Types of test to be performed
- Date of test
- Room number and bed (if applicable)
- Physician's name and/or code
- Test status (timed, stat, fasting, etc.)
- Billing information (optional)
- Special precautions (potential bleeder, faints easily, etc.)

Equipment Selection and Preparation

Supplies for Venipuncture

Supplies for venipuncture differ according to the method used (i.e., syringe method, evacuated tube system). All methods of venipuncture involve the use of disposable gloves, a tourniquet, alcohol pads or disinfectants, cotton balls, bandages or gauze pads, glass microscope slides, needles, syringes, or evacuated tube holders.

Vacuum (Evacuated) Tube Systems

Venipuncture with a **vacuum (evacuated) tube** is the most direct and efficient method for obtaining a blood specimen. The evacuated tube system requires three components:

- The evacuated sample tube
- The double-pointed needle
- Plastic holder

One end of the double-pointed needle enters the vein, the other end pierces the top of the tube, and the vacuum aspirates the blood. Vacuum tubes may contain silicone to decrease the possibility of **hemolysis**. This system eliminates the need for syringes and consists of disposable needles and tubes. Tubes have premeasured amounts of vacuum to collect a precise amount of blood. It is imperative that the expiration date be checked before using any blood collection tube (Becan-McBride, 1999). The tubes are available in different sizes and can be purchased in glass or unbreakable plastic. Figure 8–1 demonstrates how the double-pointed needle fits into the plastic holder.

The vacutainer system tubes are color coded according to the additive contained within the tube. Refer to Table 8–2 for specimen collection tube guide. The tubes are specifically designed to be used directly with chemistry, hematology, or microbiology instrumentation. The tube of blood is identified by its barcode and is pierced by the instrument probe, and some sample is aspirated into the instrument for analyses.

NURSING FAST FACT!

Use of closed systems minimizes laboratory personnel's risk of exposure to blood. The expiration dates of tubes must be monitored carefully.

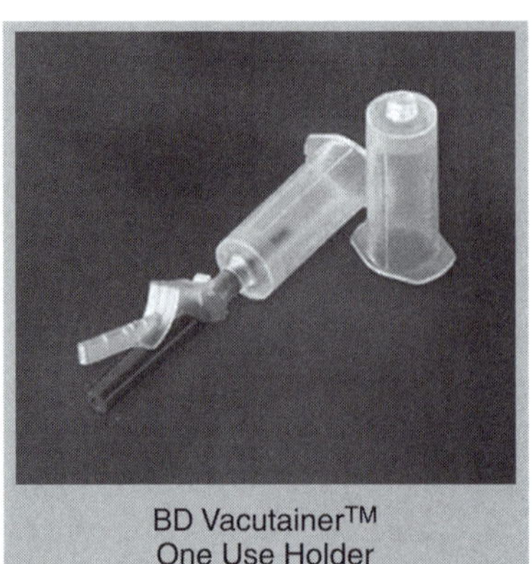

Figure 8–1 ■ BD Vacutainer™ One Use system. (Courtesy of Becton Dickinson, Franklin Lakes, NJ.)

BD Vacutainer™

Tube Guide

BD Indispensable to human health

A full line of BD Vacutainer Blood Collection Needles, Needle Holders and Blood Collection Sets is also available.

BD Vacutainer™ Tubes With Hemogard™ Closure	BD Vacutainer™ Tubes With Conventional Stopper	Additive	Inversions at Blood Collection*	Laboratory Use	Your Lab's Draw Volume/Remarks
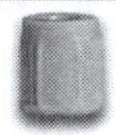 Gold	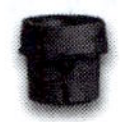 Red/ Black	• Clot activator and gel for serum separation	5	BD Vacutainer™ SST™ Tube for serum determinations in chemistry. Tube inversions ensure mixing of clot activator with blood. Blood clotting time 30 minutes.	
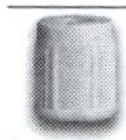 Light Green	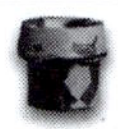 Green/ Gray	• Lithium heparin and gel for plasma separation	8	BD Vacutainer™ PST™ Tube for plasma determinations in chemistry. Tube inversions prevent clotting.	
 Red	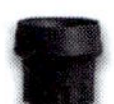	• None (glass) • Clot activator (plastic tube with Hemogard closure)	0 5	For serum determinations in chemistry and serology. Glass serum tubes are recommended for blood banking. Plastic tubes contain clot activator and are **not** recommended for blood banking. Tube inversions ensure mixing of clot activator with blood and clotting within 60 minutes.	
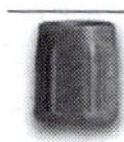 Orange	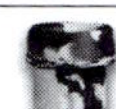 Gray/ Yellow	• Thrombin	8	For stat serum determinations in chemistry. Tube inversions ensure complete clotting which usually occurs in less than 5 minutes.	
 Royal Blue		• Sodium heparin • Na_2EDTA • None (serum tube)	8 8 0	For trace-element, toxicology and nutritional-chemistry determinations. Special stopper formulation provides low levels of trace elements (see package insert).	
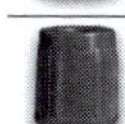 Green	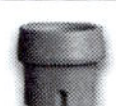	• Sodium heparin • Lithium heparin	8 8	For plasma determinations in chemistry. Tube inversions prevent clotting.	
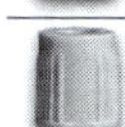 Gray	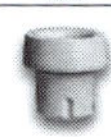	• Potassium oxalate/ sodium fluoride • Sodium fluoride/Na_2 EDTA • Sodium fluoride (serum tube)	8 8 8	For glucose determinations. Oxalate and EDTA anticoagulants will give plasma samples. Sodium fluoride is the antiglycolytic agent. Tube inversions ensure proper mixing of additive and blood.	
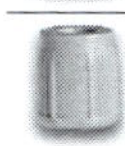 Tan		• Sodium heparin (glass) • K_2EDTA (plastic)	8 8	For lead determinations. This tube is certified to contain less than .01 µg/mL(ppm) lead. Tube inversions prevent clotting.	

(Continued on following page)

> Table 8–2 VACUTAINER TUBE GUIDE *(Continued)*

Tube	Additive	Inversions*	Laboratory Use
Yellow	• Sodium polyanethol sulfonate (SPS)	8	SPS for blood culture specimen collections in micro-biology. Tube inversions prevent clotting.
	• Acid citrate dextrose additives (ACD): **Solution A -** 22.0g/L trisodium citrate, 8.0g/L citric acid, 24.5g/L dextrose	8	ACD for use in blood bank studies, HLA phenotyping, DNA and paternity testing.
	Solution B - 13.2g/L trisodium citrate, 4.8g/L citric acid, 14.7g/L dextrose	8	
Lavender	• Liquid K_3EDTA (glass) • Spray-dried K_2EDTA (plastic)	8 8	K_3EDTA for whole blood hematology determinations. K_2EDTA for whole blood hematology determinations and immunohematology testing (ABO grouping, Rh typing, antibody screening). Tube inversions prevent clotting.
NEW Pink	• Spray-dried K_2EDTA	8	For whole blood hematology determinations and immunohematology testing (ABO grouping, Rh typing, antibody screening). Designed with special cross-match label for required patient information by the AABB. Tube inversions prevent clotting.
Light Blue	• .105M sodium citrate/ (3.2%) • .129M sodium citrate/ (3.8%) • Citrate, theophylline, adenosine, dipyridamole (CTAD)	3-4 3-4 3-4	For coagulation determinations. NOTE: Certain tests may require chilled specimens. Follow your institution's recommended procedures for collection and transport. CTAD for selected platelet function assays and routine coagulation determination. Tube inversions prevent clotting.
Partial-draw Tubes / Small-volume Pediatric Tubes			
Red	• None	0	For serum determinations in chemistry and serology. Glass serum tubes are recommended for blood banking. Plastic tubes contain clot activator and are not recommended for blood banking. Tube inversions ensure mixing of clot activator with blood and clotting within 60 minutes.
Green	• Sodium heparin • Lithium heparin	8 8	For plasma determinations in chemistry. Tube inversions prevent clotting.
Lavender	• Liquid K_3EDTA (glass) • Spray-dried K_2EDTA (plastic)	8 8	K_3EDTA for whole blood hematology determinations. K_2EDTA for whole blood hematology determinations and immunohematology testing (ABO grouping, Rh typing, antibody screening). Tube inversions prevent clotting.
Light Blue	• .105M sodium citrate (3.2%) • .129M sodium citrate (3.8%)	3-4	For coagulation determinations. Tube inversions prevent clotting. NOTE: Certain tests may require chilled specimens. Follow your institution's recommended procedures for collection and transport of specimen.

BD Vacutainer Systems
Preanalytical Solutions

1 Becton Drive
Franklin Lakes, NJ 07417 USA

BD Technical Services:
800.631.0174

*** Invert gently, do not shake**

Courtesy of Becton Dickinson and Company © 2004.

Evacuated tubes can also be used for transferring blood from a syringe into the tubes. The syringe needle is simply pushed through the top of the tube, and blood is automatically pulled into the tube because of the vacuum. Place the vacuum tube in a rack before pushing the needle into the tube top. A safety syringe shielded transfer device needs to be used to avoid possible exposure to the patient's blood. See Figure 8–2 for an example of a safety collection device.

NOTE > Refer to Chapter 6 to review needleless and needle protector equipment.

The following are protective equipment for blood withdrawal:

- BD Vacutainer Systems have a protective shield so that blood collector can slide the protective shield over the needle and lock it in place after the needle is withdrawn from the puncture site.
- BD Eclipse is a single-use blood collection needle that allows the user to shield the needle after use.
- SIMS Venipuncture Needle-Pro (SIMS Portex Inc., Keene, NH) provides immediate containment of a used needle.
- Vanishpoint (Retractable Technologies, TX) is a safety blood collection tube holder that provides for the needle to automatically retract into it after blood collection.
- Proguard II (Care Medical Products, Ontario, CA) is a single-use vacuum tube/needle holder.
- Sarstedt, Inc. has the S Monovette (Sarsdt, Inc., Newton, NC) Blood Collection System, which is a safety device for vacuum collection or a syringe collection.

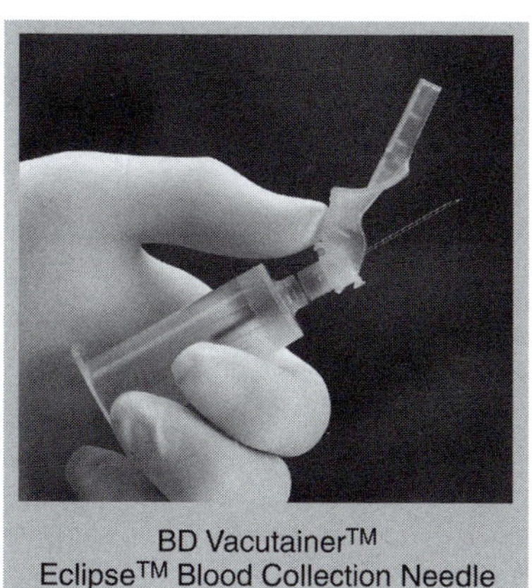

Figure 8–2 ■ BD Vacutainer Eclipse™ Blood Collection Safety Needle. (Courtesy of Becton Dickinson, Franklin Lakes, NJ.)

Summary of Tube Types and Their Uses

ANTICOAGULANTS AND BLOOD COLLECTION TUBES

Most clinical laboratories use serum, plasma, or whole blood to perform various **assays**. Many coagulation factors are involved in blood clotting, and coagulation can be prevented by the addition of different types of anticoagulants. These anticoagulants often contain preservatives that can extend the metabolism and life span of the red blood cell. Refer to Figure 8–3 for examples of Vacutainer tubes.

Coagulation of blood can be prevented by the addition of oxalates, citrates, **ethylenediaminetetraacetic acid (EDTA)**, or heparin. **Oxalates**, citrates, and **EDTA** prevent coagulation of blood by removing calcium and forming insoluble calcium salts. These three anticoagulants cannot be used in calcium determinations; however, citrates are frequently used in coagulation blood studies. EDTA prevents platelet aggregation and is used for platelet counts and platelet function tests. Heparin prevents blood clotting by inactivating the blood-clotting chemicals thrombin and thromboplastin.

NURSING FAST FACT!

It is important to choose the correct anticoagulant tube for a specific laboratory assay, along with using the correct amount or dilution of anticoagulant in the blood specimen.

TUBES WITHOUT ADDITIVES

Red-topped, royal blue-topped, and brown-topped tubes. Red-topped tubes indicate a tube without an anticoagulant; therefore blood collected

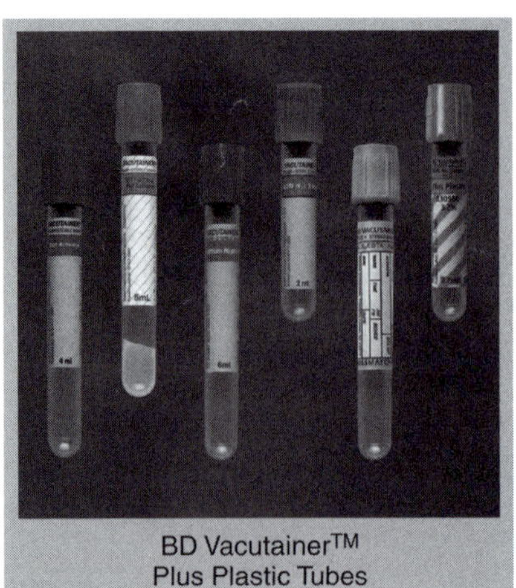

Figure 8–3 ■ BD Vacutainer™ Plastic Tubes. (Courtesy of Becton Dickinson, Franklin Lakes, NJ.)

in this tube will clot. The royal blue–topped tubes are used to collect samples for nutritional studies, therapeutic drug monitoring, and toxicology. The royal blue–topped tube is the trace element tube. The brown-topped tube contains no additive or heparin and is used for blood lead values.
Yellow-topped tubes. Yellow-topped tubes are used for blood cultures. The blood must be collected in a sterile container (vacuum tube, vial, or syringe) under aseptic conditions.

NURSING FAST FACTS!

Clotted specimens should not be shaken.

Some yellow color-coded tubes contain ACD (acid–citrate–dextrose) and are used for specialty blood banking.

TUBES WITH ADDITIVES

Green-topped tubes. The anticoagulants sodium heparin, ammonium heparin, and lithium heparin are found in green-topped vacuum tubes.
Gray-topped tubes. Gray-topped vacuum tubes usually contain either potassium oxalate and sodium fluoride or lithium iodoacetate and heparin. This type of collection tube is primarily used for glycolytic inhibition tests. Gray-topped tubes are not used for hematology studies.
Purple-topped tubes. Purple-topped vacuum tubes contain EDTA and are used for hematology procedures.
Light blue–topped tubes. Tubes with light blue tops contain sodium citrate and are used for coagulation procedures. The sodium citrate comes in a concentration of 3.2 or 3.8 percent. It is preferable to use the 3.2 percent concentration to reduce false-negative or false-positive results (Adcock, Kressin, & Marlar, 1997).
Mottled-topped, speckled-topped, and gold-topped tubes. These tubes contain a polymer barrier that is present at the bottom of the tube. The specific gravity of this material lies between the blood clot and the serum. During **centrifugation**, the polymer barrier moves upward to the serum–clot interface, where it forms a stable barrier, separating the serum from fibrin and cells.
Pink-topped tubes. These tubes recently received FDA approval for blood bank collections. They contain EDTA.

Safety Syringes

Veins that are too fragile for collection may collapse with vacuum tubes; therefore, safety syringes are generally used. Syringes are sometimes used for collecting blood from central venous catheter (CVC) lines.

NOTE > The procedure for blood sampling from a central line is discussed in Chapter 12.

The barrel of the syringe is in graduated measurements, usually milliliters. Sizes range from 0.2 to 50.0 mL; however, for specimen collection purposes, 5- to 20-mL syringes are most often used.

Needles

The gauge and length of a needle used on a syringe or a vacuum tube is selected according to specific tasks. Larger 18-gauge needles are used for collecting donor units of blood, and smaller 21- or 22-gauge needles are used for collecting specimens for laboratory assays. Needles are sterile and packaged by vendors in sealed shields that maintain sterility.

Different types of needles are used with vacuum collection tubes and the holder to allow for multiple tube changes without blood leakage within the plastic holder. The multiple-sample needle has a rubber cover over the tube-top puncturing portion of the needle; this cover creates a leakage barrier. The single-sample needle is usually used for collecting blood with a syringe.

Winged/Butterfly Needle Collection Sets

The winged infusion set or butterfly needle is the most commonly used intravenous device used for blood collection. The most common butterfly needle sizes are 21-, 23-, and 25-gauge. The butterfly needle is used to collect blood from patients whose veins are difficult to access with conventional method Refer to Figure 8–4 for an example of a blood collection butterfly collection set.

NURSING FAST FACT!

It is important to use Luer adapters on all safety blood collection sets to avoid possible blood leakage and exposure.

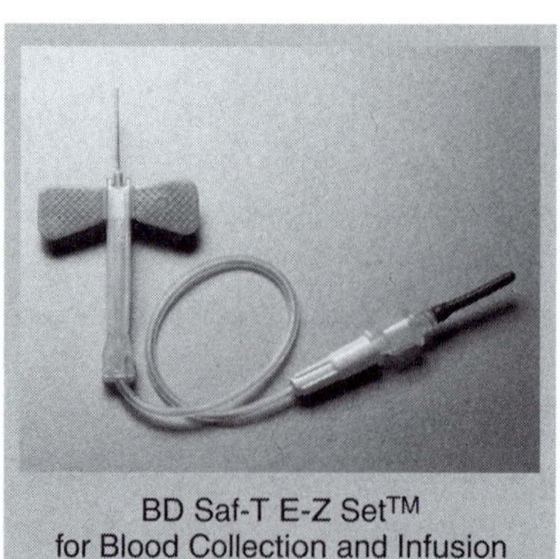

Figure 8–4 ■ BD Saf-T E-Z ™ Set for Blood Collection. (Courtesy of Becton Dickinson, Franklin Lakes, NJ.)

Microcollection Equipment

LANCETS AND TUBES

Skin puncture blood-collecting techniques are used on infants. Skin puncture collection is indicated for adults and older children when they are severely burned, or have veins that are difficult to access because of their small size or location. The volume of plasma or serum that generally can be collected from a premature infant is approximately 100 to 150 μL, and about two times that amount can be taken from a full term newborn Refer to Figure 8–5 for an example of a lancet.

Lancets for these sticks are available for two different incision depths, depending on the needs of the infant; the teal-colored Quikheel by BD Quickheel has a depth of 1.0 mm and width of 2.5 mm, and the purple-colored Quickheel Preemie lancet has a preset incision depth of 0.85 mm and width of 1.5 mm. Most lancet blades retract permanently after activation to ensure safety for the healthcare worker.

NURSING FAST FACT!

The recommended penetration depth of lancet is no more than 2.0 mm on the heel.

The National Committee for Clinical Laboratory Standards (NCCLS) recommends penetration depth of no more than 2.0 mm on heelsticks to avoid penetrating the bone (NCCLS, 1998b).

INS Standard. For the pediatric patient the amount of blood obtained for laboratory assay should be documented in the patient's medical record. (INS, 2000, 67)

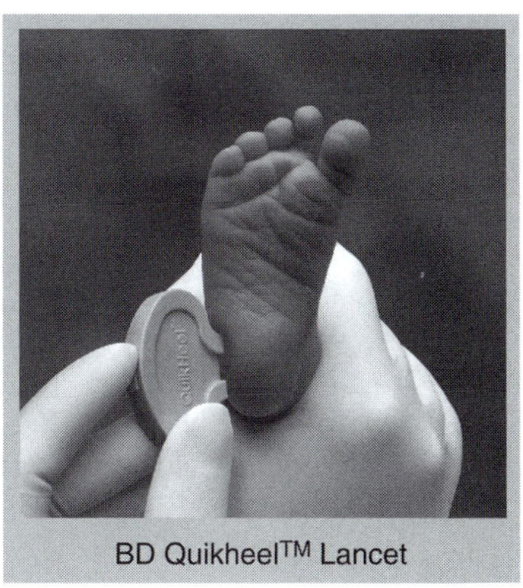

Figure 8–5 ■ BD Quikheel™ Lancet. (Courtesy of Becton Dickinson, Franklin Lakes, NJ.)

A laser-based device that is FDA approved for blood collection is the Lasette (Cell Robotics, Albuquerque, NM). The laser penetrates to a depth of 1 to 2 mm and a width of 250 μm. This is a smaller puncture hole than other devices and can provide 100 μL of blood for collection (News & Views, 1997, 689).

Websites for Suppliers of Safety Blood Collection Equipment

Baxter Healthcare Corp.: *www.baxter.com*
Becton Dickinson and Co. (BD): *www.bd.com*
Bio-Plexus, Inc.: *www.bio-plexus.com*
Erie Scientific Corp.: *www.eriesci.com*
Greiner Labortechnik: *www.vacuette.com*
Healthmark Industries Co.: *www.hmark.com*
Helena Products: *www.helena.com*
International Technidyne Corp.: *www.itcmed.com*
Kendall Co. LP: *www.kendallhq.com*
Lab Safety Supply: *www.labsafety.com*
Retractable Technologies, Inc.: *www.vanishpoint.com*
Safe Tec Clinical Products, Inc.: *www.safetec.com*
Sarstedt, Inc.: *www.sarstedt.com*
SIMS Portex, Inc.: *www.portexusa.com*

Venipuncture Site Selection

The most common site for venipuncture is in the antecubital area of the arm, where the median cubital veins lie close to the surface of the skin. The median cubital vein is most commonly used; the cephalic vein lies on the outer edge of the arm, and the basilic vein lies on the inside edge. Refer to Figure 8–6. The healthcare practitioner should palpate the veins to get an idea of the size, angle, and depth of the vein. The patient can assist in the process by closing his or her fist tightly.

NURSING FAST FACT!

Do not have patient repeatedly open and close "pump" the hand for it may alter the test results.

The dorsal side of the hand or wrist should be used only if arm veins are unsuitable. Hand veins or the veins on the dorsal surface of the wrist are preferred over foot or ankle veins because coagulation and vascular complications may occur in the lower extremities, especially for diabetic patients.

The same precautions must be taken into consideration when performing venipuncture for blood analysis on patients who have had mas-

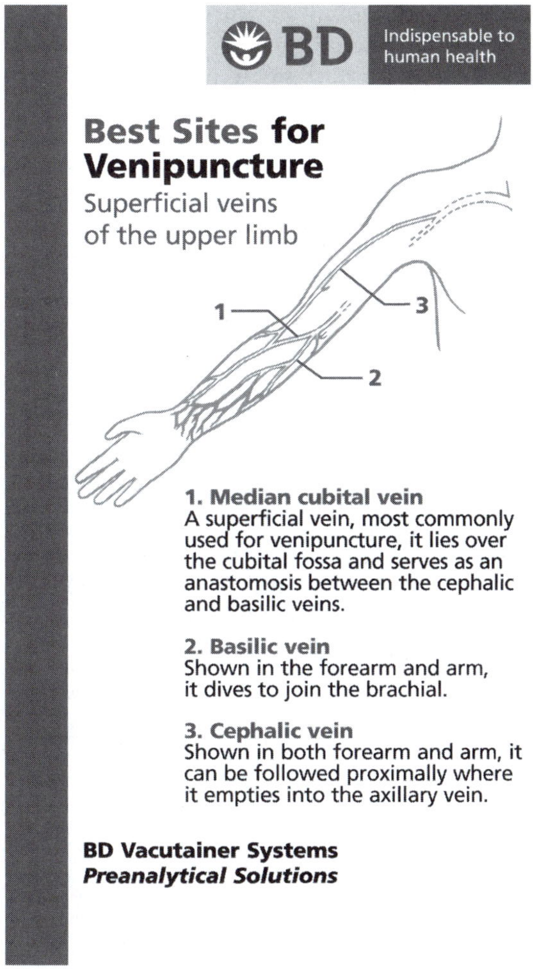

Figure 8–6 ■ Best sites for venipuncture. (Courtesy of Becton Dickinson, Franklin Lakes, NJ.)

tectomy or surgical procedures on one arm/hand, have in place a dialysis shunt, or have special problems that must be taken into consideration prior to venipuncture.

NURSING FAST FACTS!

- *Never draw above an infusing I.V.; this can alter the test results.*
- *Use caution during venipuncture; although nerve damage during venipuncture is rare, it has been known to occur as a result of excessive needle probing and sudden movement of the patient.*
- ***Never** place towels or washcloths in a microwave oven.*

The venipuncture site may be warmed to facilitate vein prominence. A surgical towel or washcloth heated to about 42°C and then wrapped around the site for 3 to 5 minutes can increase skin temperature. Encasing the towel or washcloth in a plastic bag or wrap helps to retain heat.

NOTE > Refer to Chapter 10 for techniques in working with the patient who has difficult veins to access.

Preparation of Venipuncture Site

Once the site is selected, the site should be prepped with 70 percent isopropyl alcohol or chlorhexidine (ChloraPrep® Medi-Flex). Alcohol is not recommended for use when obtaining a specimen for blood alcohol level determination. Chlorhexidine is recommended; however, check institutional policy.

Povidone-iodine (Betadine) is usually used for drawing blood for blood gas analysis and blood cultures. Remove excess povidone-iodine from the skin with sterile gauze after prepping because iodine can interfere with some laboratory tests.

NURSING FAST FACT!

Do not touch the prepared venipuncture site after prepping. The alcohol should be allowed to dry (30 to 60 seconds).

Venipuncture Methods

Venipuncture Technique

Once the venipuncture site is prepped, the healthcare worker may hold the patient's arm below the site, pulling the skin tightly with the thumb (traction). A safety syringe, butterfly, or Vacutainer system can be used for venipuncture. Procedures for each follow. The needle should be lined up with the vein and inserted smoothly and quickly at approximately a 15 to 30 degree angle with the skin. The needle should be inserted with the bevel side upward and directly above a prominent vein or slightly below the palpable vein. Sometimes a slight "pop" can be felt when the needle enters the vein. Refer to Figure 8–7 for an illustration of how needle positioning can result in failure to draw blood.

The tourniquet can be released immediately after blood begins to

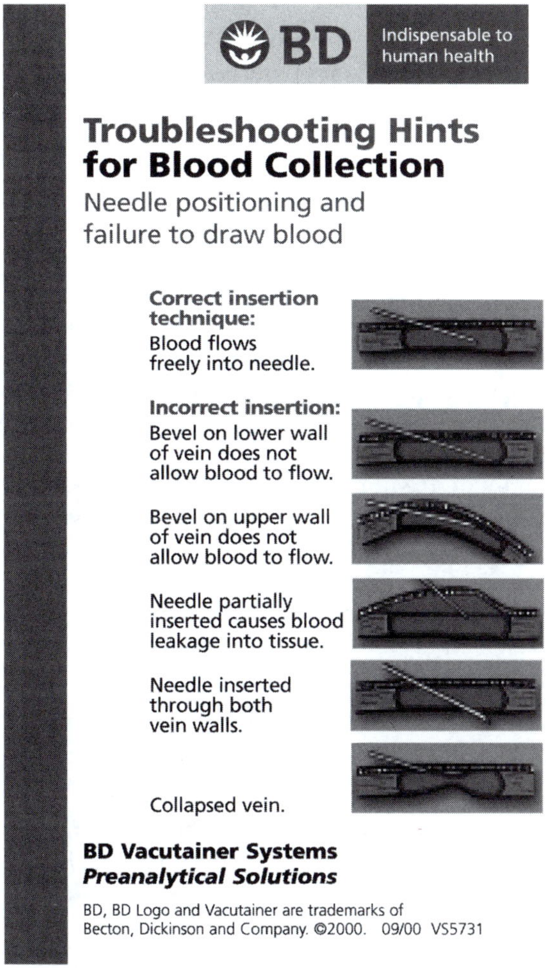

Figure 8–7 ■ Needle positioning and failure to draw blood. (Courtesy of Becton Dickinson, Franklin Lakes, NJ.)

flow so as not to collect blood that is **hemoconcentrated**. When a tourniquet is placed on the patient the tourniquet pressure forces low molecular compounds and fluid to move into the tissues from the intravascular space. Large molecules such as cholesterol and proteins cannot move through the capillary wall, and their blood levels increase as the tourniquet remains on the arm (Becan-McBride, 1999). In addition, the longer the tourniquet remains on the arm, the greater amount of potassium leakage occurs from tissue cells into the blood, increasing the chances of a false blood potassium level reading (Garza & Becan-McBride, 2002).

NURSING FACT FACTS!

- *It is recommended that the tourniquet be released as the last tube is filling, but always before withdrawing the needle from the arm.*
- *If the patient continues to bleed, the healthcare practitioner should apply pressure until the bleeding stops.*

Remove the last specimen tube from the holder prior to removing the needle from the vein. Gently but quickly remove the needle.

A dry sterile gauze or cotton ball should be applied with pressure to the puncture site for several minutes or until bleeding has stopped. Keep the patient's arm straight, or elevate above the heart, if possible. A pressure bandage should be applied and the patient should be instructed to leave it on for at least 15 minutes.

All contaminated equipment should be discarded into appropriate containers. Paper and plastic wrappers can be thrown into a wastebasket. Needles and lancets should be placed into a sturdy puncture-proof disposable container following OSHA guidelines.

Any items, such as cotton or gauze, that have been contaminated with blood should be disposed of in biohazardous disposal containers following standard precautions.

Evacuated Tube System

When the evacuated tube system is used the needle must first be threaded onto the holder, and the first test tube should be pushed carefully into the holder so that the test tube cap rests in the holder. Refer to Figure 8–8 for proper insertion of an evacuated tube. If the tube is punctured prior to entering the vein, loss of vacuum in the tube will occur.

NURSING FAST FACTS!

- *For beginners it is easier not to try to balance the tube in the holder prior to venipuncture. Access the vein and then pick up the tube and push it onto the inner needle.*
- *Vigorous handling of the blood tubes and sluggish propulsion of blood into the tube can cause hemolysis and separation of cells from liquid, which can affect the test results (Mohler et al., 1998).*
- *Some healthcare workers use the dominant hand to change tubes while the other hand keeps the needle apparatus steady.*

Refer to Procedures Display 8–1 for steps in performing the evacuated tube blood collection method.

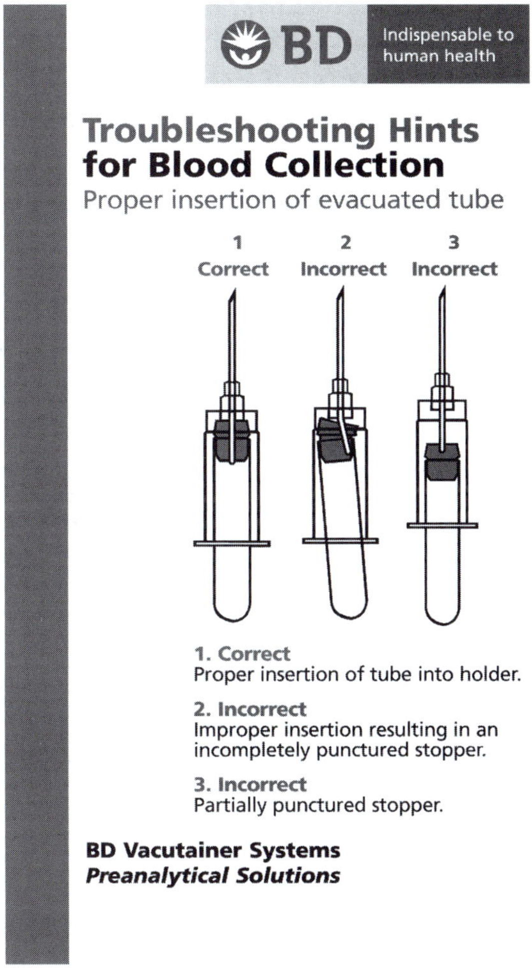

Figure 8–8 ■ Proper insertion of evacuated tube. (Courtesy of Becton Dickinson, Franklin Lakes, NJ.)

When multiple sample tubes are to be collected, each tube should be gently removed from the Vacutainer holder and replaced with the next tube. Experienced healthcare workers are able to mix a full tube in one hand while holding the needle apparatus with the other hand. Multiple tubes can be filled in less than 1 minute if the needle remains stable in the vein and the vein does not collapse. The holder must be securely held while changing tubes so the needle is not pushed further into or removed from the vein.

After collection of the blood and removal of the last tube, the entire needle assembly should be withdrawn quickly. Safety devices should be activated immediately, depending on the manufacturer's specifications.

PROCEDURES DISPLAY 8–1

Collection of Blood in an Evacuated Tube System

1. Place the patient in a position of comfort and safety, arm extended and in a dependent position if possible.
2. Arrange all supplies in an accessible place so that reaching for equipment is minimized. Line up tubes in the order of draw.
3. Locate the vein, usually the antecubital fossa.
4. Cleanse the area with 70 percent alcohol or chlorhexidine, using a circular or back and forth technique. Allow skin to air-dry or blot with sterile gauze
5. Apply the tourniquet 3 to 6 inches above the site to be used, and have patient make a fist. (Do not have patient "pump" fist.) (Do not leave tourniquet on for longer than 1 minute.)
6. Apply traction to the skin of the forearm, below the intended venipuncture site, to stabilize the vein
7. Hold the vacuum tube assembly between the thumb and last three fingers of your dominant hand. Rest the back of these fingers on the patient's arm. The free index finger rests against the hub of the needle and serves as a guide. With the needle held at an angle of 15 to 30 degrees to the arm and in line with the vein, insert the needle into the vein, with the bevel up.
8. Once you feel that you are in the vein, change your grip: the hand that was stabilizing the vein in place should now hold the hub firmly, while the index and third finger of the dominant hand grip the tube. This will prevent movement of the needle. Now use your thumb to gently but firmly push the tube onto the needle. This will allow the vacuum to pull blood into the tube.
9. If more than one tube is to be drawn, pull the filled tube out of the hub very gently with the hand that pushed it in.
10. When the last tube of blood is drawn, remove it from the hub. Release the tourniquet, during filing of the last tube, then gently remove the needle from the arm and place a cotton ball or small gauze pad over the puncture site. Ask the patient to put pressure on the area.
11. Activate the safety feature on the needle
12. Gently rotate the specimens to assure adequate mixing with tube additives
13. When bleeding has stopped, apply a pressure bandage.
14. Label all samples

NURSING FAST FACTS!

- *Occasionally a faulty tube will have no vacuum.*
- *If you notice a hematoma during venipuncture, withdraw the needle, apply local pressure, and retry in the other arm.*

Syringe Method

When using a **syringe method** the same approach to needle insertion should take place as is used for the evacuated tube method. Once the needle is in the vein, the syringe plunger can be drawn back gently to avoid hemolysis of the specimen until the required volume of blood has been withdrawn. The healthcare worker must be careful not to withdraw the needle from the vein while pulling back on the plunger.

After collection of the blood the entire needle assembly should be withdrawn quickly. Safety devices should be activated immediately, depending on the manufacturer's specifications. Refer to Procedures Display 8–2 for steps in the syringe method of blood collection.

NURSING FAST FACT!

Turn the syringe so that the graduated markings are visible.

PROCEDURES DISPLAY 8–2

Collection of Blood Using a Syringe Method

1. Place the patient in a position of comfort and safety, arm extended and in a dependent position if possible.
2. Arrange all supplies in an accessible place so that reaching for equipment is minimized.
3. Locate the vein, usually the antecubital fossa.
4. Don nonsterile gloves.
5. Cleanse the area with 70 percent alcohol or chlorhexidine. Allow skin to air-dry or blot with sterile gauze.
6. Apply the tourniquet 3 to 6 inches above the site to be used, and have the patient make a fist. (Do not leave tourniquet on for longer than 1 minute.)
7. Apply traction to the forearm to stabilize the vein.
8. The needle should be lined up with the vein and inserted smoothly and quickly at an approximately 15- to 30-degree angle with the skin. The needle should be inserted with the bevel side upward and directly above a prominent vein or slightly below the palpable vein.
9. Pull back gently on the plunger until the desired amount of blood is obtained.
10. Release the tourniquet, and then gently remove the needle from the arm and place a cotton ball or small gauze pad over the puncture site. Ask the patient to put pressure on the area.

(Continued on following page)

PROCEDURES DISPLAY 8–2

Collection of Blood Using a Syringe Method *(Continued)*

11. Activate the safety feature on the needle.
12. Gently rotate the specimens to ensure adequate mixing with tube additives.
13. When bleeding has stopped, apply a pressure bandage.
14. Transfer the sample into the desired blood tubes.
15. Label the sample.

NURSING FAST FACT!

If you notice a hematoma during venipuncture, withdraw the needle, apply local pressure, and retry in the other arm.

Winged Infusion System or Butterfly Method

A winged infusion system can be used for particularly difficult venipunctures. This method is now used with safety equipment so as to decrease the risk of needlestick injuries to the healthcare worker. This method is sometimes useful for patients with:

- Small veins, such as the hand
- Pediatric or geriatric patients
- Restrictive positions, that is, traction, severe arthritis
- Patients with numerous needlesticks
- Patients with fragile skin and veins
- Short-term infusion therapy
- Patients who are severely burned

The needles range from $^1/_2$ to $^3/_4$ inch in length and from 21- to 25-gauge in diameter. Attached to the needle is a thin tubing with a Luer adapter at the end so that it can be used on a syringe or an evacuated tube system from the same manufacturer.

NURSING FAST FACT!

Since the tubing contains air, it will underfill the first evacuated tube by 0.5 mL. This affects the additive-to-blood ratio. A red-topped nonadditive tube should be filled before any tube with additives is filled.

Healthcare workers should be extra cautious as the needle is removed from the patient to activate the safety device that is built into the system.

Use of the winged infusion or butterfly system requires training and practice. Failure to activate the safety devices correctly as described by the manufacturer may result in a higher incidence of needlestick injuries. Refer to Procedures Display 8–3 for steps in using winged needle system for blood collection.

PROCEDURES DISPLAY 8–3

Collection of Blood Using a Winged or Butterfly Collection Set

1. Place the patient in a position of comfort and safety, arm extended and in a dependent position if possible.
2. Arrange all supplies in an accessible place so that reaching for equipment is minimized.
3. Locate the vein, usually the antecubital fossa.
4. Don nonsterile gloves.
5. Cleanse the area with 70 percent alcohol or chlorhexidine. Allow skin to air-dry or blot with sterile gauze. (Drying prevents dilution of the sample with antiseptic.)
6. Connect the winged infusion system to the syringe or evacutainer system.
7. Apply the tourniquet 3 to 6 inches above the site to be used, and have patient make a fist. (Do not leave tourniquet on for longer than 1 minute.)
8. Apply traction to the forearm to stabilize the vein.
9. The needle should be lined up with the vein and inserted smoothly and quickly at an approximately 15- to 30-degree angle with the skin. The needle should be inserted with the bevel side upward and directly above a prominent vein or slightly below the palpable vein.
10. Release the tourniquet, and then gently remove the needle from the arm and place a cotton ball or small gauze pad over the puncture site. Ask the patient to put pressure on the area.
11. Activate the safety feature on the winged needle.
12. Gently rotate the specimens to ensure adequate mixing with tube additives.
13. When bleeding has stopped, apply a pressure bandage.
14. Label the sample.

NURSING FAST FACT!

If you notice a hematoma during venipuncture, withdraw the needle, apply local pressure, and retry in the other arm.

Order of Tube Collection

The National Committee for Clinical Laboratory Standards (NCCLS, 1998a) recommends the following specific order when collecting multiple tubes of blood via the evacuated method or the syringe transfer method:

1. Blood culture tubes (yellow top), or blood culture vials or bottles
2. Plain tubes, nonadditive (red/some pink top)
3. Coagulation tube (light blue top)
4. Additive tubes:
   a. Gel separator tube
   b. Heparin (green top)
   c. EDTA (purple top)
   d. Oxalate/fluoride (gray top)

Refer to Table 8–3 for order of draw for multiple tube collections.

Tips

- Be meticulous about time, type of test, and the volume of blood required (Langlois, 2000).
- Blood cultures are always drawn first to decrease the possibility of bacterial contamination.
- When drawing just coagulation studies for diagnostic purposes, it is preferable that at least one other tube of blood be drawn before the coagulation test specimen. This diminishes contamination with tissue fluids, which may initiate the clotting sequence (Yawn & Lodge, 1996). Usually a nonadditive red top is used.
- Coagulation tubes should be mixed as soon after collection as possible.
- Minimize the transfer of anticoagulants from tube to tube by holding the tube horizontally or slightly downward during blood collection.
- When a large volume (more than 20 mL) of blood has been drawn

> Table 8–3 **ORDER OF DRAW FOR MULTIPLE TUBE COLLECTIONS**

Collection Tube	Mix by Inverting
Blood Cultures - SPS	8 to 10 times
Serum Tube (glass)	—
Citrate Tube	3 to 4 times
BD SST Gel Separator Tube	5 times
Serum Tube (plastic)	5 times
Heparin Tube	8 to 10 times
BD PST Gel Separator Tube with Heparin	8 to 10 times
EDTA Tube	8 to 10 times
Fluoride (glucose) Tube	8 to 10 times

Note: *Always follow your facility's protocol for order of draw.*
Adapted courtesy of Becton Dickinson, Franklin Lakes, NJ.

using a syringe, there is a possibility that some of the blood may be clotted.

- If two syringes of blood have been withdrawn, NCCLS recommends taking blood from the second syringe for coagulation studies (NCCLS, 1998).
- Watch the "fill" rate and volume in each tube; evacuated tubes with anticoagulants must be filled to the designated level for the proper mix of blood with the anticoagulant. Note: Partial fill tubes are available when it is suspected that the blood specimen will not be adequate.

Specimen Identification and Labeling

Specimens should be labeled immediately at the patient's bedside or ambulatory setting. Some laboratories require labels to be placed so that the label does not obscure the entire specimen. This allows the specimen to be observed for proper clotting and handling.

All specimens should contain the following label information:

- Patient's full name
- Patient's identification numbers
- Date of collection
- Time of collection
- Healthcare worker's initials
- Patient's room number, bed assignment, or outpatient status are optional information.

NURSING FAST FACT!

Placing the label with the patient name toward the top (by the stopper) allows easier identification when the tube is in the specimen rack.

Tubes should not be prelabeled.

NURSING PLAN OF CARE

COLLECTION OF BLOOD SPECIMENS

Focus Assessment

Subjective

- Assess patient's understanding of the blood test.
- Assess patient's degree of anxiety about the procedure.
- Assess the infant's or child's need for restraint and reassurance.
- Ensure that food, fluid, and medication restrictions have been followed.

(Continued on following page)

NURSING PLAN OF CARE

COLLECTION OF BLOOD SPECIMENS *(Continued)*

Objective

- Verify the patient's identity.
- Assess both arms for appropriate venipuncture site.

Patient Outcome/Evaluation Criteria

Patient will:

- Verbalize understanding of purpose of blood testing.
- Identify interventions for post–blood sampling site observations and care.
- Identify complications from blood sampling procedure.

Nursing Diagnoses

- Knowledge deficit related to purpose of blood tests.
- Risk of skin integrity impaired, related to venipuncture technique.

Nursing Management

1. Select appropriate evacuated tubes or syringe.
2. Ensure the collected sample is valid by applying the tourniquet appropriately; avoid possible invalid testing caused by prolonged use of tourniquet, excessive suction on the syringe, or vigorous shaking of specimen in a tube.
3. Use aseptic technique.
4. Apply adhesive bandage after bleeding has stopped.
5. Provide support to the client if the puncture is not successful and another must be performed to obtain the blood sample.
6. Check the venipuncture site after 5 minutes for hematoma formation.
7. If the client is immunosuppressed, check the puncture site every 8 hours for signs and symptoms of infection.
8. If the specimen cannot be transported to the laboratory within a reasonable time or if analysis is delayed, arrange for proper storage to prevent deterioration or contamination that can cause inaccurate results (Cavanaugh, 2003).
9. Document in the patient medical record; include the amount of blood used for sampling and patient's response to the procedure (INS, Policies, 2002).

Patient Education

- Explain the purpose of the test.
- Explain the procedure, including the site from which the blood sample is likely to be obtained.
- Educate regarding any limitations of movement
- Instruction to notify the nurse if puncture site begins to bleed.
- Instruct to notify the nurse if puncture site becomes red, warm to touch, or pain develops.

Website

Patient education: *www.patient-education.com*

Home Care Issues

The physical setting can affect the collection of blood in the home care setting. If specimens are to be collected in homes, all procedures are similar except that extra care must be taken for the following:

- Extra supplies and equipment, including biohazard container for disposable and a specimen transport container, should be taken into the home.
- Locate the nearest bathroom, sink, and clean towels for washing hands.
- Carefully inspect the area after the procedure to ensure that all trash and used supplies have been properly discarded before leaving the home environment.
- Specimens should be carefully labeled and placed in leakproof containers.
- Ensure that specimens are transported at appropriate temperatures.
- Reinforce patient education.

Key Points

- Specimens incorrectly acquired, labeled, or transported by the nurse can cause the laboratory tests to be useless or even cause harm to the patient
- The nurse performing phlebotomy procedures must have the following knowledge base to perform blood withdrawal procedures safely: knowledge of basic anatomy and physiology, medical terminology, sources of error, safety measures and infection control practices, fundamental biology, quality control procedures; equipment and methods, sites for blood collection.

- A two-step process must identify patient: ask name, and confirm match between patient response, the test requisition, and ID bracelet.
- The vacuum (evacuated) tube system includes the evacuated sample tube, the double-pointed needle, and plastic holder.
- Vacuumized tubes for blood include those without additives and those with anticoagulant additives.
- Safety syringes should be used when the syringe method of blood collection is used.
- The antecubital area is the most frequently used area for blood collection. The dorsal side of hand or wrist should be used only if the arm veins are unsuitable.
- The tourniquet should be released once blood begins to flow into the tube (no longer than 1 minute) to prevent hemoconcentration of the blood specimen.
- The order of tube draw is: blood culture tubes, then plain tubes (nonadditives), coagulation tubes (light blue), additive tubes (green), EDTA (purple), and then oxalate/fluoride (gray top).

Critical Thinking: Case Study

A 70-year-old Hmong, non–English-speaking woman was admitted to an acute care hospital, accompanied by her husband, who had limited English. On admission her physician had ordered a series of blood tests. When the healthcare worker arrived to collect blood for laboratory tests, she introduced herself and asked the patient her name. The patient did not respond and looked perplexed.

Questions:

1. What should the healthcare worker do next?
2. What other factors need to be considered in this scenario (i.e., safety, ethics, legal)?

Media Link: Use the enclosed CD–ROM for more critical thinking activities and the answers to this case study.

Post-Test

1. Which of the following anticoagulants is found in a green-topped collection vacuum tube?
   - **a.** EDTA
   - **b.** Sodium citrate
   - **c.** Sodium heparin
   - **d.** Ammonium oxalate

2. The color coding for tubes indicates the:
   a. Length of needle needed to access the tube
   b. Manufacturer
   c. Additive contained within the tube
   d. Amount of blood necessary to fill the tube

3. From the following list of tubes, which would be the first tube used in the evacuated tube system?
   a. Lavender-topped tube
   b. Blood culture tube
   c. Light blue–topped tube
   d. Red-topped tube

4. Containers for the disposal of needles and syringes should have which of the following features?
   a. Be puncture resistant
   b. Be labeled with a "biohazard" sign
   c. Have yellow and black markings
   d. Contain antiseptic solutions

5. Prior to venipuncture for lab sampling, which of the following is the best method of patient identification?
   a. Patient's chart
   b. Patient's family
   c. Another nurse
   d. Patient's armband

6. The most common site for venipuncture is in which of the following areas?
   a. The dorsal side of the wrist
   b. The antecubital fossa of the arm
   c. Hand veins
   d. The heel

7. All of the following tubes contain an anticoagulant additive **EXCEPT:**
   a. Lavender
   b. Pink
   c. Green
   d. Red

8. In all of the following situations, the use of a butterfly needle is beneficial **EXCEPT:**
   a. Heel puncture
   b. Veins in the hand
   c. Geriatric patients
   d. Patients who are burned
9. Which of the following solutions is used most frequently as a prep solution for venipuncture for lab collection of blood chemistry?
   a. 70 Percent isopropyl alcohol
   b. Povidone-iodine
   c. 2 Percent iodine
   d. Acetone
10. What is the minimum amount of time a pressure bandage should be left in place after a venipuncture for blood collection?
    a. 5 minutes
    b. 10 minutes
    c. 15 minutes
    d. 30 minutes

References

Adcock, D.M., Kressin, D.C., & Marlar, R.A. (1997). Effect of 3.2% vs 3.8% sodium citrate concentration on routine coagulation testing. *American Journal of Clinical Pathology*, 107, 105–110.

American Society of Clinical Pathologists (1999). *Careers in the Laboratory Series. Phlebotomists.* Chicago: ASCP Board of Registry.

Becan-McBride, K. (1999). Laboratory sampling: Does process affect the outcome? *Journal of Intravenous Nursing*, 22(3), 137–142.

Cavanaugh, B.M. (2003). *Nurse's Manual of Laboratory and Diagnostic Tests* (4th ed.). Philadelphia: F.A. Davis.

Garza, D., & Becan-McBride, K. (2002). *Phlebotomy Handbook* (6th ed.). Upper Saddle River, NJ: Prentice–Hall, pp. 183–271.

Infusion Nurses Society (2000). Revised standards of practice. *Journal of the Infusion Nurses Society*, 23(65), S71.

Infusion Nurses Society (2002). *Policies and Procedures for Infusion Nursing* (2nd ed.). Cambridge, MA: Infusion Nurses Society, p. 140.

Langlois, J.C. (2000). Laboratory sampling, alternate site perspective. *Journal of Intravenous Nursing*, 23(2), 112–114.

Mohler, M., Sato, Y., Bobick, K., & Wise, L.C. (1998). The reliability of blood sampling from peripheral intravenous infusion lines. *Journal of Intravenous Nursing*, 21, 209–214.

National Committee for Clinical Laboratory Standards (NCCLS) (1998a). *Procedures for the Collection of Diagnostic Blood Specimens by Venipuncture.* Villanova, PA: NCCLS. Approved Standard, H3-A4.

National Committee for Clinical Laboratory Standards (NCCLS) (1998b). *Evacuated Tubes and Additives for Blood Specimen Collection* (4th ed.). Villanova, PA: NCCL Approved Standard, H1-A4.

News & Views (1997). Lasers to replace lancets? *Laboratory Medicine,* 28(11), 689.

Yawn, B.P., & Lodge, C. (1996). Prothrombin time: One tube or two? *American Journal of Clinical Pathology,* 105(6), 764–797.

Answers to Chapter 8 Post-Test

1. **c**
2. **c**
3. **b**
4. **a**
5. **d**
6. **b**
7. **d**
8. **a**
9. **a**
10. **c**

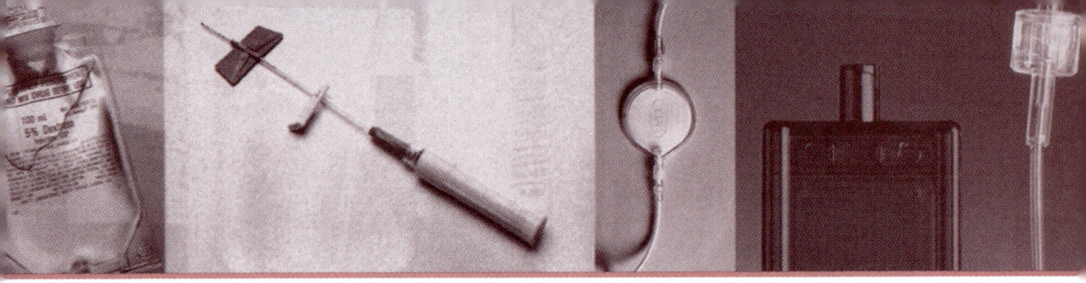

Chapter 9
Complications of Intravenous Therapy

The most important practical lesson that can be given to nurses is to teach them what to observe—how to observe—what symptoms indicate improvement—what the reverse—which are of importance—which are of none—which are the evidence of neglect—and of what kind of neglect.

—Florence Nightingale, 1859

Chapter Contents

LEARNING OBJECTIVES

Upon completion of this chapter, the reader will be able to:

1. Define terms related to the hazards associated with I.V. therapy.
2. Differentiate between local and systemic complications.

3. Describe the signs and symptoms of eight local complications.
4. Identify prompt treatment for local and systemic complications.
5. Document assessment of each local and systemic complication.
6. Identify INS Standards of practice rating infiltration.
7. List three risk factors for phlebitis.
8. Use the phlebitis scale for identifying and rating postinfusion phlebitis.
9. Identify erratic flow rates as they relate to the hazards associated with I.V. therapy.
10. Identify organisms responsible for septicemia related to infusion therapy.
11. Identify prevention techniques for the six systemic complications.
12. State the recommendations for prevention of complications involving intravascular devices.

GLOSSARY

Ecchymosis A bruise; a "black and blue spot" on the skin caused by escape of blood from injured vessels

Embolism A sudden obstruction of a blood vessel by a clot or foreign material formed or introduced elsewhere in the circulatory system and carried to the point of obstruction by the bloodstream

Extravasation Escape of fluid from a vessel into the surrounding tissue

Hematoma A localized mass of blood outside of the blood vessel usually found in a partially clotted state

Infiltration Process of seepage or diffusion of I.V. infusate into tissue

Phlebitis Inflammation of the intima of a vein associated with chemical irritation (i.e., chemical phlebitis), mechanical irritation (i.e., mechanical phlebitis), or bacterial infection (i.e., bacterial phlebitis); postinfusion inflammation of the intima of a vein within 48 to 96 hours after cannula removal

Reflex sympathetic dystrophy syndrome Chronic pain caused by trauma to nerve complexes or soft tissue

Septicemia Systemic disease caused by the presence of pathogenic microorganisms in the body

Speed shock Systemic reaction that occurs when a substance foreign to the body is rapidly introduced into the circulation

Thrombosis Formation or presence of a blood clot; venous arrest of circulation in the vein by a blood clot; also called phlebemphraxis

Vasospasm Contraction of the muscular coats of the blood vessels; also called angiospasm

Vesicant Any agent that produces blisters

Complications of I.V. Therapy

The nursing profession assumed the role of initiation of intravenous therapy in the 1940s, and since that time a large body of knowledge has been gathered about infusion therapy. Application of the nursing process in prevention of complications of infusion therapy is critical in today's complicated therapies. The fact that 90 percent of hospitalized patients receive I.V. fluids and medications puts patients at risk for developing complications associated with this form of therapy.

Complications associated with I.V. therapy are classified according to their location. A local complication is usually seen at or near the insertion site or occurs as a result of mechanical failure. These complications are more common than systemic complications. Systemic complications are those occurring within the vascular system, usually remote from the I.V. site. Although not as common as local complications, they are very serious and can be life threatening.

Local Complications

Local complications of I.V. therapy occur as adverse reactions or trauma to the surrounding venipuncture site. These complications can be recognized early by objective assessment. Assessing and monitoring are the key components in early intervention. Good venipuncture technique is the main factor related to the prevention of most local complications associated with I.V. therapy.

Local complications include hematoma, thrombosis, phlebitis, postinfusion phlebitis, thrombophlebitis, infiltration, extravasation, local infection, and venous spasm.

Hematoma

The terms **hematoma** and **ecchymosis** are used to denote formations resulting from the infiltration of blood into the tissues at the venipuncture site. Often this complication is related to nursing venipuncture technique. Patients who bruise easily can develop a hematoma when large cannulae are used to initiate I.V. therapy, owing to trauma to the vein during insertion. Patients receiving anticoagulant therapy and long-term steroid therapy are at particular risk of bleeding from vein trauma (Fig. 9–1).

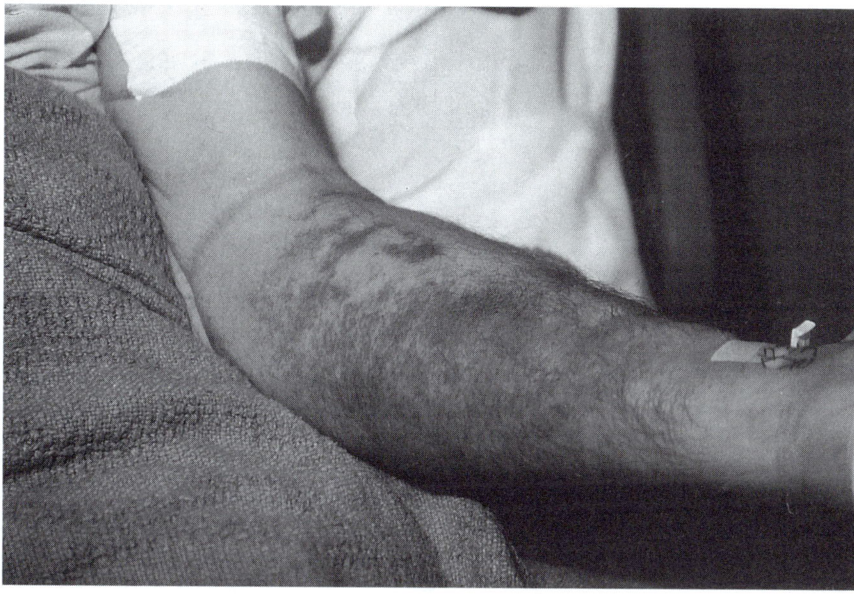

Figure 9–1 ■ Hematoma. (Courtesy of Beth Fabian, CRNI.)

Subcutaneous hematoma is the most common complication (62 percent of all local complications) and is related to nursing skills (Chukhraev & Grekov, 2000). Although not dangerous by itself, this complication can be a starting point for other complications such as thrombophlebitis and infection. Hematoma more often is caused by incorrect manipulation technique and rarely by spontaneous rupture of the vein.

Hematomas are most often related to:

- Nicking the vein during an unsuccessful venipuncture attempt
- Discontinuing the I.V. cannula or needle without pressure held over the site after removal of the cannula or needle
- Applying a tourniquet too tightly above a previously attempted venipuncture site

Signs and Symptoms

Signs and symptoms of hematoma include:

- Discoloration of the skin (i.e., **ecchymoses**) surrounding the venipuncture (immediate or slow)
- Site swelling and discomfort
- Inability to advance the cannula all the way into the vein during insertion
- Resistance to positive pressure during the lock flushing procedure

AGE-RELATED CONSIDERATIONS 9–1

Hematomas and ecchymoses are frequently seen in elderly persons. Fragile veins are easily injured.

Prevention

Techniques for prevention of hematoma formation include:

1. Use of an indirect method rather than a direct approach for starting an I.V. This decreases the chance of piercing through the vein, which then causes seepage of blood into the subcutaneous tissue. (See Chapter 7 for techniques for venipuncture.)
2. Apply the tourniquet just before venipuncture.
3. For elderly patients, patients taking corticosteroids, or patients with paper-thin skin, use a small needle or catheter, preferably 20- or 22-gauge. Use a blood pressure cuff rather than a tourniquet to fill the vein so you have better control of the pressure exerted on the vein.
4. Be very gentle when performing venipuncture.

NURSING FAST FACT!

The presence of both ecchymoses and hematomas limits future use of the affected veins (Perdue, 2001).

Treatment

1. Apply direct, light pressure using a sterile 2 × 2 inch gauze pad over the site after catheter or needle is removed for 2 to 3 minutes (Chukhraev & Grekov, 2000).
2. Have the patient elevate the extremity over his or her head or on a pillow to maximize venous return.
3. Ice may be applied to the area to prevent further enlargement of the hematoma.

Documentation

Document observable ecchymotic areas. Be sure to document the nursing interventions used for care of the site.

Thrombosis

Catheter-related obstructions can be categorized as mechanical or nonthrombotic (42 percent of all obstructions) or thrombotic (58 percent of all obstructions) (Mayo, 2001). Trauma to the endothelial cells of the venous wall causes red blood cells to adhere to the vein wall, which may lead to the formation of a clot. This clot is referred to as a thrombosis, and usually occludes the circulation of blood. Thrombus formation is manifested by the flow of the I.V. solution: the drip rate slows, or the line does not flush easily and resistance is felt, especially in a lock device. The I.V. site may appear healthy. There are two areas of great concern in assessing for a thrombosis. First, do not propel the clot into the bloodstream with pressure from a syringe; second, keep in mind that a thrombus within a vein can trap bacteria.

Thrombotic complications include the development of a thrombus either within or around the device or in the surrounding vessel. Thrombosis results when hemostasis occurs at an inappropriate time. Venous thrombi consist of fibrin and red blood cells. They are large with tapering tails that extend into larger veins and are attached to the venous intima, usually at a valve or venous bifurcation.

Common terms to describe catheter function and thrombosis are listed below (Bagnall-Reeb, 1998; Herbst, Kline, & McKinnon, 1998):

1. Persistent withdrawal occlusion: Catheter is flushed easily without resistance, but there is no blood return on aspiration.
2. Partial occlusion: Resistance to flushing or a sluggish blood return on aspiration
3. Complete occlusion: Inability to infuse or aspirate
4. Fibrin tail: Thrombotic material that has adhered to the end of a catheter. Symptoms include persistent withdrawal occlusion or partial occlusion if the tail is aspirated against the catheter opening and acting as a one-way valve.
5. Fibrin sheath: Thrombus or fibrin deposit encasing a catheter tip
6. Mural thrombosis: Formation of thrombi caused by the presence of the catheter

Thrombosis associated with central venous access devices is discussed in Chapter 12.

Thrombosis formation is most often related to:

- Blood backing up in the system of a hypertensive patient
- A low flow rate, which limits the fluid movement that is necessary to maintain patency
- The location of the I.V. cannula (e.g., a catheter placed in a flexor area may occlude when the position is changed).
- Obstruction of flow rate caused by the patient's compressing the I.V. line for an extended period of time
- Trauma to the wall of the vein by the cannula

Thrombosis, along with thrombophlebitis, can lead to a systemic embolism.

NURSING FAST FACT!

Infusion specialists must avoid injuring the vein wall, performing multiple punctures, and performing through-and-through punctures.

Signs and Symptoms

Signs and symptoms of a thrombosis include:

- Fever and malaise
- Slowed or stopped infusion rate
- Inability to flush locking device

Prevention

Techniques for the prevention of a thrombosis include:

1. Use pumps and controllers for managing rate control. Rate control devices prevent blood from backing up in the tubing and produce an alarm when the I.V. line is dry.
2. Choose microdrip tubing (60 drops/mL) when I.V. gravity flow rates are below 50 mL/h. Remember, more drops mean more movement.
3. Avoid placing an I.V. cannula in areas of flexion.
4. Use filters.
5. Avoid cannulation of lower extremities.

Treatment

1. Never flush a cannula to remove an occlusion!
2. Discontinue the cannula and restart the I.V. infusion with a new catheter in a different site.
   Apply dry sterile 2 × 2 inch gauze dressing.
3. Notify the physician and assess the site for circulatory impairment.

NURSING FAST FACT!

If an occlusion occurs, do not irrigate. Irrigation of an occluded line with saline can propel the clot into the circulatory system, causing an embolism. If there is any resistance when gentle pressure is exerted on the syringe plunger when you are attempting to flush an I.V. catheter, STOP! The application of force could dislodge the clot. Never use a syringe with a barrel size of 2 or 3 mL to flush or aspirate clots in an I.V. line. A small syringe creates excess pressure that can damage the intima of the vein.

Documentation

Document the change of infusion rate, the steps taken to solve the problem, and the end result. Be sure to chart the new I.V. site, its patency, and the size of the catheter used to restart the infusion. Also, document the appearance of the occluded site.

Phlebitis

Phlebitis is an inflammation of the vein in which the endothelial cells of the venous wall become irritated and cells roughen, allowing platelets to adhere and predispose the vein to inflammation-induced phlebitis. The site is tender to touch and can be very painful. At the first sign of redness or complaint of tenderness, the I.V. site should be checked. Phlebitis can prolong hospitalization unless treated early.

The process of phlebitis formation involves an increase in capillary permeability, which allows proteins and fluids to leak into the interstitial space. The traumatized tissue continues to be susceptible to mechanical or chemical irritation (Table 9–1).

> Table 9–1 **TYPES OF PHLEBITIS**

Mechanical Phlebitis

Mechanical irritation causing a phlebitis or inflammation of the vein can be attributed to use of too large a cannula in a small vein. A large cannula placed in a vein with a smaller lumen than the cannula irritates the intima of the vein, causing inflammation and phlebitis. Large veins with thick walls hold up better during an infusion. In addition, veins higher on the forearm are less likely to develop phlebitis. The other cause of mechanical phlebitis is improper taping, in which the catheter tip rubs the vein wall, damaging the endothelial cell. Manipulation of the catheter during infusion causes irritation of vein wall. Securely affix the catheter hub and tubing using the Chevron method to prevent wiggling of the catheter.

NURSING FAST FACT!

The technical expertise of the person inserting the cannula influences the risk for mechanical phlebitis. In comparative trials (Maki & Ringer, 1991), a twofold lower rate of infusion-related phlebitis and reduction of catheter-related sepsis occurred when experienced nurses on an I.V. therapy team inserted I.V. catheters and provided close surveillance of infusion sites.

Chemical Phlebitis

Chemical phlebitis occurs when a vein becomes inflamed by irritating or vesicant solutions or medication. This is the result of contact with infusates with high or low osmolarities or pH or if very small veins are used for venous access.

Several factors contribute to chemical phlebitis. Generally, these include administration of:

- Irritating medications or solutions
- Improperly mixed or diluted medications
- Too-rapid infusion
- Presence of particulate matter in solution

(Continued on following page)

> Table 9–1 **TYPES OF PHLEBITIS** *(Continued)*

The more acidic the I.V. solution, the greater is the risk of the patient's developing chemical phlebitis. I.V. solutions have a pH of 3 to 6, which helps to prevent them from caramelizing during sterilization and helps to maintain stability. Dextrose solutions have a pH of 3.5 to 6.5 or lower, whereas saline solutions have a pH of 5.5. The pH falls further with storage; pH values of 3.4 have been found in date-expired 5% dextrose solutions. Additives such as vitamin C, doxorubicin (Adriamycin), and cimetidine can further decrease the pH. Some drugs such as heparin, which has a pH of 5 to 7.5, can raise the pH. Hypertonic fluids such as 10% dextrose, which have a tonicity of greater than 375, increase the hazards of phlebitis. An increase in electrolytes also adds to the increased tonicity of the solution.

Additives such as potassium chloride (KCl) and various I.V. medications can produce severe venous inflammation. Perdue (2000) found that phlebitis developed in 27.2% of patients who received continuous infusion of KCl in addition to intermittent medications. It was reported that patients who received more than 30 mEq of KCl/L of solution have a greater risk of developing phlebitis.

Chemical Phlebitis

Another factor contributing to chemical phlebitis is particulate matter in a solution, such as drug particles that do not fully dissolve during mixing and are not visible to the eye. The use of a 0.5- to 1.0-micron particulate matter filter eliminates this problem.

The use of catheters for peripheral I.V. therapy can predispose patients to phlebitis. Several different materials are used in the manufacture of catheters. Catheters made of silicone elastomer and polyurethane have a smoother microsurface, are thermoplastic, are more hydrophilic, become more flexible than polytetrafluoroethylene (Teflon) at body temperature, and induce less venous irritation. Maki and Ringer (1991) showed that the incidence of phlebitis increased progressively with increasing period of cannulation. Their study revealed the risk to be 30% by day 2 and 39 to 40% by day 3.

Intermittent infusions with heparin locks cause less irritation to the vein wall over time than continuous infusions. The slower the rate of infusion, the less irritating the solution is to the vein wall because cells of the vein are exposed for a shorter period of time to solutions with less than normal pH. The fact that heparin is used to maintain the lock might have further significance in the reduction of phlebitis rates.

NURSING FAST FACT!

Examples of three common I.V. solutions and their pH and osmolarity:

Solution	pH	Osmolarity, mOsm/L
5% dextrose in water	3 to 5	252
5% dextrose in water with 0.45% sodium chloride	4	406
5% dextrose in water with Ringer's lactate	5	524

Bacterial Phlebitis

Bacterial phlebitis, also referred to as septic phlebitis, is the least common type of phlebitis. It is an inflammation of the intima of a vein that is associated with a bacterial infection. Factors contributing to the development of bacterial phlebitis include poor aseptic technique, failure to detect breaks in the integrity of the equipment, poor cannula insertion technique, inadequately taped cannula, and failure to perform site assessments.

(Continued on following page)

Bacterial phlebitis can be prevented by preparing solutions aseptically under a laminar flow hood. All solution containers should be inspected carefully before they are hung; in addition, handwashing and preparing skin carefully are necessary to prevent bacterial phlebitis.

NURSING FAST FACT!

Handwashing is the most important procedure for preventing nosocomial infections and thus bacterial phlebitis. All equipment should be inspected for integrity, particulate matter, cloudiness, and any signs indicating a break in sterility.

Shaving is not recommended because of the potential for microabrasion, which allows microorganisms to enter the vascular system.

Postinfusion Phlebitis

Postinfusion phlebitis is associated with inflammation of the vein that usually becomes evident within 48 to 96 hours after the cannula has been removed. Factors that contribute to its development are cannula insertion technique; condition of vein used; type, compatibility, and pH of solution or medication being infused; gauge, size, length, and material of cannula; and cannula indwelling time.

Postinfusion phlebitis can occur without the usual signs or symptoms. There is no way to anticipate this type of phlebitis; however, after it appears, the treatment is the same as for any other phlebitis.

The immune system causes leukocytes to gather at the inflamed site. When leukocytes are released, pyrogens stimulate the hypothalamus to raise body temperature. Pyrogens also stimulate bone marrow to release more leukocytes. Redness and tenderness increase with each step of the phlebitis (Maki & Ringer, 1991). When local inflammation is viewed under a microscope, histologic changes are marked, with loss of endothelial cells, edema, and presence of neutrophils in the vein wall. Inspection of the affected site reveals a similar appearance regardless of the underlying cause (Fig. 9–2).

Maki and Ringer (1991) showed that the incidence of phlebitis increased progressively with increasing period of cannulation. Their studies revealed the risk to be 30 percent by day 2 and 39 to 40 percent by day 3.

Factors that influence the development of phlebitis include but are not limited to:

- The insertion technique
- The condition of the patient; vein condition compatibility (type and pH) with the medication or solution; ineffective filtration
- The gauge, size, length, and material composition of the cannula
- Duration of cannulation

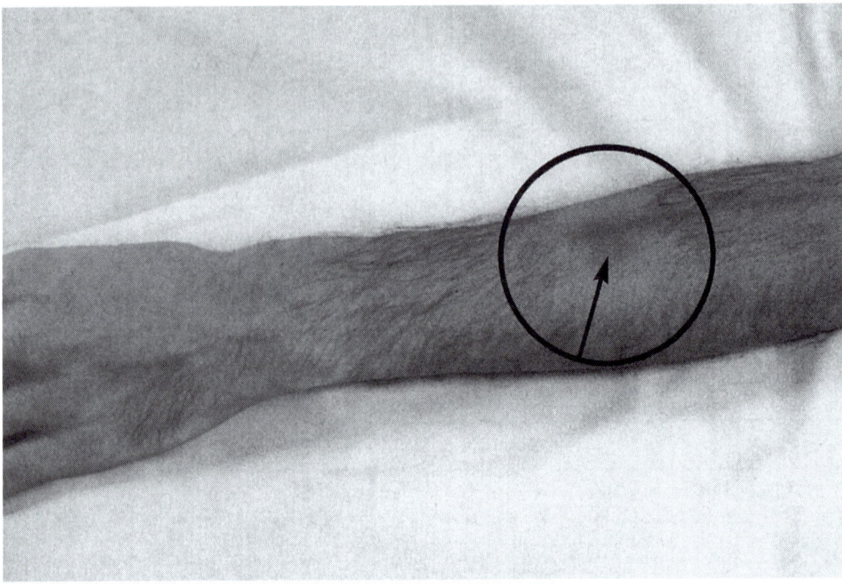

Figure 9–2 ■ Phlebitis. (Courtesy of Johnson & Johnson Medical Inc., Arlington, TX.)

- Infrequent dressing changes
- Host factors, gender, age, and presence of disease (Table 9–2)

Signs and Symptoms

Signs and symptoms associated with phlebitis include:

- Redness at site
- Site warm to touch
- Local swelling
- Palpable cord along the vein
- Sluggish infusion rate
- Increase in basal temperature of 1°C or more

INS Standard. The Infusion Nurses Society (INS) recommends a phlebitis scale to provide a uniform standard for measuring degrees of phlebitis (Table 9–3).

Phlebitis always requires corrective action and documentation. The phlebitis rate is calculated according to a standard formula (INS, 2000, 59):

$$\frac{\text{Number of phlebitis incidents x 100}}{\text{Total number of peripheral I.V. lines}} = \text{Percent of peripheral phlebitis}$$

> Table 9–2 FACTORS AFFECTING PHLEBITIS FORMATION

1. Catheter material
   Polypropylene > Teflon
   Silicone elastomer > polyurethane
   Teflon > polyurethane
   Teflon > steel needles
2. Catheter size
   Large bore > small bore
3. **Insertion in emergency room > inpatient unit**
4. **Increasing duration of catheter placement**
5. **Infusate**
   Low pH
   Potassium chloride
   Hypertonic glucose, amino acids, lipids
   Antibiotics (especially β-lactams, vancomycin, metronidazole)
   High flow rate of I.V. fluid (>90 mL/h)
6. Daily I.V. dressing changes > dressing changes every 48 hours
7. Host factors
   Poor-quality peripheral veins
   Insertion in the upper arm or wrist > hand
8. Age
   Children: older > younger
   Adults: younger > older
   Women > men
   White > Black
9. **Individual biologic vulnerability**

> denotes a significantly greater risk for phlebitis.
Terms in bold print are significant predictors of risk in this study.
Source: *Adapted from Maki, D.G., & Ringer, M. (1991). Risk factors for infusion-related phlebitis with small peripheral venous catheters: A randomized controlled trial. Annals of Internal Medicine, 114, 845–854.*

Prevention

Techniques for the prevention of phlebitis include:

1. Use larger veins for hypertonic solutions.
2. Use central lines or long-arm catheters for long-term hypertonic solutions.

> Table 9–3 PHLEBITIS SCALE

Grade	Clinical Criteria
0	No clinical symptoms
1	Erythema at access site with or without pain
2	Pain at access site, with erythema and/or edema
3	Pain at access site with erythema and/or edema, streak formation, and palpable venous cord
4	Pain at access site with erythema and/or edema, streak formation, palpable venous cord >1 inch in length, purulent drainage

Source: *Revised Standards of Practice. (2000). Cambridge, MA: Infusion Nurses Society; with permission.*

3. Choose the smallest I.V. cannula appropriate for the infusate.
4. Rotate the I.V. site every 72 hours, a practice that has been shown to significantly decrease the risk of phlebitis.
5. Stabilize the catheter to prevent mechanical irritation.
6. Use a 0.22-micron inline final filter, which removes air, bacteria, and harmful particulate matter.
7. Venipuncture should be performed only by skilled professionals.
8. Observe good handwashing practices.
9. Add a buffer to known irritating medications and to hypertonic solutions.
10. Change solution containers every 24 hours.

NURSING FAST FACTS!

BE AWARE THAT:

- *Phlebitis risk factors in I.V. therapy increase after 24 hours.*
- *All peripheral I.V.s should be changed every 48 to 72 hours.*
- *A 3+ phlebitis (see Table 9–4) takes from 10 days to 3 weeks to heal.*
- *Dextrose solutions, potassium chloride (KCl), antibiotics, and vitamin C have a lower pH and are associated with a higher risk of phlebitis.*

> Table 9–4 **INFILTRATION SCALE**

Grade	Criteria
0	No symptoms
1	Skin blan ched Edema <1 inch Cool to touch With or without pain
2	Skin blanched Edema 1 to 6 inches Cool to touch With or without pain
3	Skin blanched and translucent Gross edema >6 inches Cool to touch Mild to moderate pain Possible numbness
4	Skin blanched and translucent Skin tight, leaking Gross edema >6 inches Deep, pitting tissue edema Circulatory impairment Moderate to severe pain

Source: *Revised Standards of Practice. (1998). Cambridge, MA: Infusion Nurses Society; with permission.*

Treatment

1. Discontinue the infusion at the first sign of phlebitis (1+).
2. Apply warm or cold compresses to the affected site. Cold significantly decreases intradermal skin toxicity for 45 minutes.
3. Consult the physician if the patient has a phlebitis rating of 3+ or 4+.
4. Depending on agency policy, notify infection control.

Documentation

Documentation is critical when phlebitis has been detected. Document the site assessment, the phlebitis rating (1, 2, 3, or 4), whether the physician was notified, and the treatment provided. Document the discontinuation of the I.V. catheter, and location of new I.V. site.

Thrombophlebitis

Thrombophlebitis denotes a twofold injury: thrombosis and inflammation. A painful inflamed vein promptly develops from the point of thrombosis. Thrombophlebitis causes the patient unnecessary discomfort. Chemical or mechanical phlebitis can also precipitate a thrombophlebitis.

Thrombophlebitis is related to:

- Use of veins in the legs for infusion therapy
- Use of hypertonic or highly acidic infusion solutions
- Causes similar to those leading to phlebitis (i.e., insertion technique; condition of patient; vein condition; compatibility [type and pH of medication or solution]; ineffective filtration; and the gauge, size, length, and material of the cannula)

NURSING FAST FACT!

Thrombophlebitis is often the sequela of phlebitis.

Signs and Symptoms

Signs and symptoms of thrombophlebitis include:

- Sluggish flow rate
- Edema in the limbs
- Tender and cordlike vein
- Site warm to touch
- Visible red line above venipuncture site
- Diminished arterial pulses
- Mottling and cyanosis of the extremities

NURSING FAST FACT!

If the inflammation is the result of bacterial phlebitis, a much more serious condition leading to septicemia may develop if the patient is not treated.

Prevention

Techniques used to prevent thrombophlebitis include:

1. Use the veins in the forearm rather than in the hands when infusing any medication.
2. Do not use veins in joint flexion areas.
3. Check the infusion site for signs and symptoms of redness, swelling, or pain at the site at least every 4 hours in adults and every 2 hours in children.
4. Anchor the cannula securely to prevent mobility of the catheter tip.
5. Infuse solutions at the prescribed rate. Do not attempt to catch up on delayed infusion time.
6. Use the smallest sized catheter that meets the needs of the patient.
7. Dilute irritating medications.

Septic thrombophlebitis can be prevented with:

- Appropriate skin preparation
- Aseptic technique in the maintenance of infusion
- Following hand hygiene procedures

NURSING FAST FACT!

Thrombophlebitis can lead to a potential embolism owing to thrombus formation in the vein wall.

Discontinue the infusion, remove the cannula, and restart in a new site to prevent progression of thrombophlebitis.

Treatment

1. Remove the entire I.V. catheter and restart the infusion in the opposite extremity, using all new equipment.
2. Consult the physician.
3. Provide comfort by applying warm, moist compresses to the area for 20 minutes.

Documentation

Document all observable symptoms and the patient's subjective complaints such as "feels tender to touch" and "it hurts." State your actions to resolve the problem and the time at which you notified the physician. Document the site in which you restarted the infusion.

Infiltration

Infusion Nursing Standards of Practice (2000) defin inadvertent administration of a nonvesicant solution i sue. Infiltration occurs from the dislodgement of the intima of a vein. It can also occur from phlebitis, ca become threadlike when the lumen along the cannula ws, so fluid leaks from the site where the cannula enters the vein wall. Infiltration is second to phlebitis as a cause of I.V. therapy morbidity.

Infiltration is related to:

- Puncture of the distal vein wall during venipuncture
- Puncture of any portion of the vein wall by mechanical friction from the catheter or needle
- Dislodgement of the catheter or needle from the intima of the vein
- Poorly secured infusion device
- High delivery rate or pressure (psi) from an electronic infusion device
- Overmanipulation of an I.V. device

Signs and Symptoms

Signs and symptoms of infiltration include:

- Coolness of skin around site
- Taut skin
- Dependent edema
- Absence of blood backflow
- A "pinkish" blood return
- Infusion rate slows but the fluid continues to infuse.

Complications associated with infiltration fall into three categories:

1. *Ulceration and possible tissue necrosis:* The severity of tissue damage depends on many variables, including the drug's vesicant potential, the amount of drug infiltrated and the venipuncture site. Ulceration is not immediately apparent; the ulcer may actually take days or weeks to develop. See the section on extravasation later in this chapter.
2. *Compartment syndrome:* Muscles, nerves, and vessels are in compartments confined in inflexible spaces bound by skin, fascia, and bone. When fluid inside a compartment increases, the venous end of the capillary bed becomes compressed. If vessels cannot carry away the excessive fluid, hydrostatic pressure rises, leading to vascular spasm, pain, and muscle necrosis inside the compartment. Functional muscle changes can occur within 4 to 12 hours of injury. Within 24 hours ischemic nerve damage can result in functional loss.
3. *Reflex sympathetic dystrophy syndrome:* This complication occurs when severe infiltration occurs, and a chronic and exaggerated inflammatory process begins, leaving the patient with limited function in the affected extremity (Hadaway, 2002).

...tion

...revention of infiltration includes performing adequate and continuous assessment of the site. Checking for a blood return, or backflow of blood, is not a reliable method of determining the patency of a cannula. Blood return may be present when small veins are used because they may not permit blood flow around the cannula. Use of veins that have had previous punctures or veins that are very fragile may cause a seeping of fluid at the site above or below the vein cannula entry point; blood return may be present, yet an infiltration is occurring (Fig. 9–3).

Infiltration and swelling below the I.V. site may occur as a result of placing hands underneath the patient during turning. Occlusion

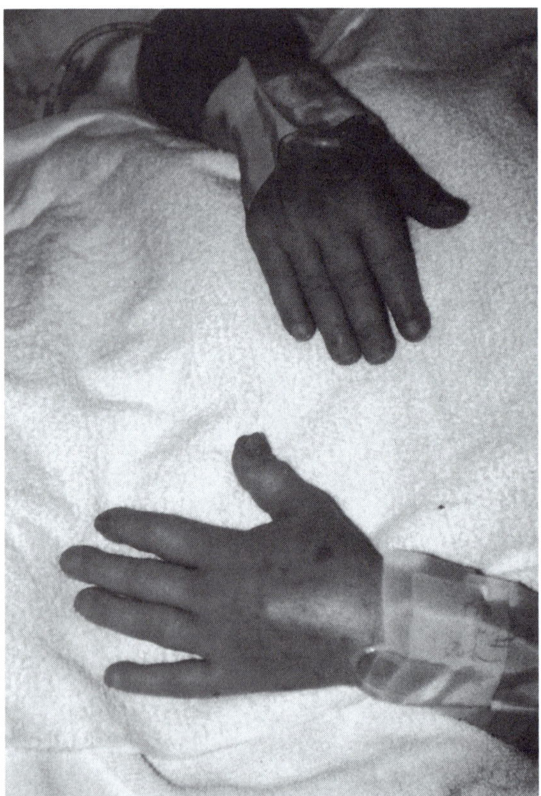

Figure 9–3 ■ Infiltration and swelling below the I.V. site occurring after hands were placed underneath the patient during turning. Occlusion or restriction of blood flow caused fluid to back up in the vessels, resulting in infiltration and dependent edema below the I.V. site rather than above. (Courtesy of Beth Fabian, CRNI.)

or restriction of blood flow causes fluid to back up in the vessels, resulting in infiltration and dependent edema below the I.V. site rather than above.

The most accurate method of checking for infiltration is assessment of the site: With infusion running, apply pressure 3 inches above the catheter site in front of the catheter tip either with digital pressure or use of a tourniquet. If the infusion continues to run, suspect infiltration. When the vein is compressed and the catheter is in proper alignment in the vein, the I.V. solution will stop because of occlusion. In addition, compare both of the patient's arms when assessing for infiltration (Fig. 9–4).

INS Standard. Use Infusion Nurses Society infiltration classification for rating infiltration on a scale of 0 to 4. (INS, 2000, 60) (Refer to Table 9–4.)

NURSING FAST FACT!

Immobilized patients and patients with muscular weakness or paralysis of an extremity may have edema of an extremity that is not related to infiltration of an I.V. site. Accurate assessment of the cannula and infusion site is the key to differentiation.

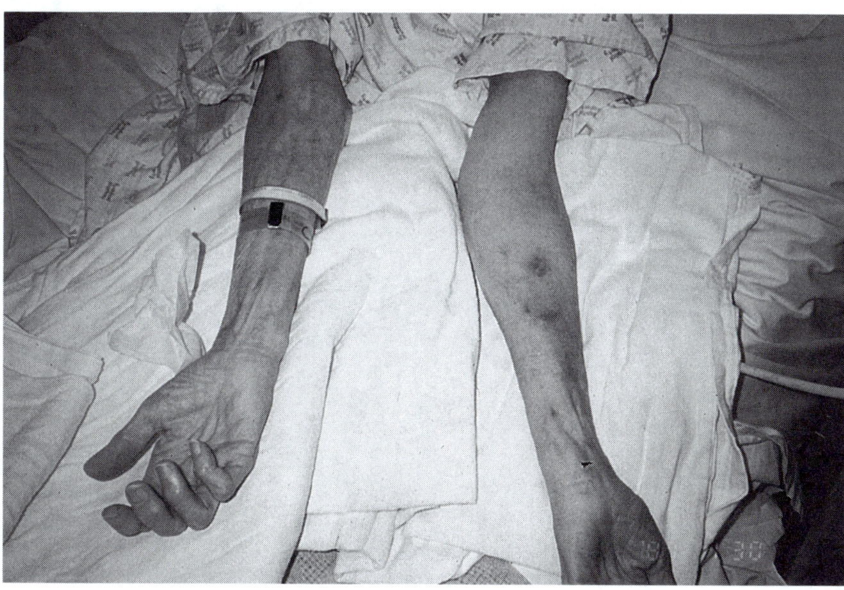

Figure 9–4 Infiltration. Compare both arms when assessing for infiltration (note that the left arm is swollen compared with the right arm).

Treatment

Use of warm compresses to treat infiltration has become controversial. It has been found that cold compresses may be better for some infiltrated infusates and warm compresses may be more effective for others. Refer to Table 9–7 for treatment options. Elevation of the infiltrated extremity may be painful for the patient. A study showed a 4-inch elevation of the extremity made no difference in the rate of fluid reabsorption. Let the patient decide on the position of comfort in this situation (Hadaway, 2002).

Documentation

Document the assessment findings, any written and verbal communications, nursing and medical interventions, and patient response patterns.

Extravasation

Extravasation, according to Infusion Nurses Society, is the inadvertent administration of a vesicant solution into surrounding tissue. A **vesicant** solution is a fluid or medication that causes the formation of blisters, with subsequent sloughing of tissues occurring from the tissue necrosis (Figs. 9–5 and 9–6).

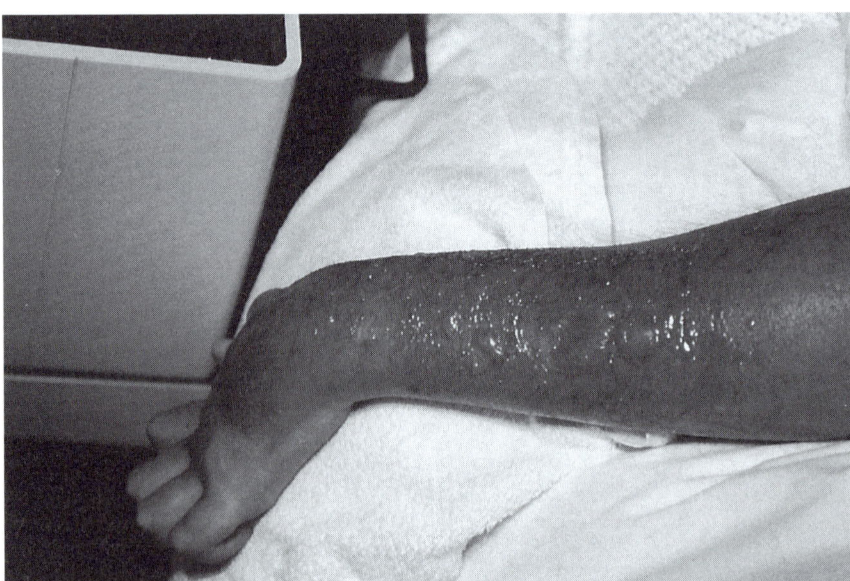

Figure 9–5 ■ Infiltration of vancomycin into subcutaneous tissue, causing blistering of skin. (Courtesy of Beth Fabian, CRNI.)

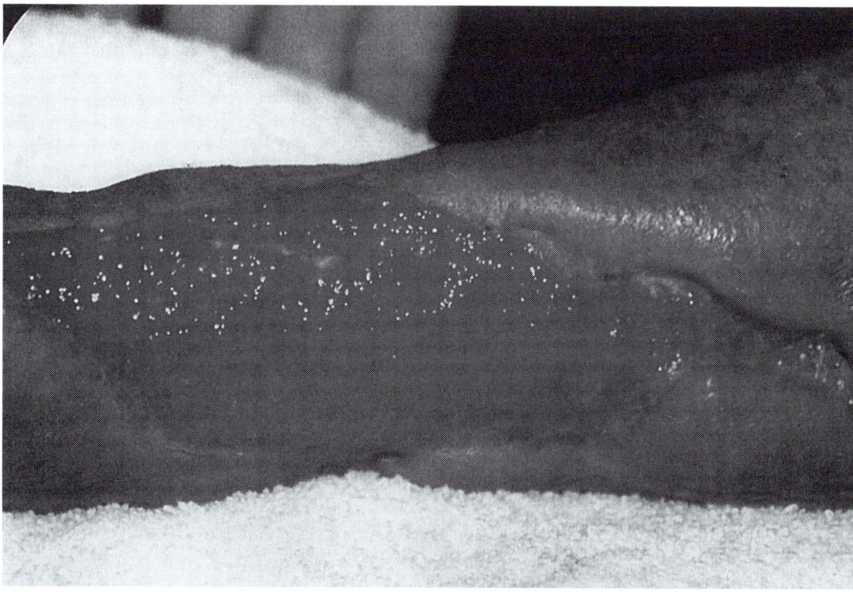

Figure 9–6 ■ Extravasation with tissue necrosis. (Courtesy of Johnson & Johnson Medical Inc., Arlington, TX.)

Patients who are at high risk for extravasation injury are presented in Table 9–5.

Extravasation injury is related to:

- Puncture of the distal vein wall during venipuncture and administration of irritating or vesicant medications or solutions
- Puncture of any portion of the vein wall by mechanical friction from the catheter or needle while infusing irritating or vesicant solutions
- Dislodgement of the catheter or needle from the intima of the vein

> Table 9–5 **FACTORS AFFECTING RISK FOR EXTRAVASATION INJURY**

Age
- Neonate
- Geriatric patient

Condition
- Oncology patient
- Comatose patient
- Anesthetized patient
- Patients with peripheral or cardiovascular disease
- Diabetic patient

Equipment
- High-pressure infusion pumps

- Poorly secured infusion device
- High delivery rate or pressure from an electronic infusion device
- Overmanipulation of the I.V. device
- Thrombus or fibrin sheath formation at the vascular access device (VAD) catheter tip

Signs and Symptoms

Signs and symptoms of extravasation (Skokal, 2001) include:

- Complaints of pain or burning
- Swelling proximal to or distal to the I.V. site
- Puffiness of the dependent part of the limb
- Skin tightness at the venipuncture site
- Blanching and coolness of the skin
- Slow or stopped infusion
- Damp or wet dressing

NURSING FAST FACT!

Never increase the flow rate to determine the infiltration of a vesicant. Checking for blood return is not a reliable method of determining an infiltration.

The severity of damage is directly related to the type, concentration, and volume of fluid infiltrated into the interstitial tissues. The endothelium is particularly sensitive to pH and osmolarity differences found in physiologic and nonphysiologic solutions. These fluids may induce cellular injury through irritation, stimulating the inflammatory process. The damaged tissue release precipitating proteins with an increase in capillary permeability, which allows fluid and protein shifts to interstitial space. Edema, ischemia, vasoconstriction, pain, and erythema are responses to these cellular changes and may lead to tissue necrosis (Hastings-Tolsma et al., 1993).

Refer to Table 9–6 for a list of vesicant medications.

Prevention

To prevent vesicant extravasations, the following should be considered:

1. The use of skilled practitioners. Registered nurses specifically trained and supervised in chemotherapy administration should administer any medications that are irritating and vesicant. Practitioners should also be skillful in venipuncture and skillful and competent in using VADs.
2. The practitioner's knowledge of vesicants. The practitioner should have an understanding of the signs and symptoms of extravasation and be able to perform appropriate management.
3. The condition of the patient's vein. Patients with small, fragile

> Table 9–6 **VESICANT MEDICATIONS**

Antibiotics	Antivirals	Antineoplastic Drugs	Vasodilators	Electrolyte Solutions	Vasopressors
Doxycycline	Acyclovir	Carmustine	Nitroprusside sodium	Calcium chloride	Dopamine
Nafcillin		Dacarbazine		Calcium gluconate	Epinephrine
Piperacillin		Dactinomycin		Potassium chloride	Metaraminol
Piperacillin/ tazobactam (Zosyn)		Daunorubicin		Sodium bicarbonate	Norepinephrine
Vancomycin		Doxorubicin			
		Epirubicin			
		Idarubicin			
		Mechlorethamine			
		Mitomycin C			
		Paclitaxel			
		Plicamycin			
		Streptozocin			
		Vinblastine			
		Vincristine			
		Vinorelbine			

Sources: *Hadaway (2002); Davis's Drug Guide (2003); Roth (2003).*

veins; limited access; long-term therapy; and multiple vein sticks are prone to infiltration.

4. The drug administration technique.
   a. Give continuous vesicant administration into a long-term VAD.
   b. Avoid giving vesicant through a VAD without a good blood return.
   c. Use a free-flowing I.V. to give push medications, when possible.
   d. Avoid using a controlled infusion device for vesicants given peripherally.
   e. Assess for blood return frequently (such as every 2 to 5 mL or hourly).
5. The site of venous access. Avoid the large veins of the forearm, especially the posterior basilic vein, and the metacarpal veins of the dorsum of the hand. Avoid the use of the antecubital fossa and avoid using the lower extremity veins. Remove dressings to fully visualize the vein during administration.
6. The condition of the patient. Vomiting, coughing, or retching can cause excessive movement, resulting in a loss of access. Sedation from antiemetics or pain medications limits a patient's ability to report pain during infusion. Patients who are unable to communicate, such as infants and obtunded patients, also need to be observed closely (Camp-Sorrell, 1998).

NURSING FAST FACT!

Restraints must be applied with extreme caution and within the guidelines established by the Joint Commission on Accreditation of Healthcare Organizations (JCAHO) and by the Food and Drug Administration (FDA). Immobilization devices should be well padded and applied so that they do not cause nerve damage, constrict circulation, or cause pressure areas; they should be removed at frequent intervals, and nurse-assisted range-of-motion exercises should be performed. Inadequate or improper use of immobilization devices can cause very serious complications; policies and procedures should be established to guide their use.

INS Standard. Treatment of infiltration should be established in organizational policy and procedure. (INS, 2000, 60)

Treatment

Treatment depends on the severity of the infiltration. Refer to Table 9–4 for the infiltration scale. Consideration should be given to the completion of an unusual occurrence report on type of infusate and severity of the infiltration (INS, 2000, 60).

INS Standard. The infiltration of any amount of blood product, irritant, or vesicant is classified as a grade 4 (INS, 2000, 60).

The most effective treatment for extravasation is prevention. However, if extravasation is suspected:

1. Stop the I.V. flow and leave the cannula in place until after any residual medication and blood are aspirated and an antidote particular to the vesicant is instilled into the tissues.
2. Administer the prescribed antidote (this cannot be delayed).
3. Remove the cannula.
4. Apply thermal manipulation to alter the temperature in the superficial skin for 24 to 72 hours. Cold topical applications are used for all extravasations except those of the vinca alkaloids.
5. Photograph the suspected area of extravasation according to institutional policy.
6. Elevate the arm 4 inches. (Note: Elevation of the extremity with infiltration or extravasation is controversial). Research shows that using small quantities of infiltrated I.V. solutions followed by magnetic resonance imaging decreases the volume of hypotonic solutions; hypertonic solutions increase in volume with elevation. A 4-inch (10-cm) elevation of the extremity made no difference in the rate of fluid reabsorption for either solution. Elevating the arm may be uncomfortable for some patients (Hadaway, 2002).

7. Consult the physician. Request a plastic surgery consultation if a vesicant drug has infiltrated.
8. Document all details of the incidence (Camp-Sorrell, 1998; Hadaway, 1998).

Antidotes

Antidotes for extravasation injury fall into four categories: (1) those that alter local pH, (2) those that alter DNA binding, (3) those that chemically neutralize, and (4) those that dilute extravasated drug (Table 9–7).

If you are going to instill an antidote, do so through the existing I.V. catheter or use a 1-mL tuberculin syringe, injecting small amounts subcutaneously in a circle around the infiltrated area (Camp-Sorrell, 1998).

> Table 9–7 **ANTIDOTES FOR EXTRAVASATED DRUGS**

Extravasated Drug Class	Medications	Antidote, Dose*	Nursing Tip
	Adrenergic Agents		
Usually sloughing and tissue necrosis with extravasation	Amrinone (Inocor) Dobutamine (Dobutrex) Dopamine (Intropin) Epinephrine (Adrenaline) Isoproterenol (Isuprel) Metaraminol (Aramine) Methoxamine (Vasoxyl) Norepineprine (Levophed) Phenylephrine (NeoSynephrine)	5 to 10 mg phentolamine mesylate	Discontinue infusion Apply cold compresses Slightly elevate† extremity only if the elevation does not cause pain Use small intradermal needle (27- to 25-gauge)
	Alkalinizing Agents		
Usually cause ulceration, sloughing, cellulitis, and tissue necrosis	Sodium bicarbonate	Inject 1% procaine to reduce venospasm	Discontinue infusion
	Tromethamine (Tham-E)	Hyaluronidase 150 U/mL 0.2 mL × 5 SQ	Use small intradermal needle (27- to 25-gauge) Apply cold compresses Elevate slightly†

(Continued on following page)

> Table 9–7 **ANTIDOTES FOR EXTRAVASATED DRUGS** *(Continued)*

Extravasated Drug Class	Medications	Antidote, Dose*	Nursing Tip
	Alkylating Agents		
Usually causes sloughing and tissue necrosis	Carmustine (BCNU) irritant	Inject longacting dexamethasone or other corticosteroid	Discontinue infusion Apply cold compress Elevate slightly†
	Stretptozocin (Zancosar)	Dimethyl sulfoxide (DMSO) applied topically	Apply every 3, 4, 6, or 8 hours for 7 to 14 days
	Mechlorethamine (nitrogen mustard) vesicant	Sodium thiosulfate Dilute 4 mL with 6 mL of sterile water inject 1 to 4 mL through existing cannula; give 1 mL for each milliliter extravasated	Use ice compresses for 20 min/h until inflammation dissipates
	Antihypertensive Agents		
	Nitroprusside sodium (Nipride)	Sodium thiosulfate Dilute 4 mL with 6 mL of sterile water inject 1 to 4 mL through existing cannula; give 1 mL for each milliliter extravasated	Discontinue infusion Use cool compress Elevate slightly†
	Dobutamine (Dobutrex) Dopamine (Dopastat) Epinephrine Metaraminol (Aramine) Norepinephrine	Phentolamine (Regitine), 5 to 10 mg SQ diluted in 10 to 15 mL of sodium chloride	Treatment must start immediately Use cool compresses
	Antineoplastic Agents		
(DNA/RNA inhibitors or mitotic inhibitors) Usually causes severe tissue sloughing and necrosis	Dacarbazine (DTIC) vesicant Etoposide (VePeside) irritant Vinblastine (Velban) vesicant Vincristine (Oncovin) vesicant Vindesine (Eldisine) vesicant	Inject long-acting dexamethasone or other corticosteroid	Discontinue infusion Apply warm compress Elevate slightly†

(Continued on following page)

Extravasated Drug Class	Medications	Antidote, Dose*	Nursing Tip
	Antibiotic Antineoplastic Agents		
Generally cause stinging, burning, severe cellulitis, and tissue necrosis	Dactinomycin (Actinomycin D) vesicant Daunorubicin (Daunomycin) vesicant Doxorubicin (Adriamycin) vesicant	Flush the extravasated area with 0.9% sodium chloride Inject long-acting OR Inject hyaluronidase (15 U/mL 0.2 mL × 5 SQ throughout the area)	Discontinue infusion Use small gauge (27 to 25-gauge) needle Apply cold compresses Elevate slightly†
	Idarubicin (Idamycin) vesicant	Aspirate as much of drug as possible from tissue Flush with 0.9% sodium chloride Inject long-acting OR Inject hyaluronidase 15 U/mL 0.2 mL × 5 SQ	Discontinue infusion Apply ice compresses Elevate slightly†
	Mitomycin C (Mutamycin) vesicant Plicamycin (Mithramycin) vesicant	Inject long-acting dexamethasone	Discontinue infusion after sodium bicarbonate (neutralizing agent is instilled into cannula) Apply cool compresses
Vein irritants that generally cause necrosis, sloughing, cellulitis, and tissue necrosis	Calcium salts Calcium carbonate Calcium chloride Calcium gluconate Calcium lactate Calcium gluceptate Potassium solutions	Inject hyaluronidase through 150 U/mL 0.2 mL × 5 SQ	Discontinue infusion Apply cool compresses Elevate slightly†
Hypertonic (>10%) solutions	Dextrose solutions	Inject hyaluronidase through 150 U/mL 0.2 mL × 5 SQ	Discontinue infusion Apply cool compresses Elevate slightly†

**Side effects of antidotes:*

Dimethyl sulfoxide (DMSO): Mild side effects, mild burning, skin scaling and unpleasant garlic odor. Use with local cooling measures

Hyaluronidase (Wydase): Rash, urticaria

Phentolamine (Regitine): Hypotension, tachycardia, flushing, nausea and vomiting

Sodium thiosulfate: Rash, hypersensitivity

Hydrocortisone sodium or dexamethasone: Delayed wound healing, various skin eruptions

†Research on small quantities of infiltrated I.V. solutions followed by magnetic resonance imaging found that hypotonic solutions decreased in volume and hypertonic solutions increased in volume with elevation. A 4-inch (10-cm) elevation of the extremity made no difference in the rate of fluid reabsorption for either solution. Elevating the arm may be uncomfortable for some patients.

> Table 9–8 **FACTORS IN FLOW-RATE CONTROL**

Patient-Related	**Vein-Related**
Patient or family intervention	Infiltration
Patient blood pressure	Phlebitis
Tubing-Related	Venous spasm
"Cold flow" of plastic tubing	**Clot formation needle or catheter position**
Drop formation rate	**Other**
Final in-filters kinked or pinched tubing	Height of I.V. standard
Rate of fluid flow	Bed position
Slipping of roller clamp	
Electronic infusion device malfunction	

Source: *Adapted from Steele, J. (1983). Too fast or too slow: The erratic I.V. American Journal of Nursing, 6, 898–900, with permission.*

NOTE > Table 9–8 may be reproduced and posted in the medication area for quick reference.

Documentation

Documentation of an extravasation event in the patient's medical record must be comprehensive. Document assessments and interventions include the vascular access device type, insertion site, name of medication or solution, and how it was infused (push or infusion, with or without pump). Assess the status of circulation at, above, and below the insertion site, including skin color capillary refill and circumference of both the extremities at the site. Estimate how much solution entered the subcutaneous tissue by noting the time of the first complaint, the time the infusion was stopped, and the rate of the infusion. Multiply the length of time by the hourly rate. Document the treatment of the infiltrated site, the antidote used, and the procedure for injection of the antidote. Document site checks and record the condition of the site before and after treatment. At the time of infiltration photo document for the chart according to facility policy. Notify the patient's primary care provider. Arrange a plastic surgery consult, if applicable. File an unusual occurrence report according to facility policy (Hadaway, 2002).

NURSING FAST FACT!

Soft tissue damage from extravasation can lead to prolonged healing, potential infections, necrosis, multiple débridement surgeries, cosmetic disfiguration, loss of limb function, and amputation.

There can be legal ramifications to venous extravasation events; the occurrence of extravastion does not of itself constitute negligence; rather it is the failure to take special precautions to minimize the potential for extravasation that may prove a successful cause of legal action (Roth, 2003).

Websites

National Association of Vascular Access Networks: *www.navannet.org*

Other sites:

Local Infections

Infections related to the use of I.V. therapy consist of those related to microbial contamination of the cannula or infusate. One of the most serious forms of intravascular device–related infection occurs when intravascular thrombus surrounding the cannula becomes infected. This causes septic thrombophlebitis (suppurative phlebitis) (Maki & Mermel, 1998).

Local infections are preventable by maintaining aseptic technique and following guidelines established by the INS or Centers for Disease Control and Prevention for the duration of infusion, length of time of catheter placement, and tubing change criteria.

Local infections are related to:

- Catheters left in place for more than 72 hours
- Field sticks that are not changed after 24 hours
- Poor technique in placing the catheter
- Poor technique in maintaining and monitoring the peripheral site

NURSING FAST FACT!

In any patient with an intravascular catheter who develops high-grade bloodstream infection that persists after an infected cannula has been removed, it is likely the patient has an infected thrombus in recently cannulated vein (Maki & Mermel, 1998).

Signs and Symptoms

Signs and symptoms of local infection include:

- Redness and swelling at the site
- Possible exudate of purulent material

- Increased quantity of white blood cells
- Elevated temperature (chills are not associated with local infection)

The ways a catheter tip may acquire bacteria are:

- During introduction of catheter
- During removal of stylet
- From colonization from skin
- From contaminated I.V. solutions
- From air inlet filter malfunction
- From microorganisms entering system at the catheter or administration set junction

Prevention

Techniques used to prevent local infections include:

1. Inspect all solution containers for cracks and leaks before hanging.
2. Change solution containers every 24 hours.
3. Maintain aseptic technique during cannula insertion, I.V. therapy, and catheter removal (Perdue, 2001).

The choice and preparation of site affect the risk of local infection. The venipuncture site should be scrubbed with 70 percent alcohol to remove blood or dirt, which can interfere with disinfectant prepping solution. Then for excellent bactericidal activity, perform a 20-second circular preparation with 1 to 2 percent tincture of iodine, iodophor, or 70 percent isopropyl alcohol or chlorhexidine, and allow the site to dry. If the patient is allergic to iodine, use 70 percent alcohol for a 1-minute vigorous scrub. Chlorhexidine is associated with the lowest incidence of infection (Maki & Mermel, 1998). Contamination of I.V. cannulae by microorganisms on the hands of hospital personnel during the time of insertion contributes significantly to local infections. Washing hands with soap and water using mechanical friction for at least 15 seconds removes most transient acquired bacteria (INS, 2000, 25).

NOTE > See Chapter 2 for further information on infections at cannula sites.

The Centers for Disease Control and Prevention (CDC) and Association for Professionals in Infection Control and Epidemiology (APIC) standard for infection rate calculation is:

$$\frac{\text{Number of infected I.V. lines}}{\text{Total number of catheter days}} \times 1000 = \text{Number of infected I.V. lines per 1000 catheter days}$$

Treatment

1. Consult with the physician.
2. Remove the cannula.
3. Culture the cannula tip and insertion site, and prepare at least two separate cultures of blood samples (one drawn percutaneously) before antibiotic therapy is initiated (Mermel et al., 2001).
4. Apply a sterile dressing over the site.
5. Use systemic antibiotic therapy, which may be necessary.
6. Monitor the site.

Documentation

Document the assessment of the site, culture technique, sources of culture, notification of the physician, and any treatment initiated. Culture techniques are discussed in Chapter 2.

Venous Spasm

A spasm is a sudden, involuntary contraction of a vein or an artery resulting in temporary cessation of blood flow through a vessel. Venous spasm can occur suddenly and for a variety of reasons. The spasm usually results from the administration of a cold infusate, an irritating solution, or a too-rapid administration of I.V. solution or viscous solution such as a blood product.

Venous spasm is related to:

- Administration of cold infusates
- Mechanical or chemical irritation of intima of vein

Signs and Symptoms

Signs and symptoms of venous spasms include:

- Sharp pain at the I.V. site that travels up the arm, which is caused by a piercing stream of fluid that irritates or shocks the vein wall
- Slowing of the infusion

Prevention

Venous spasm can be prevented. Techniques used to prevent vasospasm include:

1. Dilute the medication additive adequately.
2. Keep the I.V. solution at room temperature.
3. Wrap the extremity with warm compresses during the infusion.
4. Give the solution at the prescribed rate.

5. Consider using a fluid warmer for rapid transfusions of potent cold agglutinins.
6. All refrigerated medications and parenteral solutions should be allowed to reach room temperature before they are administered (Perdue, 2001).

NURSING FAST FACT!

If a rapid infusion rate is desired, use a larger cannula.

Treatment

1. Apply warm compresses to warm the extremity and decrease flow rate until the spasm subsides.
2. Restart the I.V. if venous spasm continues.

Documentation

Document the patient complaints, duration of complaints, treatment, and length of time to resolve the problem. Also document whether the I.V. site needed to be rotated to resolve the problem.

Systemic Complications

Systemic complications can be life threatening. Such complications include septicemia, circulatory overload, pulmonary edema, air embolus, speed shock, and catheter embolus.

Septicemia

Septicemia is a febrile disease process that results from the presence of microorganisms or their toxic products in the circulatory system (Guyton & Hall, 2001). The incidence of nosocomial bloodstream infections has increased twofold to threefold in the past decade, with central catheter infections accounting for 90 percent of the catheter-related infections. These infections have a case-fatality rate of more than 20 percent (Maki & Mermel, 1998).

The microorganism most frequently implicated in hospital-acquired catheter-related bloodstream infections (BSI) is coagulase-negative staphylococcus, followed by enterococci. Coagulase-negative staphylococci accounted for 37 percent and *S. aureus* for 12.6 percent of reported hospital-acquired BSIs. Enterococci accounted for 13.5 percent of BSIs, an increase from 8 percent reported during the 1986–1989 statistics. *Candida* spp. caused 8 percent of hospital-acquired BSIs reported in both data collection periods. The resistance of *Candida* spp. to commonly used antifungal agents is increasing (CDC, 2002).

Nurses must be aware of risk factors, prevention techniques, and the presence of an infected catheter tip because bacteremia, fungemia, or septicemia could occur. Risk factors associated with septicemia include:

- Patient factors: age, alteration in host defense, underlying illness, presence of other infectious processes
- Infusion factors: solution container, stopcocks, catheter material and structure, insertion site, hematogenous seeding, manipulation of the infusion system, certain transparent dressings, and duration of cannulation
- Practitioner-related factors: lack of handwashing, break in sterile technique, inexperience of the professional inserting the cannula, inadequately prepared or maintained insertion sites, repeated manipulation of infusion system (Perdue, 2000)

Signs and Symptoms

Signs and symptoms of septicemia include:

- Fluctuating fever, tremors, chattering teeth
- Profuse, cold sweat
- Nausea and vomiting
- Diarrhea (sudden and explosive)
- Abdominal pain
- Tachycardia
- Increased respirations or hyperventilation
- Altered mental status
- Hypotension

As the organisms overcome the host, vascular collapse, shock, and death can occur (Jackson, 2001).

Prevention

Techniques used to prevent septicemia include:

1. Good hand hygiene. Handwashing and sterile technique are imperative to minimize the risk of technique-induced septicemia.
2. Carefully inspect solutions for abnormal cloudiness, cracks, and pinholes.
3. Use only freshly opened solutions.
4. Protein solutions, such as albumin and protein hydrolysates, should be used as soon as the seal is broken.
5. Rather than using alcohol-containing antiseptics, use iodine-containing antiseptics, as the latter have a superior spectrum of antimicrobial activity. They are also inexpensive, well tolerated, and highly reliable.
6. Use Luer-Lok connections when possible.

7. Cover infusion sites with a sterile dressing.
8. Limit use of add-on devices.
9. Inspect the site and assess the patient routinely to ensure early recognition of symptoms.
10. Change peripheral cannulae according to the INS standards of practice.

NURSING FAST FACT!

The key to prevention of septicemia is staff education.

Treatment

It is sometimes difficult to differentiate between infusion-associated sepsis and septicemia from other causes, unless associated with phlebitis (Maki & Mermel, 1998).

The steps in treating suspected septicemia based on patient signs and symptoms are:

1. Consult the physician.
2. Restart a new I.V. system in the opposite extremity.
3. Obtain cultures from the administration set, container, and catheter tip site, as well as the patient's blood.
4. Initiate antimicrobial therapy as ordered.
5. Monitor the patient closely.
6. Determine whether the patient's condition requires transfer to the ICU.

Documentation

Document the signs and symptoms assessed, the time the physician was notified, and all treatments instituted. Document the time of transfer to ICU, the time the new I.V. infusion and system was started, and how the patient is tolerating interventions.

Fluids temporarily discontinued to administer blood components should be discarded and fresh solutions restarted after the transfusion is terminated.

Websites

Association of Professionals in Infection Control: *www.apic.org*

Other sites:

Fluid Overload and Pulmonary Edema

Overloading the circulatory system with excessive I.V. fluids causes increased blood pressure and central venous pressure. Circulatory overload is caused by infusing excessive amounts of isotonic or hypertonic crystalloid solutions too rapidly, failure to monitor the I.V. infusion, or too-rapid infusion of any fluid in a patient compromised by cardiopulmonary or renal disease.

Fluid overload can lead to pulmonary edema. Fluids infused too rapidly increase venous pressure and lead to pulmonary edema. Pulmonary edema is an abnormal accumulation of fluid in the lungs. In pulmonary edema, fluid leaks through the capillary wall and fills the interstitium and alveoli. "The pulmonary vascular bed has received more blood from the right ventricle than the left ventricle can accommodate and remove. The slightest imbalance between inflow on the right side and outflow on the left side may have drastic consequences" (Smeltzer & Bare, 2004).

Patients at risk for pulmonary edema are those with cardiovascular disease, those with renal disease, and elderly patients. It is important to identify patients at risk for pulmonary edema and provide nursing care that decreases the heart's workload. Sodium chloride given to correct profound sodium deficits can lead to pulmonary overload and must be monitored closely (Metheny, 2000).

Fluid overload and pulmonary edema are related to:

- Overzealous infusion of parenteral fluids, especially those that contain sodium
- Patients with compromised cardiovascular or renal systems

AGE-RELATED CONSIDERATIONS 9–2

The risk of fluid overload and subsequent pulmonary edema is especially increased in elderly patients with cardiac disease.

Signs and Symptoms

Signs and symptoms of circulatory overload include:

- Restlessness, headache
- Increase in pulse rate
- Weight gain over a short period of time
- Cough
- Presence of edema (eyes, dependent, over sternum)
- Hypertension
- Wide variance between intake and output
- Rise in central venous pressure (CVP)
- Shortness of breath and crackles in lungs
- Distended neck veins

As fluid builds in the pulmonary bed, later signs and symptoms include hypertension, severe dyspnea, gurgling respirations, coughing up frothy fluid, and moist crackles. If the condition is allowed to persist, congestive heart failure, shock, and cardiac arrest can result.

Prevention

Techniques used to prevent circulatory overload leading to pulmonary edema include:

1. Monitor the infusion, especially sodium chloride, and know the solution's physiologic effects on the circulatory system.
2. Maintain flow at prescribed rate.
3. Do not "catch up" on I.V. solutions that are behind schedule; instead, recalculate all infusions that are not on time.
4. Monitor the intake and output on all patients receiving I.V. fluids.
5. Know the patient's cardiovascular history.

Treatment

Consult the physician if you suspect circulatory overload.

1. Decrease the I.V. flow rate.
2. Place the patient in the high Fowler position.
3. Keep the patient warm to promote peripheral circulation.
4. Monitor vital signs.
5. Administer oxygen as ordered.
6. Consider changing the administration set to a microdrip set.

Documentation

Document patient assessment, notification of physician, and treatments instituted by physician order. Monitor the patient and record vital signs on an interval flow sheet.

Air Embolism

Air embolism is a rare but lethal complication, especially involving VADs. The problem is treatable with prompt recognition, but prevention is the key. The pathophysiologic consequences of air emboli are a result of air entering the central veins, which is quickly trapped in the blood as it flows forward. Trapped air is carried to the right ventricle, where it lodges against the pulmonary valve and blocks the flow of blood from the ventricle into the pulmonary arteries. Less blood is ejected from the right ventricle, and the right heart overfills. The force of right ventricular contractions increases in an attempt to eject blood past the occluding air pocket. These forceful contractions break small air bubbles loose from the air pocket. Minute air bubbles are subsequently pumped into the pulmonary circulation, causing even greater obstruction to the forward flow of blood as well as local pulmonary tissue hypoxia. Pulmonary hypoxia results in vasoconstriction in the lung tissue, which further increases the workload of the right ventricle and reduces blood flow out of the right heart. This leads to diminished cardiac output, shock, and death.

The same intrathoracic pressure changes that allow for pulmonary ventilation are responsible for air emboli associated with subclavian line removal. Pressure in the central veins decreases during inspiration and increases during expiration. If an opening into a central vein exposes the vessel to the atmosphere during the negative inspiratory cycle, air can be sucked into the central venous system in much the same manner that air is pulled into the lungs.

The causes of air embolism include:

- Allowing the solution container to run dry
- Superimposing a new I.V. bag to a line that has run dry without clearing the line of air
- Loose connections that allow air to enter the system
- Poor technique in dressing and tubing changes for central lines
- Presence of air in administration tubing cassettes of electronic infusion devices

Signs and Symptoms

Initial signs and symptoms of air embolism include:

- Patient complaints of palpitations
- Lightheadedness and weakness
- Pulmonary findings: dyspnea, cyanosis, tachypnea, expiratory wheezes, cough, and pulmonary edema
- Cardiovascular findings: "mill wheel" murmur; weak, thready pulse; tachycardia; substernal chest pain; hypotension; and jugular venous distention
- Neurologic findings: change in mental status, confusion, coma, anxiousness, and seizures

If untreated, these signs and symptoms lead to hemiplegia, aphasia, generalized seizures, coma, and cardiac arrest.

Prevention

Techniques used to prevent air embolism include:

1. Remove air from administration sets. To do so, wrap tubing around a pencil to force air bubbles upward into drip chamber infusing.
2. Vent air from port using a syringe attached to needleless system.
3. Use a 0.22-micron air-eliminating filter.
4. Follow the protocol for dressing and tubing changes of central lines.

5. Superimpose I.V. solutions before the previous solution runs completely dry.
6. Attach piggyback medications to the injection port closest to the drip chamber so that the check valve will prevent air from being drawn into the line after the infusion of medication.
7. Use Luer-Lok connectors whenever possible.
8. Do not bypass the "pump housing" of electric volumetric pumps.

Treatment

If you suspect an air embolus, do the following:

1. Call for help.
2. Place the patient in the Trendelenburg position on left side (left lateral decubitus position) with the head down. This causes the air to rise in the right atrium, preventing it from entering the pulmonary artery.
3. Administer oxygen.
4. Monitor vital signs.
5. Call for emergency equipment.
6. Notify the physician immediately.

NURSING FAST FACT!

A pathognomonic indicator of an air embolism is a loud, churning, drumlike sound audible over the precordium, called a "mill wheel murmur." This symptom may be absent or transient.

Documentation

Document patient assessment, nursing interventions to correct the cause of embolism if apparent, notification of physician, and treatment. If emergency treatment was necessary, use an interval flow sheet to document the management of the air embolism, record interval vital signs, and indicate patient response.

Speed Shock

Speed shock occurs when a foreign substance, usually a medication, is rapidly introduced into the circulation. Rapid injection permits the concentration of medication in the plasma to reach toxic proportions, flooding the organs rich in blood—the heart and the brain. Syncope, shock, and cardiac arrest may result.

Speed shock is related to administration of I.V. medications or solution at a rapid rate.

Signs and Symptoms

Signs and symptoms of speed shock include:

- Dizziness
- Facial flushing
- Headache
- Tightness in the chest
- Hypotension
- Irregular pulse
- Progression of shock

Prevention

Techniques used to prevent speed shock include:

1. Reduce the size of drops by using microdrop sets for medication delivery.
2. Use an electronic flow control with high-risk drugs.
3. Monitor the infusion rate for accuracy before piggybacking in the medication.
4. Be careful not to manipulate the catheter; cannula movement may speed up the flow rate.

NURSING FAST FACT!

Prevention of speed shock is the key. When giving I.V. push drugs, give slowly and according to the manufacturer's recommendations.

Treatment

If you suspect speed shock, do the following:

1. Get help.
2. Give an antidote or resuscitation medications as needed.
3. Have naloxone (Narcan) available on the unit if giving I.V. narcotics.

NOTE > See Chapter 11 for appropriate steps in delivery of I.V. push medications.

Documentation

Document the medication or fluid administered and the signs and symptoms the patient reported and those assessed. Also document the physician notification, the treatment initiated, and the patient response.

Catheter Embolism

Catheter embolism is an infrequent systemic complication of over-the-needle catheters. In this situation, a piece of the catheter breaks off and travels through the vascular system. It may migrate to the chest and lodge in the pulmonary artery or the right ventricle.

Catheter embolism is related to:

- Reinsertion of the same catheter that was used in an unsuccessful venipuncture
- Removing a stylet and reinserting it, shearing off the catheter tip
- Pressure directly over the catheter during discontinuation of therapy
- Placement of the catheter in a joint flexion

Signs and Symptoms

Signs and symptoms include:

- Sharp, sudden pain at the I.V. site
- Minimal blood return
- Rough and uneven catheter noted on removal
- Cyanosis
- Chest pain
- Tachycardia
- Hypotension

Pulmonary embolism, cardiac dysrhythmia, sepsis, endocarditis, thrombosis, and death may result if the catheter embolism migrates to the chest and lodges in the pulmonary artery or the right ventricle.

Prevention

Techniques used to prevent catheter embolism include:

1. Never reinsert a needle in a catheter (over-the-needle) after removal.
2. Avoid inserting the catheter over joint flexion when movement causes catheter to bend back and forth.
3. Splint the arm if the patient is restless.
4. Do not apply pressure over the site while removing a catheter.

NURSING FAST FACT!

Always use radiopaque catheters, so the catheter will be detectable on radiograph.

Be sure to assess the circulation of the extremity while the tourniquet is on the arm.

Treatment

If the patient is cooperative, have him or her apply digital pressure on the vein above the insertion site. This may prevent the catheter from migrating. Other techniques include:

1. Applying a tourniquet above the elbow
2. Contacting the physician and radiologist
3. Starting a new I.V. line
4. Preparing the patient for radiographic examination
5. Measuring the remainder of the catheter tip to determine the length of the embolized tip

Documentation

Document the patient's subjective complaints, using the patient's exact words and recording them in quotes. Document the discontinuation of the catheter, the technique used, and the length of catheter removed. State the nursing interventions and the time the physician was notified.

Erratic Flow Rates

There are many factors to consider in determining flow rate (Table 9–8). These include body size, fluid type, patient's age and condition, physiologic responses as reflected by urinary output, pulmonary status, and specific drugs being infused. The very young and the very old often need a slower rate of infusion and small volumes of solution. Patients with cardiac or renal diseases may also have problems tolerating large fluid volumes or fast rates. Situations in which flow rates have been poorly regulated can have serious consequences, especially with I.V. solutions containing medications such as epinephrine, theophylline, meperidine, lidocaine, sodium bicarbonate, amphotericin B, potassium chloride magnesium, and heparin (ECRI, 1994).

Accurate flow rate is imperative when a drug level must be kept constant. If the rate is too slow:

- The patient is not receiving the desired amount of drug or solution.
- It can lead to a clogged I.V. needle or catheter and perhaps the loss of a premium vein.

If the rate is too fast:

- Hypotonic solutions can lead to the development of pulmonary edema or congestive heart failure.
- Rapid infusion of hypertonic glucose can result in osmotic diuresis, leading to dehydration.
- Hypertonic solutions are also irritating and phlebitis can result.
- Free-flow administration of drugs can cause serious cardiovascular and respiratory complications.

NURSING FAST FACTS!

- *A fast rate is considered more dangerous than a rate that is too slow.*
- *In addition, notify the product evaluation committee or central services if cause of erratic flow is an electronic infusion device.*

Prevention

Measures to prevent erratic flow rates and the complications they cause include:

1. Allowing only experienced nurses to set up, adjust, or remove I.V. administration sets
2. Using pumps that provide free-flow protection; checking with each manufacturer
3. Properly closing clamps if removing administration set from pump
4. Checking or recalculating infusion rates
5. Providing or attending staff development education on electronic infusion devices
6. Reporting all free-flow incidents

Treatment

Treatment techniques for erratic flow rates include the following:

1. Stopping the flow and recalculating the drip rate
2. Treating the patient symptomatically
3. Consulting the physician
4. Recalculating the infusion rate

Table 9–9 presents a summary of the complications of peripheral I.V. therapy.

> Table 9–9 **COMPLICATIONS OF PERIPHERAL I.V. THERAPY**

Complication	Signs and Symptoms	Treatment	Prevention
		Local	
Hematoma	Ecchymoses Swelling Inability to advance catheter Resistance during flushing	Remove catheter if indicated Apply pressure with 2 × 2 inch gauze Elevate extremity	Use indirect method of venipuncture Apply tourniquet just before venipuncture
Thrombosis	Slowed or stopped infusion Fever and malaise Inability to flush device	Discontinue catheter Apply cold compresses to site Assess for circulatory impairment	Use pumps Choose microdrip sets with gravity flow if rate is below 50 mL/h Avoid flexion areas

(Continued on following page)

Complication	Signs and Symptoms	Treatment	Prevention
Phlebitis	Redness at site Site warm to touch Local swelling Palpable cord along vein Sluggish infusion rate	Discontinue catheter Apply cold compresses initially, then warm Consult physician if 3+	Use larger veins for hypertonic solutions Choose smallest I.V. cannula that is appropriate for infusion Good handwashing practices Add buffer to irritating solutions Change solution containers every 24 h Rotate infusion sites every 48 to 72 h
Infiltration (extravasation)	Coolness of skin around site Taut skin Dependent edema Backflow of blood absent Infusion rate slowing	Discontinue catheter Apply cool compresses Elevate extremity slightly Follow guidelines if extravasation occurs Have antidote chart available	Stabilize the catheter Place catheter in appropriate site Avoid antecubital fossa
Local infection	Redness and swelling at site Possible exudate of purulent material Increased WBC count Elevated temperature	Discontinue catheter and culture site and cannula Apply sterile dressing over site Administer antibiotics as ordered	Inspect all solutions Good technique during venipuncture and site maintenance
Venous spasm	Sharp pain at I.V. site Slowing of infusion	Apply warm compress to site with infusion still running Restart infusion if spasm continues	Dilute medications Keep I.V. solution at room temperature
Hypersensitivity reactions	Vary depending on reaction Rashes, itching, bronchial spasm, anaphylaxis	Stop infusion and keep I.V open with sodium chloride DO NOT use DC cannula Have emergency equipment available Administer drugs according to agency policy	Thorough history Verify allergies Proper patient identification

(Continued on following page)

> Table 9–9 **COMPLICATIONS OF PERIPHERAL I.V. THERAPY** *(Continued)*

Complication	Signs and Symptoms	Treatment	Prevention
		Systemic	
Septicemia	Fluctuating fever Profuse sweating Nausea and vomiting Diarrhea Abdominal pain Tachycardia Hypotension Altered mental status	Restart new I.V. system Obtain cultures Notify physician Initiate antimicrobial therapy ordered Monitor patient closely	Good handwashing technique Careful inspection of solutions Use Luer locks Cover infusion sites with sterile dressings Follow standards of practice related to rotation of sites and hang time of infusions Use iodine-based prepping solutions
Fluid overload	Weight gain Puffy eyelids Edema Hypertension Changes in I & O Rise in CVP Shortness of breath Crackles in lungs Distended neck veins	Decrease I.V. flow rate Place patient in high Fowler position Keep patient warm Monitor vital signs Administer oxygen as ordered Consider changing to microdrip set	Monitor infusion Maintain flow at prescribed rate Monitor I & O Know patient's cardiovascular history Do not "catch up" infusions; instead, recalibrate
Air embolism	Lightheadedness Dyspnea, cyanosis, tachypnea, expiratory wheezes, cough Mill wheel murmur, chest pain, hypotension Change in mental status, confusion coma, seizures	Call for help Place patient in Trendelenburg position Administer oxygen Monitor vital signs Notify physician	Remove all air from administration sets Use locks Attach piggyback
Speed shock	Dizziness Facial flushing Headache Tightness in chest Hypotension Irregular pulse Progession of shock	Get help Give antidote or resuscitation medications	Reduce the size of drops by using a microdrip set Use electronic infusion device Monitor infusion rate Dilute I.V. push medications if possible
Catheter embolism (Note: Use only radiopaque catheters)	Sharp sudden pain at I.V. site Rough, uneven catheter noted on removal Chest pain Tachycardia	Apply tourniquet above elbow Contact physician Start a new I.V. line Measure remainder of catheter	Do not apply pressure over site Never reinsert a stylet that has been removed from sheath Avoid joint flexions

CVP = central venous pressure; I & O = Intake and Output.

NURSING PLAN OF CARE

PREVENTION OF COMPLICATIONS

Focus Assessment

Subjective

Patient verbalizes discomfort at the I.V. site

Objective

- Assess infusion site for signs and symptoms including redness, swelling, exudate, tenderness, dressing integrity.
- Evaluate patient for anxiety or fear.
- Assess intake and output ratios.
- Assess cardiac and renal functions.
- Assess for age-related risks.
- Determine baseline weight.
- Assess vital signs, blood pressure, pulse, respirations, and temperature.

Patient Outcome/Evaluation Criteria

Patient will:

- Express fears related to infusion therapy.
- Remain free of complications related to the administration of I.V. therapy.
- Report any changes in comfort of I.V. site.
- Demonstrate care in maintaining the I.V. system.

Nursing Diagnoses

- Anxiety (mild, moderate, severe) related to threat to or change in health status; misconceptions regarding therapy
- Altered tissue perfusion (peripheral) related to infiltration of fluid or medication
- Decreased cardiac output related to sepsis contamination; infusion of isotonic or hypertonic fluids
- Fear related to insertion of catheter; fear of needles
- Hyperthermia related to increased metabolic rate, illness, dehydration
- Impaired gas exchange related to ventilation–perfusion imbalance; embolism
- Impaired skin integrity related to I.V. catheter, irritating I.V. fluids, inflammation, infection, infiltration
- Impaired tissue integrity related to altered circulation; fluid deficit or excess; irritating I.V. fluids; inflammation; infection; infiltration
- Impaired physical mobility related to pain or discomfort resulting from placement and maintenance of I.V. infusion
- Alteration in comfort, pain, related to physical trauma (e.g., catheter insertion)
- Risk of infection related to broken skin or traumatized tissue

(Continued on following page)

NURSING PLAN OF CARE

PREVENTION OF COMPLICATIONS *(Continued)*

Nursing Management

1. Maintain strict aseptic technique.
2. Examine the solution for type, amount, expiration date, character of the fluid, and lack of damage to container.
3. Select and prepare an electronic infusion device as indicated.
4. Administer fluids at room temperature.
5. Administer I.V. medications at prescribed rate and monitor for results.
6. Monitor I.V. for
   a. flow rate.
   b. infusion site.
   c. intake and output.
   d. serial weights.
7. Follow CDC hand hygiene procedures.
8. Replace the peripheral I.V. cannula, administration set, and dressing every 72 hours.
9. Maintain occlusive dressing.
10. Perform I.V. site checks and document at regular intervals.
11. Be aware of vesicant and irritating drugs and solutions that have a potential for tissue damage.
12. Radiographic studies are needed to determine the exact location of the catheter tip.

Patient Education

- Instruct the patient to perform routine activities: bathing, movement in bed, and ambulation to maintain I.V. system.
- Instruct the patient to report any signs or symptoms of common local complications (e.g., redness, swelling, pain at site).
- Instruct the patient to report any interruption in flow rate.
- Instruct the patient on the purpose of the electronic infusion device.

Home Care Issues

Home care practitioners must be aware of the potential danger that exists in I.V. drug administration and must be able to handle emergency situations. Adverse reactions, such as drowsiness, dizziness, nausea, diarrhea, and local and systemic complications, can occur with delivery of medications in the home setting.

(Continued on following page)

Allergic reactions from hypersensitivity to a specific antigen can also occur. An emergency kit, including epinephrine, diphenhydramine (Benadryl), and dexamethasone (Decadron) or hydrocortisone (Solu-Cortef), should be available to clinicians delivering medication in the home setting. The emergency kit should also include an airway, unused tubing, and additional catheters in the event that a new I.V. access must be established.

Potential problems and complications encountered in home infusion therapy include:

- Mechanical problems
- Nonrunning I.V. lines
- Inability to flush lines
- Malfunction of electronic infusion devices (EID)

Key Points

- After reading this chapter, you have increased your awareness about the risks to patients receiving I.V. therapy. Remember, you have observation skills to assess for local complications, as well as cognitive skills to assess for systemic complications.
- There are two divisions of complications, local and systemic.
- Local complications can become dangerous systemic adverse processes.
- Prevention is the best intervention for avoiding complications of infusion therapy.
- Key tips for preventing local complications:
  - Maintain INS guidelines regarding tubing change, cannula change, and length of time I.V. solutions remain hanging.
  - Follow aseptic technique in skin preparation and venipuncture techniques.
  - Follow CDC hand hygiene guidelines.
  - Choose appropriate dressings.
  - Secure tubing and cannula with good taping technique.
  - Use a 0.22-micron inline filter as an extra safeguard.
  - Keep solutions at the prescribed rate.
  - Document observed I.V. site every 4 hours for adults and every 2 hours for infants and children.
- Phlebitis (bacterial, chemical, or mechanical) is a frequently encountered problem associated with infusion therapy and can lead to cellulitis, thromboembolic complications, or sepsis.
- Key tips for preventing systemic complications:
  - Follow hand hygiene procedures.
  - Inspect solutions and equipment for breaks in integrity.

- Use Luer-Lok connectors.
- Limit the use of add-on devices.
- Maintain flow rates at the prescribed rate.
- Use a 0.22-micron filter when appropriate.
- Use electronic infusion devices.

Critical Thinking: Case Study

A 40-year-old woman with insulin-dependent diabetes mellitus is familiar with her disease, but does not take care of herself. She is currently admitted with an infected plantar ulcer and had a transmetatarsal amputation. She was discharged home on a regimen of I.V. antibiotics via a PICC, with home care follow-up.

What potential complications would the home care nurse be alert for? What documentation needs to be addressed at every visit?

What patient education needs to be reinforced at home?

Media Link: Answers to this critical thinking exercise and additional exercises are on the CD–ROM.

Post-Test

1. Which of the following are local complications associated with I.V. therapy?
   - **a.** Speed shock, septicemia, and venous spasm
   - **b.** Phlebitis, venous spasm, and hematoma
   - **c.** Septicemia, thrombophlebitis, and hematoma
   - **d.** Phlebitis, pulmonary edema, and speed shock
2. All of the following are ways to prevent the formation of a thrombosis **EXCEPT:**
   - **a.** Use of pumps or controllers for managing rate control
   - **b.** Avoid placing the cannula in areas of flexion
   - **c.** Use of needleless systems
   - **d.** Use of filters
3. A patient states that his I.V. site is sore. You assess the site and note redness and swelling but no signs of palpable cord or streak. Using the criteria for infusion phlebitis, what is the severity of this phlebitis?
   - **a.** 3+
   - **b.** 2+
   - **c.** 1+
   - **d.** 0

4. All of the following patients are at risk for developing phlebitis **EXCEPT:**
   a. Immunosuppressed patient
   b. Neonate
   c. Patient receiving antibiotics
   d. Patient receiving heparin

5. While a solution is infusing, which of the following is a treatment for venous spasm?
   a. Apply a cold pack to the site.
   b. Increase the flow rate of the solution.
   c. Apply a warm compress to the site.
   d. Administer pain medication.

6. An air embolism can be caused by:
   a. Severed I.V. line
   b. I.V. administration set that is improperly primed
   c. Bypassing the pump housing
   d. All of the above

7. You check an infusion site on a patient and find swelling and cool skin temperature. Also, the patient's skin appears blanched and feels rigid, and the infusion rate has slowed. These are signs of:
   a. Phlebitis
   b. Catheter embolus
   c. Hematoma
   d. Infiltration

8. You are performing a venipuncture and an ecchymosis forms over and around the insertion area, which has become raised and hardened. You are unable to advance the cannula into the vein. These are signs of:
   a. Phlebitis
   b. Infiltration
   c. Hematoma
   d. Occlusion

9. What is the one MOST important nursing intervention that is key to the prevention of many I.V.-related complications?
   a. Reading the policy and procedure manuals
   b. Hand hygiene procedures
   c. Using microdrip sets
   d. Competency testing

10. To prevent damage to the intima of the vein wall, which of the following syringe barrels should be used on a peripheral I.V. line?

  a. 1 mL or smaller

  b. 3 mL or smaller

  c. 3 mL or larger

  d. 10 mL or larger

References

Bagnall-Reeb, H. (1998). Diagnosis of central venous access device occlusion. *Journal of Intravenous Nursing,* 21(5S), 116–121.

Camp-Sorrell, D. (1998). Developing extravasation protocols and monitoring outcomes. *Journal of Intravenous Nursing,* 21(4), 232–241.

Chukhraev, A.M., & Grekov, I.G. (2000). Local complications of nursing interventions on peripheral veins. *Journal of Intravenous Nursing,* 23(3), 167–169.

Emergency Care Research Institute (ECRI) (2004). IV free flow still a cause for alarm. www.mdsr.ecri.org

Guyton, A.C., & Hall, J.C. (2001). *Textbook of Medical Physiology* (10th ed.). Philadelphia: W.B. Saunders.

Hadaway, L. (1998). Infiltration vs extravasation: Identification and interventions. Annual Conference, Intravenous Nurses Society, May, 1998.

Hadaway, L. (2002). I.V. infiltration: Not just a peripheral problem. *Nursing 2002,* 32(8), 36–42.

Hastings-Tolsma, M.T., Yucha, C.B., Tompkins, J., et al. (1993). Effect of warm and cold applications on the resolution of I.V. infiltration. *Research in Nursing & Health,* 16, 171–178.

Herbst, S., Kline, L., & McKinnon, B. (1998). Vascular access device: Managing occlusions and related complications in home infusion. *Infusion* 4 (8 Suppl), 1–32.

Intravenous Nursing Society (2000). *Revised Infusion Nursing Standards of Practice.* Philadelphia: Lippincott-Williams & Wilkins.

Jackson, D. (2001). Infection control principles and practices in the care and management of vascular access devices in the alternate care setting. *Journal of Intravenous Therapy,* 24(3S), S29–S34.

Joint Commission on Accreditation of Health Care Perspective (2002). Joint Commission perspectives: Interpretations: Limitations on hospital patient movement that constitute restraint. *Joint Commission on Accreditation of Health Care Organizations,* 2(7), 11–12, 15–16.

Maki, D.G., & Mermel, L.A. (1998). Infections due to infusion therapy. In Bennett, J.V., & Brachman, P.S. (eds.). *Hospital Infections* (3rd ed.) Philadelphia: Lippincott-Raven.

Maki, D.G., & Ringer, M. (1991). Risk factors for infusion-related phlebitis with small peripheral venous catheters. *Annals of Internal Medicine,* 114, 845–854.

Mayo, D.J. (2001). Catheter-related thrombosis. *Journal of Intravenous Therapy,* 24 (3S), S13–S21.

Mermel, L.A., Farr, B.M., & Sherertz, R.J. (2001). Guidelines for the management of intravascular catheter related infections. *Journal of Intravenous Nursing* 24(3), 180–201.

Metheny, N.M. (2000). *Fluid and Electrolyte Balance: Nursing Considerations* (4th ed.). Philadelphia: J.B. Lippincott.

Miserly, S. (2003). Extravasation injuries associated with the use of central vascular access devices. *Journal of Vascular Access Devices,* 8(1) 21–27.

Nightingale, F. (1859). *Notes on Nursing: What It Is, And What It Is Not.* London: Harrison, 59, Pall Mall, 59.

Perdue, M. (2000). Intravenous complications. In Hankins, J., Lonsway, R.A., Hedrick C., & Perdue, M. (eds.). *Infusion Therapy in Clinical Practice* (2nd ed.). The Infusion Nurses Society and Philadelphia: W. B. Saunders, pp. 418–446.

Skokal, W.A. (2001). Extravasation. *RN,* 64(9), 57.

Smeltzer, S.C., & Bare, B.G. (2004). *Brunner and Suddarth's Textbook of Medical-Surgical Nursing* (10th ed). Philadelphia: J.B. Lippincott.

U.S. Centers for Disease Control and Prevention (2002). *Guidelines for Prevention of Intravascular Infections.* Atlanta: US Department of Health and Human Services.

White, S.A. (2001). Peripheral intravenous therapy related phlebitis rates in an adult population. *Journal of Intravenous* Nursing 24(1), 19–24.

Answers to Chapter 9 Post-Test

1. **b**
2. **c**
3. **b**
4. **d**
5. **c**
6. **d**
7. **d**
8. **c**
9. **b**
10. **c**

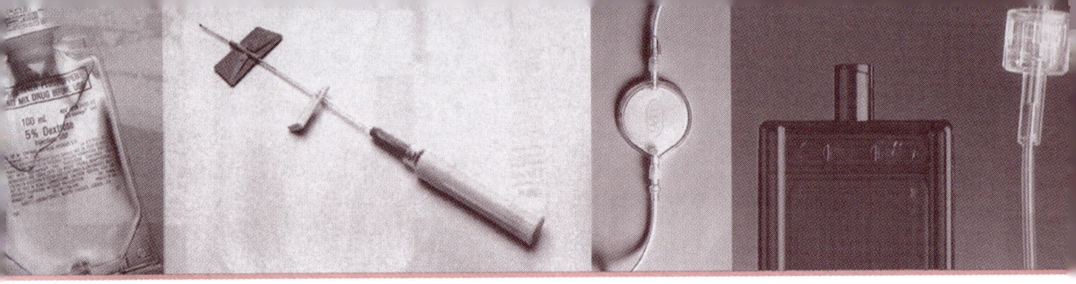

Chapter 10
Special Considerations Related to Intravenous Therapy: The Pediatric and Geriatric Populations

Children are not little adults.
—Virginia Turner, 1995

Chapter Contents

LEARNING OBJECTIVES

Upon completion of this chapter, the reader will be able to:

1. Describe terms related to delivery of infusion therapy to pediatric and geriatric patients.
2. Identify physiologic characteristics of neonates, infants, children, and geriatric patients related to their venous structure.
3. Locate common sites for venipuncture in pediatric and geriatric patients.
4. Identify common reasons for neonate and infant infusions.
5. List the formulas available for calculating the fluid needs of an infant.
6. Contrast the stages of development and fears through the life span as related to the performance of invasive procedures.
7. Identify the types of needles and catheters available for pediatric patients.
8. Describe special considerations for successful venipuncture of neonates, infants, and geriatric patients.
9. Describe the use of intraosseous infusions in pediatric patients.
10. Identify the complications related to intraosseous infusions.
11. List the risk factors associated with infusions in pediatric and geriatric patients.
12. Describe techniques for venipuncture in patients with sclerotic veins, alterations in skin integrity, obesity, and edema.

GLOSSARY

Body surface area Surface area of the body determined through use of a nomogram

Caloric method Calculation of metabolic expenditure of energy

Infant Child younger than age 2 years

Intraosseous infusion Infusion within the bone marrow cavity

Meter square method Use of a nomogram to determine surface areas of a patient
Neonate Infant in the period of extrauterine life up to the first 28 days after birth
Oncotic Tissue pressure within the tissue
Purpura Condition in which spontaneous bleeding occurs in the subcutaneous tissue, causing purple patches to appear on the skin
Tangential lighting Light touching a curve; indirect lighting
Weight method Formula based on weight in kilograms to estimate the fluid needs

Children, older adults, and persons with certain disorders can create challenges to the safe administration of I.V. therapy. Understanding these problems and ways to overcome them can help I.V. nurses ensure safe delivery with minimal risk to patients.

Pediatric I.V. Therapy

Intravenous therapy for pediatric patients requires special considerations to safeguard children. When assessing a child before administration, the practitioner must be aware of the body composition of an infant and the homeostatic differences between children and adults. In addition, the calculation of small doses, low infusion rates, and choice of appropriate venipuncture site and equipment need to be taken into consideration.

Physiologic Characteristics

A **neonate** is a child in the period of extrauterine life up to the first 28 days after birth. Low-birth-weight and premature infants have decreased energy stores and increased metabolic needs compared with those of full-term, average-weight newborns.

A premature infant's body is made up of approximately 90 percent water; the newborn infant's is 70 to 80 percent, and the adult's is about 60 percent. **Infants** have proportionately more water in the extracellular compartment than do adults. Therefore, any depletion in these water stores may lead to dehydration. As an infant becomes older, the ratio of extracellular to intracellular fluid volume decreases.

Although infants have relatively greater total body water content, this does not protect them from excessive fluid loss. Infants are more vulnerable to fluid volume deficit because they ingest and excrete a relatively greater daily volume of water than adults (Metheny, 2000). Any condition that interferes with normal water and electrolyte intake or that produces excessive water and electrolyte losses will produce a more rapid depletion of water and electrolyte stores in an infant than it will in an adult.

CULTURAL AND ETHNIC CONSIDERATIONS: NEWBORN INFANTS 10–1

Newborn body proportions differ among racial groups. It has been thought that newborn body proportions appear to be genetically programmed to conform to the pelvic shape of the mother (Giger & Davidhizar, 2004).

Illness, increased muscular activity, thermal stress, congenital abnormalities, and respiratory distress syndrome influence metabolic demands as well. The metabolic demand of an infant is two times higher per unit of weight than that of adults (Hockenberry, 2003).

In most cases, 100 to 120 cal/kg per day maintains a normal infant and provides sufficient calories for growth. For high-risk infants who require increased handling for procedures, the calorie requirement is up to 100 percent higher than that of a normal newborn. Heat production increases calorie expenditure by 7 percent per degree of temperature elevation. Infants and young children cannot store protein as well as adults; therefore, preventive nutritional support is needed.

Young children have immature homeostatic regulating mechanisms that need to be considered when water and electrolyte replacement is needed. Renal functioning, acid–base balance, body surface area differences, and electrolyte concentrations all must be taken into consideration when planning fluid needs.

Newborns' renal functions are not yet completely developed. Infants' kidneys appear to become mature by the end of the neonatal period. An infant's kidneys have a limited concentrating ability and require more water to excrete a given amount of solutes. Infants are less likely to be able to regulate fluid intake and output.

The buffering capacity to regulate acid–base balance is lower in newborns than in older children. Neonates, with an average pH of 7.0 to 7.38, are slightly more acidotic than adults. This base bicarbonate deficit is thought to be related to high metabolic acid production and to renal immaturity.

The integumentary system in neonates is an important route of fluid loss, especially in illness. This must be considered when determining fluid balance in infants and young children because their body surface area is greater than those of older children and adults. Any condition that produces a decrease in intake or output of water and electrolytes affects the body fluid stores of the infant. Because the gastrointestinal (GI) membranes are an extension of the body surface area, relatively greater losses occur from the GI tract in sick infants (Hockenberry, 2003).

Plasma electrolyte concentrations do not vary strikingly among infants, small children, and adults. The plasma sodium concentration changes little from birth to adulthood. The potassium and chloride concentrations are higher in the first few months of life than at any other time.

Magnesium and calcium levels are both low in the first 24 hours after birth. The serum phosphate level is elevated in the early months of infancy, which contributes to a low calcium level. Newborn infants are vulnerable to disrupted calcium homeostasis when stressed by illness or by an excess phosphate load and are at risk for hypocalcemia (Metheny, 2000). Table 10–1 provides normal laboratory values in newborns.

CULTURAL AND ETHNIC CONSIDERATIONS: DECISION MAKING 10–2

In many cultures, women can express an option regarding the care of a child; however, many others consider women to be subservient to men; and the men (e.g., the husband or the eldest son) make all decisions. Be sure to be sensitive to lines of communication.

> Table 10–1 **NORMAL LABORATORY VALUES FOR CHILDREN**

Laboratory Value	Neonate	Infant	2–5 years	6–12 years	Adolescent
Blood Count					
Red blood cells (million/μL)		2.7–5.4	4.27	4.31	4.60
Whole blood cells (per μL)		6000–17,000	5000–15,500	4500–13,500	4500–11,000
Platelet count (per μL)	84,000–479,000	150,000–400,000/mm all remaining ages <17 s			
Partial thromboplastin time and prothrombin time				18–22s	
Hemoglobin (g/dL)	14.5	9.0–14.0		11.5–15.5	Male 13–16 Female 12–16
Serum Electrolytes					
Sodium (mEq/L)		139–146	138–145		136–146
Potassium (mEq/L)		4.1–5.3		3.4–4.7	3.5–5.1
Magnesium (mEq/L)			1.4–1.9 … same for all ages		
Calcium (mg/dL)	7.5–11	8.8–10.8			8.4–10.8
Chloride (mEq/L)			98–106 … same for all ages		
Phosphorus (mg/dL)	4.0–10.5		5.0–7.8		

Physical Assessment

A physical assessment should be performed on pediatric patients before I.V. therapy is begun. Table 10–2 presents the components of a pediatric assessment.

Risk factors that must be considered during the assessment phase include prematurity, catabolic disease state, hypothermia, hyperthermia, metabolic or respiratory alkalosis or acidosis, and other metabolic derangements.

Candidates for neonatal I.V. therapy include those with:

- Congenital cardiac disorders
- GI defects
- Neurologic defects

Candidates for infant I.V. therapy include those with:

- Fluid volume deficit (dehydration)
- Electrolyte imbalance (diarrhea)
- Antibiotic therapy for treatment of serious infections
- Need for nutritional support for maintenance of growth and development
- Antineoplastic therapy for treatment of cancer

Assessment of Fluid Needs

There are three methods for assessment of 24-hour maintenance of fluids: meter square, caloric, and weight.

Meter Square Method

A nomogram is used to determine the body surface area (BSA) of the patient in the **meter square method**. To use a nomogram in this method, draw a straight line between the point representing the patient's height on

> Table 10–2 COMPONENTS OF THE PEDIATRIC PHYSICAL ASSESSMENT

Measurement of head circumference (up to 1 year)
Height or length
Weight
Vital signs
Skin turgor
Presence of tears
Moistness and color of mucous membranes
Urinary output
Characteristics of fontanelles
Level of child's activity related to growth and development

the left vertical scale to the point representing the patient's weight on the right vertical scale. The point at which the line intersects indicates the body surface area in square meters.

ADVANTAGES

- Provides calculation of body surface area to help determine the amount of fluid and electrolytes to be infused and assists with computing rate of infusion.
- Helps to calculate adult and pediatric dosages of I.V. medications.
- Is simple to calculate.

DISADVANTAGE

- Difficulty in accessibility to visual nomogram

To calculate the maintenance of fluid requirements, use the following:

$$\text{Formula: } 1500 \text{ mL/m}^2 \text{ per 24 hours}$$

Example: If child's surface area is 0.5 m^2, then 1500 mL $\times$ 0.5 m^2 = 750 mL/24 h.

Weight Method

The weight method uses the child's weight in kilograms to estimate fluid needs. This method uses 100 to 150 mL/kg for estimating maintenance fluid requirements and is most useful in children weighing less than 10 kg. (Use of the square meter method is recommended for children weighing more than 10 kg.)

ADVANTAGE

- Simple to use

DISADVANTAGE

- Inaccurate in children who weigh more than 10 kg

Example: For a child weighing 10 kg, 100 $\times$ 10 kg = 1000 mL in 24 hours.

Caloric Method

The caloric method calculates the usual metabolic expenditure of fluid. It is based on the following metabolic expenditure:

- Child weighing 0 to 10 kg expends approximately 100 cal/kg per day.
- Child weighing 10 to 20 kg expends approximately 1000 calories plus 50 cal/kg for each kilogram over 10 kg.
- Child weighing 20 kg or more expends approximately 1500 calories, plus 20 cal/kg for each kilogram over 20 kg.

ADVANTAGE

- Simple to calculate

DISADVANTAGE

- Not totally accurate unless actual calorie requirements and energy intake are continuously assessed

The formula for calculating fluid requirement is:

100 to 150 mL/100 calories metabolized

Example: If the weight of the child is 30 kg and the child expends 1700 cal/day, fluid requirement is 1700 to 2550 mL/24 h.

Factors Affecting Fluid Needs in Pediatric Patients

The most common cause of increased fluid and calorie needs in children is temperature elevation. An increase in temperature of 1 degree increases a child's calorie needs by 12 percent. Fluid requirements of a child who is hypothermic decrease by 12 percent (Hockenberry, 2003). In children, loss of GI fluids, ongoing diarrhea, and small intestinal drainage can seriously affect fluid balance.

NURSING FAST FACT!

To ensure accuracy in determining fluid needs, most pediatric patients should be on strict intake and output monitoring, including diaper weighing. When weighing an infant's diaper, consider the weight of the diaper before it was wet. The weight difference between a dry and a wet piece of linen represents the amount of liquid that it has absorbed. The weight of the fluid measured in grams is the same as the volume measured in milliliters (Hockenberry, 2003).

Site Selection

When selecting the venipuncture site, keep in mind that the main goal of I.V. therapy is to provide the treatment with safety and efficiency while meeting the child's emotional and developmental needs (Frey, 2001). Consider the following factors before selecting a site for venipuncture:

- Age of child
- Size of child
- Condition of veins
- Reason for therapy
- General patient condition
- Mobility and level of activity of child

- Gross and fine motor skills (e.g., sucks fingers, plays with hands, holds bottle, draws)
- Sense of body image
- Fear of mutilation
- Cognitive ability of the child (i.e., can understand and follow directions) (Frey, 2001)

Peripheral Routes

Peripheral routes for pediatric I.V. therapy include scalp veins and the veins in the dorsum of the hand, forearm, and foot (Fig. 10–1).

SCALP VEINS

The major superficial veins of the scalp can be used. Scalp veins can be used in children up to age 18 months; after that age, the hair follicles mature and the epidermis toughens. There are four scalp veins used most commonly for I.V. access: frontal (best access), preauricular, supraorbital, and occipital.

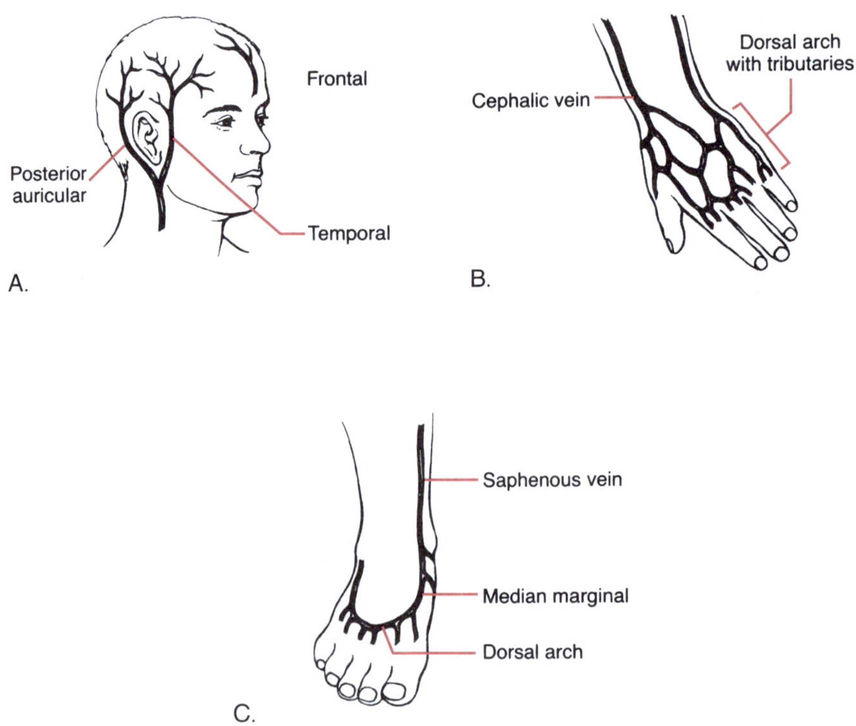

Figure 10–1 ■ Superficial veins of the scalp (*A*) and dorsum of hand (*B*) and foot (C). (From Kuhn, M.: *Pharmacotherapeutics: A Nursing Process Approach,* 4th ed. Philadelphia: F. A. Davis, with permission.)

NURSING FAST FACT!

The choice of a scalp vein for placement of I.V. therapy is often traumatic for the parents because removal of hair may have cultural as well as religious significance. In addition, maintaining patency of this site can be difficult at times.

ADVANTAGES

- Easily visualized
- Readily dilates because it has no valves
- Hands kept free
- Head easily stabilizes

DISADVANTAGES

- Need to shave hair
- Infiltrates easily
- Disfigurement with infiltration
- Difficult to secure device
- Increased family anxiety
- Cultural considerations

The I.V. needle must be placed in the direction of blood flow to ensure that the I.V. fluid will flow in the same direction as that of the blood returning to the heart. In the scalp, venous blood generally flows from the top of the head down.

NURSING FAST FACT!

A rubber band with a piece of tape attached can be used as a tourniquet (or pressure can be applied with the finger to distend the vein). Place the rubber band low on the forehead like a headband. It is also recommended that the rubber band be cut to decrease the chances of dislodging the I.V. after cannulation (Frey, 2001).

Shaving is not recommended; if necessary, clip the hair on infants.

CULTURAL AND ETHNIC CONSIDERATIONS: USING SCALP VEINS 10–3

People in the Hmong culture believe the spirit (soul) of the child can be released from the head. Be sure to check with an elder family member before choosing a site for venipuncture.

DORSUM OF THE HAND AND FOREARM

Because the veins over the metacarpal area are mobile and not well supported by surrounding tissue, the limb must be immobilized with a splint and tape before cannulation. This site can be used in children of all ages.

The antecubital fossa should not be routinely used because of the use of the antecubital area for blood drawing and the mobility problems resulting from use of this site. However, the antecubital area can be used for placement of peripherally inserted central catheters (PICCs).

ADVANTAGES

- Easily accessible
- Readily visible
- Large enough for a larger-gauge cannula
- Bones act as natural splints.

DISADVANTAGES

- Increased nerve endings
- Difficult to anchor cannula on infant
- Interferes with child's activity

DORSUM OF THE FOOT

The foot is used as a venipuncture site for infants and toddlers but should be avoided in children who are walking. The curve of the foot, especially around the ankle, makes entry and cannula advancement difficult. The veins used are the saphenous, median, and marginal dorsal arch. Because neonates have very little subcutaneous adipose tissue, the veins are easily identified and cannulated just beneath the skin.

NURSING FAST FACT!

The foot should be secured on a padded board with a normal joint position.

ADVANTAGES

- Readily dilates
- Hands kept free
- Less rolling of vein
- Increased visibility in chubby infants
- Easy to splint

DISADVANTAGES

- Decreased mobility in walking
- Limited to smaller-gauge cannulas
- Located near arteries
- Difficult to advance cannula

Selecting the Equipment

A nurse must be aware of the special needs of pediatric patients when selecting appropriate equipment for administering fluids and medication. When choosing administration equipment, the safety of the child requires that the activity level, age, and size of the patient be considered. For safe delivery of I.V. therapy in pediatric patients, the following equipment is recommended:

- An electronic infusion device for administration of therapy
- A solution container with a volume based on the age, height, and weight of the patient containing no more than 500 mL of fluid (preferably 250 mL)
- Special pediatric equipment, such as volume control chamber for the delivery of therapy.
- Plastic fluid containers (preferable to glass because of possible breakage)
- Microdrip tubing (60 gtt/min)
- Visible cannula site
- A 0.2-micron air-eliminating filter set (Fig. 10–2) is available for neonates and infants to provide 96-hour bacterial and associated endotoxin retention for patient protection.

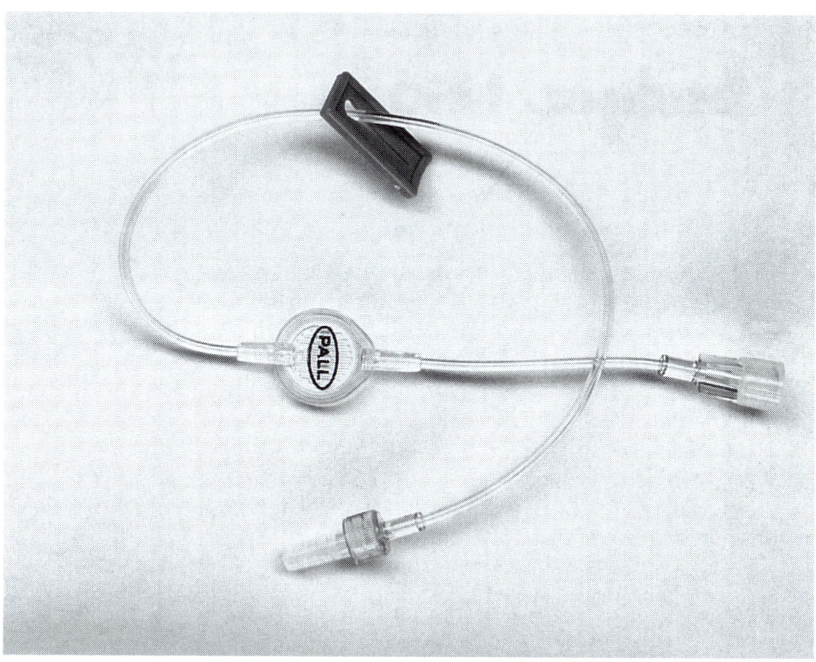

Figure 10–2 ■ Neonatal and infant 0.2-micron air-eliminating filter set. (Courtesy of Pall Corporation, Port Washington, NY.)

It is necessary to monitor at least every 2 hours and more frequently, depending on patient's age and size or type of therapy.

Needle Selection

The choice of needle depends on the site selected. Peripheral cannulas, gauges 26 to 21, can be used in children. A 27- to 19-gauge scalp vein (butterfly) needle is easy to insert but has the risk of infiltrating easily. Over-the-needle catheters, 26- to 14-gauge, are now used more frequently than metal needles. For neonates, 26- to 24-gauge needles are used; for children, 24- to 22-gauge are most common. Over-the-needle cannulas usually last longer than scalp vein needles. These catheters are also easier to stabilize.

Venipuncture Techniques

The methods for venipuncture are the same for children as for adults (see Chapter 7); a direct or indirect method can be used. Keep in mind the following safety guidelines when setting up an I.V. for a child.

- A child's I.V. container should contain no more than 500 mL of I.V. fluid. A 250 mL solution container should be used for children younger than age 12 months.
- Obtain a volume control chamber. Connect it to the infusion container.
- Fill the cylinder with enough fluid to prime the tubing plus fluid for a *maximum* of 2 hours.

Tips

The following tips on technique are unique to pediatric patients:

1. Venipuncture should be performed in a room separate from the child's room. The child's room is his or her "safe space."
2. Use a pacifier for neonates and infants.
3. Use mummy and clove-hitch immobilizers as needed. Infants should be covered with a blanket to minimize cold stress. If the dorsum of the hand is used, place the extremity on an armboard before venipuncture.
4. A flashlight or transilluminator device placed beneath the extremity helps to illuminate tissue surrounding the vein; the veins are then outlined for better visualization (Frey, 2001).
5. Warm hands by washing them in hot water before gloving.
6. Omit tourniquet use if possible. Use a rubber band to dilate scalp veins.
7. Use a saline-filled syringe with a scalp vein infusion device.
8. Minimizing pain during venipuncture is a goal of nursing care.

Two commonly used methods are the use of a topical cream (EMLA or Numby Stuff) or ethyl chloride spray (an assistant is needed to spray).

9. Flush the needle immediately with saline if a backflow of blood occurs.
10. Use surgical lubricating jelly to help secure the tape around a scalp I.V. by applying a small amount under the tape.
11. Use only hypoallergenic or paper tape. When you are ready to remove the tape, apply warm water; the tape will then lift off easily (Frey, 2001).
12. Stabilize the cannula with a padded tongue blade. Collect laboratory specimens at the time of I.V. insertion.
13. Use colored stickers or drawings on the I.V. site as a reward.
14. Always have extra help.

INS Standard. The site selected should be readily visible and roller bandages should never be used around the cannula site. (INS, 2000, 49)

NURSING FAST FACTS!

- *When securing a child's extremity to an armboard, use clear tape for visualization of the I.V. site and digits or skin immediately adjacent to the site.*
- *Use of a paper cup to cover the infusion site on the scalp is not recommended. A clear medicine cup can offer the needed protection.*

Stabilizing and maintaining the patency of I.V. cannula sites can be a challenge. Poorly secured I.V. access sites may result in dislodgements or infiltrations requiring I.V. restarts. Products are available to help stabilize pediatric I.V.s, while maintaining visualization. The I.V. House (Progressive IVs, Inc.) is a clear, one-piece unit that protects any I.V. site (Figs. 10–3 and 10–4).

For children, illness and hospitalization constitute major life crises. Children are vulnerable to the crises of illness and hospitalization because stress represents a change from the usual state of health and environmental routine and because children have a limited number of coping mechanisms to resolve the stressful events.

Children's understanding of, reaction to, and methods of coping with illness or hospitalization are influenced by the significance of individual stressors during each developmental phase. The major stressors are separation, loss of control, and bodily injury. Table 10–3 summarizes the principal behavioral responses to each stressor as related to the function of I.V. therapy.

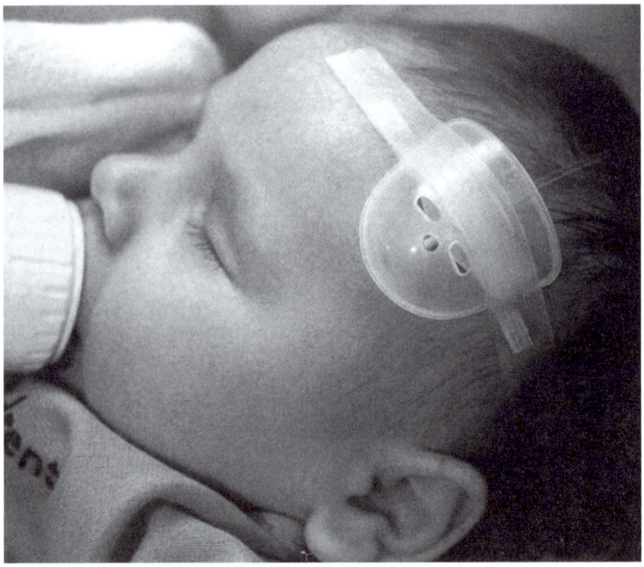

Figure 10–3 ■ Site protector for scalp vein catheter. (Courtesy I.V. House, Inc., Hazelwood, MO.)

Medication Administration

Delivering medication to children requires that the nurse have expert knowledge of the techniques for the delivery of medication and for the calculation of formulas. The most common methods of calculation are covered in the beginning of this chapter: body weight and body surface area are most frequently used. Dosages of pediatric medications are usually recommended in terms of body weight. The dose and volume can be different in children, and drugs are frequently calculated to the tenth of a milligram or milliliter (Frey, 2000).

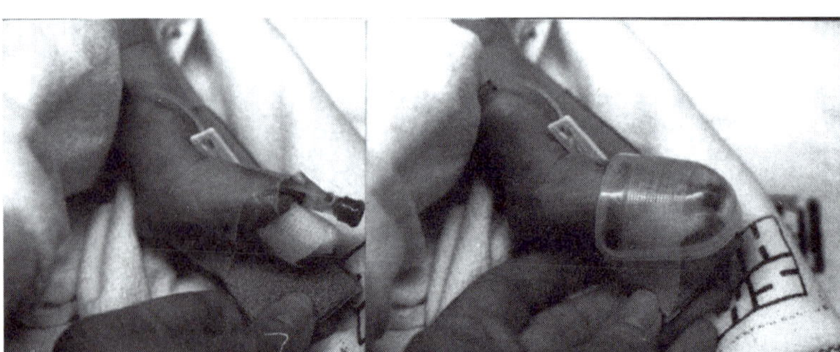

Figure 10–4 ■ I.V. site protector for neonate's foot catheter. (Courtesy I.V. House, Inc., Hazelwood, MO.)

> Table 10–3 **NURSING INTERVENTIONS FOR THE CHILD REQUIRING I.V. THERAPY AS RELATED TO PHYSICAL AND PSYCHOLOGICAL DEVELOPMENT**

Age	Development/ Stressor	Behavior	Intervention
Infant	Trust versus mistrust *Stressor:* Pain	Cries, screams, clings in protest Neonate: easily distracted—total body reaction Infant: localized reaction; often uncooperative	Consistency in assigning caregivers Encourage parents to assist with care Explain I.V. to parents Have assistance starting I.V.
Toddler	Autonomy versus shame and doubt *Stressor:* Loss of control Physical restriction Loss of routine and rituals Bodily injury and pain	Protests verbally Cries for parents Kicks, bites, tries to escape to find parents Resists Verbally uncooperative	Allow to express feelings Encourage parental help Allow as much mobility as possible in securing I.V. Encourage presence of favorite toy or blanket during procedure Use comfort after procedure
Preschool	Initiative versus guilt *Stressor:* Loss of control Sense of own power Bodily injury—intrusive procedure, mutilations	Protests less directly Anxiety, guilt, shame, physiologic responses Immature behavior	Allow child to express protest Provide play and diversional activity Encourage to play out feelings and fears Allow as much mobility as possible; limit invasive procedures Explain procedure in simple terms; start pretend I.V. on doll
School-age	Industry versus inferiority *Stressor:* Loss of control Enforced dependency Altered family roles Bodily injury and pain Illness and death—intrusive procedures in genital area	Loneliness, boredom, isolation, hostility, and frustration Depression and displaced anger Seeks information Passively accepts Communicates about pain	Allow to express feelings both verbally and nonverbally Involve in starting I.V. by tearing tape or holding tubing Encourage peer contacts Use diversional activities
Adolescent	Identity versus role diffusion *Stressor:* Loss of control Loss of identity Enforced dependency Bodily injury and mutilation	Rejection Uncooperativeness Self-assertion Overconfidence Boredom	Explore feelings regarding hospitalization Help to adjust to authority Explain all procedures Allow choices in sites Provide privacy

Source: *From Wong, D.L. (2003). Whaley and Wong's Essentials of Pediatric Nursing, (7th ed). St. Louis: Mosby, Inc. Reprinted with permission.*

Most infusion complications in pediatric patients are attributed to dosing, fluid administration, or both. A nurse administering infusion therapy to pediatric patients must possess the knowledge necessary to verify, calculate, administer, and accurately control the rate of the prescribed therapy.

INS Standard. Consideration should be given to the use of smaller volume containers in infants and premature infants because of complications of fluid volume overload and special pediatric equipment for the delivery of therapy. (INS, 2000, 2)

Prevention strategies for delivering medication to children include:

- Purchase and use only scales that measure weight in kilograms.
- Have a method (flow sheets) of documenting weight changes. Include weight changes in shift reports.
- Perform annual checks of competency in weighing children, using scales on the unit.
- Collaborate with biomedical engineers regarding the frequency of quality assurance and calibration checks of scales.
- Require nurses to verify accuracy in dose recommendations and calculations on original drug and I.V. fluid prescription forms.
- Have available a current medication manual that provides necessary information for safe administration of I.V. medications.
- Develop charts of frequently used drugs that provide practical information of medication concentrations, drug dosing, and administration requirements.

Intermittent Infusions

The inline calibrated chamber is commonly used in the general pediatric setting. The medication is injected into the inline chamber and infused at a prescribed rate.

ADVANTAGE

- Simplicity

DISADVANTAGES

- Not practical for small infants
- Necessity of drug compatibility with primary solution or requirement of a second tubing setup
- Flushing of the chamber with a certain volume is insufficient to clear the chamber of medication.

Retrograde Infusion

Retrograde infusion is used in the general pediatric area and neonatal intensive care units and often in infants or children who cannot tolerate rapid infusion rates or additional fluid volume. A specific retrograde administration set is required for this purpose. The tubing volume varies but generally holds less than 1 mL. A three-way stopcock or access port is at each end of the tubing. To use retrograde infusion, follow these steps:

1. Attach the retrograde tubing and prime along with the primary administration set. The tubing functions as an extension set when it is not used to administer medication.
2. To administer the medication, attach a medication-filled syringe to the port proximal to the patient and connect an empty syringe to the port most distal from the patient.
3. Make sure the clamp between the port and the child is closed and then inject the medication distally up the tubing. The fluid in the retrograde tubing is displaced upward into the tubing and the empty syringe.
4. Remove both syringes and open the lower clamp. The medication is then infused into the patient at the prescribed rate.

Syringe Pump

Using syringe pumps is an increasingly popular and accurate method of delivery of I.V. medications in children. They can be connected by an extension set into a primary line. (See Chapter 6 for information on syringe pumps.)

NURSING FAST FACT!

Parenteral nutrition and transfusion therapy are also frequently administered to the pediatric client; special considerations for the delivery of blood products and parenteral nutrition are discussed in Chapters 13 and 15.

Formulas for Delivery of Pediatric Therapies

The following are formulas used in calculating the delivery of pediatric therapies.

Body Weight

Doses of drugs based on kilograms of body weight require that nurses use the weight (in kg) of the child in dosage administration (1 kg = 2.2 lb). Many drugs are ordered as milligram per kilogram of body weight. Multiply the milligrams of the drug by the kilograms of body weight.

$$\text{mg of drug} \times \text{kg of child's body weight} = \text{Child's dose}$$

Body Surface Area (BSA)

Doses of drugs based on BSA are determined by multiplying the child's BSA (m^2) times the recommended adult dose, divided by the adult's BSA (1.73 m^2).

$$\frac{\text{BSA of child } (m^2) \times \text{Recommended adult dose}}{\text{BSA of adult } (1.73\ m^2)} = \text{Child's dose}$$

Bastedo's Rule

This rule determines the child's dose based on the child's age plus 3, times the average adult dose, divided by 30.

$$\frac{\text{Age (years)} + 3 \text{ x Average adult dose}}{30} = \text{Child's dose}$$

Clark's Rule

This rule determines the child's dose based on the child's weight in relation to the average adult body weight and dose.

$$\frac{\text{Weight (lb)} \times \text{Average adult dose}}{(\text{Average adult weight} = 150 \text{ lb})} = \text{Child's dose}$$

Cowling's Rule

This rule determines the child's dose based on the child's age and the average adult dose, divided by 24.

$$\frac{\text{Age (years on next birthday)} \times \text{Average adult dose}}{24} = \text{Child's dose}$$

Fried's Rule

This rule determines the infant's dose based on the infant's age in relation to the average adult body weight and dose.

NURSING FAST FACTS!

- *Fried's Rule is effective only for infants younger than 1 year of age.*
- *Using a calculator is advisable for all pediatric doses; always double-check calculations with another licensed nurse (Buchholz, 2003).*

Young's Rule

This rule determines the child's dose based on the child's age and average adult dose, divided by the child's age plus 12.

$$\frac{\text{Age in years x Average adult dose}}{\text{Age (in years)} + 12} = \text{Child's dose}$$

Alternative Administration Routes

Alternative routes for administration of I.V. therapy in pediatric patients are intraosseous and umbilical veins and arteries.

Intraosseous Route

The intraosseous route is a safe alternative for fluid and drug administration in infants and children. From 1940 to 1950, the **intraosseous infusion** for both adults and children was widely used. By the late 1950s, it was replaced by plastic catheters and newer infusion techniques.

The American College of Surgeons (1999) provides guidelines for emergency vascular access in children. Intraosseous infusion is recognized as an effective route for the administration of emergency medications or fluids to children age 6 years or younger. These guidelines further emphasize the importance of establishing and maintaining an infusion route during the resuscitation of critically ill children.

This method of access does not replace conventional methods of venous access. Instead, the intraosseous route provides immediate vascular access in emergency situations when access by the I.V. route is unattainable (usually after 5 minutes of attempts), and fluid and medication administration is essential to sustain life.

Intraosseous infusion uses the rich vascular network of the long bones to transport fluids and medications from the medullary cavity to the circulation. The medullary cavity is composed of a spongy network of venous sinusoids that drain into a central venous canal. Blood exits the venous canal by the nutrient and emissary veins into the circulation. Fluids infused into the medullary space diffuse a short space and then are absorbed into the venous circulation; the distribution is similar to that in I.V. injection (Smith, 1998) (Fig. 10–5).

ADVANTAGES

- Provides quick access in emergency cases when life-sustaining medication must be administered.
- In patients with difficult venous access, provides alternative access for delivery of volume resuscitation.
- Useful in patients with cardiac arrest, shock, trauma, or any situation in which the potential benefits of rapid venous access outweigh the low incidence of complications.

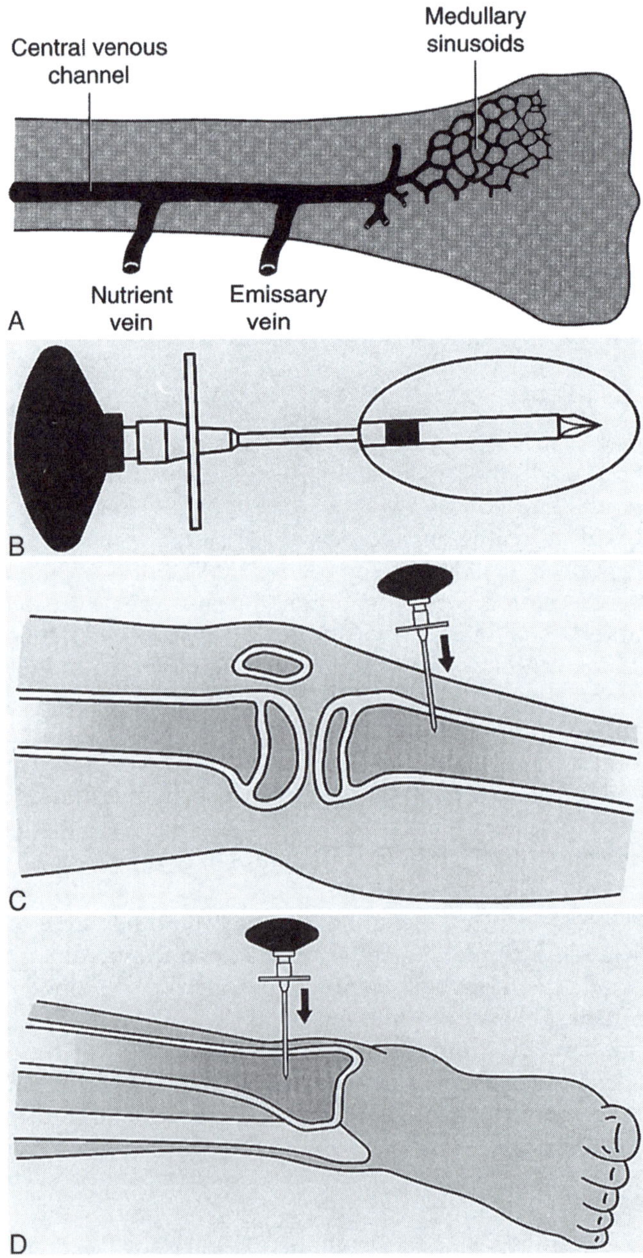

Figure 10–5 ■ Intraosseous infusion. (*A*) Intramedullary venous system. (From Spivey, W.H., [1987]. Intraosseous infusions. *Journal of Pediatrics 111*, 639. Used with permission.) (*B*) Intraosseous needle, (*C*) placement of intraosseous needle in proximal tibia, (*D*) placement of intraosseous needle in distal tibia. (Courtesy of Cook Critical Care. Ellettsville, IN.)

DISADVANTAGES

- Potential for compartment syndrome
- Potential for osteomyelitis (low incidence reported)
- Potential for cellulitis; however, studies have reported only a 0.6 percent incidence of cellulitis
- Potential damage to the epiphyseal plate
- Potential embolus caused by fat dislodged from the marrow cavity

Intraosseous needles shall be removed within 6 hours (American College of Surgeons, 1999).

INS Standard. Intraosseous ports are removed within 30 days or immediately if complications develop. (INS, 2000, 68)

CONTRAINDICATIONS

Patients who have areas of cellulitis or infected burns or those with recently fractured bones should not undergo intraosseous infusion. Patients with osteogenesis imperfecta or osteoporosis are not good candidates for this route.

Umbilical Vein and Arteries

There are three vessels in the umbilical cord: one vein and two arteries. These vessels provide alternative routes for vascular access in neonates. These routes are reserved for emergency access in the delivery room and for hemodynamic monitoring in the neonatal intensive care unit.

The goals of arterial catheterization are different from those of venous catheterization. The main goals of arterial umbilical catheterization are:

- Monitoring arterial pressure
- Obtaining blood samples for arterial pH and blood gases
- Performing aortography
- Performing exchange transfusions

The vein of the umbilicus can be catheterized at up to 4 days of life. However, it is usually inserted in the delivery room in a compromised infant. The goals of venous catheterization include:

- Administering emergency medications and fluids
- Obtaining venous blood sampling
- Performing exchange transfusion (Frey, 2001)

Umbilical catheterization carries a risk of vascular compromise, hemorrhage, air embolism, infection, thrombosis, and vascular perforation. The risk of infection is greater with the venous catheter and becomes a significant risk after 24 hours. The umbilical venous catheter is removed as soon as an alternative access route has been established (usually within 48 to 72 hours).

Websites

Society of Pediatric Nurses: *www.pednurse.org*
American Academy of Pediatrics: *www.aap.org*
Intravenous Nurses Society: *www.ins1.org*
Transcultural Nursing Society: *www.tcns.org*

Other sites:

Geriatric I.V. Therapy

According to the National Center for Health Statistics, life expectancy has risen dramatically over the past century. According to the data from the National Vital Statistics System (2000), in 1998 a 75-year-old man could be expected to live until the age of 85, and a 75-year-old woman could be expected to live until the age of 87. By 2030, people older than 65 years of age will account for 22 percent of the population, compared with 13 percent in 2001. Health practitioners need a heightened awareness and understanding of the special care needs of elderly clients.

Physiologic Changes

Aging occurs on all levels of bodily function: cellular, organic, and systemic. "Loss of cells and loss of physiologic reserve make up the dominant processes of aging" (Smeltzer & Bare, 2004). The major system changes the nurse must be aware of related to infusion therapy are homeostatic changes, immune system and cardiovascular changes, and skin and connective tissue changes.

Homeostasis is the body's ability to maintain a stable internal environment. As a person ages, his or her homeostatic mechanism become less efficient, and reserve power is lost. For example, when external stressors such as trauma or infection occur, there is minimal reserve capacity. This creates a situation in which the person is more vulnerable to disease.

Two immune processes change with aging:

1. The immune system becomes hyporesponsive to foreign antigens (e.g., decreased numbers of circulating lymphocytes and cells have fewer receptors to decrease ability to generate energy).
2. The immune system becomes hyperresponsive to itself.

Cardiovascular changes related to arteriosclerosis become clinically recognizable. With aging, three functions of the heart are affected: (1) the ability to oxygenate the cardiac muscle decreases, (2) diastolic filling decreases, and (3) left ventricular wall thickness increases. Arteries show progressive chemical and anatomic changes, with an increase in cholesterol, other lipids, and calcium. The intima increases, which increases resistance and decreases compliance of veins and arteries. The elastic fibers progressively straighten, fray, split, and fragment. There is an increase in density and amount of collagen fibers in the vessel walls, along with decreasing elasticity of these walls.

The skin is one of the first systems to show signs of the aging process. The epidermis and dermis are visible markers of aging and greatly affect the placement of peripheral catheters. As a person ages, a loss of subcutaneous supporting tissue and resultant thinning of the skin occur. The turnover rate for the production of new cells slows: at the age of 20 years, turnover of new cells takes 3 weeks; at age 30 years, 6 weeks; and after age 30 years, 2 months. Folds, lines, wrinkles, and slackness appear as the skin ages. **Purpura** and ecchymoses may appear owing to the greater fragility of the dermal and subcutaneous vessels and the loss of support for the skin capillaries. Minor trauma can easily cause bruising.

A common symptom in older people is pruritus or "itchiness." This is usually caused by dry skin and by medications and should be considered when preparing the patient for parenteral therapy.

NURSING FAST FACT!

Alcohol as a preparatory aid will add to the drying effect on the skin.

The dermis becomes relatively dehydrated and loses strength and elasticity. This layer has underlying papillae that hold the epidermis and dermis together; this means that as one ages, the older skin loosens. Older skin has decreased flexibility in the collagen fibers, increased fragility of the capillaries, and fewer capillaries. Older skin feels dryer because of loss of subcutaneous fat and decreased production of sebum and sweat (Smeltzer & Bare, 2004).

Fluid Balance in Elderly Persons

Fluid balance in elderly persons is affected by the physiologic changes associated with aging. Older people do not possess the fluid reserves of younger individuals or the ability to adapt readily to rapid changes. Alterations in fluid and electrolyte balance frequently accompany illness.

Renal structural changes associated with the aging process result in a decreased glomerular filtration rate. When fluid is restricted for any reason, nurses must be aware that there will be a slower conservation of fluids in response to the fluid restriction.

The total body water is reduced by 6 percent, which creates a potential for fluid volume deficit. GI changes such as decreased volumes of saliva and gastric juice as well as decreased calcium absorption cause the mouth to be drier in the aged, in addition to the potential for sodium and potassium deficit during episodes of vomiting and gastric suction, and calcium deficit.

Cardiovascular and respiratory changes combine to contribute to a slower response to the stress of blood loss, fluid depletion, shock, and acid–base imbalances (Metheny, 2000). Elderly patients should be assessed for potential fluid volume disturbances (Table 10–4).

Careful assessment and monitoring of elderly patients for complications related to infusion therapy can help avoid systemic complications. Monitor electrolyte, blood urea nitrogen (BUN), and creatinine levels throughout therapy. Assess regularly signs and symptoms of fluid overload: distended neck veins, full bounding pulse, elevated blood pressure, and moist crackles. Weigh the patient daily (Powers, 1999).

NURSING FAST FACT!

Dextrose administered without a pump to elderly patients can lead to cerebral edema more rapidly than in younger patients.

Many elderly patients take digoxin for cardiac problems. Be careful with administering to elderly patients over a lengthy period of time fluids that do not contain potassium. Hypokalemia can potentiate the action of digitalis glycosides, causing toxicity.

> Table 10–4 **ASSESSMENT GUIDELINES FOR FLUID VOLUME DISTURBANCES IN THE ELDERLY**

Skin turgor of forehead or sternum
Temperature (normal body temperature often below 98.6°F)
Rate and filling of veins in hand or foot
Daily weight possibly a more accurate measure of patient's fluid balance
Intake and output
Tongue—center should be moist, with observable pool of saliva beneath the tongue (even though the aged have decreased saliva, this method is useful in evaluating hydration)
Orthostatic (postural) blood pressure changes
Swallowing ability
Functional assessment of patient's ability to obtain fluids

Venipuncture Techniques

Special venipuncture techniques are required to successfully place and maintain I.V. therapy in elderly patients. The potential complications associated with trauma, surgery, and illness in elderly people, along with the physiologic changes mentioned previously, require that nurses be knowledgeable in the special skills associated with delivery of care.

> **INS Standard.** Geriatric patients may be at greater risk for potential complications related to infusion therapy and may require more frequent monitoring. (INS, 2000, 3)

Vascular Access Device Selection

Consider the skin and vein changes of older adults before initiating I.V. therapies. Also, consider catheter design and gauge size. Softer, more flexible materials and those that soften after insertion into the vein may allow increased indwelling time and prevent or reduce complications. The bevel-tip design of the peripheral catheter's needle may help to decrease trauma to vein.

NURSING FAST FACT!

To reduce insertion-related trauma use a 22- to 24-gauge catheter.

Selecting Administration Equipment

Because of the risk of over-administration or under-administration of I.V. therapy, the type of infusion equipment selected should provide safe, consistent delivery of medication and fluids. Advanced technology provides uses of stationary and ambulatory electronic monitoring devices. Monitoring devices must have safety features to protect high-risk patients from fluid volume overload.

NURSING FAST FACT!

To prevent fluid overload, use a microdrip administration set when appropriate. Because of the fragile nature of the veins of elderly patients, be aware of the potential complications associated with pressures generated from mechanical infusion devices (see Chapter 6 for a discussion of safety features associated with programmable pumps).

Selecting a Vein

Selecting a vein that can support I.V. therapy for at least 72 hours can be a challenge for nurses. Initial venipuncture should be in the most distal portion of the extremity, allowing for subsequent venipunctures to move progressively upward. However, in older adults, the veins of the hands may not be the best choice for the initial site because of the loss of subcutaneous fat and thinning of the skin. Physiologic changes in the skin and veins must be considered when a site is selected. Areas for I.V. access should have adequate tissue and skeletal support. Avoid flexion areas and areas with bruising because the oncotic pressure is increased in these areas and causes vessels to collapse.

NURSING FAST FACT!

To enhance vein location, use adequate lighting. Bright, direct overhead examination lights may have a "washout" effect on veins. Instead, use side lighting, which can add contour and "shadowing" to highlight the skin color and texture and allow visualization of the vein shadow below the skin.

Use a tourniquet to help distend and locate appropriate veins, but avoid applying it too tightly because it can cause vein damage when the vein is punctured. During venous distention, palpate the vein to determine its condition. Veins that feel ribbed or rippled may distend readily when a tourniquet is applied, but these sites are often impossible to access, causing pain for the patient.

NURSING FAST FACTS!

- *Place a tourniquet over a gown or sleeve to decrease the sheering force on fragile skin (Walther, 2000).*
- *To thread a catheter through an inflexible valve, reduce the catheter size by several gauges.*

Valves become stiff and less effective with age. Bumps along the vein path (i.e., valves) may cause problems during attempts at vein access. Venous circulation may be sluggish, resulting in slow venous return, distention, venous stasis, and dependent edema. A catheter may not thread into a vein with stiff valves.

Small surface veins appear as thin tortuous veins with many bifurcations (Fig. 10–6). Appropriate catheter gauge and length selection is critical to successful I.V. access placement in these veins.

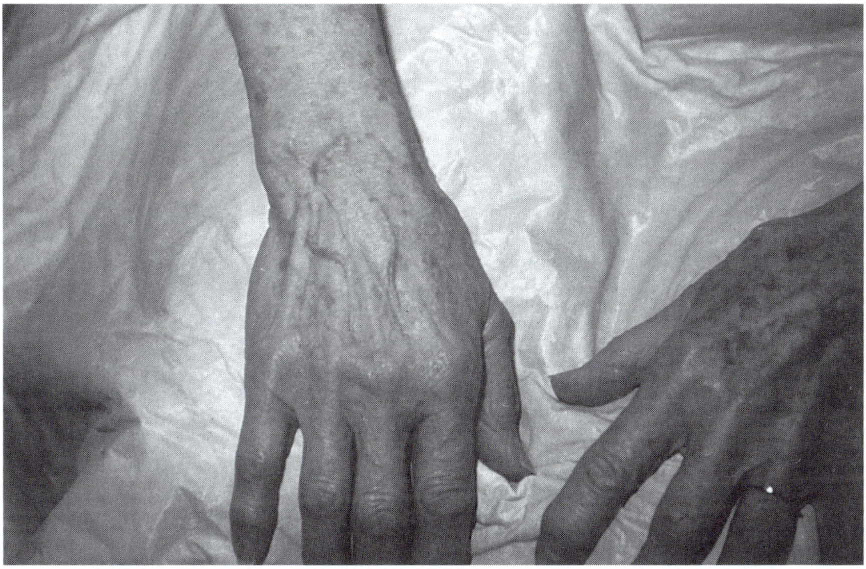

Figure 10–6 ■ Fragile veins of the elderly patient.

Cannulation Techniques

In elderly patients, stabilization of the vein is critical. The vessels may lack stability as a result of the loss of tissue mass and may tend to roll. Techniques to perform a venipuncture in elderly patients include:

1. Use of traction by placing the thumb directly along the vein axis about 2 to 3 inches below the intended venipuncture site. The palm and fingers of the traction hand serve to hold and stabilize the extremity. Using the index finger of the hand, provide traction to further stretch the skin above the intended venipuncture site. Maintain traction throughout venipuncture.
2. Insert the catheter, using either the direct or indirect technique. When the direct technique is used, insert the catheter at a 20- to 30-degree angle in a single motion, penetrating the skin and vein simultaneously. Do not stab or thrust the catheter into the skin; this could cause the catheter to advance too deeply and accidentally damage the vein. Use the indirect method (two-step) for patients with small, delicate veins. An alternative method is to have another nurse apply digital pressure with the hand above the site of venipuncture and release it after the vein has been entered.
3. For patients with very small, spidery veins, preflush the catheter before access is attempted. Preflushing enhances the backflow.

NURSING FAST FACT!

If the veins are fragile or if the patient is taking anticoagulants, avoid using a tourniquet; constricted blood flow may overdistend fragile veins, causing vein damage, vessel hemorrhages, or subcutaneous bleeding.

Tips for Fragile Veins

The following are tips for elderly patients with fragile veins:

- To prevent hematoma, avoid overdistention.
- Avoid multiple tapping of the vein.
- Use the smallest gauge needle necessary.
- Lower the angle of approach.
- Pull the skin taut and stabilize the vein throughout venipuncture.
- Use the one-handed technique: advance the catheter off the stylet into the vein.

Other Special Problems

Before initiating infusion therapy, the nurse must know the patient's diagnosis and allergies, in order to meet the special challenges of patients with difficult venous access. Conditions involving alterations in skin surface (e.g., in patients with systemic lupus erythematosus, dermatitis, skin lesions, and burns); hard sclerosed veins (e.g., in patients with renal failure or sickle cell disease, and those who are I.V. drug abusers), obesity, and edema affect the technique that the therapist will use for a successful venipuncture.

Alterations in Skin Surfaces

Take precautions in patients with alterations in skin surfaces caused by lesions, burns, or a disease process. Patients with altered skin integrity are often photosensitive and need additional protection of their already damaged tissue. **Tangential lighting** is recommended (Fig. 10–7). This indirect lighting does not flatten veins or cause damage to the skin. Use a light directed toward the side of the patient's extremity to illuminate the blue veins and provide a guide for venipuncture. This technique can also be used on dark-skinned individuals.

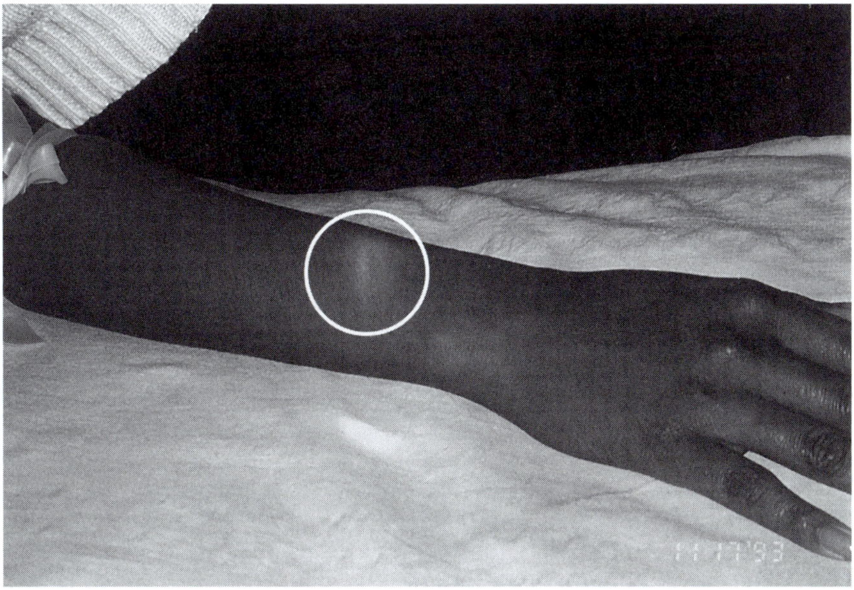

Figure 10–7 ■ Tangential lighting.

CULTURAL AND ETHNIC CONSIDERATIONS: SKIN COLOR 10–4

Skin color is the most significant biological variation in terms of nursing care. When caring for clients with highly pigmented skin, establish the baseline color by daylight. Give dark-skinned individuals a window to provide access to sunlight (Giger & Davidhizar, 2004).

Hard Sclerosed Vessels

If the peripheral vessels are hard and sclerosed because of a disease process, personal misuse, or frequent drug therapy, venous access is difficult. The practitioner should assess for collateral circulation. To find collateral veins, a nurse can use the multiple tourniquet technique (Procedures Display 10–1). By increasing the **oncotic** pressure inside the tissue, blood is forced into the small vessels of the periphery (Fig. 10–8).

The multiple tourniquet technique helps novices learn the differences between collateral veins and sclerosed vessels. Usually, veins appear in the hand when this approach is used.

PROCEDURES DISPLAY 10–1

Multiple Tourniquet Technique

Equipment Needed

- I.V. start equipment and fluids

Instructions to Patient

Explain reasons for use of multiple tourniquet technique and that there may be some pressure discomfort. Verify the patient's understanding of the explanation.

Procedure

1. Place one tourniquet high on the arm for 2 minutes and leave in place. The arm should be stroked downward toward the hand.
2. After 2 minutes, place a second tourniquet at midarm just below the antecubital fossa for 2 minutes.
3. If soft collateral veins do not appear in the forearm, place a third tourniquet at the wrist.
4. Tourniquets must not be left on longer than 6 minutes.

Documentation

Chart the site, needle type and size, type of fluid and medication, and patient response to the treatment.

Obesity

In patients with excessive adipose tissue, the veins in the extremities react one of two ways to the subcutaneous fat:

- The vessels will be buried deep in the tissue, thereby requiring a 2 inch catheter to access the vein.
- The vasculature will be forced to the surface because the veins have been displaced by the adipose tissue. A vessel can usually be located below the antecubital site on the lateral dorsum of the forearm.

CULTURAL AND ETHNIC CONSIDERATIONS: OBESITY 10–5

African-Americans have heavier bones and muscle mass than European-Americans. Usually African-American women are heavier in every age group than their European-American counterparts.

(Continued on following page)

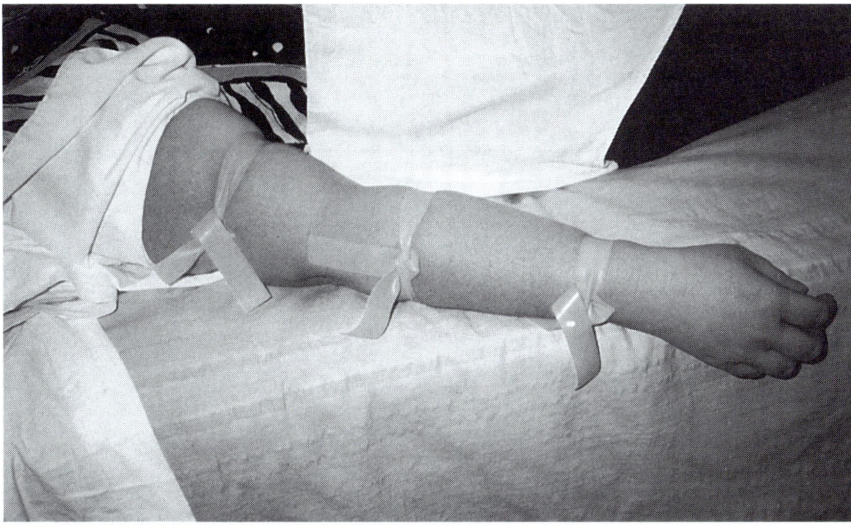

Figure 10–8 ■ Multiple-tourniquet technique.

Although ethnicity does appear to have an influence on body weight, a predictor of obesity is socioeconomic status. Average obesity is more pronounced in individuals in a low socioeconomic class, less pronounced in the middle class, and even less pronounced in the upper class (Giger & Davidhizar, 2004).

NURSING FAST FACT!

Use of a blood pressure cuff is not recommended for obese patients because increased pressure from the cuff can cause a backflow of blood.

Edema

In locating accessible vasculature in a patient with edema, the nurse must displace tissue fluid with digital pressure. Often this will allow visualization of an accessible vein. Care must be taken not to contaminate the site after the area is prepared. Venipuncture must be done quickly after the area is prepped to prevent the edematous fluid from obscuring the site.

Edematous fluid causes an increase in oncotic pressure. Therefore, if the fluid is not infusing after the catheter is in place, suspect that the vein may have collapsed as a result of the oncotic pressure in the tissue.

NURSING PLAN OF CARE

PEDIATRIC PATIENTS

Focus Assessment

Subjective

- Interview the patient's parents for the patient's current health status.

Objective

- Measure height and weight for calculation of body surface area and drug dosage.
- Note developmental level.

Patient Outcome/Evaluation Criteria

Pediatric patient will:

- Maintain hydration status, with decreased edema.
- Demonstrate beneficial effects from I.V. therapy.
- Return to preillness weight.
- Have normal vital signs for his or her age.
- Participate in activities appropriate to his or her age.
- Demonstrate reduced fear behaviors.
- Participate in decision-making process about self-care when appropriate.

Nursing Diagnoses

- Impaired skin integrity related to I.V. infiltration, diarrhea, edema, or dry skin
- Alteration in comfort or pain related to the position of the I.V.
- Risk of infection related to invasive procedures
- Potential anxiety related to the procedure of I.V. therapy
- Altered body image related to the placement of I.V. therapy equipment
- Alteration in family process related to the hospitalization of family member
- Parental role conflict related to illness or hospitalization of a child
- Sensory and perceptual alterations related to fluid imbalances
- Ineffective thermoregulation related to newborn transition to extrauterine environment
- Fear related to loss of control, autonomy, independence, competence, and self-esteem
- Diversional activity deficit related to environmental lack of activity; frequent, lengthy treatments; long-term hospitalization.
- Fluid volume deficit related to vomiting, diarrhea, burns, hemorrhage, wound drainage

(Continued on following page)

Nursing Management

1. Monitor for
   a. Intake and output.
   b. I.V. site every 2 hours and document
   c. Fluid overload
   d. Alterations in vital signs
2. Explain procedures and equipment.
3. Provide opportunities for non-nutritive sucking in infants.
4. Encourage parents to provide daily care of the child.
5. Instruct the parents in performing special care for the child.
6. Inform the parents about the child's progress.
7. Explain the rationales for treatment and procedures to parents and pediatric patient when appropriate.
8. Comfort infant after painful procedures.
9. Maintain daily routine during hospitalization.
10. Provide quiet, uninterrupted environment during nap time and nighttime as appropriate.
11. Immobilize when appropriate for venipuncture.
12. Use appropriate equipment for delivery of safe I.V. therapy.
13. Maintain standard precautions.
14. Calculate drug dosage correctly and double check with another licensed nurse before administration

Patient Education: Pediatric and Elderly Patients

Pediatric Patients

- Provide age-appropriate instructions.

Infants

- Encourage parents to keep in infant's line of vision and encourage parents to comfort child.

Toddlers

- Allow the child to participate during instruction; give simple explanations; explain procedures in relation to what the child sees, hears, tastes, smells, and feels; emphasize the aspects of procedures that require cooperation (e.g., lying still).
- Communicate using behaviors; use play by demonstrating with dolls and small replicas of equipment.
- Limit teaching sessions to 5 to 10 minutes.
- Prepare immediately before the procedure.

(Continued on following page)

Patient Education: Pediatric and Elderly Patients *(Continued)*

Preschoolers

- Explain procedures in simple terms and in relation to how they affect the child.
- Demonstrate the uses of and allow child to play with equipment.
- Encourage "playing out" on a doll.
- Avoid overestimating the child's comprehension; encourage the child to verbalize.
- Limit each teaching session to 10 to 15 minutes.
- Explain unfamiliar situations such as noises and lights.

School-Age Children

- Explain procedures using correct terminology; explain reasons for procedures using anatomic drawings.
- Explain function and operation of equipment in clear terms.
- Allow manipulation of and practice with equipment.
- Allow for questions and discussion.
- Limit teaching sessions to 20 minutes.
- Instruct in advance of procedures.
- Use small groups or encourage teaching of peers.
- Instruct parents.
- Provide ways to maintain control (e.g., deep breathing, counting, relaxation).

Adolescents

- Involve patient in all decisions.
- Discuss how procedure may affect physical appearance.
- Be aware of adolescent's difficulty with accepting authority.
- Instruct in groups and encourage peer instruction.
- Teaching session can be as long as 45 minutes (Wong, 2003).
- Be sensitive to cultural issues, especially related to nursing care of children in the home care setting:
  - Communication channels
  - Spatial behaviors (tactile and visual space)
  - Social (family system) organization
  - Perception of time
  - Use of folk medicine and health-seeking behaviors of the parent (Giger & Davidhizar, 2004)
  - Remember that in most Asian cultures, nursing care must be directed to the family as a whole as well as to the individual family member.

Elderly Patients

- Speak slowly, clearly, and directly to elderly patients with sensory deficits.
- Address the patient by his or her proper name.
- Explain the steps of any procedure to increase cooperation and decrease anxiety.
- Do not use terminology that is unfamiliar.

Home Care Issues: Pediatric and Elderly Patients

Pediatric Patients

The home care environment must be assessed to be sure that I.V. therapy can be carried out safely. In the home children are more mobile and active. The parents must be educated about the use and care of I.V. therapy and accept involvement in and responsibility for the treatment regimen.

Focus on the psychosocial and developmental needs of the child and family in planning home infusion therapy.

The best infusion device is one that is portable and easy for the child and family to operate. A syringe pump and positive-pressure devices such as an elastomeric infusion device are examples of easy-to-use equipment.

Keep in mind that parents need support from a home care agency in case the hospital unit nurses are not available; this may increase anxiety and fear.

Identify alternate caregivers.

Elderly Patients

Educating older adults in the administration of home infusion therapy can present challenges. The patient may be less ready to adapt to environmental changes, especially relating to independence.

The teaching of complex drug admixtures, tubing connections, I.V. maintenance, I.V. pump programming, and accessing and deaccessing devices requires patience and step-by-step approaches. All equipment should be user friendly. Written teaching materials, video programs, and demonstrations, including return demonstrations, can be helpful.

Evaluation of language or cultural differences can dramatically affect understanding of necessary healthcare concepts.

Sensory changes occur with aging (e.g., in vision, hearing, and manual dexterity). Observe the patient while working with various devices (the needleless system may eliminate the risk of needlestick injuries) to ensure proficiency.

Key Points

Pediatric Infusion Therapy

- Children are not small adults. Physiologic differences must be kept in mind with particular focus on total body weight (85 to 90 percent water) and heat production (increases caloric expenditure by 7 percent for each degree of temperature), and immature renal and integumentary systems important in regulation of fluid and electrolyte needs.
- Physical assessment of a pediatric patient includes measuring the head circumference (for patients up to 1 year of age) and checking height or length, vital signs, skin turgor, presence of tears, moistness and color of membranes, urinary output, characteristics of fontanels, and level of child's activity.

- Dehydration is a common cause of fluid and electrolyte imbalance; assessment of fluid needs includes the meter square weight or caloric method.
- Peripheral routes include the four scalp veins, dorsum of the hand and forearm, and dorsum of the foot.
- Selection of I.V. equipment must keep in mind safety, activity, age, and size.
- Needle selection depends on the age of child: 26- to 24-gauge for neonates; 24- to 22-gauge for children.
- Use small volumes of solutions (250 or 500 mL). Use a volume control chamber and, when indicated, infusion pumps.
- Always have extra help when starting an I.V. in a child.
- Perform venipuncture in a separate room, use a pacifier for neonates and infants, warm hands before applying gloves, use a rubber band to dilate scalp veins, use surgical lubricating jelly under adhesive tape, and use stickers or drawing as rewards.
- Delivery of medications to children can be by intermittent infusion, retrograde infusion, or syringe pump.
- Alternate routes include intraosseous and umbilical vein and arteries.
- Intraosseous route: use only for 6 hours; use for children younger than 6 years of age. Contraindicated in patients with cellulitis or infected burn, fractured bone, osteoporosis, or osteogenesis imperfecta.

Geriatric Infusion Therapy

- Physiologic changes include homeostatic mechanisms becoming less efficient; immune system becoming hyporesponsive to foreign antigens; cardiovascular changes, including a change in elasticity of the vein walls; skin losses; subcutaneous support; and thinning of skin.
- Assessment guidelines include skin turgor, temperature, rate and filling of veins in hand or foot, daily weight, intake and output, center of tongue should be moist, postural blood pressure, swallowing ability, and functional assessment of patient's ability to obtain fluids if not NPO.
- Venipuncture techniques should take into consideration the skin and vein changes of elderly persons; use small-gauge catheters, use blood pressure cuff, or place loose tourniquet over clothing. Use warm compresses to visualize veins. Consider microdrip administration sets.

Other Special Problems

- Alterations in skin surfaces: Use tangential lighting.
- Hard sclerosed vessels: Use multiple tourniquet technique.

- Obesity: Use 2-inch catheter, lateral veins, and multiple tourniquet technique.
- Edema: Displace edema with digital pressure.
- Fragile veins: Maintain traction using one-handed technique. Be gentle.

Critical Thinking: Case Study

An 85-year-old man is admitted to the hospital with dehydration. He also has Alzheimer's disease and has been residing in a residential care facility for about 1 year. He is disoriented and does not recognize his wife who accompanies him to your unit. He is restless, combative, and very anxious. The emergency room personnel inserted an I.V. of 5 percent dextrose in water at 50 mL per hour into his right forearm and secured his hands with wrist restraints.

His lab work on admission reads:

Sodium 150 mEq/L
BUN 54 mg/dL
Creatinine 1.5 mg/dL

What does his lab work reflect? Is the I.V. solution correct? What else should be considered in this case?

Media Link: Answers to this case study and additional critical thinking activities are on the CD–ROM that accompanies this textbook.

Post-Test

1. The preferred choice for peripheral infusion site in the young infant younger than age 9 months is the:
   a. Frontal vein in the scalp
   b. Dorsum of the foot
   c. Dorsum of the hand
   d. Occipital vein on the head
2. The weight method of estimating fluid requirements in a child refers to:
   a. Weighing diapers and estimating output to replace sensible losses
   b. A formula based on weight in kilograms to estimate fluid needs
   c. A calculation of metabolic expenditure of energy based on weight
   d. Use of a nomogram

3. In a dark-skinned person, the best method for locating an accessible vein is:
   a. Multiple tourniquets
   b. Tangential lighting
   c. Direct overhead lighting
   d. Light application of a tourniquet
4. Which of the following is the most appropriate cannula size for use on a 2-month-old infant?
   a. 18-gauge over-the-needle catheter
   b. 23- to 25-gauge scalp vein needle
   c. 16-gauge scalp vein needle
   d. 22- to 24-gauge over-the-needle catheter
5. The most common site for intraosseous infusion is the:
   a. Proximal humerus
   b. Distal humerus, 6 cm below the acromion process
   c. Anterior tibia, 1 to 3 cm below the tibial tuberosity
   d. Proximal posterior femur
6. When performing an I.V. on a toddler, methods that can be used to assist the therapist in this invasive procedure based on developmental age include:
   a. Letting the child express feelings and scream
   b. Encouraging the child to hold a favorite toy or blanket
   c. Performing the procedure quickly with assistance from other staff or parents
   d. All of the above
7. The most appropriate equipment for an infant receiving I.V. fluids includes:
   a. Microdrip tubing connected to a 50-mL infusate container
   b. Microdrip volume control cylinder attached to a 250-mL infusate container
   c. Macrodrip tubing connected to a volume control cylinder
   d. Any tubing or container as long as it is regulated with an electronic infusion device
8. The three methods for assessment of 24-hour fluid needs in an infant are:
   a. Meter square, diaper weight, and urinary output
   b. Meter square, weight, and caloric methods
   c. Meter square, specific gravity, and head circumference

9. Complications of intraosseous infusions include all of the following **EXCEPT:**
   a. Osteomyelitis
   b. Cellulitis
   c. Damage to the epiphyseal plate
   d. Fractured humerus

10. Techniques to dilate a vein for venipuncture in an elderly person with fragile veins include all of the following **EXCEPT:**
   a. Apply the tourniquet loosely over the patient's sleeve.
   b. Apply multiple tourniquets.
   c. Use digital pressure to enhance vein filling.
   d. Use warm compresses before venipuncture.

Media Link: Additional test questions and rationales are contained on the CD–ROM that accompanies this textbook.

References

American College of Surgeons (1999). Emergency vascular access in children. American College of Surgeons Committee on Trauma. September 1999. Internet: *www.facs.org/commerce/2003/trauma*

Buchholz, S. (2003). Henle's *Med-Math* (4th ed.). Philadelphia: Lippincott Williams & Wilkins, pp. 241–257.

Frey, A.M. (2001). Intravenous therapy in children. In Hankins, J., Lonsway, R.A., Hedrick, C., & Perdue, M.B. (eds.). *Infusion Therapy: Clinical Principles and Practice* (2nd ed.). Infusion Nurses Society and Philadelphia: W.B. Saunders.

Giger, J.N., & Davidhizar, R. (2004). *Transcultural Nursing Assessment & Intervention* (4th ed.). St. Louis: Mosby.

Hockenberry, M.J. (2003). *Whaley & Wong's Nursing Care of Infants and Children* (7th ed.). St. Louis: Mosby-Year Book.

Infusion Nursing Society (2000). Revised standards of practice. *Journal of Intravenous Nursing*, 21 (1S).

Metheny, N.M. (2000). *Fluid and Electrolyte Balance: Nursing Considerations* (4th ed.). Philadelphia: J.B. Lippincott.

Nugent, K., Chernecky, C., & Macklin, D. (2002). Using focus groups to evaluate the patient's involvement in decision-making associated with their vascular access device. *Journal of Vascular Access Devices*, 7(2), 33–37.

Powers, F.A. (1999). Your elderly patient needs I.V. therapy: Can you keep her safe? *Nursing, 99*, 99(7), 54–55.

Smeltzer, S.C., & Bare, B.G. (2004). *Brunner and Suddarth's Textbook of Medical-Surgical Nursing* (10th ed.). Philadelphia: J.B. Lippincott, pp. 150–165.

Smith, M.F. (1998). Emergency access in pediatrics. *Journal of Intravenous Nursing*, 21(3), 149–159.

Walther, K. (2000). Intravenous therapy in the older adult. In Hankins, J., Lonsway, R.A., Hedrick, C., & Perdue, M.B. (eds.). *Infusion Therapy: Clinical Principles and Practice* (2nd ed.). Infusion Nurses Society and Philadelphia: W.B. Saunders.

Wong, D.L. (2003). *Wheley and Wong's Essentials of Pediatric Nursing,* (7th ed). St. Louis: Mosby, Inc.

Answers to Chapter 10 Post-Test

1. **c**
2. **b**
3. **b**
4. **d**
5. **c**
6. **d**
7. **b**
8. **b**
9. **d**
10. **b**

Unit 3

Advanced Infusion Practice

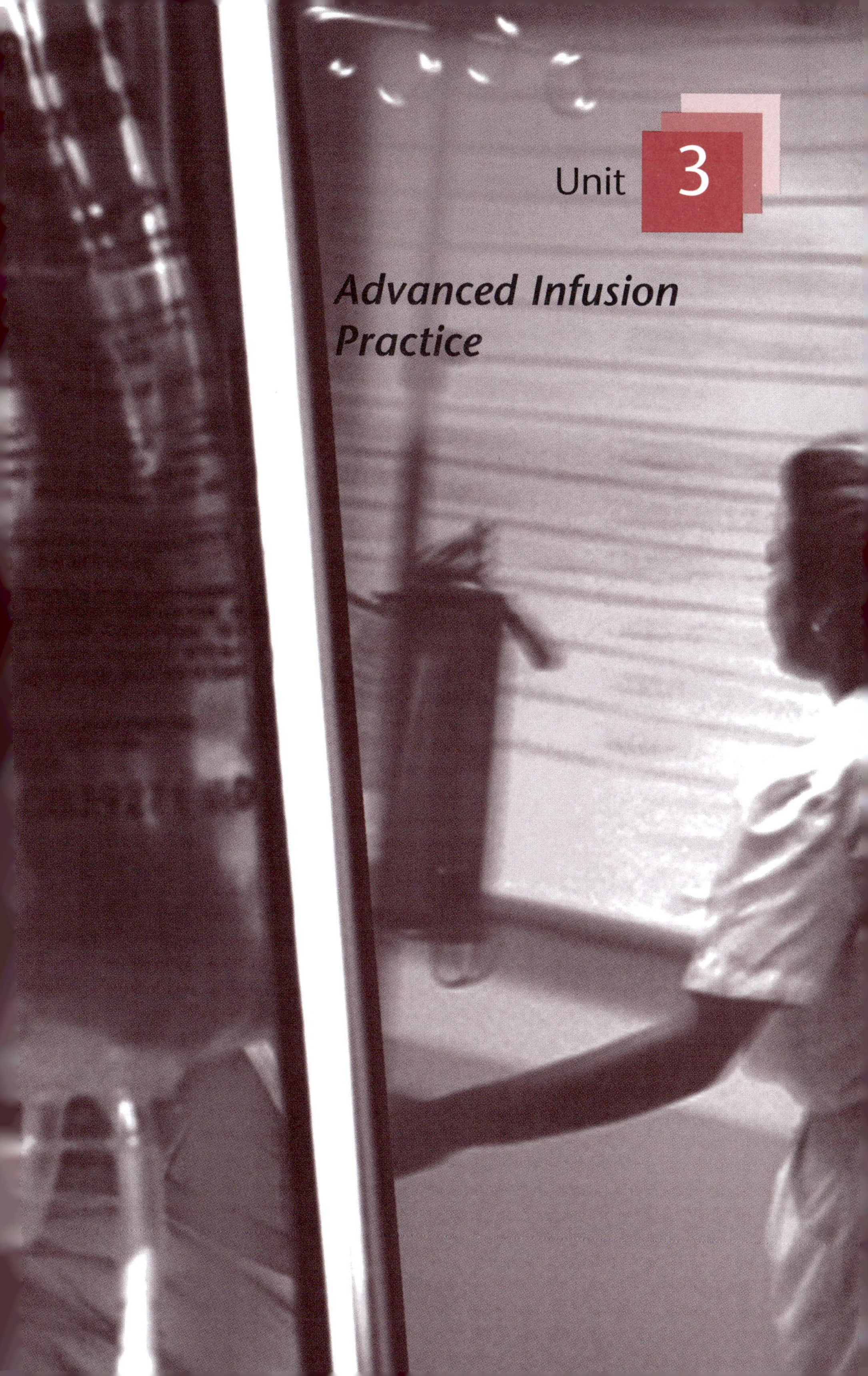

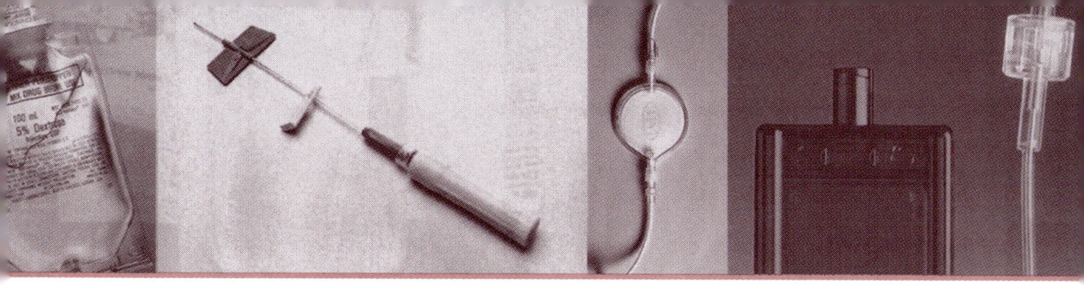

Chapter 11
Administration of Intravenous Medications

In the future, which I shall not see, for I am old, may a better way be opened! May the methods by which every infant, every human being will have the best chance of health, the methods by which every sick person will have the best chance of recovery, be learned and practiced! Hospitals are only an intermediate state of civilization never intended, at all events, to take in the whole sick population.

—Florence Nightingale, 1860

Chapter Contents

LEARNING OBJECTIVES

Upon completion of this chapter, the reader will be able to:

1. Define the glossary terms related to nursing care of the patient receiving medications by infusion.
2. Identify the advantages and hazards of delivering medications by the intravenous route.
3. Discuss the three incompatibilities related to intravenous therapy.
4. Describe the proper technique in delivery of a medication by the intravenous bolus route.
5. Describe the treatment of adverse side effects of intravenous medications.
6. State the precautions to be followed when medication is infused via the epidural route.
7. List the key steps in dressing management of an intraspinal catheter.
8. Describe the method of delivery and nursing considerations for intraperitoneal therapy.
9. Discuss the purpose of delivery of fluids and medications by the intraventricular route.
10. List the key points in delivery of fluids by the intraosseous route.
11. Discuss the key points for delivery of anti-infective agents.
12. Describe nurses' roles in the delivery of investigational drugs.

GLOSSARY

Admixture Combination of two or more medications

Adsorption Attachment of one substance to the surface of another

Bolus Concentrated medication or solution given rapidly over a short period of time; may be given by direct I.V. injection or I.V. drip

Chemical incompatibility Change in the molecular structure or pharmacologic properties of a substance, which may or may not be visually observed

Clinical trial Planned experiment that involves patients and is designed to evoke an appropriate treatment of future patients with a given medical condition

Compatibility Capable of being mixed and administered without undergoing undesirable chemical or physical changes or loss of therapeutic action

Delivery system A product that allows for the administration of medication

Distribution Process of delivering a drug to the various tissues of the body

Drug interaction An interaction between two drugs; also, a drug that causes an increase or decrease in another drug's pharmacologic effects

Epidural Situated on or over the dura mater

Incompatibility Chemical or physical reaction that occurs among two or more drugs or between a drug and the delivery device

Intermittent drug infusion I.V. therapy administered at prescribed intervals

Intraspinal Spaces surrounding the spinal cord, including the epidural and intrathecal spaces

Intrathecal Within a sheath, surrounded by the epidural space and separated from it by the dura mater; contains cerebrospinal fluid

Intravenous push Manual administration of medication under pressure over 1 minute or as manufacturer of medication recommends

Multiple-dose vial Medication bottle that is hermetically sealed with a rubber stopper and designed to be entered more than once; usually contains a preservative.

Physical incompatibility An undesirable change that is visually observed

Single-dose vial Medication bottle that is hermetically sealed with a rubber stopper and is intended for one-time use; usually does not contain a preservative.

Therapeutic incompatibility Undesirable effect occurring within a patient as a result of two or more drugs being given concurrently

Principles of Intravenous Medication Administration

Advantages

The advantages of I.V. medication administration include the fact that it provides (1) direct access to the circulatory system, (2) a route for administration of fluids and drugs to patients who cannot tolerate oral medications, (3) a method of instant drug action, and (4) a method of instant drug administration termination. This route offers pronounced advantages over the subcutaneous (S.Q.), intramuscular (I.M.), and oral routes (Table 11–1).

Drugs that cannot be absorbed by other routes because of the large molecular size of the drug or destruction of the drug by gastric juices can be administered directly to the site of **distribution**, the circulatory system, with I.V. infusion. Drugs with irritating properties that cause pain and trauma when given by the intramuscular or subcutaneous route can be given intravenously. When a drug is administered intravenously, there is instant drug action, which is an advantage in emergency situations. The I.V. route also provides instant drug termination if sensitivity or adverse reactions occur. This route provides for control over the rate at which drugs are administered; prolonged action can be controlled by administering a dilute medication infusion intermittently over a prolonged time period.

Intravenous medications are provided for rapid therapeutic or diagnostic responses or a delivery route for solutions or medications that cannot be delivered by any other route. Nurses administering the solution or medication are accountable for achieving effective delivery of prescribed therapy and for evaluating and documenting deviations from an expected outcome, including the implementation of corrective action.

> Table 11–1 **ADVANTAGES AND DISADVANTAGES OF INTRAVENOUS MEDICATION ADMINISTRATION**

Advantages
1. Provides a direct access to the circulatory system 2. Provides a route for drugs that irritate the gastric mucosa 3. Provides a route for instant drug action 4. Provides a route for delivering high drug concentrations 5. Provides for instant drug termination if sensitivity or adverse reaction occurs 6. Provides for better control over the rate of drug administration 7. Provides a route of administration in patients in whom use of the gastrointestinal tract is limited
Disadvantages
1. Drug interaction because of incompatibilities. 2. Adsorption of the drug is impaired, which is caused by leaching into I.V. container or administration set. 3. Errors in compounding (mixing) of medication 4. Speed shock 5. Extravasation of a vesicant drug 6. Chemical phlebitis

INS Standard. Nurses are responsible for assessing the appropriateness of prescribed therapy, including patient assessment; patient age and condition; appropriateness of solution and medication prescribed; and appropriateness of drug and its dose, route, and rate. Before administration of the solution or medication, the nurse must be knowledgeable in indications, actions, use, side effects, and adverse reactions associated with the solution or medication. (INS, 2000, 73)

Disadvantages

Despite the many advantages of I.V. medication, there are also disadvantages associated with this venous route; these disadvantages are not found with other drug therapies (refer to Table 11–1).

The number of drug combinations, along with the ever-increasing production of drugs and parenteral fluids, has compounded these disadvantages. The disadvantages specific to the administration of I.V. drugs include **drug interactions**; drug loss via **adsorption** of I.V. containers and administration sets; errors in mixing techniques; and the complications of speed shock, extravasation of vesicant drugs, and phlebitis.

Drug Interactions

Drug interactions are not always clear cut. Many factors affect drug interactions, including drug solubility and drug **compatibility.** Mixing of two drugs in a solution can cause an adverse interaction called drug **incompatibility.** Factors affecting drug solubility and compatibility include:

- Drug concentration
- I.V. fluid or drug
- Type of administration set
- Preparation technique, duration of drug–drug or drug–solution contact
- pH value
- Temperature of the room and light

Drugs can be compatible when mixed in certain solutions but incompatible when mixed with others. Mixing two incompatible drugs in solution in a particular order may be enough to avoid a potentially adverse interaction (Gahart & Nazareno, 2004).

The pH of both the solution and the drug must be considered when compounding medications. Drugs that are widely dissimilar in pH values are unlikely to be compatible in solution. For example, dextrose solutions are slightly acidic, with a pH of 4.5 to 5.5. Several antibiotics on the market have an acidic pH that is stable in dextrose; however, alkaline antibiotics, such as carbenicillin, are unstable when mixed with dextrose. Dextrose, with a pH of 4.5 to 5.5, should be used as a base for acidic drugs; sodium chloride solution, with a pH value of 6.8 to 8.5, should be used for alkaline medication dilution.

NURSING FAST FACT!

When in doubt about I.V. drug compatibilities, a good practice is to flush the I.V. administration set with sodium chloride before and after medications are infused.

Adsorption

Adsorption is the attachment of one substance to the surface of another. Many drugs adsorb to glass or plastic. The disadvantage associated with adsorption is that the patient receives a smaller amount of the drug than was intended. The amount of adsorption is difficult to predict and is affected by the drug concentration, solution of the drug, amount of surface contacted by the drug, and temperature changes.

An example of adsorption is the binding of insulin to plastic and glass containers. The insulin rapidly adsorbs to I.V. containers and tubing until all potential adsorption sites are saturated. During the initial part of an infusion, very little insulin may reach the patient; later, after adsorption sites are saturated, more of the insulin in the solution is delivered to the patient. To prevent this from occurring, injecting the drug as close to the I.V. insertion site as possible will promote better therapeutic drug effects.

Polyvinyl chloride (PVC) in plastic flexible I.V. bags promotes drug adsorption. A phthalate (DEHP) is a plasticizer that is added to PVC that allows PVC to be flexible. Some drug formulations leach this plasticizer out of the plastic matrix and into the solution. DEHP is fat-soluble, I.V. fat emulsion products can extract the plasticizer from the PVC bags and tubing. DEHP is also leached from PVC bags by organic solvents and surfactants contained in some drugs, which may result in DEHP-induced toxicity. In the package inserts, many drug manufacturers recommend nonphthalate **delivery systems**. Many companies are manufacturing nonphthalate I.V. bags and tubing to prevent this problem. (Chapter 6 provides further information on DEHP leaching and a list of nonphthalate products.)

NURSING FAST FACTS!

- *When mixing medications into glass or plastic systems, refer to the manufacturer's guidelines to prevent adsorption.*

(Continued on following page)

- *Burning at the I.V. site from a presumably dilute drug is a warning that the concentration of the drug is too high and needs to be diluted further.*
- *Many hospitals allow only registered pharmacists to prepare admixtures.*

Errors in Mixing

Drug toxicity, subtherapeutic infusion, or erratic therapeutic effects can result from inadequate mixing of a drug into the infusion container. Inadequate mixing can contribute to a **bolus** of medication being delivered to the patient, which may cause adverse effects.

Factors that contribute to inadequate mixing include:

- Length of time required to adequately mix drugs in flexible bags
- Addition of a drug to a hanging flexible bag
- Additives injected at a slow rate into the primary bag (the turbulence of fast flow promotes mixing, especially in glass containers)
- Inadequate movement of the additive from the injection port (e.g., the long, narrow sleeve-type additive ports on some flexible bags, as opposed to the button type, hinder effective mixing)
- Tendency of very dense drugs to settle at the bottom of infusion container

Ten key recommendations for adequate mixing of I.V. medications are presented in Table 11–2.

Intravenous Drug Safety

Getting the right solution or medication to a patient is often a complicated, error-prone process. The order has to be properly written on the correct medical record, read, and properly interpreted and transcribed. The drug has to be retrieved and labeled correctly. The proper patient has to be identified and the infusion rate correctly set.

Infusion Nurses Society (INS, 2000, 73) practice criteria for medication and solution administration include the following:

1. Aseptic technique and standard precautions should be used in the administration of medications and solutions.
2. A list of approved medications and solutions should be established in organizational policies and procedures.
3. Orders should be reviewed for appropriateness of prescribed therapy for patient's age and condition, access device dose, route of administration, and rate of administration.

Table 11–2 TEN KEY RECOMMENDATIONS FOR ADEQUATE MIXING OF I.V. MEDICATIONS

1. Gently invert the I.V. container several times to adequately mix the medication with the solution, taking care to avoid foaming the solution.
2. When inversion is impossible, gently swirl or rotate to mix to prevent the drug from settling to the bottom of the container.
3. When agitating an intermittent infusion set, clamp off the air vent; if the vent becomes wet, the solution will not infuse properly after mixing.
4. Vacuum devices can facilitate mixing in plastic flexible bags by creating a vacuum and drawing any drug left in the port into the body of the bag.
5. When possible, use premixed solutions from the manufacturer; for example, using premixed heparin or potassium chloride solutions can save time and avoid dose errors as well as preclude mixing problems.
6. Add one drug at a time to the primary I.V. solution. Mix and examine thoroughly before adding the next drug.
7. Add the most concentrated or most soluble drug to the solution first because some incompatibilities, such as precipitates, require a certain concentration or amount of time to develop. Mix well, and then add the dilute drugs.
8. Add colored additives last to avoid masking possible precipitate cloudiness.
9. Always visually inspect containers after adding and mixing drugs; hold the container against a light or a white surface and check for particulate matter, obvious layering, or foaming.
10. If you do not have a clear understanding of the compatibility or stability of the admixtures you are using, check the manufacturer's recommendation of consult a pharmacist.

4. The nurse administering medications and solutions should have knowledge of indications for therapy, side effects, and potential adverse reactions and appropriate interventions.
5. Prior to administration of medications and solutions, the nurse should appropriately label all containers, vials, and syringes; identify the patient; and verify contents, dose, rate, route, expiration date, and integrity of the solution.
6. The nurse should be accountable for evaluating and monitoring effectiveness of prescribed therapy; documenting patient response, adverse events, and interventions; and achieving effective delivery of the prescribed therapy.
7. Medications or solutions should be discarded within 24 hours after being added to an administration set.

Preventing Medication Administration Errors

In 1999 the Institute of Medicine released a report, "To Err Is Human: Building a Safer Health System," and according to this report between 44,000 and 98,000 deaths may result each year from medical errors in hospitals alone. More than 7,000 deaths each year are related to medication errors. Error reduction strategies and strengthening checks and balances to prevent errors is now part of the U.S. health system (IOM, 1999). In addition, the Department of Health and Human Services (HHS) and other federal agencies formed the Quality Interagency Coordination Task Force in 2000 and issued an action plan for reducing medical errors. In 2001, HHS announced a Patient Safety Task Force to coordinate a joint effort to improve data collection on patient safety. The lead agencies include FDA, CDC, Medicare and Medicaid Services, and the Agency for Healthcare Research and Quality.

The following is a list of strategies implemented to reduce medication errors.

1. Bar Code Label Rule: In March of 2003, the FDA published regulations on barcode labeling on certain drug and biological product labels. The rule takes effect in 2006 and applies to prescription drugs; biological products such as vaccines, blood, and blood components; and over-the-counter drugs that are commonly used in hospitals.
2. Drug name confusion: To minimize confusion between drug names that look or sound alike, the FDA reviews about 300 drug names a year before they are marketed.
3. Drug labeling: New regulation requires a standardized "Drug Facts" label on more than 100,000 OTC drug products.
4. Error tracking and public education: On March 13, 2003, the FDA announced a proposed rule that would revamp safety reporting requirements. The FDA reviews medication error reports that come from drug manufacturers and through MedWatch. However, a recent Institute for Safe Medication Practices (ISMP) survey on medication error reporting practices showed that health professionals submit reports more often to internal reporting programs such as hospitals than to external programs such as the FDA.

NURSING FAST FACT!

In December of 2002 an analysis of medication errors captured in 2001 found that of 105,603 errors, 3,361 (3.2 percent) involved children. Most of the errors were corrected before causing harm, but 190 caused patient injury and of those, two resulted in death. In January of 2003 USP released recommendations for preventing drug errors in children (FDA, 2003b).

The American Hospital Association lists the following as some common types of medication errors:

- Incomplete patient information (not knowing about patient's allergies, other medicines the patient is taking, previous diagnoses, and lab results)
- Unavailable drug information
- Miscommunication of drug orders, which can involve poor handwriting, confusion between drugs with similar names, misuse of

zeroes and decimal points, confusion of metric and other dosing units, and inappropriate abbreviations
- Lack of appropriate labeling as a drug is prepared and repackaged into smaller units; and environmental factors, such as lighting, heat, noise, and interruptions, that can distract healthcare professionals from their medical tasks (FDA, August, 2003)

Table 11–3 provides nursing guidelines for drug safety.

AGE-RELATED CONSIDERATIONS: OLDER ADULTS AND THE EFFECTS OF GENDER 11–1

Almost 60 percent of older adults fear adverse drug reactions or overmedication, which leads to noncompliance in taking their medications (Kuhn, 1999). Drug side effects in elderly persons are often mistaken for signs of aging. Gender can have a profound effect on metabolism of drugs. For example, women have the potential for higher blood plasma levels of psychotropic drugs, especially when used with oral contraceptives. Also, women have a greater likelihood of adverse reactions to antipsychotic agents.

Websites: Agencies that Track Medication Errors:

The Food and Drug Administration: Through MedWatch
www.fda.gov/medwatch/how.htm
Institute for Safe Medication Practices: Publishes Safe Medicine, a consumer newsletter on medication errors. 1-215-947-7797
www.ismp.org

> Table 11–3 Nursing Guidelines for Drug Safety

1. Don't store vials of concentrated electrolyte solutions (such as potassium chloride concentrate) in patient-care units.
2. Eliminate unnecessary multiple concentrations of all drugs and solutions.
3. Avoid using drug samples for inpatients; keep samples for outpatients in a secure area that's inaccessible to patients and where the pharmacy can tightly control them.
4. Minimize drug calculations and the need to admix drugs in patient-care areas. Use standard concentrations of premixed solutions and dosing or infusion rate charts to determine rates without calculations.
5. Eliminate excessive unit-drug stock and use of multiple-dose vials.
6. Institute standard drug administration times and dosing windows: Once the first dose of a medication is available and has been administered, you need safe, predetermined time frames for a standard dosing schedule.
7. Prevent nonpharmacists from having access to the pharmacy. Only the nursing supervisors should have access to a segregated, secured cabinet outside the pharmacy when it is closed.

***Source:** Smetzer (2001).*

National Coordinating Council for Medication Error Reporting and Prevention: *www.nccmerp.org*
U.S. Pharmacopeia: *www.usp.org*

Drug Compatibility

Compatibility is required for a therapeutic response to prescribed therapy. Chemical, physical, and therapeutic compatibility must be identified before admixing and administering I.V. medications.

An incompatibility results when two or more substances react or interact and change the normal activity of one or more components. Incompatibility may be manifested by harmful or undesirable effects and is likely to result in a loss of therapeutic effects. Incompatibility may occur when:

- Several drugs are added to a large volume of fluid to produce an **admixture**.
- Drugs in separate solutions are administered concurrently or in close succession via the same I.V. line.
- A single drug is reconstituted or diluted with the wrong solutions.
- One drug reacts with another drug's preservative.

Specific incompatibilities fall into three categories: physical, chemical, and therapeutic.

Physical Incompatibility

A **physical incompatibility** is also called a pharmaceutical incompatibility. Physical incompatibilities occur when one drug is mixed with other drugs or solutions to produce a product that is unsafe for administration.

Insolubility and absorption are the two types of physical incompatibility. Insolubility occurs when a drug is added to an inappropriate fluid solution, creating an incomplete solution or a precipitate. This risk occurs more frequently with multiple additives, which may interact to form an insoluble product. Signs of insolubility include visible precipitation, haze, gas bubbles, and cloudiness. Some precipitation may be microcrystalline (i.e., smaller than 50 microns) and not apparent to the eye. The use of micropore filters is intended to prevent such particles from entering the vein. The use of a 0.22-micron inline filter reduces the amount of microcrystalline precipitates.

The presence of calcium in a drug or solution usually indicates that a precipitate might form if mixed with another drug. Ringer's solution preparations contain calcium, so check carefully for incompatibility before adding any drug to this solution.

Other physical incompatibilities caused by insolubility include the increased degradation of drugs added to sodium bicarbonate and the formation of an insoluble precipitate when sodium bicarbonate is combined with other medications in emergency situations.

The following are important recommendations regarding physical drug incompatibilities:

- Never administer a drug that forms a precipitate.
- Do not mix drugs prepared in special diluents with other drugs.
- When administering a series of medications, prepare each drug in a separate syringe. This will lessen the possibility of precipitation. Insolubility may also result from the use of an incorrect solution to reconstitute a drug.
- Follow the manufacturer's directions for reconstituting drugs (Kuhn, 1998).

Chemical Incompatibility

A **chemical incompatibility** is a reaction of a drug with other drugs or solutions, which results in alterations of the integrity and potency of the active ingredient. The most common cause of chemical incompatibility is the reaction between acidic and alkaline drugs or solutions, resulting in a pH level that is unstable for one of the drugs. A specific pH or a narrow range of pH values is required for the solubility of a drug and for the maintenance of its stability after it has been mixed.

Therapeutic Incompatibility

A **therapeutic incompatibility** is an undesirable effect occurring in a patient as a result of two or more drugs being given concurrently. An increased therapeutic or a decreased therapeutic response is produced.

This incompatibility often occurs when therapy dictates the use of two antibiotics. For example, in the use of chloramphenicol and penicillin, chloramphenicol has been reported to antagonize the bacterial activity of penicillin. If prescribed, penicillin should be administered at least 1 hour before the chloramphenicol to prevent therapeutic incompatibility.

Therapeutic incompatibility may go unnoticed until the patient fails to show the expected clinical response to the drug or until peak and trough levels of the drug show a lack of therapeutic levels. If an incompatibility is not suspected, the patient may be given increasingly higher doses of the drug to try to obtain the therapeutic effect.

When more than one antibiotic is prescribed for intermittent infusion, stagger the time schedule so that each can be infused individually.

CULTURAL AND ETHNIC CONSIDERATIONS: I.V. DRUG ADMINISTRATION 11–1

In ethnic and cultural groups (i.e., African-Americans and Asian-Americans) with a high incidence of glucose-6-phosphate dehydrogenase (G6PD) deficiency, some drugs may impair red blood cell metabolism, leading to anemia. Caffeine, a component of many drugs, is excreted more slowly by Asian-Americans. Asian-Americans may require smaller doses of certain drugs (Giger & Davidhizar, 2004).

Intravenous Medication Administration

General Guidelines

Several methods are used to administer I.V. medications, including continuous, intermittent infusions, and I.V. push. Nursing responsibilities of I.V. drug administration include:

- Identifying whether a prescribed route (i.e., continuous, intermittent, or push) is appropriate
- Using aseptic technique and Standard Precautions when preparing an admixture
- Identifying the expiration date on solutions and medications
- Following the manufacturer's guidelines for the preparation and storage of the medication
- Monitoring the patient for therapeutic response to the medication

NURSING FAST FACTS!

- *Be knowledgeable of the pharmacologic implications relative to patient clinical status and diagnosis.*
- *Verify that all solution containers are free of cracks, leaks, and punctures.*

Guidelines for I.V. Medication Delivery

1. Check all labels (drugs, diluents, and solutions) to confirm appropriateness for I.V. use.
2. Use a filter needle when withdrawing I.V. medications from ampules to eliminate possible pieces of glass.
3. Do not use bacteriostatic diluents containing benzyl alcohol in treating neonates.
4. Ensure adequate mixing of all drugs added to a solution.
5. When combining drugs in solution (additives) always consider the required rate adjustment of each drug.
6. Examine solutions for clarity and any possible leakage.
7. Frozen infusion solutions should be thawed at room temperature

(25°C or 77°F) or under refrigeration. All ice crystals must be melted before administration. Do not refreeze.

8. Prepackaged syringes for use in specific pumps is now available for many drugs.
9. Controlled room temperature (CRT) is considered to be 25°C (77°F). Most medications tolerate variations in temperature from 15° to 30°C (59° to 86°F) (Gahart & Nazareno, 2004).

NURSING FAST FACT!

Do not force thawing by immersion in water baths or in a microwave oven.

Methods of Administration

Continuous Infusion

Continuous infusion occurs when large-volume parenteral solutions of 250 to 1000 mL of infusate are administered over 2 to 24 hours. Medications added to these large-volume infusates are administered continuously. Continuous infusion is used when a medication must be highly diluted, constant plasma concentrations of the drug maintained, or large volumes of fluids and electrolytes administered. Electronic infusion devices are used to ensure an accurate flow rate.

ADVANTAGES

- Admixture and bag changes can be performed every 8 to 24 hours.
- Constant serum levels of the drug are maintained.

DISADVANTAGES

- Monitoring the drug rate can be erratic if not electronically controlled.
- There is a higher risk of drug incompatibility problems.
- Accidental bolus infusion can occur if medication is not adequately mixed with the solution.

NURSING FAST FACT!

When adding medication to an infusion container, use single-dose vials instead of multiple-dose vials to decrease the potential for infection, complications, and medication errors.

AGE-RELATED CONSIDERATIONS: PEDIATRIC PATIENTS 11–2

Continuous infusions in pediatric patients should have inline volume-control chambers and be controlled by infusion pumps. No more than 1 to 2 hours' worth of solution should be placed in the chamber at any one time.

INS Standard. After an administration set is added, a solution or medication container must be infused or discarded within 24 hours. (INS, 2000, 73)

Intermittent Infusion

Intermittent infusion is any administration of a medication or an infusion that is not continuous. A medication is added to a small volume of fluid (25 to 250 mL) and infused over 15 to 90 minutes at intervals (Douglas & Hedrick, 2001). Types of intermittent infusions are piggybacked through the established pathway of the primary solution, simultaneous infusion, use of volume control set, and intermittent infusions through a locking device.

SECONDARY INFUSION THROUGH THE PRIMARY PATHWAY

A secondary I.V. line used intermittently is commonly called a piggyback set. Secondary infusion through an established pathway of the primary solution is the most common method for drug delivery by the intermittent route. A secondary set includes a small I.V. container, short administration set without ports, and a macrodrip system. The drug is diluted in 25 to 250 mL of 5 percent dextrose in water or 0.9 percent sodium chloride and administered over 15 to 90 minutes (Douglas & Hedrick, 2001). When infusing medications with this method, the secondary infusion is administered via the Y port with the backcheck valve on the primary administration set (Fig. 11–1A).

This Y port is located on the upper third of the primary line. Although the primary infusion is interrupted during the secondary infusion, the drug from the intermittent infusion container comes in contact with the primary solution below the injection port; therefore, the drug and the primary solution should be compatible. Electronic infusion devices may be used to maintain constant infusion rates and maintain accurate titration of drug dosages.

ADVANTAGES

- Risk of incompatibilities is reduced.
- Larger drug dose can be administered at a lower concentration per milliliter than with the I.V. push method.
- Peak flow concentrations occur at periodic intervals.
- There is a decreased risk of fluid overload.

DISADVANTAGES

- The administration rate may not be accurate unless electronically monitored.
- The high concentration of drug in the intermittent solution may cause venous irritation.
- I.V. set changes can result in wasting a portion of the drug.

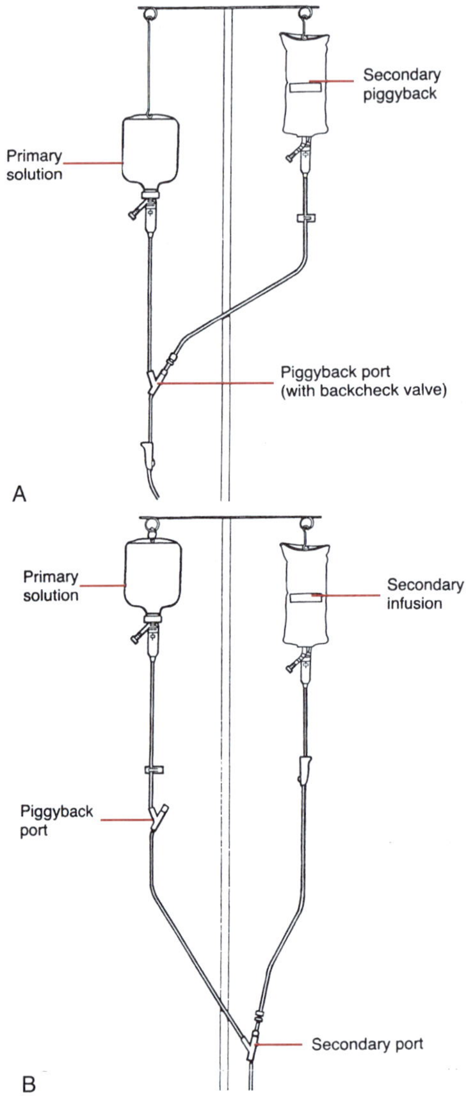

Figure 11–1 ■ Methods of delivery of secondary infusions. *(A)* Secondary piggyback infusion. *(B)* Simultaneous infusion.

- If the patient is not properly monitored, fluid overload or speed shock may result.
- Drug incompatibility can occur if the administration set is not adequately flushed between medication administrations.

INS Standard. When preparing solutions or medications for administration, single-use medication vials or ampules are recommended. The use of multiple-dose vials increases the potential for infection, complications, and medication errors. If multiple-dose vials are used, they should be labeled with date and time the vial is initially entered. (INS, 2000, 73)

NURSING FAST FACT!

Consider the volume of fluid delivered with a secondary infusion as part of the patient's overall intake when calculating intake.

SIMULTANEOUS INFUSION (PRIMARY AND SECONDARY)

Secondary infusions can be infused concurrently with the primary solution. Rather than connecting the intermittent infusion at the piggyback port (closest to the primary infusion bag), it is attached to the lower Y site (Fig. 11–1B). Disadvantages of administration of secondary concurrent with primary solution include the tendency for blood to back up into the tubing after the secondary infusion has been completed, causing occlusion of the venous access device and increased risk of drug incompatibility.

NURSING FAST FACT!

Drug incompatibility is a greater risk with the simultaneous infusion method.

VOLUME CONTROL CHAMBER

The volume control chamber method of intermittent delivery of medication is used most frequently with pediatric patients or when the delivery of a small amount of well-controlled drug needs to be administered to critical care patients. Medication is added to the volume control chamber and diluted with I.V. solution. The infusion is generally over 15 minutes to 1 hour. Volumes delivered vary from 25 to 150 mL per drug dose (Fig. 11–2).

ADVANTAGES

- Runaway infusions are avoided without the use of electronic infusion devices.
- The volume of fluid in which the drug is diluted can be adjusted.

DISADVANTAGES

- Medication must travel the length of the tubing before it reaches the patient, causing a significant time delay.
- A portion of the medication can be left in the tubing after the chamber empties.

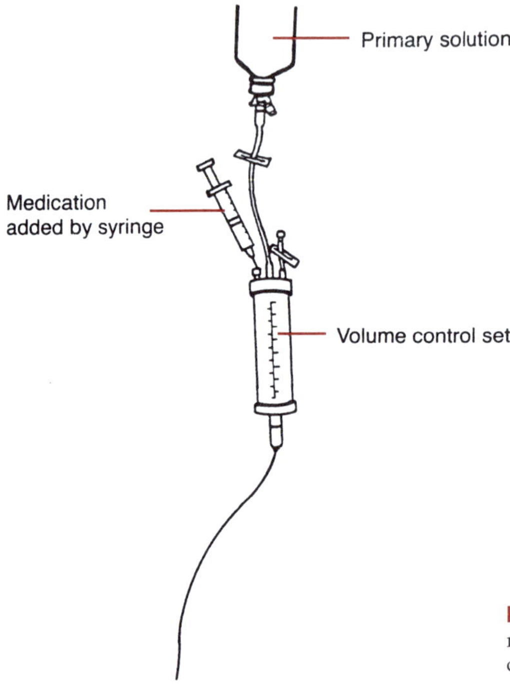

Figure 11–2 ■ Administration of medication via a volume control chamber.

- Incompatibilities may develop when the chamber, which is usually within the primary line, is used for multiple drug deliveries.
- Labeling of the chamber must coincide with the drug being delivered. If multiple drugs are delivered, this could present a problem.

Direct Injection (I.V. Push)

Intravenous push administration of a medication provides a method of administering high concentrations of medication. Administration through this route can be accomplished by direct venipuncuture, using a scalp vein infusion set or over-the-needle infusion device, or by access of low injection port of primary administration sets. The purpose is to achieve rapid serum concentrations. Refer to Procedures Display 11–1.

Direct injection requires that the drug be drawn into a syringe before administration or that the drug be available in a prefilled syringe. Needle protector or needle-free systems can be connected to the venous access device or used with administration sets to deliver the medication.

ADVANTAGES

- Barriers of drug absorption are bypassed.
- Drug response is rapid and usually predictable.
- The patient is closely monitored during the full administration of the medication.

PROCEDURES DISPLAY 11–1

Direct Administration (I.V. Push)

Verify the physician's order, educate the patient regarding the purpose of therapy, and document the procedure and any patient teaching that you may have performed. Wash hands and observe Standard Precautions.

Step 1. Check the compatibility of the drug with the primary solution (if drug is to be administered via a continuous infusion).
Step 2. Dilute opioid analgesics and follow the recommendation of the manufacturer for administration.
Step 3. Cleanse the lowest Y port if using primary line; or the resealable lock on the locking device with antiseptic solution. If the drug is incompatible with the primary solution, flush the catheter with 0.9 percent sodium chloride before and after administration of the medication (INS, 2000, 73).
Step 4. Insert the syringe into the medication port.
Step 5. Pinch the tubing to the primary solution if using primary line.
Step 6. Inject one fourth of the medication into the patient over a 15- to 20-second period.
Step 7. Observe the patient for any adverse effects.
Step 8. Repeat steps 5 to 7, delivering one fourth of the drug each time for three more times.
Step 9. When the entire desired drug is delivered, remove the syringe.

NURSING FAST FACTS!

Direct I.V. push method should take at least 1 minute; however, always follow the recommendations of the manufacturer for the delivery of the drug. For example, drugs such as phenytoin and diazepam must be delivered over a lengthy period of time; the manufacturer provides specific guidelines for administration.

Heparin is no longer routinely recommended for intermittent flushing of peripheral lines (Hadaway, 2003).

DISADVANTAGES

- Adverse effects occur at the same time and rate as therapeutic effects.
- The I.V. push method has the greatest risk of adverse effects and toxicity because serum drug concentrations are sharply elevated.
- Speed shock is possible from too-rapid administration of medication.

Adverse effects that can occur during administration of a medication directly into a vein include changes in the patient's level of consciousness, vital functions, and reflex activity. There may be an increased risk of phlebitis if a medication that is irritating to the vein is injected (Perdue, 2001).

NURSING FAST FACT!

If adverse effects occur, supportive care is the basis for treatment of most symptoms because specific antidotes are available for only certain drugs.

Continuous Subcutaneous Medication Administration

Continuous subcutaneous infusion is a practical and simple approach to pain management. Two factors that contribute to unsatisfactory pain management are (1) inadequate dosage and titration of available pain medications and (2) limited resources to properly educate and advise physicians and nurses on pain management. Patients who require parenteral narcotics are candidates for continuous subcutaneous infusion. This type of infusion therapy can be established for the following types of patients who require intermittent injection, usually longer than 48 hours:

- Patients unable to take medications by mouth
- Patients who require parenteral opioid analgesics but have poor venous access

Refer to Procedures Display 11–2.

ADVANTAGES

- Easy care for home management of pain
- Decreased number of times tissue is traumatized by repeated injections
- Better home management of pain, which decreases hospital time
- Decrease in central nervous system (CNS) side effects associated with intermittent drug therapy, such as nausea, vomiting, and drowsiness
- Decrease in pain breakthrough

DISADVANTAGES

- Local irritation at infusion site
- Rapidly escalating pain of dying patients requiring larger volumes of drug; this route is inappropriate for volumes larger than 1 mL/h

PROCEDURES DISPLAY 11–2

Administration of Continuous Subcutaneous Infusion (Hypodermoclysis)

Verify the physician's order, educate the patient regarding the purpose of therapy, and document the procedure and any patient teaching you may have performed. Wash hands, don gloves, and follow Standard Precautions.

Step 1. Establish baseline vital signs.
Step 2. Have the patient rate his or her pain on a scale of 1 to 10.
Step 3. Establish subcutaneous access per facility policy and use continuous infusion guidelines.
Step 4. Use a 27-gauge butterfly needle or a Soft-set (MiniMed Technologies) which is a 24-gauge catheter with a 26-gauge insertion needle and 42-inch microbore tubing attached to the infusion device, which can then be attached to a PCA pump. This system has a Luer-Lok hub. The tubing is made of polyolefin. Subcutaneous sites that can be used are the right or left subclavicular areas, the thighs, or the right, left or mid-abdomen, but not within two inches of the umbilicus (Gorski & Czaplewski, 2001).
Step 5. Prime tubing if needed.

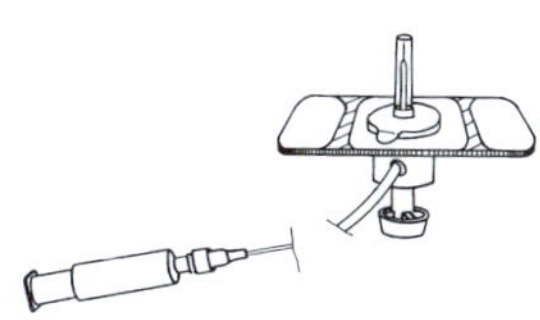

1. Fill syringe and Sof-set. TM

Step 6. Cleanse site with povidone-iodine or chlorhexidine swab stick.

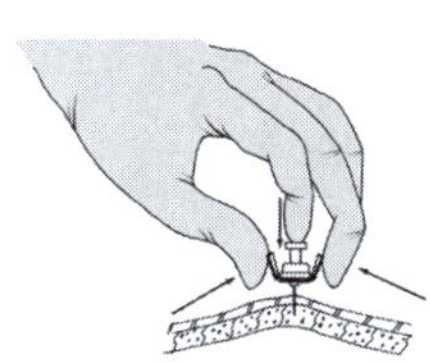

2. Cleanse and pinch skin.

(Continued on following page)

PROCEDURES DISPLAY 11–2

Administration of Continuous Subcutaneous Infusion (Hypodermoclysis) *(Continued)*

Step 7. Insert the 27-gauge butterfly needle at a 45-degree angle into the subcutaneous site. If using a Soft-set insert the needle perpendicular to the skin.

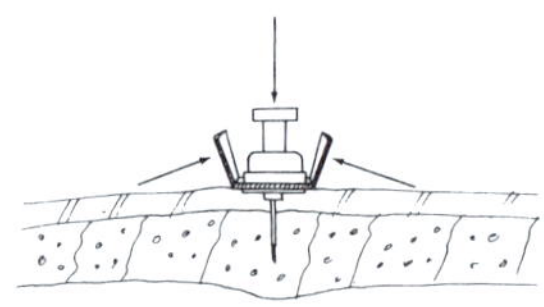

3. Insert needle.

Step 8. Stabilize the needle or catheter following manufacturer recommendations. Use a transparent dressing over the device to keep the insertion site visible.

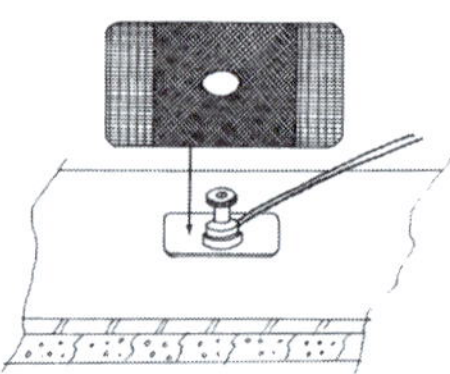

4. Place tape over Sof-set.™

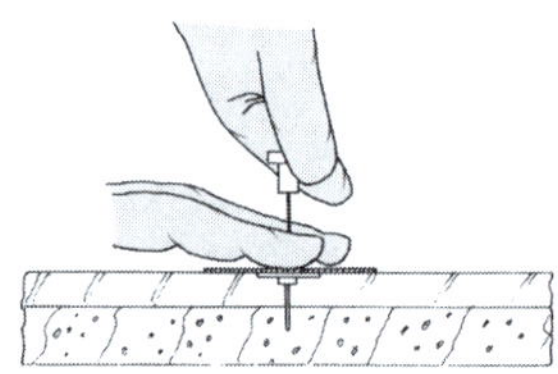

5. Remove introducer needle.

Step 9. Administer the prescribed bolus dose and immediately begin the continuous infusion at a rate not to exceed 3 mL/h. Electronic infusion devices should be considered when administering fluids and/or medications via the subcutaneous infusion route (INS, 2000, 69).

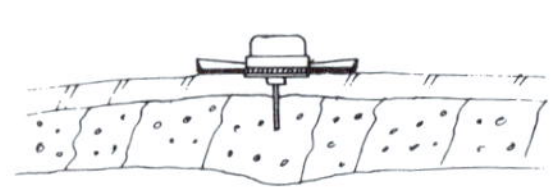

6. Begin pumping.

Step 10. Obtain vital signs and assess neurologic status and pain level every 30 minutes (four times) and as needed.

NURSING FAST FACT!

The character of the skin is important; the skin surface must be dry, and body hair may need to be clipped, not shaved. Use an adhesive bandage to secure subcutaneous device.

Figures courtesy of MiniMed Technologies, Sylmar, CA.

INS Standard. Rates higher than 3 mL/h should be defined by organizational policies and procedures. To reduce the risk of complications, the subcutaneous access site should be rotated a minimum of every 3 days or as clinically indicated. Consideration should be given to use of additives that enhance absorption and diffusion of the medication or solution. (INS, 2000, 69)

Intraperitoneal Medication Administration

An intraperitoneal catheter has been developed for the treatment of patients with intra-abdominal malignant tumors. A Tenckhoff dialysis catheter or port is surgically placed and chemotherapeutic agents are instilled directly into the intraperitoneal cavity. Access to the peritoneal cavity can be achieved through the use of a temporary catheter. Ovarian and colorectal cancers often have a high incidence of peritoneal seeding when a patient undergoes surgical treatment for intra-abdominal adenocarcinoma or sarcoma (Malloy, 2001). (The intraperitoneal route is discussed in further detail in Chapter 14.)

Intraosseous Medication Administration

Intraosseous infusion, or the administration of drugs or solutions through a needle inserted into the bone marrow of children younger than age 6 years, is common practice in the emergency room setting. This route is used when conventional routes cannot be used. Indications for the use of the intraosseous route include patients with extensive burns or trauma in whom diffuse edema causes difficult peripheral access; profound shock resulting in poor circulatory system; and combative behavior, making any catheter insertion difficult. (The intraosseous route is discussed in further detail in Chapter 10.)

Intraventricular Medication Administration

Intraventricular access sites using an Ommaya reservoir are used for:

1. The delivery of antifungal agents to treat fungal meningitis and brain abscesses
2. The delivery of antibacterial drugs for the treatment of chronic CNS infections
3. The delivery of chemotherapy for treatment of meningeal leukemia and neoplastic infiltration of the CNS
4. Intrathecal administration of methotrexate to patients who have primary intraocular lymphoma with CNS spread

5. Intractable pain control in patients with advanced head and neck cancer
6. Administration of medications through a temporary ventriculostomy to relieve rapid increases in intracranial pressure
7. In patients with unresectable tumors as a means to drain excessive fluid accumulation caused by cystic brain tumors
8. The regular intrathecal removal of cerebrospinal fluid (CSF) to monitor drug levels in patients receiving antibiotic therapy

The intraventricular route related to administration of chemotherapeutic agents is discussed in Chapter 14.

Intra-arterial Medication Administration

The intra-arterial route is used for the delivery of chemotherapy through the blood supply to a tumor. The arteries most commonly used are the hepatic artery (for colorectal metastasis to the liver), the celiac artery (for liver tumors), and the carotid artery (for tumors of the head, neck, and brain). The pelvic arteries have been used to infuse high concentration of antineoplastic medications to treat patients with advanced cervical cancer. (The intra-arterial route is discussed in Chapter 14.)

Pain Management

Pain management begins with complete assessment of the patient's pain, including location, intensity, quality, frequency, onset, duration, aggravating and alleviating factors, associated symptoms, and coping mechanisms. Pain perception and tolerance are highly individual responses. According to McCaffery and Pasero (1999), the definition of pain is "whatever the experiencing person says it is, existing whenever he says it does."

Many therapeutic approaches are available for pain including behavioral approaches, application of heat and cold, massage, physical therapy, management with narcotics and non-narcotics by oral, subcutaneous, or I.V. routes, neurosurgery, and anesthetics.

The American Pain Society (1999) has grouped analgesia into three types: opioids, non-opioids, and adjuvants. Opioids include agonists and antagonists. Non-narcotic analgesics, nonopioids, and nonsteroidal anti-inflammatory drugs (NSAIDs) provide relief of mild to moderate pain. Adjuvants are drugs that have additive or independent analgesic effects, such as antidepressants, anticonvulsants, neuroleptics, antihistamines, biphosphonates, and corticosteroids (McCaffery & Pasero, 1999).

The Joint Commission on Accreditation of Healthcare Organizations (JCAHO, 2001) standards integrate pain assessment and management into the JCAHO accreditation standards. The standards call on accredited hospitals, home care agencies, long-term care facilities, behavioral health facilities, outpatient clinics, and health plans to:

- Recognize the right of patients to appropriate assessment and management of their pain.
- Assess pain in all patients.
- Record the results of the assessment in a way that facilitates regular reassessment and follow-up.
- Educate relevant providers in pain assessment and management.
- Determine competency in pain assessment and management during the orientation of all new clinical staff.
- Establish policies and procedures that support appropriate prescription or ordering pain medications.
- Ensure that pain does not interfere with participation in rehabilitation.
- Educate patients and their families about the importance of effective pain management.
- Include the patient's needs for symptom management in the discharge planning process.

Opioid Analgesics

Parenteral opioids can be delivered by continuous infusion or by intermittent dosing. The routes for continuous infusion include the I.V., subcutaneous, and intraspinal (epidural or intrathecal) routes.

Nursing Points-of-Care: Opioid Medications

- All opioids are kept under double locks.
- The use of all opioid drugs must be recorded on a special record and on the client's chart.
- Lost or contaminated doses must be signed for by two nurses.
- Opioids are counted by two nurses, one from the oncoming shift and one from the departing shift. Both nurses sign the record (Pasero, 2002).
- The nurse must be aware of the hospital policy for stop time on opioid orders (Reiss & Evans, 2002).

Continuous Infusion

Morphine is the narcotic most commonly used for continuous infusion for pain management. Continuous infusions lead to a continuous level of pain control without the peaks of side effect development and the troughs of breakthrough pain. A smaller amount of the drug is generally needed to prevent the recurrence of the pain. Continuous infusions of opioids are appropriately used in trauma, postsurgical, and terminal care settings.

Intermittent Dosing (Patient-Controlled Analgesia)

The concept of patient-controlled analgesia (PCA) began in 1970. PCA is a pain management strategy that allows a patient to self-administer I.V. narcotic pain medication by pressing a button that is attached to a computerized pump. Patients may receive intermittent doses of narcotics when they state that the pain is episodic. It is desirable to treat pain only when experienced, with fast-acting narcotics that are effective for short periods. The goal of PCA is to provide the patient with a serum analgesia level for comfort with minimal sedation. Putting patients in charge of their own pain management makes sense because only the patient knows how much he or she is suffering.

It is more desirable to use small doses of narcotics frequently than large doses of narcotics infrequently.

Nursing Points-of-Care: Patient-Controlled Analgesia

- Patient-controlled analgesia is a philosophy of treatment, rather than a single method of drug administration.
- A pump infuser can be used to administer intravenous bolus doses of analgesics for the relief of acute pain.
- When patient-controlled analgesia is used, the nurse retains responsibility for assessing the patient's level of comfort and for addressing the deficient knowledge related to this method of pain relief.
- Patient-controlled analgesia has been shown to be both safe and effective in relieving pain (Reiss & Evans, 2002).

Candidates for whom PCA should be considered include:

1. Patients who are anticipating pain that is severe yet intermittent (e.g., patients suffering from kidney stones)
2. Patients who have constant pain that worsens with activity
3. Pediatric patients who are older than age 7 years who are capable of being taught to manage the PCA machine
4. Patients who are capable of manipulating the dose button
5. Patients who are motivated to use PCA

(Continued on following page)

Key concepts of PCA include:

1. In the first 24 hours after surgery, the patient has the greatest need for pain control.
2. Studies have shown that the best results for PCA occur when the patient can administer a bolus every 5 to 10 minutes.
3. When patients have control of their opioid doses, they will keep the opioid within therapeutic levels.
4. When patients are in control and know they can get more immediate pain relief by pushing a button, they are more relaxed.
5. Analgesia is most effective when a therapeutic serum level is consistently maintained.
6. Postoperative patients can easily titrate doses according to need and avoid peaks and troughs associated with conventional I.V. and intramuscular administration of opioid.
7. Studies have found that orthopedic patients seemed more tolerant of repositioning when on PCA.
8. Patients with abdominal surgery ambulate sooner after surgery.
9. Patients whose pain is controlled are better able to cough and deep breathe.

Websites

American Academy of Pain Management: *www.aapainmanage.org*
American Pain Society: *www.ampainsoc.org*

Other sites:

Epidural and Intrathecal Medication Administration

Anatomy of the Epidural and Intrathecal Spaces

The spinal anatomy consists of two spaces, the **epidural** space and the **intrathecal** space. **Intraspinal** is the term used to encompass both the epidural and intrathecal spaces surrounding the spinal cord. The intrathecal space is surrounded by the epidural space and separated from it by the dura mater; the intrathecal space contains cerebrospinal fluid (CSF), which bathes the spinal cord. The epidural and intrathecal spaces share a common center, the spinal cord. The epidural space surrounds the spinal cord and intrathecal space and lies between the ligamentum flavum and the dura mater. This is a potential space because the ligamentum flavum and the dura mater are not separated until medication or air is injected between them. This potential space contains a network of veins that are large and thin walled and has a strong leukocytic activity to reduce the risk of infection. Dividing epidural and intrathecal spaces is a tough, fatty membrane called the dura. The dura's permeability is important in determining how fast epidural drugs cross into the intrathecal space and how long they remain there to be active. The epidural space also contains fat in proportion to a person's body fat. Opiate receptor sites are cells contained in the dorsal horn of the spinal cord, at which point opioids combine with their respective receptor site to generate analgesia.

Local anesthetic agents are frequently used with opioids, and are instrumental in controlling pain and reducing postoperative complications. When a patient experiences acute pain, the sympathetic system (part of the autonomic nervous system) is activated, increasing the workload of the heart. When intraspinal local anesthetic agents are administered, a sympathetic block results, which produces a decrease in blood pressure, pulse, and respirations. The advantages of adding local anesthetic agents to an epidural opioid are that it produces a sympathetic block, resulting in decreased workload on the heart, and decreases the incidence of thrombophlebitis and paralytic ileus (St. Marie, 2001).

Epidural Medication Administration

The epidural route can be used for acute, chronic, and cancer pain management. There are various approaches to the administration of narcotics by the epidural route: a single-bolus injection of opioid or local anesthetic, a continuous infusion of opioid with or without local anesthetics, or a continuous infusion of opioid with a patient-activated bolus.

A single injection of epidural opioid may be used for procedures that produce a short course of postoperative pain. This method may be appropriate for a patient having a cesarean section or vaginal hysterectomy, or same-day surgical procedures. Care must be taken to avoid the inadvertent administration of additional opioids by another route that may oversedate the patient, causing respiratory depression. Continuous epidural infusion is administered for short or long periods of time. Patients with pain from surgery, trauma, and acute medical disorders creating severe pain may benefit from short-term continuous infusions. This method can also be employed for the cancer patient with acute exacerbation of pain. Epidural pain control can be safely administered by patient control in the postoperative setting. This allows the patient to administer medications beyond their low infusion rate to accommodate pain.

See Figure 11–3 for various methods of epidural administration.

External Catheters

A temporary or permanent epidural catheter may be used externally for a short period. A temporary catheter is used from 3 days up to 1 week. Manufacturers do not guarantee a temporary catheter's integrity for long-term use. An advantage of the temporary catheter is its ease and speed of insertion. A disadvantage is that it cannot be easily secured.

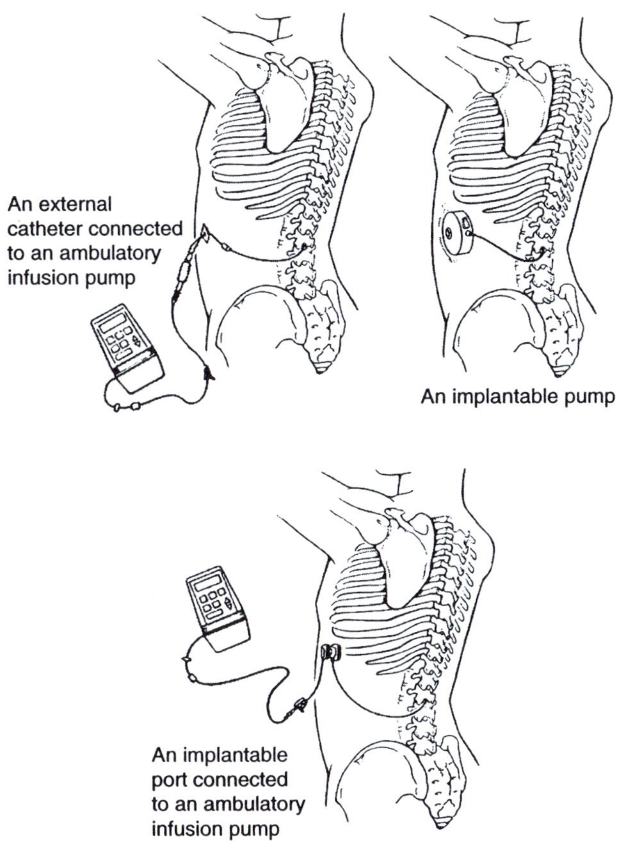

Figure 11–3 ■ Methods of epidural administration. (Courtesy of Deltec, Inc., St. Paul, MN.)

Permanent epidural catheter use for long-term therapy threads between the spinous processes and is tunneled subcutaneously until it exits around the rib, where it can be intermittently accessed. An advantage to the permanent external catheter is the length of dwell time. Permanent epidural catheters have been left in place and functional or more than a year (St. Marie, 2001).

Internal Catheters

The epidural catheter connected subcutaneously to an implanted port has the advantage in that it is under the skin and cannot be easily dislodged. There are no external components to trail bacteria into the epidural space. The disadvantage of the portal system for patients who have continuous infusion is that the metal needle may be irritating to the skin or become dislodged.

Common Epidural Medications

Medications commonly administered through the epidural route include:

- Preservative-free morphine (Astromorph and Duramorph)
- Sublimaze (Fentanyl)
- Sufentanil (Sufenta)
- Bupivacaine (Marcaine)
- Lidocaine
- Tetracaine

NURSING FAST FACTS!

- *Adding epinephrine increases the duration of lidocaine and tetracaine by 50 percent (Kreger, 2001).*
- *Preservatives in narcotics or local anesthetics used in the epidural or intrathecal space need to be avoided to prevent nerve damage.*
- *Preservative-free morphine, which is water soluble and has a slower onset of action and longer duration of action, therefore is a better choice for patients who need more prolonged analgesia. Lipid-soluble fentanyl and sufentanil penetrate the dura mater faster than water-soluble opioids, providing a faster onset of action but a shorter duration of action (Kreger, 2001).*

Advantages of Epidural Medication Administration

- Permits control or alleviation of severe pain without the sedative effects
- Permits delivery of smaller doses of a narcotic to achieve desired level of analgesia
- Prolongs the analgesia (average about 14 hours)

- Allows for continuous infusion, if needed
- Allows terminal cancer patients treated with epidural narcotics to be more comfortable and mobile
- Can be used for short-term or long-term therapy
- Does not produce motor paralysis or hypotension

Disadvantages of Epidural Medication Administration

- Nurses' lack of understanding of pharmacologic agents; nurses must be educated in the use of these agents.
- Only preservative-free opioids can be used.
- Complications such as paresthesia, urinary retention, and respiratory depression (greatest 6 to 10 hours after injection) can occur.
- Catheter-related risks (e.g., infection, dislodgement, and leaking) can occur.
- Pruritus can occur on the face, head, and neck or may be generalized.
- Unless the epidural catheter and medication are clearly labeled, an intravenous infusion could be inadvertently given via the intraspinal route which could cause serious complications or death (St. Marie, 2001).

INS Standard. Placement of an epidural catheter, port, or pump is a medical act. Administration of medication by a registered nurse (RN) shall be in accordance with the state Nurse Practice Act. (INS, 2000, 67)

NURSING FAST FACT!

Ineffective pain control should be reported to the physician or anesthesiologist who is managing care of the epidural catheter.

INS Standard. The epidural device should be aspirated to ascertain the absence of spinal fluid before administration of medication. (INS, 2000, 67)

Monitoring

A flowsheet (Fig. 11–4) should be used to monitor the patient's response to epidural medication. This allows tracking of the patient's analgesia and any side effects. Included on the flow sheet are the following items:

- Evaluation of mental status
- Respiratory status
- Indication of numbness in the lower extremities
- Signs of infection
- Bowel function

Nursing Points-of-Care: Epidural Catheter Management

The insertion of the epidural catheter is a sterile procedure and is a function performed by a physician or anesthesiologist. Administration of medication by a nurse through an epidural catheter must be in accordance with each state's Nurse Practice Act. Nursing responsibilities include: (1) patient and family education, (2) site and dressing management, (3) medication administration (depending on State Practice Acts), and (4) evaluation of pain relief.

Key points in epidural catheter management include:

1. Avoid the use of preservatives (mainly alcohol, phenol, sodium metabisulfite) in medications because they have a destructive effect on neural tissue.
2. After insertion, lay the exposed catheter length cephalad along the spine and over the shoulder.
3. Tape the entire length of the exposed catheter in place to provide stability and protection. The end of the catheter and the filter are generally placed on the patient's chest wall and taped securely in a position that allows the patient or family member to access the catheter for use.
4. To prevent particulate matter from infusing into the spinal fluid, a 0.2-micron surfactant-free inline filter should always be used when accessing any intraspinal catheter (INS, 2000, 62).
5. Clearly label the epidural catheter after placement to prevent accidental infusion of fluids or medications.
6. Understand the lipid and water solubility properties of the drugs being administered. (This better prepares the nurse to work with patients receiving epidural or intrathecal analgesic agents through the various methods of administration.)
7. Evaluate the effects of the drug on the patient's alertness; caregivers should also be taught to observe for levels of sedation.
8. Site care must be done carefully to avoid dislodgement of the catheter.
9. Alcohol must not be used on the skin or on the hub of the catheter since alcohol has neurotoxic effects.

- Bladder function
- Integrity of the epidural system
- Narcotic dose
- Patient's pain rating
- Site care

Refer to Procedures Display 11–3.

ENLOE
MEDICAL CENTER

EPIDURAL FLOWSHEET
INTERMITTENT OR CONTINUOUS INFUSION

DATE ________________ MEDICATION ______________________________

EDUCATION: CHART ON BACK OF FLOW SHEET

1) INTERMITTENT INJECTIONS: VS Q 15" X 2 THEN Q 4 HOURS
2) CONTINUOUS INFUSION: VS Q 15" X 2 THEN Q 4 HOURS
A) RESP., SEDATION LEVEL, MOTOR RESPONSE, DERMATOMES (ANESTHETICS) Q 1 HOUR X 4, THEN Q 2 HOURS X 24 HOURS. CONTINUE AT EVERY 4 HOURS.

FOR ANY INFUSION RATE CHANGE RETURN TO INITIAL ASSESSMENT FREQUENCIES

TIME															
TEMPERATURE															
BLOOD PRESSURE															
PULSE															
RESPIRATIONS: RATE															
DEPTH / QUALITY															
SEDATION LEVEL/RAP SCORE															
PAIN SCALE															
SITE ASSESS .Q8°															
MOTOR RESPONSE NO DEFICIT															
DERMATOMES LEVEL/RESPONSE															
PT C/O															
INTERVENTIONS															
INITIALS															

ASSESS PAIN Q 4 HOURS FOR ALL TYPES OF EPIDURAL ANALGESIA

RAP (Revised Aldrete Protocol): Add all 3 columns for total score

	LOC	**RESP**	**S & M**
2 =	Awake & oriented	Normal resp. & awake	Full function X 4
1.5 =	Drowsy & oriented or awake	Normal respiration & asleep	Full motor return with nearly complete sensory return
1 =	Responds to verbal stimuli	Labored respiration oral or nasal airway	Sensory & motor block with decreasing levels
.5 =	Responds only to noxious stimuli	N/A	N/A
0 =	Non-responsive	Apnea or ET tube	No spontaneous movement or sensory motor block with stable level

PT C/O
A. Circumoral tingling
B. Muscle twitching
C. "Metallic" taste/tinnitus
D. Nausea
E. Urinary Retention
F. Breakthrough Pain
G. Blurred Vision
H. Epidural Site Pain
I. Itching
J. Light Headedness
K. None

PAIN
0 – 10 scale
0 – no pain
10 – worst pain

RESPIRATIONS: DEPTH / QUALITY
Regular
Unlabored
Deep
Irregular
Labored
Shallow

DERMATOMES
(Anesthetics only)

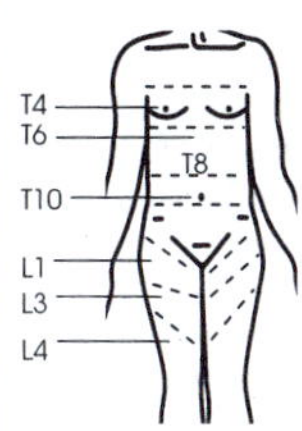

INTERVENTIONS
1. Cont. Pulse Ox
2. Position Checked
3. Line and Bag Changed
4. Dressing Changed
5. Dose Increased
6. Dose Decreased
7. Med for Breakthrough Pain
8. See MAR
9. See Nurses Notes

Signatures
(07–15) ______________________
(15–23) ______________________
(23–07) ______________________

Addressograph

Figure 11–4 ■ Example of continuous or intermittent epidural flowsheet. (Courtesy of Enloe Medical Center, Chico, CA.)

INS Standards. Mask and sterile gloves are worn for access and maintenance procedures (INS, 2000, 67). A 0.2-micron filter without surfactant should be utilized for medication administration. (INS, 2000, 67).

Dressing Management of Epidural Catheters

Temporary epidural catheters should be handled carefully during the site care because they are easily dislodged. Permanent external epidural

PROCEDURES DISPLAY 11–3

Administration of Medication via an Epidural Catheter

Verify the physician's order, educate the patient regarding the purpose of therapy, and document the procedure, including any patient teaching you may have performed. Wash hands, don mask and gloves, use aseptic technique, and follow Standard Precautions.

Step 1. Verify patient identity. Check the anesthesiologist's order, narcotic dosage, and route. Ensure that naloxone (Narcan) or ephedrine is readily available. Double check for correct medication (preservative-free diluent), dose, and route before administration.

Step 2. Verify that the estimated level of the catheter tip and the initial dose are documented by the anesthesiologist. Mark the catheter/port/pump, administration tubing, and infusion pumps clearly to prevent accidental injections of medications through the epidural catheter/port/pump.

Step 3. Inform the patient of the procedure.

Step 4. Assemble the equipment; wash hands with antimicrobial cleanser.

Step 5. Complete a patient assessment including inspection of the catheter site for signs of injection and cerebral spinal fluid drainage; pain level; baseline vital signs; response to previous injection; and urinary bladder fullness. Observe exit site for redness, cerebrospinal fluid drainage, swelling, or pain.

Step 6. Secure the entire hub apparatus by sandwiching with transpore tape.

Step 7. Draw up the dose into a 10-mL or larger size syringe using a filter needle.

Step 8. Attach pulse oximetry monitor to the patient.

Step 9. Don gloves, scrub the injection port with antimicrobial swab, and allow 2 minutes of contact time. Wipe with sterile 2 × 2 gauze to remove any excess antimicrobial solution.

Step 10. Enter the injection cap using a noncoring needle attached to a 10-mL empty syringe. Gently aspirate to verify catheter location by observing that less than 1 mL of clear fluid returns.

NURSING FAST FACT!

If the aspirate is blood, blood-tinged fluid, or greater than 1 mL of fluid, notify the anesthesiologist and do not continue the procedure. Save the aspirated fluid.

(Continued on following page)

Step 11. Rescrub the injection cap with a antimicrobial solution without alcohol for 20 seconds. Wipe with a sterile 2 × 2 gauze to remove any excess solution. Enter the injection port with the 10-mL syringe that contains the prescribed preservative-free analgesia through a 0.22-μm filter, surfactant-free. Slowly inject the narcotic at a rate of approximately 5 mL/min.
Step 12. Check the catheter cap and hub assembly connection for fluid leakage.
Step 13. Closely monitor the patient's vital signs, and pain level every 15 minutes for 2 hours, then every 4 hours.
Step 14. Document initial and ongoing assessments in the nurses' notes; any changes in the patient's condition; all communication with the physician; and education provided to the patient.

NURSING FAST FACT!

Have naloxone (Narcan) available, 0.4 mg, to treat respiratory depression or increased sedation.

catheters require dressing changes. Permanent epidural catheters have a Dacron cuff that acts as a protective barrier against bacterial migration and secures the catheter placement.

The frequency with which epidural catheter dressings should be changed is dependent on the dressing material, age and condition of the patient, infection rate reported by the organization, environmental conditions, and manufacturer's guidelines (INS, 2000, 67). During the dressing change, the nurse must carefully stabilize the epidural catheter. This is a sterile procedure.

1. Wash hands with antimicrobial soap and water. Don gloves.
2. Secure the temporary catheter close to the exit site with a piece of tape. Remove old dressing. Use a cotton ball soaked in sterile water to assist in lifting the edge of dressing.
3. Don sterile gloves. Apply antimicrobial solution without alcohol in a circular motion, starting at the exit site and working outward. Allow the solution to air dry.
4. Apply a new dressing, gauze or transparent, making sure that the catheter is well secured and cannot dislodge accidentally.
5. The catheter should be coiled near the insertion site to prevent accidental dislodgement.
6. Document the dressing change, reporting the inspection of the exit site and how the patient tolerated the procedure (St. Marie, 2001).

NURSING FAST FACT!

Do not use alcohol on skin or at dressing site because of the risk of migration of alcohol into the epidural space and the possibility of neural damage.

Complications Associated with Epidural Pain Management

Side effects of epidural opioid are excessive somnolence and confusion, nausea, vomiting, urinary retention, and pruritus. Urinary retention is a common side effect and may occur 10 to 20 hours after the first injection of intraspinal narcotic. This may require either administration of bethanecol (Urecholine) or intermittent catheterization. Pruritus is caused by the opiate's interacting with the dorsal horn and not by a histamine release. This is best treated with an antagonist rather than with diphenhydramine (Benadryl). After an epidural injection, 8.5 percent of all patients experience pruritus; after an intrathecal injection, 46 percent experience pruritus.

Complications are not common, however, they may arise from several sources. Patients may have a reaction or side effect to the medication being administered or a problem resulting from the placement or displacement of the catheter.

Conditions requiring **immediate** physician notification include:

- Inadequate pain relief. This can occur for three reasons: epidural catheter migration, insufficient dosages of opioid and local anesthetics, and undetermined surgical complication.
- Respiratory depression from epidural or intrathecal narcotic administration. Vital signs should be assessed and naloxone should be available to reverse the depressant effects of a narcotic.
- Extreme dizziness as a result of inadequate orthostatic hypotension or excessive opioid effect
- New onset of paresthesia or paresis
- Difficulty or inability to infuse epidural medication
- Pain at the insertion site
- Displacement or migration of the epidural catheter. Catheter migration may occur in two ways: (1) the catheter may migrate through the dura mater into the intrathecal space, creating an overdose of opioid, or (2) the catheter may migrate into an epidural vein or subcutaneous space, creating inadequate pain relief.
- Infections. These are rare from epidural catheters, but precautions should be instituted to keep the catheter insertion process and exit site sterile. If an infection develops elsewhere in the body, the patient should be evaluated for removal of the epidural catheter (St. Marie, 2001).
- Excessive drowsiness or confusion occurring when too much narcotic is being administered. This is usually improved by decreasing

the amount of epidural narcotic infusion. Titrating an opioid antagonist, such as naloxone (Narcan), 0.2 mg I.V., or an agonist/antagonist, such as nalbuphine (Nubain), 5 to 10 mg subcutaneously, may reverse side effects without eliminating the analgesia (St. Marie, 2001).

- Signs and symptoms of coagulopathies
- Inability to remove the catheter
- Circumoral tingling
- Tremulousness
- Tinnitus
- Metallic taste
- Ascending loss of sensation in patients receiving an anesthetic medication

Other complications that may not warrant immediate physician notification but need to be reported at the earliest convenience include the inability to urinate and pruritus, which may be treated with parenterally administered medication while the epidural infusion continues.

NURSING FAST FACT!

If catheter migration is suspected, the physician should be notified and the placement check should be verified by an anesthesiologist.

Intrathecal Medication Administration

Intrathecal opioid infusions can be considered for cancer patients who have a life expectancy of more than a few months; who do not receive adequate pain relief with systemic narcotics, tricyclic antidepressants, or NSAIDs; and who have pain located below the midcervical dermatomes. Intrathecal narcotic infusions require an implanted infusion pump, not an external pump, because of the risk of infection (St. Marie, 2001).

The intrathecal injection of an opioid requires approximately 10 times **less** medication than is needed in the epidural space. The intrathecal space, however, is associated with a greater risk for infection.

Intrathecal opioids given as a single injection are commonly used for postoperative pain management, for cesarean surgeries, vaginal hysterectomies, and some orthopedic surgeries.

ADVANTAGES

- There is no external catheter creating a risk of dislodgement or infection.
- Prolonged analgesia is offered.
- The catheter is relatively simple to access.

DISADVANTAGES

- High levels of pain may be experienced as the opioid wears off.
- Respiratory depression may occur.
- The risk of infection is greater than that with epidural delivery due to cerebrospinal fluid is a good medium for bacterial growth.
- Spinal headache (3 days) may occur, especially in young women.

Guidelines for monitoring, site care, and managing complications and side effects are the same as those for epidural infusions.

Implanted Pumps

Implantable infusion pump technology is available as a specialty of anesthesiology and neurosurgery. Infusion pumps technology varies, some pumps may be programmed from outside the body by using a laptop computer with a telemetry device that can be placed over the implanted pump. Refer to Figure 11–5.

Another type of implanted infusion pump may provide a set rate of opioid infusion, and as the concentration of the opioid is changed inside the pump, the dosage the patient receives is changed and the rate stays the same. Design features of an implanted pump include a pump reservoir designed to continuously infuse a specific volume of medication over a specific period of time. A pump access kit is used specificly to access the septum on the port using aseptic technique. The implanted pump is

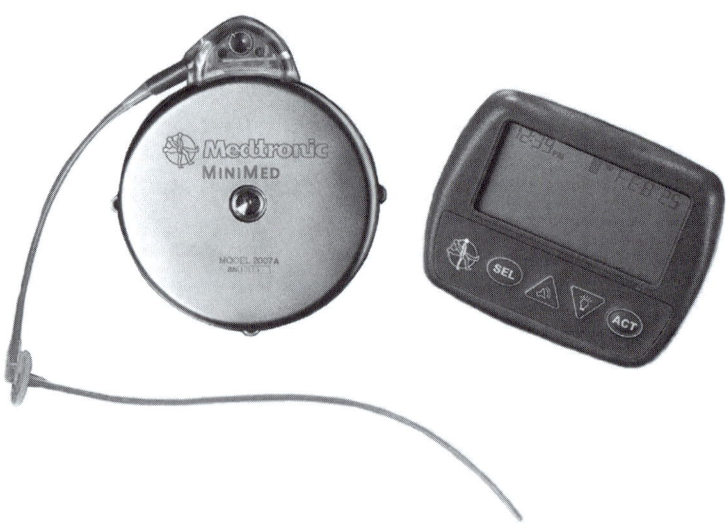

Figure 11–5 ■ Implantable infusion pump, programmable from outside the body. (Courtesy of Medtronic MiniMed, Northridge, CA.)

accessed with a noncoring (Huber) needle and any remaining drug in the pump is removed by aspirating with a syringe. The new medication is then injected into the pump and the needle is removed. A sterile occlusive dressing should be placed over the noncoring needle.

ADVANTAGES

- Risk of infection is low.
- The catheter can be placed epidurally or intrathecally.
- Pump reservoir holds 10 to 20 mL of fluid; refills are required only every 1 to 3 months.
- Infusion rates can be changed either by computer or by changing the concentration of the medication.

DISADVANTAGES

- The initial cost of the equipment is high.
- The complexity of the technology requires healthcare professionals who can adapt well to computer technology and internal pump access.
- Each fill necessitates a needlestick.
- There are concerns about long-term epidural or intrathecal infusions within the spinal canal.
- The life of the pump may be shorter than the patient's life expectancy; it may have to be surgically replaced (St. Marie, 2001).

More research is needed to document outcomes over long periods of implantable pump use.

Special Drug Administration Considerations

Anti-Infectives

Before administering antibiotic, antifungal, and antiviral agents intravenously, it is essential to understand the pharmacotherapeutics related to these drugs. Manufacturer recommendations for administration should be followed carefully. Anti-infectives are administered to achieve therapeutic coverage based on culture and sensitivity reports.

Key Questions

1. Has the infecting organism been identified (suspected or confirmed by culture)?
2. Is the organism resistant to any antimicrobials?
3. Is the site of infection identified?
4. What is the status of the host (patient) defenses?
5. Is the nurse familiar with the antimicrobial pharmacokinetics?

6. What is the status of the patient's renal and hepatic function?
7. Is monitoring the patient's blood levels necessary to avoid toxicity of dosage?
8. Does the patient have an allergy to the anti-infective agent?

Antibiotics

The action of antibiotics is bacteriostatic, inhibiting bacterial cell wall synthesis and producing a defective cell wall, or bactericidal, altering intracellular function of the bacteria. Knowledge of each antibiotic administered is essential for safe delivery of the medication.

Nursing Points-of-Care: Antibiotics

1. Be knowledgeable of the antibiotic ordered, its normal dosage, side effects, and compatibilities, and the purpose of the antibiotic in treatment of the patient's infection.
2. Be sure the drug has not expired.
3. Be familiar with reconstitution, dilution, and storage information.
4. Correctly label the admixture with drug name, concentration, diluent, date, time, and initials.
5. Be familiar with potential adverse effects of the drug, including properties such as pH and osmolarity, that can cause irritation of the vein (INS, 2001).
6. Use strict aseptic technique throughout administration.
7. Be aware that the drug must be delivered at specified times to ensure maintenance of the proper drug levels and to identify therapeutic, subtherapeutic, and toxic drug levels.
8. Use assessment skills to monitor functions of the organ or organs that metabolize the antibiotic.
9. Evaluate the patient every shift for sensitivity to the drug.
10. Be prepared to respond to anaphylaxis.

Antifungals

The method of action of antifungal agents is injury to the cell wall of the fungi. The drugs in this classification are specifically targeted for fungi. Antifungals administered by the I.V. route are amphotericin B, caspoifungin acetate, fluconozol, and itraconazole (Gahart & Nazareno, 2004).

Nursing Points-of-Care: Antifungals

- Most antifungals are infused as a suspension.
- These agents should not be filtered.
- These agents should be administered slowly over 2 to 6 hours.
- Never reconstitute amphotericin with saline or water containing a bacteriostatic agent.
- Use only sterile water for injection.
- I.V. amphotericin should be added to infusions of dextrose and water only.
- Monitor the vital signs and intake and output of all clients receiving antifungal infusions.
- Observe the client for fever, nausea, chills, and headaches and for hypokalemia if the client is receiving amphotericin.
- Observe site for phlebitis (Reiss & Evans, 2002).

Antivirals

Antiviral agents are selectively toxic to viruses. A safe, broad-spectrum antiviral drug has yet to be discovered. Most chemicals administered by the I.V. route to combat virus growth are antimetabolites or are related to the antimetabolites used in treating malignant tumors. These drugs tend to be toxic and usefulness is limited. They are administered in selected situations. For all antivirals, avoid use in patients with a previous hypersensitivity reaction. Use cautiously in patients with renal impairment, in pregnant patients, and in children. Antiviral agents that are infused by the I.V. route include acyclovir, cidofovir, foscarnet, ganciclovir, and zidovudine (Gahart & Nazareno, 2004).

Nursing Points-of-Care: Antivirals

- Monitor I.V. site for phlebitis.
- Fatal complications may occur in immunocompromised clients.
- With cidofovir, a full course of probenecid and I.V. saline prehydration must be taken with each dose.
- Zidovudine must be administered around the clock, and multiple drug interactions can occur.

Investigational Drugs

Administration of investigational medications shall be in accordance with state and federal regulations. Signed informed patient consent is required before patient participation in the investigation.

Investigational drugs are defined as medications that are not approved for general use by the Food and Drug Administration (FDA). Many **clinical trials** are conducted as a form of planned experiment that evoke appropriate treatment of future patients with a given medical condition. Clinical trials are designed to discover a drug's efficacy in selected patient populations.

Following are the phases of FDA drug studies:

Phase I: Clinical pharmacology and therapeutics

- Researchers test a new drug or treatment in a small group of people (20 to 80) for the first time to evaluate its safety, determine a safe dosage range, and identify side effects.
- Determine an acceptable single drug dosage for levels of patient tolerance for acute multiple dosing.

Phase II: Initial clinical investigation for therapeutic effect

- Evaluate drug efficacy.
- Conduct a pilot study.
- The study drug or treatment is given to a larger group of people (100 to 300) to see if it is effective and to further evaluate its safety.

Phase III: Full-scale evaluation of treatment

- The study drug or treatment is given to large groups of people (1,000 to 3,000) to confirm its effectiveness, monitor side effects, compare it to commonly used treatments, and collect information that will allow the drug or treatment to be used safely.
- Evaluate the patient population for which the drug is intended.

Phase IV: Postmarketing surveillance

- Postmarketing studies delineate additional information including the drug's risks, benefits, and optimal use.

The role of the registered nurse in investigational drugs is to assist the investigator (physician) in conducting the study.

Key points in the role of the nurse in investigational drugs include:

1. Assisting patients to find clinical trials
2. Communicating with the Institutional Review Board (IRB); being familiar with their policies and federal regulations. (Copies of communication between the investigator and the IRB should be given to the sponsor.)
3. Ensuring signed informed consent. Explaining to patient, and obtaining signature, validating the patient's understanding of the goals, risks, and benefits

4. Communicating with the hospital's legal counsel and ethics committee to complete protocols
5. Making sure the patient is eligible to receive the study drug
6. Basic knowledge of the drug's indication, desired pharmacologic response, route of administration, precautions, and common adverse events
7. Administering the investigational drug by the I.V. route (or as indicated)
8. Monitoring for any adverse reactions to the study drug
9. Participating in collection of data
10. Assisting with blood and/or urine sampling when required
11. Assisting with final study report, which is a requirement of the U.S. federal regulations for the sponsor (Brown, 2001)

General ethical requirements of clinical research worldwide are outlined in the Declaration of Helsinki, issued by the World Medical Association in 1960 and revised in 1975. This document has been accepted internationally as the basis for ethical research.

NURSING PLAN OF CARE

ADMINISTRATION OF I.V. MEDICATIONS

Focus Assessment

Subjective

- Review present illness.
- Review current drug therapy.
- Review previous drug therapy and side effects.
- Review lifestyle for home care.
- Note any allergies before starting medication.

Objective

- Observe the patient's ability to ingest and retain fluids.
- Assess vital signs.
- Weigh the patient.
- Assess patient-related factors that may alter the patient's response to drug, such as age or renal, liver, and cardiovascular function.
- Assess current medications for clues to drug interaction and incompatibility.

Patient Outcome/Evaluation Criteria

Patient will:

- Respond therapeutically to the drug.
- Demonstrate improved fluid balance.

(Continued on following page)

NURSING PLAN OF CARE

ADMINISTRATION OF I.V. MEDICATIONS *(Continued)*

- Verbalize understanding of the purpose of the medication.
- Demonstrate absence of complications associated with I.V. therapy.
- Rate pain on scale of 1 to 2 while receiving patient-controlled analgesia
- Demonstrate early ambulation.

Nursing Diagnoses

- Altered health maintenance related to limited skills of family members with I.V. medications
- Anxiety (mild, moderate, and severe) related to threat to or change in health status; misconceptions regarding therapy
- Diarrhea related to side effects of medication
- Impaired physical mobility related to pain and discomfort resulting from placement and maintenance of I.V. catheters
- Risk for injury related to altered electrolyte balance resulting from drug administration
- Fluid volume deficit related to inadequate oral intake secondary to nausea and vomiting
- Impaired tissue integrity related to adverse reaction to medication

Nursing Management

1. Develop and use an environment that maximizes safe and efficient administration of medications.
2. Follow the six rights of medication administration.
3. Verify the prescription or medication order before administering the drug.
4. Select the appropriate sizes of syringes and needles.
5. Determine the correct dilution, amount, and length of administration time as appropriate.
6. Monitor for:
   a. drug infusion at regular intervals.
   b. irritation, infiltration, and inflammation at the infusion site.
   c. therapeutic range of drug levels.
   d. therapeutic response.
   e. renal function for adequate excretion of drug through the kidneys.
   f. allergies, drug interactions, and drug incompatibilities.
   g. intake and output.
   h. need of pain relief medications, as needed.
7. Maintain I.V. access.
8. Administer drugs at selected times.
9. Note the expiration date on the medication container.

(Continued on following page)

10. Administer medication using the appropriate technique.
11. Dispose of unused or expired drugs according to agency policy.
12. Maintain strict aseptic technique.
13. Sign for opioids and other restricted drugs according to agency protocol.
14. Document medication administration and patient responsiveness.

Patient Education

- Patient education on I.V. medication administration is vital for the acute care and alternative settings. When possible, patient education should begin before a patient's discharge from the hospital to facilitate a smooth transition to home care.
- The education should begin with instructions outlining the insertion of the I.V. catheter and step-by-step details of the procedure for all peripheral, midline, and peripherally inserted central catheter (PICC) line insertions. All potential complications after insertion and the patient or responsible party should sign an informed consent.
- Routine maintenance care involved in central line management for medication infusions should be provided.
- Fully instruct the patient about the infusion pump; written step-by-step instruction with diagrams or pictures and manufacturer manuals are excellent tools. Include troubleshooting instructions and telephone numbers to call for 24-hour assistance.
- Instructions on proper hand hygiene, setting up the infusion pump with medication, flushing the catheter, and self-administration of the medication must be included in patient training sessions.
- Instruct the patient on the expected actions and adverse effects of medication.
- The patient or caregiver must be taught the procedure of drug administration clearly and in simple terminology.
- Provide a checklist to help evaluate the steps in the learning process; this also provides a method of documenting the completion of self-drug administration.
- Instruct the patient on administration of anti-infectives around the clock to maintain blood levels (Lonsway, 2001).

Patient-Controlled Analgesia

- How to use patient-controlled analgesia
- When to push the bolus button
- When to communicate with the nurse (e.g., pain not controlled with PCA, feeling of sedation)
- Discussion of fears (of addiction to medication, receiving too much medication)
- Discuss expected outcomes for the patient—pain 1 or 2, early ambulation

Home Care Issues

The rapidly growing home care infusion industry now provides many therapies in alternative settings. Therapies that are now being delivered in the home include antibiotics, parenteral nutrition, hydration therapy, chemotherapy, pain management, cardiovascular medications, blood transfusions, chelation therapy clotting factors, Prolastin therapy, and immune globulin I.V. (IVIG).

Individuals can receive medical therapies outside the hospital to maximize their independence. A number of methods exist for delivery of medication intravenously in the home environment: gravity, I.V. push, or ambulatory pump.

Safety

Patients who are able to care for themselves are the best candidates for using ambulatory pumps and usually adjust quickly to home infusion.

Effectiveness

To ensure effective treatment, coordination of care among the patient, nurse, physician, and pharmacist is essential.

Acceptance

Unless the patient understands the treatment, procedure, and administration regimen and accepts them into his or her lifestyle, home drug therapy will not be successful.

Cost

Reimbursement varies depending on the source. Coverage of infusion therapies by Medicare is complex and restrictive (Gorski & Eichelberger, 2001).

Anti-Infectives

Computerized ambulatory infusion devices (drug pumps) have enabled antimicrobial therapy to be safely and effectively administered in the home with minimal disruption in the patient's life. When administering antimicrobials in the home, safety, effectiveness, acceptance, and cost need to be considered.

NURSING FAST FACT!

To prevent medication errors home infusion pharmacy standards of practice state that the pharmacist is responsible for programming the pump and locking the program into the pump. The pump program is checked a second time before the pump is packed for delivery. The nurse must also review the program to verify that the program matches the medical order. There are some cases when a nurse will need to change a pump program, but this should be done by

(Continued on following page)

calling the pharmacy on the telephone and verifying the correct program together with the pharmacy. Nurses often program pumps differently without contacting the pharmacy and this also creates a potential error.

The I.V. push method in the home for anti-infective drug delivery has become a safe and effective route with properly trained staff using standardized policies and procedures. Low incidences of complication exist with all types of access device using the I.V. push method. It was found that there was no significant difference in phlebitis rates among delivery methods. The I.V. push method was found to be cost efficient for delivery of anti-infectives in the alternative setting (Markel-Poole, Nowobilski-Vasilios, & Free, 1999).

NURSING FAST FACT!

As with any I.V. medication delivery, emergency drugs should be readily available and protocols established for their use. Clinical assessment of the patient on anti-infectives is based on the same standards regardless of the treatment environment, including monitoring for adverse reactions, disease processes, and laboratory tests.

Pain Management

For home use, the subcutaneous, intravenous, and epidural routes are used for pain management. The epidural catheter may be attached to a preprogrammed infusion pump containing a medication cassette that requires replacing on a weekly basis. The implanted epidural infusion pump (Medtronic Synchromed) can be refilled by specially trained home infusion nurses using a special computerized transponder and refill kits. Teach the patient and caregiver on how the intraspinal catheter works and the importance of keeping appointments for pump refills.

When the Patient Should Call the Home Care Nurse

- Side effects from the drug are observed by the caregiver or reported by the patient.
- Particles are observed floating in the medication.
- The medication appears discolored.
- The medication bag is leaking.
- The medication schedule must be altered for any reason.
- The pump malfunctions.
- Problems occur with the intravenous line (e.g., inability to flush, bleeding at site, pain, redness, swelling).
- The dressing becomes loose.
- The medication label does not match the orders from the physician.

Key Points

- Advantages of I.V. medications include the fact that they provide a direct access to the circulatory system, a route for drugs that irritate the gastric mucosa, a route for instant drug action, a route for delivering high drug concentrations, instant drug termination if sensitivity or an adverse reaction occurs, and a route of administration in patients in whom use of the GI tract is limited.
- Disadvantages of I.V. medications include drug interaction because of incompatibilities, adsorption of the drug being impaired because of leaching into the I.V. container or administration set, errors in compounding of medication, speed shock, extravasation of a vesicant drug, and chemical phlebitis.
- Common errors in administering medications include lack of knowledge about drugs, errors in drug identity checking, mistakes in calculations, and improper use of pumps and controllers.
- Drug incompatibilities fall into three broad categories: physical, chemical, and therapeutic.
- I.V. medication can be delivered by continuous infusion, intermittent infusion, and I.V. push through a locking device.
- The subcutaneous infusion route is used for patients unable to take medications by mouth and who have poor venous access.
- The intraventricular route via an Ommaya reservoir can be used for delivery of medications directly to the brain.
- There are two types of intraspinal catheters: epidural and intrathecal.
- Epidural and intrathecal administrations provide superior pain control, require small doses, and produce longer periods of relief between doses while preventing many systemic side effects.
- Alcohol must **NEVER** be used for site preparation or for accessing an intraspinal catheter. Only preservative-free medications can be delivered by the intraspinal routes.
- The intraperitoneal route is used when high concentrations of medication need to be delivered directly into the peritoneal cavity.
- Administration of investigational medications must be in accordance with state and federal regulations
- Phases of FDA drug studies:
  - Phase I: Clinical pharmacology and therapeutics
  - Phase II: Initial clinical investigation
  - Phase III: Full-scale evaluation and treatment
  - Phase IV: Postmarketing surveillance

Critical Thinking: Case Study

Mrs. Robertson is one day postoperative from an abdominal hysterectomy. She has an epidural catheter in place. Her baseline vitals are 110/80, R 18,

P. 72. Your assessment finds her difficult to arouse, but she does respond to simple commands. She is able to move her legs and squeezes your fingers. Her BP is 90/60, P. 100, R. 14. She is moaning in pain, unable to rate her pain on the pain scale.

What further assessments need to be done? What further actions should the nurse initiate? What could be the reason for her change in status?

Media Link: Answers to the case study and additional critical thinking exercises are on the enclosed CD–ROM.

Post-Test

1. Which of the following are potential incompatibilities of medication admixtures?
   a. Intermittent, physical, and biotransformation
   b. Drug interaction, drug synergism, and drug tolerance
   c. Physical, chemical, and therapeutic
2. Which of the following are advantages of I.V. medications?
   a. Provide a route for irritating substances, has instant drug action, and has better control administration.
   b. Encourage speed shock, has a rapid onset of action, and allows for absorption of drugs in gastric juices.
   c. Prevent errors in compounding of medication, has a low risk of infiltration, and has a low risk of phlebitis.
   d. Allow for uninterrupted control of rate, has a low risk of side effects, and has a low risk of adsorption.
3. The key point(s) in infusion of I.V. antifungal drugs is (are):
   a. Most are infused as a suspension.
   b. They should not be filtered.
   c. They should be administered slowly.
   d. All of the above
4. The American Pain Society has grouped analgesics into which three categories?
   a. Opioids, nonopioid, and adjuvants
   b. Anesthetics, nonopioid, and NSAIDS
   c. Adrenergics, opioids, and opiates
5. I.V. push medications should be administered according to the manufacturer's recommendations, but delivered over no less than:

a. 10 minutes
b. 5 minutes
c. 1 minute
d. 30 seconds

6. The goal of patient-controlled analgesia is to provide the patient with:
   a. A serum analgesia level for comfort without sedation
   b. A serum analgesia level to achieve sedation
   c. A method of euthanasia
   d. Limited control over pain management

7. Which of the following agencies is involved in investigational drug protocols?
   a. FDA
   b. CDC
   c. IRB
   d. EPA

8. Which of the following are side effects of epidural pain medication?
   a. Urinary retention, pruritus, and respiratory depression
   b. Respiratory depression, peptic ulcer, and hemiparesis
   c. Pruritus, nausea, and urinary incontinence

9. Clear fluid in the syringe after aspiration of an epidural catheter is an indication of catheter:
   a. Patency
   b. Kinking
   c. Migration
   d. Damage

10. All of the following are key points in the delivery of epidural infusions **EXCEPT:**
    a. Use only alcohol swabs to prepare site.
    b. Use only antimicrobial swabs to prepare site.
    c. Use a 0.2-micron filter without surfactant for medication administration.
    d. Aspirate the catheter to ascertain the presence of spinal fluid.

11. Pain management may be provided by all of the following **EXCEPT** the:

a. Systemic route
b. Subcutaneous route
c. Intraspinal route
d. Intraperitoneal route

12. To reduce the hazards of vascular irritation with delivery of medication, nurses should:
    a. Use the largest cannula possible
    b. Use a cannula smaller than the lumen of a vessel
    c. Administer most medications via the intramuscular route
    d. Use electronic infusion devices with a PSI of 10 or above

13. In the alternative-setting, responsibility for infusion pump settings primarily belongs to:
    a. The patient
    b. The nurse
    c. The pharmacist
    d. The physician

14. Common errors in administering medications include all of the following **EXCEPT**:
    a. Nurse's lack of knowledge about drugs
    b. Using a drug book to verify route
    c. Errors in drug identity checking
    d. Mistakes in calculations
    e. Improper use of pump

Media Link: Rationales for answers to these questions and additional test questions are on the enclosed CD–ROM.

References

American Pain Society (1999). *Principles of Analgesic Use in the Treatment of Acute Pain and Chronic Cancer Pain. A Concise Guide to Medical Practice* (4th ed.). Skokie, IL: American Pain Society.

Brown, K. (2001). *Chemotherapy and Biotherapy Guidelines and Recommendations for Practice.* Pittsburgh: Oncology Nursing Press.

Douglas, J.B., & Hedrick, C. (2001). Pharmacology. In Hankins, J., Lonsway, R.A., Hedrick, C., & Perdue, M. (eds.). *Intravenous Therapy: Clinical Principles and Practice* (2nd ed.). Philadelphia: W.B. Saunders, pp. 176–183.

Deglin, J.H., & Vallerand, A.H. (2005). *Davis's Drug Guide for Nurses* (9th ed.). Philadelphia: F.A. Davis.

Gahart, B.L., & Nazareno, A.R. (2004). *Intravenous Medications* (20th ed.). St. Louis: Mosby.

Giger, J.N., & Davidhizar, R.E. (2004). *Transcultural Nursing: Assessment & Intervention (2nd ed.)* St. Louis: Mosby.

Gorski, L., & Czaplewski, L. (2001). Basic concepts of infusion therapy. In Gorski, L. (ed.). *Best Practices in Home Infusion Therapy.* Gaithersburg, MD: Aspen, pp. 7–37.

Gorski, L., & Eichelberger, D. (2001). Reimbursement. In Gorski, L. (ed.). *Best Practices in Home Infusion Therapy*. Gaithersburg, MD: Aspen, pp. 1–10.

Hadaway, L. (2003). Skin flora and infection. *Journal of Infusion Therapy,* 26(1), 44–45.

Infusion Nurses Society (2000). Infusion nursing standards of practice. *Journal of Infusion Nursing* (Suppl), 6S.

Institute of Medicine (1999). *To Err Is Human. Building a Safer Health System.* Washington, D.C.: National Academy Press.

Joint Commission on Accreditation of Health Care Organizations (2001). *JCAHO Pain Assessment and Management Standards.* Available: *www.jcaho.org/standard/pm-frm.html*

Kreger, C. (2001). Getting to the root of pain: Spinal anesthesia and analgesia. *Nursing 2001,* 31(6), 37–41.

Lonsway, R. (2001). Intravenous therapy in the home. In Hankins, J., Lonsway, R., Hedrick, C., & Perdue, M. (eds.). *Infusion Therapy in Clinical Practice* (2nd ed.). Philadelphia: W.B. Saunders, p. 180.

Malloy, J. (2001). Administration of intraperitoneal chemotherapy—A new approach. *Nursing 2001,* 31(4), 49–53.

Markel-Poole, S., Nowobilski-Vasilios A., & Free, F. (1999). Intravenous push medications in the home. *Journal of Intravenous Nursing,* 22(4), 209–215.

McCaffery, M., & Pasero, C. (1999). *Pain: Clinical Manual* (2nd ed.). St. Louis: Mosby.

Nightingale, F. (1860). *Notes on Nursing.* New York: Appleton & Co.

Pasero, C. (2002). Subcutaneous opioid infusion. *American Journal of Nursing,* 102 (7), 61–62.

Perdue, M. (2001). Intravenous complications. In Hankins, J., Lonsway, R., Hedrick, C., & Perdue, M. (eds.). *Infusion Therapy in Clinical Practice* (2nd ed.). Philadelphia: W.B. Saunders, pp. 418–445.

Reiss, B.S., & Evans, M. (2002). *Pharmacological Aspects of Nursing Care.* Albany: Delmar, pp. 236–239.

Smetzer, J. (2001). Take 10 giant steps to medication safety. *Nursing 2001,* 31(11), 49–61.

St. Marie, B. (2001). Pain management. In Hankins, J., Lonsway, R., Hedrick, C., & Perdue, M. (eds.). *Infusions Therapy in Clinical Practice* (2nd ed.). Philadelphia: W.B. Saunders, pp. 276–295.

U.S. Food and Drug Administration (2003a). Strategies to reduce medications errors. Department of Health and Human Services Internet: *www.fda.gov/fdac/featrus/2003/303* meds.html

U.S. Food and Drug Administration (August, 2003b). Medication Errors. Internet: *www.fda.gov/cder/drug/MedErrrors/default.htm.* September 1, 2003.

Answers to Chapter 11 Post-Test

1. **c**
2. **a**
3. **d**
4. **a**
5. **c**
6. **a**
7. **c**
8. **a**
9. **a**
10. **a**
11. **d**
12. **b**
13. **c**
14. **b**

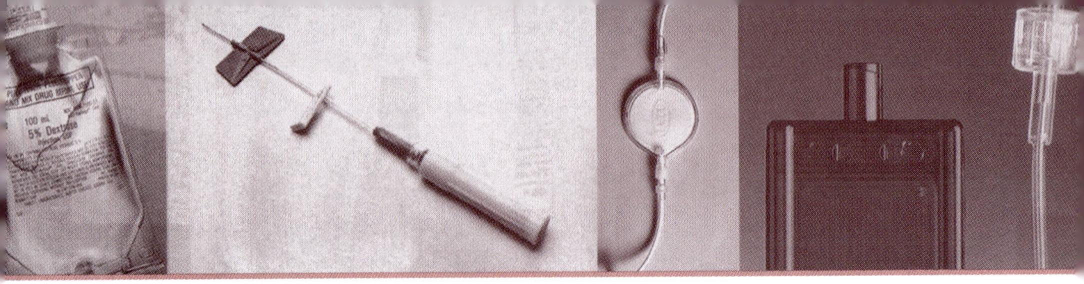

Chapter 12
Central Venous Access

Julie Eddins, RN, MSN, CRNI

As long as the beginner pilot, language learner, chess player, or driver is following rules, his performance is halting, rigid, and mediocre. But with the mastery of the activity comes the transformation of the skill, which is like the transformation that occurs when a blind person learns to use a cane. The beginner feels pressure in the palm of the hand, which can be used to detect the presence of distinct objects such as curbs. But, with mastery the blind person no longer feels pressure in the palm of the hand, but simply feels the curb. The cane has become an extension of the body.

—Expert Performance, Dreyfus and Dreyfus, 1997

A similar transformation occurs with the expert nurse clinician's tools.

Chapter Contents

LEARNING OBJECTIVES

Upon completion of this chapter, the reader will be able to:

1. Define the glossary of terms as related to nursing care of the patient with a central venous catheter (CVC).
2. Discuss the impact of healthcare worker interventions in reducing the risk of catheter-related bloodstream infections (CRBSI) during insertion and dwell.
3. Recognize two potential hazards associated with the placement of a percutaneous CVC.
4. Discuss evidence-based rationale for the insertion of a peripherally inserted central catheter (PICC).
5. Assess potential complications related to improper anatomical tip location and tonicity of infusates.
6. State tip location for a properly placed PICC and a midclavicular device.
7. Examine the relationship between catheter biomaterial and insertion site and the length of dwell and potential patient complications.
8. Explore the impact of federal and professional nursing guidelines when articulating policy and procedures for care.
9. Identify advantages and disadvantages of different types of CVCs.
10. List the steps for dressing management of CVCs, with an emphasis on aseptic technique.
11. Identify nursing management of CVC insertion complications.
12. Identify nursing management of CVC dwell complications.
13. Compare and contrast advantages and disadvantages of tunneled CVC and implanted CVCs.
14. Explore the impact on catheter integrity and syringe size when maintaining patency of a CVC.
15. Discuss the procedure for declotting of thrombotic and nonthrombotic occlusions of a CVC.

GLOSSARY

Anthropometric measurement Measurement of the size, weight, and proportions of the human body

Biocompatibility The quality of not having toxic or injurious effect on biological systems

Broviac catheter Tunneled venous catheter with one Dacron cuff with an outer diameter of 1.0; useful for infusion of nutrient solutions, commonly used in the pediatric patient population.

Central venous catheter (CVC) Location of final tip in the superior vena cava (SVC)

Central venous tunneled catheter (CVTC) Catheter inserted into a centrally located vein with tip residing in the vena cava via tunneling subcutaneously from site between sternum and nipple on chest wall to subclavian vein

Distal Farthest from the heart; farthest from the point of attachment; below previous site of cannulation

Extravascular malpositioning Introducer of the central venous percutaneous catheter is passed out of the vessel and into the pleural space or the mediastinum

Groshong® catheter Surgically implanted, long-term tunneled Silastic catheter; unique in that it has a two-way valve adjacent to the closed tip, which prevents backflow of blood

Hickman catheter Long-term tunneled Silastic catheter inserted surgically

Implanted port Catheter surgically placed into a vessel, body cavity, or organ and attached to a reservoir, which is placed under the skin

Infraclavicular Situated below a clavicle

Intravascular malpositioning Catheter tip of a percutaneous, tunneled, or implanted port coils in the vessel, which advances into a venous tributary other than the superior vena cava or does not reach the superior vena cava.

Iontophoresis Method of delivering anesthesia via an electronic device without injection through the skin

Lymphedema Swelling of an extremity caused by obstruction of lymphatic vessels

Midline catheter Catheter with tip placement in or at the junction of the axillary vein

Peripherally inserted central venous catheter (PICC) Long (20- to 24-inch) I.V. access device made of a soft flexible material (silicone or a polymer); PICCs are usually inserted into one of the superficial veins of the peripheral vascular system with the tip location in the superior vena cava

Silicone Material containing silicone carbon bond; used as lubricants, insulating resins, and waterproofing materials

Thrombogenicity Generation or production of thrombosis

Trendelenburg position Position in which the head is lower than the feet; used to increase venous distention

Tunneled catheter A central catheter designed to have a portion lie within a subcutaneous passage before exiting the body

Vascular access device (VAD) Catheter used to access the vascular system

Valsalva maneuver The process of making a forceful attempt at expiration with the mouth, nostrils, and glottis closed

Anatomy of the Vascular System

To understand the placement of central venous catheters (CVCs), it is important to understand the anatomy of the upper extremity venous system, arm, and axilla. These structures impact successful placement and tip location and ultimately the successful dwell time of the CVC. The important veins include the basilic, cephalic, axillary, subclavian, internal and external jugular, right and left innominate (brachiocephalic) veins, and superior vena cava (SVC). It is also imperative that registered nurses are fully aware of the anatomic position and structures of the arm and axilla venous system.

Venous Structures of the Arm

The superficial veins of the upper extremities lie in the superficial fascia and are visible and palpable. Superficial veins include the cephalic and the basilic veins. The cephalic vein ascends along the outer border of the biceps muscle to the upper third of the arm. It passes in the space between the pectoralis major and deltoid muscles. The vein decreases in size just a few inches above the antecubital fossa and may terminate in the axillary vein or pass above or through the clavicle in a descending curve. Normally, the cephalic vein turns sharply (90 degrees) as it pierces the clavipectoral fascia and passes beneath the clavicle. Near its termination, the cephalic vein may bifurcate into two small veins, one joining the external jugular vein and one joining the axillary vein. Valves are located along the cephalic vein's course (Gray, 1998).

The basilic vein is larger than the cephalic vein. From the posterior–medial aspect of the forearm, it passes upward in a smooth path along the inner side of the biceps muscle and terminates in the axillary vein. The origins of these veins in the lower arm are most often used for short-term peripheral devices. At and above the antecubital fossa, these veins are appropriate for the placement of **PICCs** and arm ports (CDC, 2002).

Valves are present in the venous system until approximately 1 inch before the formation of the brachiocephalic vein. The presence of valves within veins helps to prevent the reflux of blood and is especially important in the lower extremities, where venous return is working against gravity (Fig. 12–1).

Venous Structures of the Chest

The main venous structures of the chest include the subclavian, the internal and external jugular, and brachiocephalic veins (formerly called the innominate veins), and the SVC. Large veins in the head, neck and chest do not have valves. Gravity helps blood to flow properly from the head and neck, and negative intrathoracic pressure promotes flow from the head and neck and the inferior vena cava (Sansivero, 1998).

The subclavian vein extends from the outer border of the first rib to the sternal end of the clavicle and measures about 4 to 5 cm in length; the right brachiocephalic vein measures about 2.5 cm and the left brachiocephalic vein measures about 6 to 6.5 cm. The external jugular lies on the

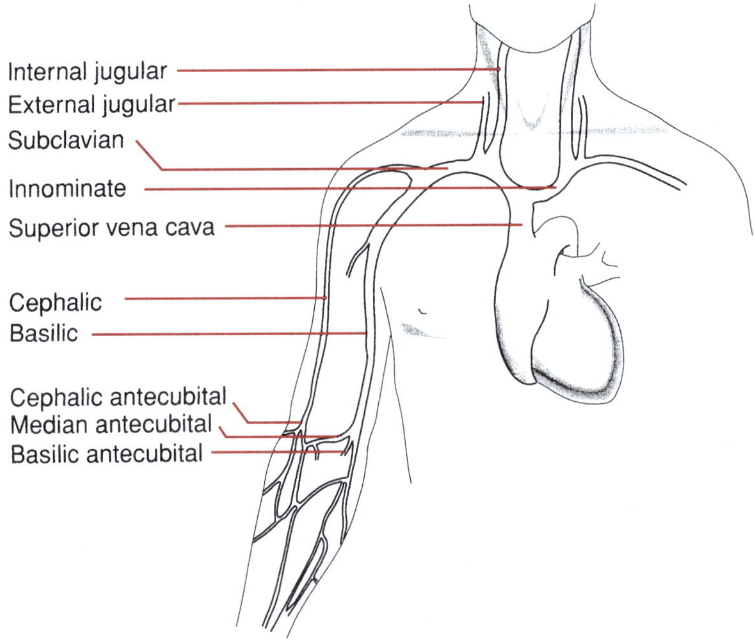

Figure 12–1 ■ Anatomic venous structures of the arm and chest. (From Markel, S., & Reynan, K. [1980]. Impact on patient care: 2652 PIC catheter days. *Journal of Intravenous Nursing,* 13[6], 349. Copyright 1990 by the *Journal of Intravenous Nursing*.)

side of the neck and follows a descending inward path to join the subclavian vein along the middle of the clavicle. The internal jugular vein descends first behind and then to the outer side of the internal and common carotid arteries; it joins the subclavian vein at the root of the neck.

The right brachiocephalic (innominate) vein is about 1 inch long and passes almost vertically downward to join the left brachiocephalic (innominate) vein just below the cartilage of the first rib. The left brachiocephalic vein is about 2.5 inches long and is larger than the right vein. It passes from left to right in a downward slant across the upper front of the chest. It joins the right brachiocephalic vein to form the SVC. The SVC receives all blood from the upper half of the body. It is composed of a short trunk 2.5 to 3.0 inches long. It begins below the first rib close to the sternum on the right side, descends vertically slightly to the right, and empties into the right atrium of the heart. The right atrium receives blood from the upper body via the SVC and from the lower body via the inferior vena cava. The venae cavae are referred to as the great veins. Table 12–1 summarizes the **anthropometric measurements** of the upper extremity veins.

NURSING FAST FACTS!

- *Blood flow in the SVC in the average adult is approximately 1.5 to 2.5 L/minute.*

Poiseuille's law (fourth power law) states that flow through a single vessel is most affected by the vessel diameter, and as vessel diameter increases, the flow rate increases by a factor of 4. For example, when the diameter doubles, flow rate increases 16 times; when the diameter increases by 4, the flow rate increases 256 times (44). The amount of blood flow in the veins follows this law:

Cephalic and basilic veins: 45 to 95 mL/min
Subclavian veins: 150 to 300 mL/min
Superior vena cava: 2000 mL/min

> Table 12–1 **ANTHROPOMETRIC MEASUREMENTS OF VENOUS ANATOMY**

Vein	Length, cm	Diameter, mm
Cephalic	38	6
Basilic	24	8
Axillary	13	16
Subclavian	6	19
Right brachiocephalic	2.5	19
SVC	7	20

SVC = superior vena cava.

Central catheters should never be placed in the right atrium. When CVCs are placed in the right atrium, there is a risk of dysrhythmias, pericardial puncture, and fluid entry into the pericardial space, and these can cause cardiac tamponade, a complication with a mortality rate of 78 to 98 percent.

Choosing the Venous Access Device

Choosing the most appropriate **venous access device (VAD)** for a patient is a collaborative process involving the patient, the practitioner placing the device, and the patient's referring physician. Knowledge of venous anatomy and physiology, VAD technology, and the patient's current health status and infusion plan are important aspects in this process. The goal of VAD selection and placement should be to deliver safe, efficient therapy that maximizes the patient's quality of life, with minimal risk of complication.

Assessment Parameters

Assessment parameters that must be considered before device selection and placement include patient characteristics, therapy characteristics, and device characteristics.

Patient characteristics include the suitability of target vessels that should be evaluated for size and patency. The vein must be large enough to accommodate the selected VAD to minimize the risk of phlebitis and thrombosis. The smallest device in the largest vein allows for maximal hemodilution of the infusate. The vein should fill when a tourniquet is applied, feeling firm but pliable to palpation. Patients who are very thin may benefit from the newer "low-profile" devices.

Patient preference of the nondominant arm for ease of self-care should be considered if appropriate. The patient's lifestyle is an important consideration in choosing an implanted versus an external device. Take into consideration activity restrictions, maintenance requirements, body image distortion, and ease of use. The patient's usual occupational and recreational activities need to be included in the assessment process.

The ability of the patient or designated caregiver to manage day-to-day VAD care and infusions should be assessed before device selection and placement. The ability to see, hear, perform fine motor tasks, read and understand written instructions, and emotionally cope with the demands of site care and therapy are important considerations. In patients who will transition from acute care to home care, the home environment and caregiver support should be taken into consideration.

Conditions That Limit VAD Placement

Conditions that may limit VAD site placement are listed in Table 12–2. These challenges can be overcome with careful device selection and placement.

Knowledge of the type of therapy can help identify the desired VAD and the number of lumens that will be necessary to deliver safe infusions. The number of concurrent and intermittent infusions along with drug compatibility and stability need to be considered (Sansivero, 1998). Nutritional solutions with final concentrations of 10 percent dextrose or 5 percent protein (or both) should be infused through a central line with the tip in the distal one third of the SVC (INS, 2000, 37). Continuous vesicant therapy, solutions with extremes of pH (less than 5 or greater than 9) or medications with osmolarity greater than 500 mOsm/L also should be given through a CVC (INS, 2000, 37). Infusion of caustic, hypertonic fluids without the benefit of hemodilution in the SVC can result in thrombosis and loss of the vessel for future use.

> Table 12–2 **CONDITIONS AFFECTING VASCULAR ACCESS DEVICE SITE PLACEMENT**

Previous surgical interventions	Lymph node dissections Subclavian vein stenting or resection Vena cava filters Myocutaneous flap reconstruction Skin grafts Previous vein harvesting Presence of A–V grafts and hemodialysis fistulas Presence of intravascular stents
Cutaneous lesions in proximity to VAD exit or puncture site	Herpes zoster and skin tears Malignant cutaneous lesions Bacterial or fungal lesions and non-intact skin Burns Extensive scarring or keloids
Disease process or conditions	Severe thrombocytopenia (<50,000 platelets) Other coagulopathy (i.e., hemophilia, idiopathic thrombocytopenia purpura, thrombotic thrombocytopenia purpura) Concurrent anticoagulation therapy Lymphedema Allergies Extremity paraplegia Preexisting vessel thrombosis or stenosis
Other considerations	Site within current radiation port Infection near exit site (e.g., tracheostomy) Morbid obesity Patient inability to position desired site for placement Patient inability to tolerate insertion procedure

Selection of Device

Selection of a device is influenced by the cost, risk factors, and benefits of various VADs in relation to any conditions that could limit VAD access, as well as patient and therapy characteristics.

The least expensive and invasive device is not necessarily the most appropriate selection, depending on the risks associated with peripheral infusions of irritant or vesicant agents. Using a venous access device selection algorithm along with a thorough patient assessment can help with device selection (Fig. 12–2).

Central Venous Catheter Materials

Most VADs are made of silicone elastomers, thermoplastic urethane (TPU), or polyvinyl chloride (PVC). Over the past 10 years, many technical advances in polymer research have provided medical manufacturers with a wide variety of new materials for catheter manufacturer. All catheters, whether they are used for short- or long-term access, should have a radiopaque lateral strip or a radiopaque distal end for visualization on radiography.

Polyvinyl Chloride

Polyvinyl chloride is a carbon chain polymer and was the first catheter material. The material is stiff, can cause damage to the tunica intima, and carries with it a risk of platelet aggregation and subsequent thrombus formation. Current technology has provided other materials for CVCs that are less thrombogenic.

Silicone Elastomers

Silicone elastomers (Silastic®) are soft and pliable and cannot be inserted by the conventional over-the-needle technique. Catheters made of Silastic® require special insertion procedures with or without guidewires. Because of its soft, flexible nature, silicone is less likely to damage the intima of the vein wall and is reported to be less thrombogenic than PVC or Teflon®. Many PICCs are made of this biocompatible material.

Although **silicone** rubber possesses a wide range of desirable properties, it is not well suited to blood-contacting applications because of its high degree of thrombogenicity. The surface "tackiness" and high coefficient of friction typical of silicone often result in difficulty with device insertion and a possibility of catheter fragmentation. Fibrin sheath formation can occur when particulate matter is present.

Polyurethane

Polyurethane catheters may be emerging as the most commonly used catheters because of the material's versatility, malleability (i.e., tensile

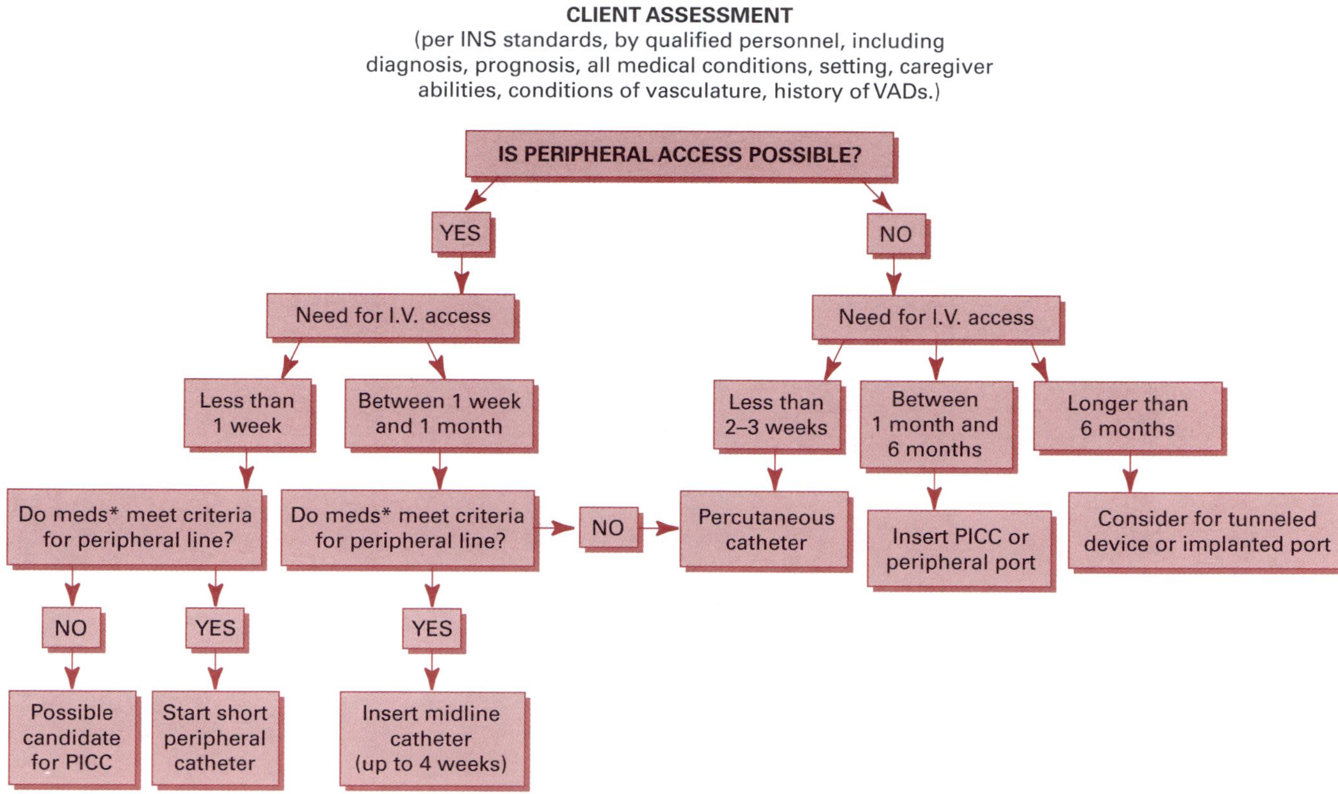

Medication criteria: Final osmolarity < 500 mOsm/L, pH between 5.0 and 9.0, not an irritant or vesicant.

Figure 12–2 ■ Venous access device selection algorithm.

strength and elongation characteristics), and **biocompatibility**. Polyurethane catheters do not have any plasticizers or other harmful additives that can be readily extracted. Polyurethane is a commonly used material for short-term percutaneously placed CVCs and is more frequently being used in long-term CVCs and PICCs. Polyurethane is stiffer than silicone, making threading of the catheter easier, and softens with increased temperature. Polyurethane catheters have thinner walls than silicone catheters owing to greater tensile strength and allow greater flow volume. Polyurethane is similar to silicone in biocompatibility and is thrombus resistant (Mayer & Wong, 2002).

Coatings

To further decrease the risk of complications inherent with even the most biocompatible materials, catheters coated or bonded with hydrophilic materials, antiseptic substances, antibiotics, or heparin are available and have been shown to reduce the risk for catheter-related bloodstream infections (CRBSI) (CDC, 2002). The quest for bacteria-resistant materials has led to studies in which antibiotics were bonded to the catheter. Central catheters, such as the ARROWgard™ were developed that have a colonization-resistant chlorhexidine and silver sulfadiazine antiseptic surface molecularly bonded into the polyurethane catheter along its entire indwelling length. CVCs impregnated on both the external and internal surfaces with minocycline/rifampin (SPECTRUM©) are available and have been associated with lower rates of CRBSI with the beneficial effects occurring after day 6 of catheterization (Darouche, Raad, & Heard, 1999).

The VitaCuff® is a stand-alone add-on device made of silver ions in a biodegradable collagen matrix that is placed around the catheter (Fig. 12–3). The cuff works in conjunction with the Dacron cuff, an inherent component of some catheters, and is positioned beneath the skin surface during catheter placement.

The device's collagen band is impregnated with silver ions that are released over several weeks, creating a physical barrier to bacteria. Silver ions have broad-spectrum activity against many of the bacteria and fungi that are related to catheter infections.

The CDC states that "the decision to used chlorhexidine/silver sulfadiazine or minocycline/rifampin impregnated catheters should be based on the need to enhance prevention of CRBSI after standard procedures have been implemented (e.g., educating personnel, use of maximal sterile barrier precautions, and using 2 percent chlorhexidine skin antiseptics) and then balanced against the concern for the emergence for resistant pathogens and the cost implementing this strategy" (CDC, 2002).

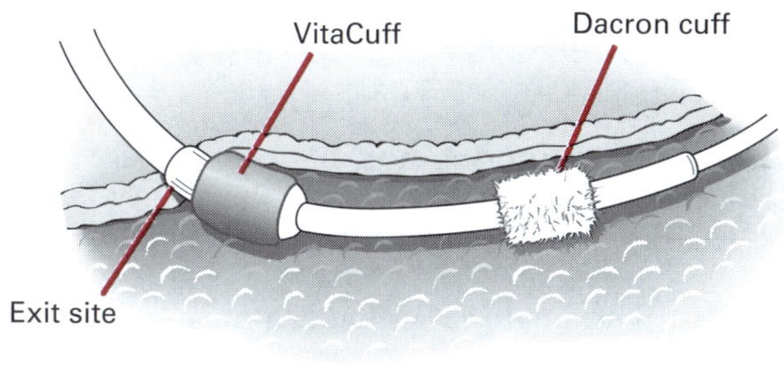

Figure 12–3 ■ Positioning of VitaCuff® antimicrobial cuff. (Courtesy of BARD Access Systems, Salt Lake City, UT.)

Lumens

Catheters are available with single, double, triple, and the recently created quadruple lumens. The diameter of each lumen varies, allowing for the administration of hypertonic or viscous solutions. Refer to each particular manufacturer's information to ascertain which lumen is the largest if rapid administration is needed. If you are administering vesicant or hypertonic solution through one lumen (Fig. 12–4) ensure that the final tip location is in the SVC.

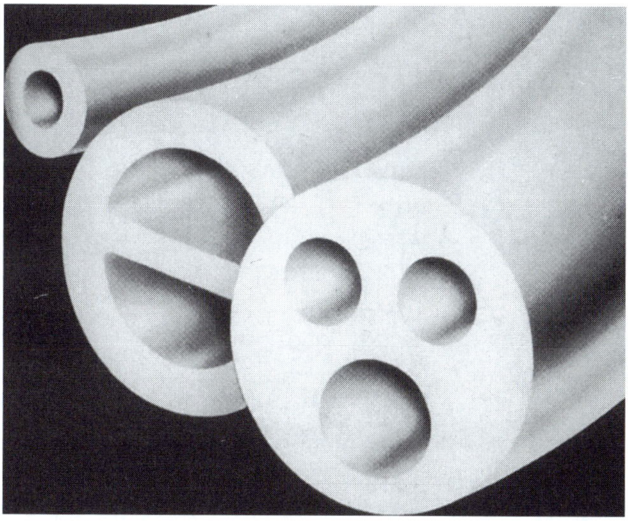

Figure 12–4 ■ Single, double, and triple lumens. (Courtesy of BARD Access Systems, Salt Lake City, UT.).

A catheter with staggered lumens opens at different points on the catheter (Fig. 12–5). Port (lumen) protocols currently used are based on the following:

- Distal port: CVP monitoring and high-volume or viscous fluids, colloids, or medications. (Distal port is the largest lumen.)
- Medial port: Reserved exclusively for total parenteral nutrition (TPN).
- Proximal port: Blood sampling, medications, or blood component administration
- Fourth port: Infusion of fluids or medications

NURSING FAST FACT!

The CDC (2002) recommends using a single-lumen CVC unless multiple ports are essential for the management of the patient and recommends a TPN-designated lumen.

Table 12–3 compares the features, advantages, and disadvantages of CVCs, and Table 12–4 discusses the care and maintenance of CVCs.

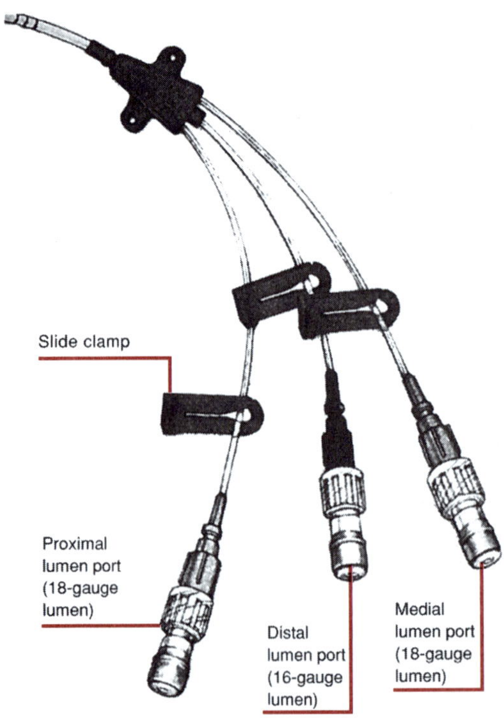

Figure 12–5 ■ Injection ports of the triple-lumen catheter include the proximal lumen port, distal lumen port, and medial lumen port. The distal port *(middle line)* is usually the largest of the three lines.

> Table 12–3 COMPARING CENTRAL VENOUS CATHETERS

Type and Use	Features	Advantages	Disadvantages
		Short-Term	
Percutaneous Up to several weeks Intended for days to several weeks	Material: Polyurethane (most common), Silicone elastomer Length: 6–30 cm Gauge: 14–27 Available features: Heparin, hydromere, antibiotic and antiseptic coatings and antimicrobial cuff available Preattached extensions with clamps Multiple lumens	Inserted at bedside; cost effective, easy to remove, easy to exchange over guidewire	Placement time limited (usually 7 days) Requires sterile dressing changes; requires daily heparin flushes; catheter may break; requires activity restrictions
PICC Up to several months	Material: Polyurethane, Silicone elastomer (most common) Length: 33.5–60.0 cm Gauge: 14–25 Lumen: Double Groshong® valve	Insertion trays, spare needles, spare catheters, and repair kits available Preattached extension with clamps Inserted at bedside by specially trained RN; cost effective; easy to remove; reliable for long-term use; eliminates risks associated with chest or neck insertion; preserves integrity of peripheral vascular system Low rate of CRBSI	Requires sterile dressing changes; requires routine heparin flushes except with Groshong® valve in place; catheter may break; requires activity restrictions; may experience restrictions in blood sampling (i.e., small gauge, certain blood samples)
		Long-Term	
Tunneled Long-term intermittent continuous or daily I.V. access	Material: Silicone elastomer Length: 55–90 cm Gauge: 2.7–19.2 French Lumen: Multiple Groshong® valve Detachable hub Antimicrobial collagen cuff	Can remain in place indefinitely; requires aseptic dressing changes; clean when site is healed; can be repaired externally; self-care possible; lower rate of infection	May require routine heparin flushes, except with Groshong® valve; catheter may break; daily to weekly site care; may be difficult to remove Surgical placement or placement in vascular interventional radiology

(Continued on following page)

> Table 12–3 **COMPARING CENTRAL VENOUS CATHETERS** *(Continued)*

Type and Use	Features	Advantages	Disadvantages
Implanted ports Long-term intermittent, continuous or daily I.V. access	Material: Silicone elastomer Catheter: Polyurethane Port: Titanium, stainless steel, plastic Height: 9.8–17.0 mm Width of base: 24–50 mm Lumen: Dual Groshong® valve	Can access dome port from any angle Preattached catheter or port or two-piece system Several catheter/port locking devices available No dressing changes required, monthly heparin flushes, no activity restrictions, reduced risk of infection	Requires noncoring needle to access; expensive; requires minor surgery to remove

> Table 12–4 **CARE OF CENTRAL VENOUS CATHETERS**

Type of Catheter	Flushing	Tubing Change	Dressing Change
Short-Term			
Percutaneous	1:10 to 1:100 U heparin equal to twice the volume capacity of tubing plus any extensions	Primary and secondary sets every 48 h; every 24 h with TPN Tubing Aseptically prep hub/connection prior to use with alcohol.	Change every 48 h for gauze dressing. Every 3–7 days or PRN for TSM dressing Use chlorhexadine 2%, wiping from site outward to cleanse site.
PICC	1:10 to 1:100 U heparin in volume equal to twice the volume capacity of tubing (1 mL) plus any extensions daily	Same as above	Same as above Remove dressing by pulling upward to avoid dislodging the catheter
Long-Term			
Tunneled	1:10 to 1:100 U heparin in volume equal to twice the volume capacity of tubing (4 mL) plus any extensions; daily to weekly With Groshong® tip, use 5 mL of 0.9% sodium chloride flush weekly	Same as above	Same as above

(Continued on following page)

Type of Catheter	Flushing	Tubing Change	Dressing Change
Implanted port	1:10 to 1:100 U heparin in volume equal to twice the volume capacity of tubing (3 mL) plus any extensions	Same as above	Same as above No dressing is needed after the incision is healed Stabilize device with Steri-Strips® when accessed Change noncoring needle at least weekly Use safty noncoring needle when accessing.

PRN = as needed; TPN = total parenteral nutrition; TSM = transparent semipermeable membrane.

Preventing Catheter-Related Infections

New research is challenging the well-known thought that "bacteria migrate from the skin down to the catheter surface and colonize the catheter." Current research is pointing to the development of a biofilm during insertion and dwell of intravascular devices. When the number of organisms exceeds a certain level, the patient develops a CRBSI. Biofilm development occurs when, immediately after insertion, plasma proteins attach to the catheter. Within 5 minutes, the layer of proteins that are attached to the catheter surface and the proteins in the bloodstream have equalized. Platelets and white blood cells also adhere to the catheter surface. The coagulation cascade is initiated with vessel wall injury, and within a few hours, the catheter is coated with a fibrin sheath from all these substances. Microbes from the skin surface and dermal layers are introduced and flushed through the catheter. The microbes interact with the platelet–protein layer, and bacteria and fungi easily attach themselves to this protein layer. Some organisms produce a slimy matrix and encapsulate themselves loosely on the surface. The biofilm cell can naturally detach from shearing forces of blood flow, detach during flushing, and move to other sites for attachment and is generally resistant to host defense mechanisms of the immune system. Because of the presence and nature of biofilm adherence, aseptic technique during the insertion care and maintenance of the device is essential to prevent the morbidity and mortality associated with CRBSIs (Hadaway, 2003). Refer to Table 12–5, Strategies to Prevent CRBSI.

A recent tool to reduce the potential for CRBSIs is a dressing consisting of a synthetic and biopolymer composite foam impregnated with an antimicrobial agent. The Biopatch® dressing consists of a foam material imbedded with chlorhexidine gluconate, an antiseptic with broad-spectrum antimicrobial and antifungal activity. The Biopatch® foam disk provides a level of action for up to seven days (Banton & Banning, 2002; Maki, Mermel, & Kugar, 2000).

> Table 12–5 **STRATEGIES TO PREVENT BLOODSTREAM INFECTIONS IN CENTRAL LINES**

During Insertion	During Catheter Dwell Time
1. Maximal sterile barrier: Sterile gown, caps, masks, and large drapes 2. Skin antisepsis with chlorhexidine gluconate 3. Experienced inserter 4. Placement of a PICC if applicable 5. Sterile technique during insertion 6. Use of antibiotic-impregnated catheters	1. Specialized infusion team caring for the catheter 2. Provide site care with chlorhexidine gluconate. 3. Avoid the use of stopcocks. 4. Administration set changes and fluid change concurrently. 5. Use Biopatch® dressing. 6. Minimize length of stay in the ICU. 7. Control glycemia. 8. Manage neutropenia. 9. Ensure an adequate RN-to-patient ratio. 10. Healthcare workers should use hand hygiene and a waterless hand gel before and after caring for each patient. 11. Minimize catheter hub contamination by prepping before entering the closed system.

Short-Term Access Devices

Short-term access devices are intended to be used for days to weeks. These devices can be single- or multiple-lumen catheters made of various materials. They are inserted by a percutaneous venipuncture and are not tunneled under the skin. The infraclavicular, jugular, or femoral veins are the sites if the insertion is performed by a physician, and the veins of the antecubital area are used if the insertion is performed by a registered nurse specially trained for peripheral central venous access.

Percutaneous Catheters

In 1961, the first I.V. catheter for accessing the central circulation was introduced. Subclavian catheterization was initially inserted using surgical cutdown technique such as that advocated by Heimback and Ivey (1976). However, percutaneous introduction into the subclavian vein using the Seldinger through-the-needle guidewire technique is now generally preferred. The percutaneous short-term catheter is secured by suturing, and the catheter is not tunneled. This catheter may remain in place for 7 days.

The most common site for insertion of percutaneous catheters is the infraclavicular approach to the subclavian vein (Fig. 12–6). However, because of the need for preservation of the subclavian vasculature, it is important to avoid in certain patients. Subclavian vein catheterization for temporary access should be avoided in all patients with kidney failure and in patients with a history of renal failure or impending renal failure because of the risk of stenosis of the central veins. Use of central venous

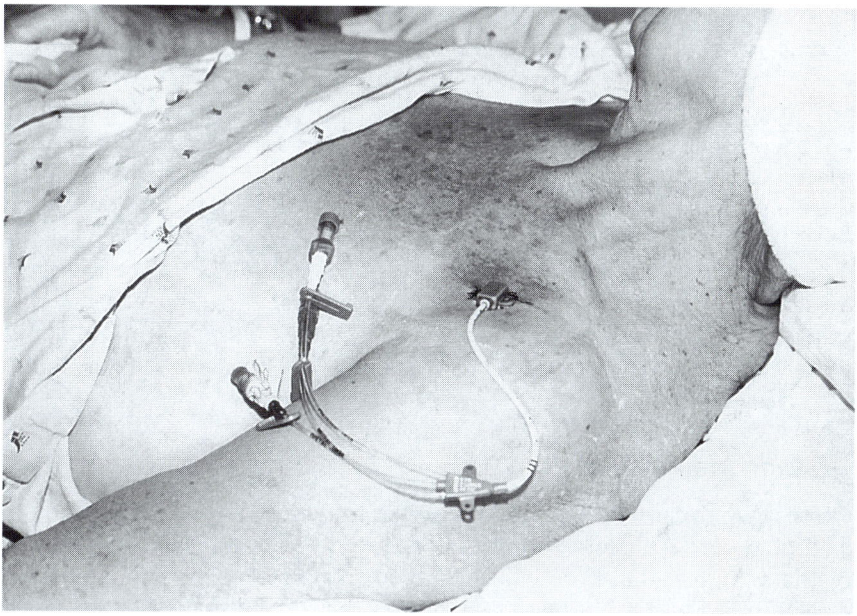

Figure 12–6 ■ Placement of intraclavicular percutaneous catheter.

catheters is associated with a high degree of central venous stenosis, particularly in the subclavian vein, and placement of venous catheters may damage target vasculature necessary for dialysis access (National Kidney Foundation, 2002).

During subclavian insertion, the patient is placed in the Trendelenburg position with a rolled bath blanket or towel between his or her shoulders. The patient should be instructed to perform a **Valsalva maneuver** during the venipuncture procedure to increase the size of the veins.

This exit site on the upper chest is well suited for many types of dressings, and care of the site is not complex.

NURSING FAST FACTS!

- *The infraclavicular approach site requires a well-hydrated patient.*
- *After insertion of the catheter, final verification by chest radiography must be obtained before any infusion. Chest x-ray confirmation should occur prior to the administration of vesicant chemotherapy and whenever tip location is questioned. After placement, the catheter can be maintained as a closed, patent device with an injection cap and heparinized while the catheter tip location is verified by radiologic examination. Do not infuse any solution prior to this radiographic-confirmation.*

The internal jugular vein is an accessible site for the physician; however, care of this site is more difficult. The motion of the neck, a beard on men, long hair, and close proximity of respiratory secretions prevent the adequate use of transparent occlusive dressings. The femoral veins are not recommended for this type of therapy because of the difficulty of placement of the catheter tip. It is also impossible to maintain an occlusive dressing on the femoral exit site.

Many practitioners use ultrasound guidance in the placement of percutaneous and peripherally inserted central catheters. This technique is designed to help identify blood vessels and thereby avoid the inadvertent puncture of an artery prior to inserting a catheter. Ultrasound also allows for needle guidance and visual confirmation of catheter insertion within the selected vessel.

Dressing Management

Percutaneous catheters can be dressed in one of two ways, depending on agency policy. An occlusive gauze or tape (preferred if the site is oozing or the patient is diaphoretic) or a transparent semipermeable membrane (TSM) dressing may be used. In today's practice, the TSM dressing has gained popularity because of its occlusive nature and ability to visualize the site. TSM dressings over a CVC should be replaced when it becomes damp, loosened, or soiled or at least every 7 days (CDC, 2002). Gauze dressings should be changed every 48 hours or if the site requires visual inspection (INS, 2000, 44; CDC, 2002) and the frequency of change should always be based on agency policy. The entire surface of a gauze dressing and all edges must be secured with tape to ensure that the dressing is closed and intact (Perrucca, 2001); tape should not be applied to a TSM dressing, as it impairs the adhesiveness of the dressing.

The use of a chlorhexidine-impregnated sponge (Biopatch™) placed over the site of short-term CVCs reduced the risk for catheter colonization and CRBSI (Maki & Mermel, 2000).

Peripherally Inserted Central Catheters

Peripherally inserted central catheters were introduced in the late 1970s as a means to administer infusates when traditional routes of venous access were unachievable. The PICC is a percutaneous I.V. line composed of silicone elastomers or polyurethane. It may have a single or multiple lumens with ranges in lengths from 33 to 60 cm and diameters of 14 to 25 gauge (4 Fr/18 gauge). Insertion may be through the needle, through a peel-away introducer, through an intact catheter, or with a guidewire, and it can be inserted with or without ultrasound guidance.

The placement of PICCs by registered professional nurses requires specialized education and demonstrated competency. PICCs are designed for delivery of therapies extending beyond 7 days to several months. The

PICC was developed for use in neonates because of the catheter's small diameter and the material's flexibility.

Indications for PICC Use

The following indications for PICC use include medical-based and specific prescribed therapies.

MEDICAL DIAGNOSES

Medical-based indications for PICC use include infectious diseases (e.g., osteomyelitis, endocarditis, delayed wound healing secondary to infection, meningitis, multiple abdominal fistulae), oncologic diseases, gastrointestinal (GI) diseases (e.g., pancreatitis, hyperemesis gravidarum, malabsorption syndromes), and low birth weight neonates. PICCs are also indicated when preexisting illness prevents the placement of a percutaneous device (low platelet count, neutropenia, inability to tolerate Trendelenburg position for placement of the device).

THERAPIES

Specific prescribed therapies for PICC use include drugs or infusates with extreme variations in osmolarity; parenteral nutrition formulations with dextrose contents greater than 10 percent or osmolarity more than 500; irritating anti-infective agents such as vancomycin, nafcillin, and amphotericin B; vesicant or irritant therapies; and prolonged duration of therapy (more than 7 days), such as with pain management or chronic vasopressor infusions (INS, 1999).

ADVANTAGES

1. Peripheral insertion eliminates the potential complication of pneumothorax or hemothorax; significant reduction in risk of CRBSI as compared to percutaneous catheters.
2. Decreases risk of air embolism owing to the ease of maintaining the insertion site below the heart.
3. Decreases pain and discomfort associated with frequent venipunctures for peripheral sites.
4. Preserves peripheral vascular system of upper extremities.
5. Is cost effective and time efficient.
6. Is appropriate for home placement and home I.V. therapy.
7. Risk of infiltration and phlebitis is reduced.
8. Allows preservation of peripheral veins.
9. Appropriate for individuals of all ages.

DISADVANTAGES

1. Special training is required to perform the procedure.
2. Forty-five minutes to 1 hour is needed to complete procedure.
3. Daily care is required.
4. Strict catheter maintenance guidelines is necessary to prevent clotting of the catheter.

5. Small-lumen PICCs may cause difficulty in obtaining blood samples because of possible collapse of the catheter on aspiration.
6. Contraindicated in patients whose lifestyles or occupations involve being in water; those with preexisting skin infections in the antecubital fossa; those with anatomic distortions related to injury, surgical dissection, or trauma; and those with coagulopathies.
7. Requires chest radiography for placement verification before initiation of therapy.

Vein Selection

The peripheral veins in the antecubital fossa (ACF) in both adults and children are the usual sites for PICC access (Fig. 12–7). Other veins that may be used include the basilic, cephalic, median–cephalic, and median–basilic veins. The cephalic and median–cephalic veins are usually avoided if possible because of the higher incidence of tip malposition with placement.

NURSING FAST FACT!

All these sites are acceptable; however, the basilic vein and the median antecubital veins are the preferred insertion sites. Each should be assessed immediately above and below the antecubital space by palpation and ultrasound if applicable.

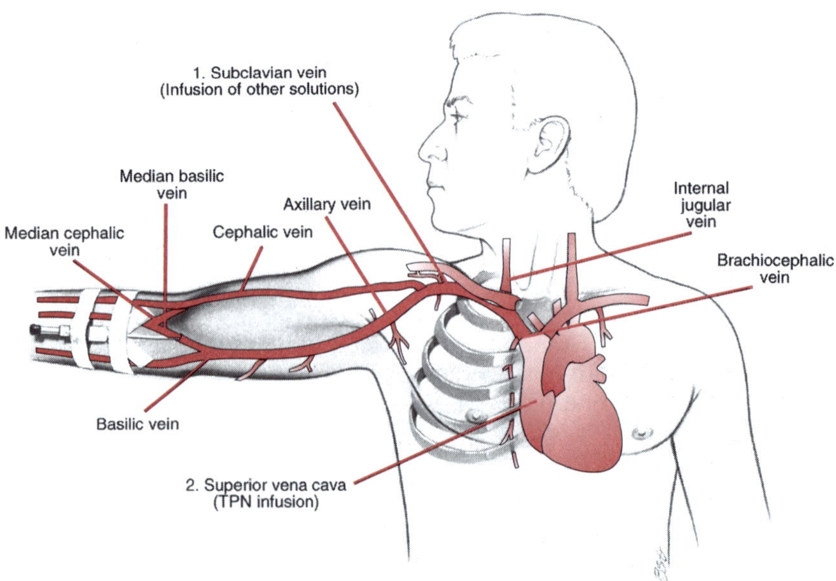

Figure 12–7 ■ Anatomical placement of peripherally placed central catheter. (Courtesy of Medivisuals, Dallas, TX.)

AGE-RELATED CONSIDERATIONS: PICC VEIN SELECTION 12–1

In the neonatal and pediatric population, the external jugular, axillary, long and short saphenous, temporal, and posterior auricular veins may be appropriate site considerations (INS, 1997a).

Placement

According to the recommendations of the Food and Drug Administration (FDA) Central Venous Catheter Working Group (1994) and the INS Standards of Practice 2000, PICCs should be placed in patients under sterile conditions by a specially trained registered nurse in settings such as a patient's room, outpatient area, or the patient's home. Various PICC designs are available for insertion, including the breakaway needle introducer, the peel-away sheath, the guidewire, or a slotted needle on a drum cartridge. PICCs are commonly inserted with the aid of ultrasound guidance, allowing visual inspection of the vasculature and assessment of the size and location of the vessel.

NURSING FAST FACT!

Catheter tip placement for PICCs is the SVC (INS, 2000, 44).

INS Standard. The responsibilities of the registered nurse should include ascertainment of product integrity, vein selection and assessment, and use of aseptic technique. (INS, 2000, 48)

Procedure

Although the actual procedure varies with different manufacturer's products, Procedures Display 12–1 provides a guideline for inserting a PICC.

Key Insertion Techniques

Threading is often the most difficult aspect of PICC insertion. Key points in overcoming difficulties in threading of a PICC line include the following:

- If you meet resistance or advancement stops, do not force advancement. Try flushing while threading, have the patient open and close his or her fist.
- During threading, if the flexible catheter tip kinks over onto itself, pull back on the catheter and flush. If flushing is ineffective, another vein may need to be used. Never force a kinked guidewire because it could puncture the catheter.

PROCEDURES DISPLAY 12–1

Insertion of a PICC Without Ultrasound Guidance

Verify the physician's order, obtain history of allergies, obtain an informed consent, and conduct patient education before beginning procedure. Use strict aseptic technique, and follow Standard Precautions. Don mask and gloves.

Equipment Needed

- One nonsterile measuring tape
- One nonsterile tourniquet
- Two pairs of sterile gloves (powderless)
- Gown and goggles or face shield
- Tamperproof, nonpermeable sharps container
- One catheter insertion kit (write down the lot number and expiration date); select the correct PICC size according to the access needs of the patient
- One local anesthetic (bacteriostatic normal saline and 1% lidocaine with or without buffering; Elamax™ or ECCA™, Numby Stufff™)
- One sterile injection cap

Procedure

PREINSERTION STEPS

1. Perform preinsertion assessment: Determine the site to be used for PICC insertion.
2. Wash the patient's arm with soap and water or chlorhexidine gluconate, rinse well, and dry thoroughly.
3. Wash hands with an antibacterial agent; chlorhexidine gluconate is the preferred agent (CDC, 2002).
4. Set up supplies and sterile field.
5. Position the patient with the arm to be accessed extended at 45 to 90 degrees from the trunk of the body.
6. Measure the arm with nonsterile tape. For PICC placement in the SVC, measure from the antecubital insertion site up the arm to the shoulder and across the shoulder, following the anatomical vein path. Continue to the sternal notch and down to the third intercostal space to the right of the sternum. Note the length of catheter to be inserted.

CANNULATION

1. Scrub hands for 60 seconds, using antiseptic soap.
2. Don mask and prepare work area.

(Continued on following page)

3. Position protective covering under the patient's arm.
4. Place a tourniquet on the mid upper arm for final vein assessment.
5. Select the vein and release the tourniquet.
6. Apply nonpowdered sterile gloves.
7. Prepare the site with chlorhexidine gluconate (ChloraPrep™) with friction (reaches resident organisms deep in the layers of the epidermis) in a back-and-forth motion for 30 seconds; then allow to dry for 30 seconds.
8. Anesthetize the anticipated venipuncture site. Assess for allergies before using any of these methods:
   a. Intradermal injection: 0.1 to 0.3 mL of 1 percent lidocaine without epinephrine, using a small-gauge needle. Perform after skin preparation and immediately before venipuncture.
   b. Topical application of anesthetic after venous site selection and before skin preparation; follow the manufacturer's recommendations for contact time
   c. Iontophoresis: Method of delivering anesthesia without injection through the skin via an electronic device. Perform before skin preparation. Allow sufficient time to achieve anesthetic effect (approximately 10 to 30 minutes).
9. Remove and discard gloves.
10. Apply tourniquet snugly.
11. Don goggles, sterile gown, and new pair of sterile powder-free gloves.
12. Drape arm with sterile towels, creating a sterile field and maximal sterile barrier.
13. Flush entire cannula according to the manufacturer's recommendations.
14. Make venipuncture while applying reverse traction with the nondominant hand to stabilize the vein.
15. On confirmation of blood return, advance the introducer unit about ¼ to ½ inch further into the lumen of the vein.
16. While gently pressing proximally on the tip of the introducer cannula to decrease blood spillage, remove the introducer stylet and activate the safety mechanism.
17. Insert the catheter through the introducer device, slowly and in small (1- to 2-mm) increments.
18. Release the tourniquet.
19. Continue to advance the catheter. When the catheter is inserted approximately halfway, instruct the patient to turn his or her head toward the affected arm with his or her chin tucked and pointed downward toward the clavicle or chest.
20. Remove the introducer.
21. Slowly advance the remaining catheter to the measured length.
22. Gently remove the guidewire from the catheter.

(Continued on following page)

PROCEDURES DISPLAY 12–1

Insertion of a PICC Without Ultrasound Guidance *(Continued)*

23. Prime and attach the extension tubing and injection cap.
24. Flush with 0.5 mL of 0. 9 percent sodium chloride solution.
25. Aspirate with 0.9 percent sodium chloride to check for blood return.
26. Assess blood for type of flow, color, consistency, and pulsation.
27. Flush vigorously with remaining sodium chloride, followed by heparinized saline.
28. Secure the catheter with:
    a. Tape with sterile wound closure strips
    b. Tape supplied in manufacturer's insertion tray
    c. Catheter securement device
    d. Suture
29. Dress with sterile 2 × 2 gauze and transparent dressing, according to organizational policy and procedure.
30. Obtain a chest radiograph for catheter tip placement.
31. Document the procedure, catheter lot number, and patient response. Obtain the arm circumference as a baseline.
32. After 24 hours, assess the insertion site and upper arm by changing the initial dressing according to organizational policy and procedure.

Sources: *Perucca (2001); INS (2000).*

- During threading of the catheter through the subclavian vein, have the patient turn his or her head before threading into the innominate vasculature. This is necessary to prevent threading the PICC into the internal jugular vein. Continue to flush while threading the catheter until the insertion length is reached.
- If threading progresses to a point at which the catheter abruptly stops (this may be caused by a valve, vessel narrowing, or thrombus), attempt to flush and thread past the valve or narrowing.
- If a venous spasm occurs during threading, flush to attempt to open the vein or wait up to 10 minutes while flushing intermittently before beginning a rethreading attempt.

NURSING FAST FACT!

Some PICCs are designed for suture placement to stabilize the catheter (or Steri-Strip™ skin closure may be used to close the exit site).

INS Standard. The length of time a PICC may indwell is dependent on factors related to the patient, clinical environment, skill of the inserter, skill of all caregivers, the composition of the infusate, and the VAD. With ongoing analysis of these factors, consideration may be given to leaving a PICC in place for up to 1 year. (INS, 1997a)

Dressing Management

A small amount of bleeding from the insertion site occurs for the first 24 hours after insertion. After 24 hours, the original dressing should be replaced with a TSM that can remain in place up to 7 days. Dressings have two functions: (1) as a protective environment for the VAD and (2) to prevent catheter migration via stabilization. Dressing change is a sterile procedure. Refer to Procedures Display 12–2.

INS Standard. The dressing should be changed every 7 days or if soiled or nonocclusive. After removal, the site should be assessed every 24 hours until the site is epithelialized. (INS, 2000, 55)

PICC dressing should be changed at intervals similar to those for other central line dressings. Transparent dressings are safe and effective up to 7 days (Maki & Mermel, 1998). Patients who are very active or perspire profusely will need more frequent dressing changes. I.V. tubing junctions must be secured with Luer locking connections, and cleansed with an antiseptic agent prior to disconnecting or changing.

PROCEDURES DISPLAY 12–2

Dressing Change PICC

Educate the patient on the purpose of the procedure. Use sterile technique. Observe hand hygiene procedures. Observe Standard Precautions.

Equipment Needed

- Gloves
- TSM dressing
- Sterile gloves
- 70 Percent alcohol swabs
- 2 Percent Chlorhexidine
- Steri-Strips®

(Continued on following page)

PROCEDURES DISPLAY 12–2

Dressing Change PICC *(Continued)*

Procedure

1. Wear nonpowdered gloves for the dressing removal.
2. Remove the transparent dressing gently by pulling in an upward direction to prevent dislodging or pulling the catheter out. Stabilize the insertion site while removing the dressing to prevent inadvertent dislodgment.
3. Assess the insertion site, the arm, and the track of the vein for redness, tenderness, edema, and drainage.
4. Remove gloves and put on a new pair of sterile nonpowdered gloves to clean the skin around the insertion site.
5. Use 2 percent chlorhexidine and alcohol (ChloraPrep®); allow to dry.

   If the catheter is not sutured, place Steri-Strips® over the insertion site to prevent migration of the catheter.
6. Apply a new transparent dressing over the exposed catheter, including the hub.
7. Initial and date the dressing.
8. Document the procedure in the patient record (Fig. 12–8).

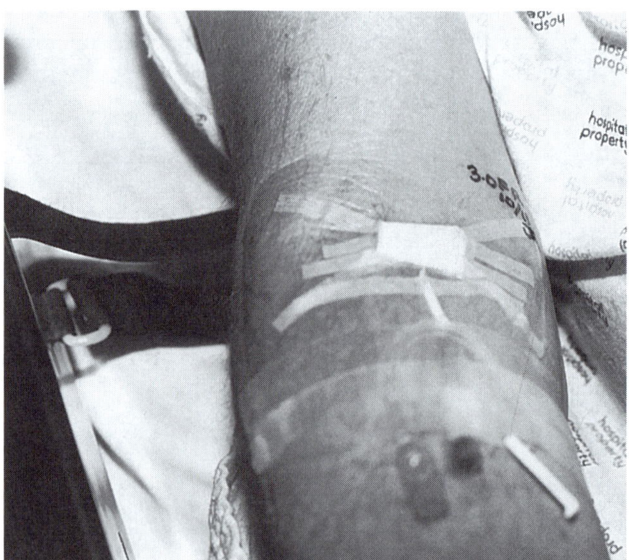

Figure 12–8 ■ Initial PICC dressing. The newly placed PICC has Steri-Strips® to secure the line and a gauze pad under the transparent dressing for the first 24 hours.

Nursing Points-of-Care: Site Care

- Avoid stretching the catheter during dressing changes and catheter removal. Stretching or excessive pressure can cause the catheter to rupture.
- When removing the old PICC dressing lift it from the catheter hub toward the patient's head, taking care not to pull the catheter out of the insertion site (Ellenberger, 2002).
- Document the following daily:
  - Solution infusing and type of administration set
  - Flow rate
  - Use of electronic infusion device
  - Location of insertion site
  - Condition of catheter tract and surrounding tissue
  - Type of I.V. site dressing
  - Patient response to catheter and patient education

Flushing Procedure

Flushing is done routinely using 0.9 percent sodium chloride followed by heparin (except for catheters with closed distal tip and three-position valve). As with many venous access devices, flushing the PICC involves administering the saline–medication–saline–heparin method (SASH):

S: 0.9 Percent sodium chloride
A: Administer medication
S: 0.9 Percent sodium chloride
H: Heparin

NURSING FAST FACT!

For best results and to prevent catheter complications, flush the I.V. catheter using the pulsatile "push–pause" method.

This flushing procedure is recommended to eliminate problems with incompatible drugs. The flushing volume is two times the internal fill volume of the catheter. The recommended heparin concentration is 10 to 100 U/mL (approximately 2 to 3 mL depending on the fill volume). Refer to Procedures Display 12–3.

INS Standard. Flushing with a heparin flush solution to ensure and maintain patency of an intermittent central venous cannula shall be performed at established intervals. The concentration of

PROCEDURES DISPLAY 12–3

Flushing PICC

Verify the physician's order. Educate the patient on the purpose of the procedure and site observation after discontinuation. Follow hand hygiene procedures. Observe Standard Precautions.

Equipment Needed

- 10-mL syringe
- Preservative-free 0.9 percent sodium chloride
- Gloves
- Sharps container
- Antiseptic solution
- Prefilled air locked syringe with 5 mL of heparin 10 to 100 U/mL (or custom-made kits)

Procedure

1. Follow the manufacturer's guidelines for flushing certain CVADs.
2. Identify the patient.
3. Don gloves.
4. Cleanse the central venous catheter injection cap (port) with 70 percent isopropyl alcohol. Allow to air-dry. Note: Additional 2 percent chlorhexidine or povidone-iodine prep necessary with blunt needle access.
5. Attach a syringe containing 0.9 percent sodium chloride to the injection port via a needleless system.
6. Aspirate to check patency.
7. Instruct patient to perform Valsalva maneuver and open the CVC if hub-to-syringe connection.
8. Irrigate the line with 0.9 percent sodium chloride using the push–pause method.
9. Attach the syringe with the heparinized saline to the injection port (if indicated). (Most CVCs require heparin unless closed end valve such as Groshong® or PASV.)
10. Irrigate the line with heparinized saline solution using the push–pause method.
11. Document the procedure on the patient record.

NURSING FAST FACT!

A 10-mL or larger syringe must be used to maintain a psi (pounds per square inch) of approximately 7. A psi pressure exerted by a 1-mL syringe is greater than 300 psi, and that exerted by a 3-mL syringe is more than 25 psi (catheter burst pressure is 25 to 40 psi).

heparin used to flush cannulas shall not alter the patient's clotting factors. (INS, 2000, 56)

The frequency of the flushing procedure depends on organizational policy and patient condition. The recommendations are:

Every 4 to 6 hours for 2 French or smaller or after each use
Every 8 to 12 hours for larger sizes or after each use (INS, 1999)

Flushing is to be done:

1. Whenever the line needs to be locked
2. After every blood draw
3. After intermittent medication administration
4. After blood or blood component administration
5. After TPN

NURSING FAST FACT!

Pulsatile (Push-Pause) Flushing

Using a rapid succession of pulsatile push–pause–push–pause movements exerted on the plunger of the syringe barrel creates a turbulence within the catheter lumen that causes a swirling effect to move residues of fibrin, medication, lipids, or other adherents attached to the catheter lumen.

Use of Infusion Pumps

The PICC line has been used successfully with all types of infusion pumps. With 3.0-French and smaller PICCs, an infusion pump may be necessary to maintain the infusion and patency of the line.

Blood Sampling

If blood sampling is needed from the PICC, a 4-French or larger catheter may improve aspiration. The walls of the PICC line are soft, so they collapse easily when a strong vacuum is applied; therefore, a gentle touch with a syringe is recommended. Vacutainers may be used in larger catheters.

Blood Administration

Blood products may be administered through a 4-French or larger PICC. Care should be taken to flush the line thoroughly after administering a blood product. An infusion pump may be necessary to maintain the infusion if the pump is approved for the administration of blood.

Repair

A PICC that is damaged externally can be repaired with a manufacturer-specific hub repair kit. If the catheter is damaged internally, consider referring the patient to interventional radiology for an over-the-wire exchange if applicable to preserve the access site, after considering the advantages, disadvantages, and infection risks. In many cases, the I.V. nurse must advocate for the patient's vascular access needs and create new techniques to preserve what may be the only access site available.

The PICC can be replaced in one of three ways:

- Using the exchange-over-wire procedure using the Seldinger method
- Totally removing and replacing with another PICC
- Using the breakaway sheath technique

If the peripherally inserted central line is damaged, another catheter can be placed. An exchange-over-wire procedure can be used as a last resort for salvaging the line. The guidewires used for this procedure can be extremely long; therefore, strict sterile technique with gowning and maximal sterile barrier is recommended. The guidewire is inserted into the catheter to be removed, and the catheter is pulled out over the wire. A new catheter is then threaded back over the wire. After the new catheter is in place, the guidewire can be removed.

Dual-lumen PICCs cannot be repaired. A sheath exchange allows for a damaged PICC to be removed and a new dual lumen to be placed. The application of the breakaway needle exchange procedure can be extended to replacement of midclavicular catheters. A sheath exchange can be used to preserve the access site and exchange a shorter catheter for a PICC line (Fabian, 1995).

A chest radiograph should be taken to verify the placement of the new catheter tip. This procedure should be performed only by experienced I.V. nurses certified to insert a PICC (INS, 1998) in accordance with the nursing practice acts. Specific manufacturer recommendations are provided for this procedure.

Discontinuation of PICC

The discontinuation of a PICC catheter must be performed by a qualified registered nurse. Minimize the risk of air embolism by positioning the patient in a dorsal-recumbent position, and instruct the patient to perform the Valsalva maneuver while the catheter is being withdrawn. The recommended procedure is presented in Procedures Display 12–4.

Difficulty with PICC withdrawal is an uncommon but not infrequent problem, with resistance encountered in 7 to 24 percent of removals (Macklin, 2000). Catheter removal may take several hours or more to achieve venous relaxation and total removal of cannula. The most common cause of "stuck" catheters is venospasm (Marx, 1995). Other causes include phlebitis, valve inflammation, and thrombophlebitis. Refer to Figure 12–9 for an algorithm for stuck PICC catheter.

PROCEDURES DISPLAY 12-4

Discontinuation of PICC

Performed by a qualified registered nurse. Verify the physician's order. Educate the patient on the purpose of the procedure and site observation after discontinuation. Follow hand hygiene procedures. Observe Standard Precautions.

Equipment Needed

- 10-mL syringe
- Sodium chloride
- Gloves
- Suture removal set, if appropriate
- Sterile dressing

Procedure

1. Position the patient in the dorsal recumbent position and abduct the patient's arm.
2. Don gloves.
3. Flush the catheter with 0.9% sodium chloride using a 10-mL syringe.
4. Remove the dressing.
5. Remove suture if necessary.
6. Remove any other securement devices if in place.
7. Withdraw the catheter with smooth gentle pressure in small increments. (DO NOT STRETCH THE CATHETER.)
8. Cover the site with a sterile 2 × 2 gauze pressure dressing.
9. Leave pressure dressing in place for 24 hours.
10. Measure the length of the catheter and compare with the length recorded before insertion.
11. Document the procedure.

Techniques to aid in removal of catheter include:

- Apply warm moist compresses.
- Use mental relaxation exercises and distraction.
- Have the patient drink a warm beverage to increase vasomotor tone.
- Gently massage the area of the upper arm over the PICC to relax the vein.
- Start a peripheral I.V. distal to the PICC line and infuse warm normal saline to relax the vein and increase the flow/volume within the vein.

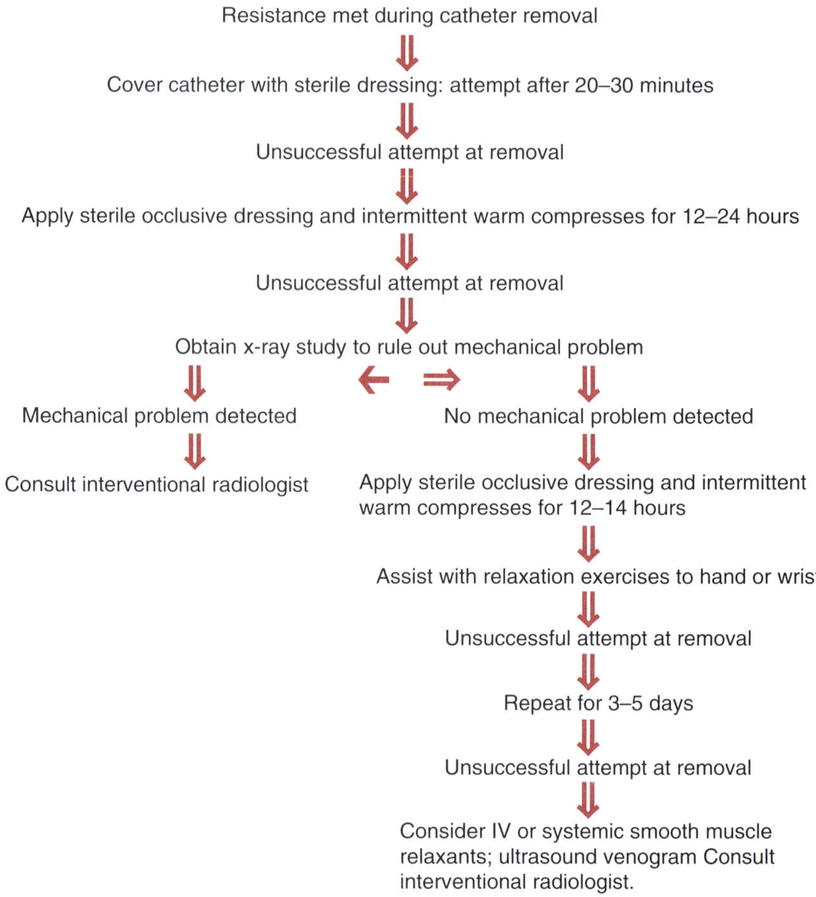

Figure 12–9 ■ Algorithm for a "stuck" peripherally inserted central catheter.

PICC-Associated Risks and Complications

The risks and complications associated with PICCs include arm edema, bleeding, tendon or nerve damage, cardiac dysrhythmias, malposition of catheter, catheter embolism, phlebitis, catheter sepsis, thrombosis, air embolism, and Twiddler's syndrome.

Nerve damage is related to the median nerve, which lies parallel and medial to the brachial artery in the antecubital space. On the lateral side, the lateral cutaneous nerve is proximal to the cephalic vein. Because of the close proximity to these nerves, damage is a risk.

Cardiac dysrhythmias are related to irritation of the myocardial wall by an overinserted guidewire or catheter. Some institutions require the patient to be placed on a cardiac monitor during placement of a PICC in the SVC. Catheters positioned in the heart are at risk of causing myocardial erosion, perforation, cardiac tamponade, and endocardial abscess.

Intravascular and **extravascular** malpositioning of all types of short-term devices has been reported. Extravascular malpositioning can occur when the introducer slips out of the vein and the catheter is passed into the pleural space or the mediastinum (primarily during a subclavian catheterization). Intravascular malpositions are more common and can be seen with all approaches to the central vascular system. The catheter may coil in the vessel, advance into the right atrium or one of the smaller venous tributaries, or it may not be advanced far enough to reach the SVC from the antecubital site. The catheter must be repositioned if malpositioning occurs.

NURSING FAST FACT!

A way to avoid intravascular malpositioning of the catheter in the jugular vein is by having the patient turn his head toward the side of the venipuncture with his chin on his shoulder. This changes the angle of the catheter to move downward toward the SVC.

If placing a device with a break-away needle, extreme care should be taken to remove the break-away needle (introducer) before threading the catheter. Catheter shearing is the most common cause of catheter embolism, but it can also result from retraction of the catheter into the arm after external breakage, rupture of the catheter with forceful irrigation, or from the "pinch-off" syndrome. Managing catheter embolism involves retaining the fragment in the arm and preventing migration into the central veins, heart, pulmonary artery, or lung periphery. If the potential of catheter embolization occurs, immediately apply local pressure or a tourniquet proximal to the site. Obtain a radiograph to determine the location of the embolus. Radiographic visualization may be difficult if the catheter segment is short.

NURSING FAST FACT!

If the patient complains of pain in the shoulder, neck, or arm at insertion site, catheter placement should be checked by radiographic examination at any time during the course of therapy.

Table 12–6 presents a summary of central venous access device complications.

Table 12–6 COMPLICATIONS ASSOCIATED WITH CENTRAL VENOUS ACCESS DEVICES

Complication and Cause	Central Line Device	Signs and Symptoms	Interventions
		Insertion Complications	
Bleeding: Common with any nontunneled catheter	Percutaneous PICC Midclavicular	Oozing from site, hematoma (watch patients with thrombocytopenia), usually first 24 h after insertion Cool, mottled skin; numbness; tingling	Apply pressure dressing Consider removal if excessive bleeding persists after pressure.
Pneumothorax: Collection of air in the pleural space between the lung and chest wall; caused by puncture of the pleural covering of the lung	Percutaneous	Shortness of breath during procedure, crunching sound on auscultation, dyspnea, cyanosis, subcutaneous emphysema	Administer oxygen A chest tube may be inserted May resolve slowly without evacuation of air Monitor vital signs
Hemothorax: Blood enters the pleural cavity as a result of trauma or transection of a vein	Percutaneous PICC Midclavicular Tunneled catheter Implanted port	Sudden onset of chest pain, tachycardia, hypotension, dusky color, diaphoresis, hemoptysis	Usually noted during insertion of catheter (subclavian artery during infraclavicular placement) Remove the catheter and apply pressure to site Monitor vital signs Administer oxygen
Chylothorax: Lymph (chyle) fluid enters the pleural cavity as a result of transection of the thoracic duct on the left side where it enters the subclavian vein; chyle is a milk-like substance	Percutaneous PICC Midclavicular Tunneled catheter Implanted port	Sudden onset of chest pain, dyspnea, withdrawal of a milk-like substance into the needle Large amounts of serous drainage from insertion site.	Remove the catheter Monitor vital signs Administer oxygen Chest tube may be necessary
Brachial plexus injury: Network of nerves located in the lower cervical and upper dorsal spinal nerves that supply the arm, forearm, and hand	Percutaneous PICC Midclavicular	Tingling sensation in fingers, pain shooting down arm, paralysis	Pain medication Physical therapy Preventive measures

Complication and Cause	Central Line Device	Signs and Symptoms	Interventions
Extravascular malposition: Catheter penetrates the vessel and the tip lies outside the vascular system; occurs during threading a catheter or needle introducer	Percutaneous PICC Midclavicular	Symptoms of pneumothorax or hemothorax	Radiographic verification of catheter tip Remove catheter Monitor vital signs Oxygen, chest tube may be necessary
		Post-insertion Complications	
Air embolism: The entry of air into the circulatory system during CVC insertion, tubing changes, or caused by catheter damage or breakage; death occurs from rapid injection of air; lethal dose 70 to 150 cc	Percutaneous PICC Midclavicular Tunneled catheter Implanted port	Chest pain, dyspnea, hypotension, lightheadedness, pallor, precordial churning murmur (mill wheel), tachycardia, thready pulse, unresponsiveness	Place patient in left lateral Trendelenburg position Clamp catheter Notify physician Monitor vital signs Prepare for resuscitation Note: It takes only 1 second for 100 cc of air to be inspired by a patient sitting upright with an open 14-g CVC Always use Leur-lock connections
Catheter migration: CVC moves from its insertion placement site to another location; may result from improper suturing, disease process, changes in intrathoracic pressure, forceful catheter flushing, tumor progression, venous thrombosis; also spontaneous (no reason when patient physically active)	Percutaneous PICC Midclavicular Tunneled catheter Implanted port	Aspiration difficulties; burning sensation, discomfort, or pain during infusion; edema of chest or neck; increased external catheter length; leaking around the insertion site; cardiac dysrhythmias; palpation of catheter in external jugular vein; patient complaints of gurgling sound in ear	Radiographic verification of tip placement Assist with CVC removal and replacement Place new PICC
Local infection: Infection at insertion site as result of break in aseptic technique; a local infection may precede or occur concomitantly with sepsis; local infection includes exit site, pocket, or tunnel infections	Percutaneous PICC Midclavicular Tunneled catheter Implanted port	Cording of vein; site drainage, redness, tenderness, warmth; increased basal temperature	Notify physician Draw blood cultures from CVC Obtain peripheral blood cultures Administer antibiotics, anticoagulants Evaluate central line for removal Aseptic prep with 2% CHG after placement

(Continued on following page)

Table 12–6 COMPLICATIONS ASSOCIATED WITH CENTRAL VENOUS ACCESS DEVICES *(Continued)*

Complication and Cause	Central Line Device	Signs and Symptoms	Interventions
Septicemia (sepsis): Systemic infection caused by contaminated infusate or break in aseptic technique; the formation of a fibrin sheath increases the potential for microbial growth or other infectious processes; occurs more frequently in patients who are immunocompromised, malnourished, or undergoing steroid and TPN therapy	Percutaneous PICC Midclavicular Tunneled catheter Implanted port	Chills, cyanosis, fever, facial flushing, explosive diarrhea, headache, nausea and vomiting, positive blood culture results, tachycardia, septic shock (altered mental function), hypotension, inadequate organ perfusion, petechiae, purpuric pustules	Assess for all sources of infection Assess vital signs Draw central and peripheral blood cultures Administer antibiotics, anticoagulants, antipyretics Prepare for respiratory support and emergency resuscitation Use of 2% CNG for aseptic skin prep; and dressing changes.
Thrombosis: The formation of blood clots within the blood vessel; causes include catheter placement outside of SVC, fibrin sheath formation, platelet aggregation on the catheter, preexisting conditions (e.g., cardiovascular disease, hematopoietic pathology, limb edema), stasis and sluggish flow rate, use of thrombogenic catheter materials (PVC), vessel wall injury at the catheter insertion site, or from mechanical irritation, or infusion of irritating products	Percutaneous PICC Midclavicular Tunneled catheter Implanted port	Earache or jaw pain, insertion site edema or redness, malaise, tachycardia, tachypnea, unilateral arm or neck pain, edema, absence of pulse distal to the obstruction, coldness, cyanosis, necrosis of digits	Administer analgesics, anticoagulants Administer oxygen if needed Apply moist, warm compresses locally Apply surgical stocking Assess vital signs Avoid use of limb affected Position patient in semi- to high Fowler's position Prepare to institute emergency resuscitative measures Prepare patient for operative thromboectomy, insertion of vena cava filter if indicated Intermittent or continuous infusion of thrombolytic (tPA) Assist with catheter removal if necessary
Nonthrombolytic: Occlusion; crystallization of TPN admixtures and drug-to-drug or drug-to-solution incompatibilities	Percutaneous PICC Midclavicular Tunneled catheter Implanted port	Sluggish flow rates, total occlusion, inability to flush or obtain blood withdrawal	Attempt to restore patency using appropriate solution (HCl or sodium bicarbonate, or ethanol)

Complication and Cause	Central Line Device	Signs and Symptoms	Interventions
Thrombolytic occlusions: Deposits of fibrin and blood components within and around the CVC; intraluminal blood clot, fibrin sheath totally or partially; fibrin or precipitate accumulation can occur in portal reservoir in implanted devices	Percutaneous PICC Midclavicular Tunneled catheter Implanted port	Sluggish flow rates, total occlusion, inability to flush or obtain blood withdrawal (clinically silent), fibrin (may be able to infuse solutions), but unable to aspirate blood, "ball-valve-effect"	Attempt to aspirate clot Initiate appropriate fibrinolytic treatment with tPA
Pinch-off syndrome: CVC inserted via the percutaneous subclavian site is compressed by the clavicle and the first rib; results in mechanical occlusion; can result in complete or partial catheter transection and embolization	Percutaneous	Frequently unrecognized, catheter is positional, weak points on the catheter balloon out, difficulty in aspiration of blood, resistance to flushing or infusion (often relieved by rolling the shoulder or raising the arm), infraclavicular pain or swelling	Remove catheter Retrieve the embolized segment if necessary
SVC syndrome: Condition caused by blood clot, fibrin formation, or both that occludes the SVC	PICC Tunneled catheter Implanted port	Progressive shortness of breath; cough; sensation of skin tightness; unilateral edema; cyanosis of face, neck, shoulder, and arms; "short-cap edema" (edema of the upper extremities without edema of lower); jugular, temporal, and arm veins are engorged and distended; prominent venous pattern is present over chest	Notify physician immediately Radiographic confirmation of SVC syndrome Catheter may or may not be removed Anticoagulant therapy Place patient in semi-Fowler's position Administer oxygen Monitor fluid volume status
Damaged catheter: External: broken catheter caused by scissors, penetration with needle; internal: rupture caused by use of a smaller than 10-mL syringe, pinch-off syndrome	Percutaneous PICC Midclavicular Tunneled catheter Implanted port	External: Leakage from catheter, wet dressing, leakage at insertion site Internal: Swelling in chest area, infusion of solution into chest wall; swelling at point of catheter rupture (Note: Damaged external catheter can be an entry point of bacteria into the vascular system)	Monitor for pinholes, leaks, wet dressing External: Apply nonserrated clamp to proximal to damaged part of catheter Internal: Stop infusion, place patient on bedrest, prepare to repair or remove catheter

Long-Term Access Devices

Devices designed for long-term use can be divided into two categories: tunneled catheters and implanted ports. These catheters are made of silicone or polyurethane and are available with single or multiple lumens. They require a surgical procedure for insertion. Certain catheters and cuffs are coated or impregnated with antimicrobial or antiseptic agents can decrease the risk for CRBSI and potentially decrease hospital costs associated with treating CRBSIs.

These agents include:

- Chlorhexidine/silver sulfadiazine
- Minocycline/rifampin
- Platinum/silver
- Ionic silver

Central Venous Tunneled Catheters

The need for prolonged central venous access and a method to decrease potential infection from the skin exit site resulted in the development of central venous catheters **(CVTCs)**. CVTCs have been available since 1975, when **Broviac** catheters were introduced for long-term TPN. The Broviac catheter was followed by a modified version, the **Hickman** catheter, which could accommodate the delivery of therapies to bone marrow transplant patients. CVTCs became the prototype for a variety of tunneled catheters currently on the market for various therapies. Inserted through a subcutaneous tunnel, these catheters are often referred to as indwelling catheters, tunneled CVCs, or right atrial catheters.

CVTCs are intended to be used for months to years to provide long-term venous access for obtaining blood samples and for administering drugs, blood products, and TPN.

CVTCs are composed of polymeric silicone with a Dacron polyester cuff that anchors the catheter in place subcutaneously. This cuff is about 2 inches from the catheter's exit site, which becomes embedded with fibroblasts within 1 week to 10 days after insertion, reducing the chances for accidental removal and minimizing the risk of ascending bacterial infection. CVTCs are available with single, double, or triple lumens. They vary in size from pediatric to adult, with most internal lumens ranging from 0.5 to 1.6 mm.

One of the advantages of CVTCs is that a break or tear in the catheter is easy to repair without adhesive. Depending on the type of catheter and the type of repair needed, adhesive may be required.

An attachable cuff, VitaCuff,™ is available for CVTCs. This cuff is made of biodegradable collagen impregnated with silver ion. Subcutaneous tissue grows to the cuff, providing a mechanical barrier, and the silver ion provides a chemical barrier against organisms. This cuff has proved to be cost effective in decreasing catheter-related septicemia (Maki & Mermel, 1998).

A development in CVTCs is the application of the Groshong® valve feature, which has been marketed since 1984 (Fig. 12–10). This catheter has a few unique features that set it apart from other CVTCs. The Groshong® catheter is made of soft, flexible silicone material. The outer diameter dimensions are small. The catheter is available with single, double, or triple lumens. The silicone material has a recoil memory that returns it to its original configuration if accidentally pulled. Another unique feature of the Groshong® catheter is the two-way valve placed near the distal end, which restricts backflow of blood, but can be purposefully overridden to obtain venous blood samples. This valve eliminates the need for flushing with heparin. The valve is open inward, minimizing the risks of blood backing up the catheter lumen. The Groshong® valve feature is now available on a variety of CVCs, including PICCs and ports (Fig. 12–11).

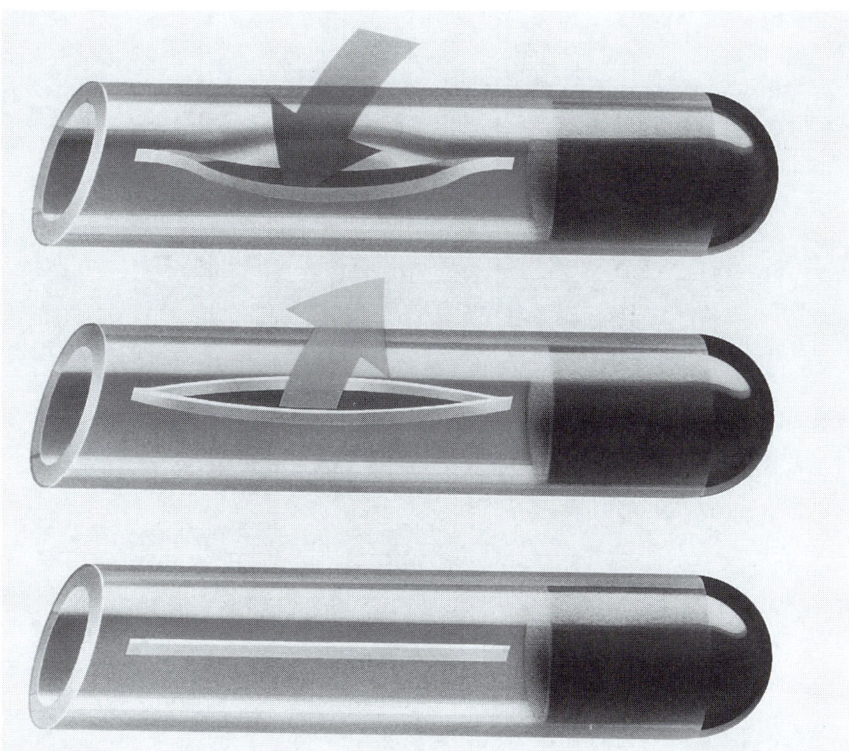

Figure 12–10 ■ Groshong® valve. (Courtesy of BARD Access Systems, Salt Lake City, UT.)

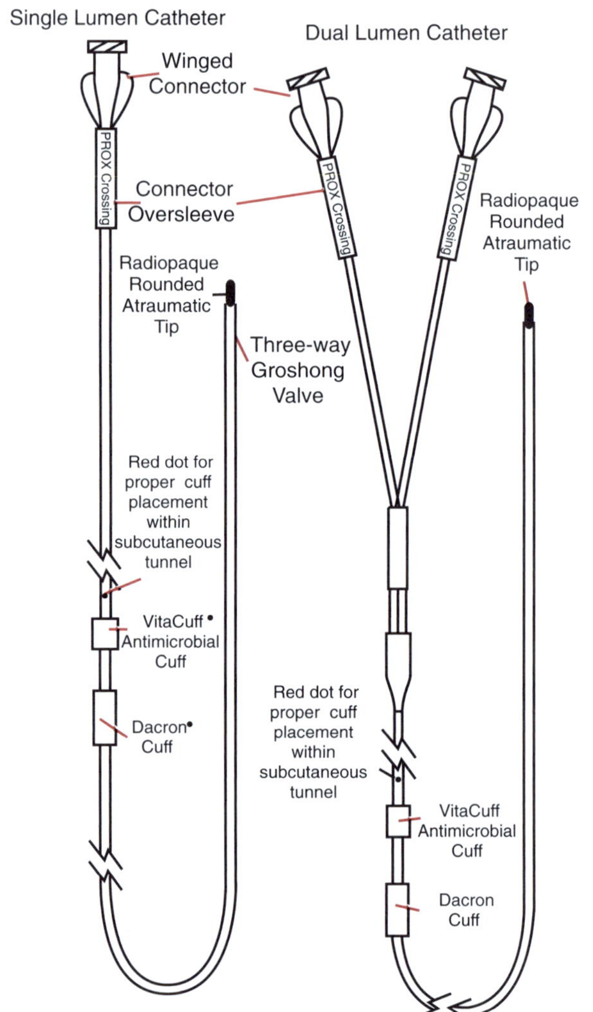

Figure 12–11 ■ Schematic of Groshong® catheters—single- and double-lumen with VitaCuff® and Dacron cuff. (Courtesy of BARD Access Systems, Salt Lake City, UT.)

ADVANTAGES

1. Can be repaired if it breaks or tears.
2. Can be used for many purposes including:
   a. Blood samples
   b. Monitoring central venous pressure
   c. Administering TPN
   d. Drug administration
3. Can be used for the patient with a chronic need for I.V. therapy.

DISADVANTAGES

1. Daily to weekly site care
2. Cost of maintenance supplies (dressings, materials, and changes; frequency of flushing and cap changing)
3. Surgical catheter insertion procedure that requires maintenance
4. Can affect the patient's body image.

Insertion of Tunneled Catheters

Central venous tunneled catheters are inserted with the patient under local or general anesthesia by surgical **cutdown** or percutaneous puncture, and the catheter is placed by locating the jugular, femoral, or subclavian vein. A separate proximal incision is made on the chest or abdominal wall, and the catheter is directed through a subcutaneous tunnel between the two incisions. The catheter is open at the distal and proximal ends and trimmed to the approximate estimated length and threaded into the SVC or in the case of the femoral insertion, the inferior

Nursing Points-of-Care: Tunneled Catheters

- Be sure the catheter is clamped or capped at all times to prevent inadvertent air embolism. To maintain patency follow the steps for flushing the catheter.
- Keep all sharp objects away from the catheter.
- Never use scissors or pins on or near the catheter.
- If the catheter leaks or breaks, take a nonserrated (without teeth) clamp and clamp the catheter between the broken area and the exit site. Cover the broken part with a sterile gauze bandage and tape it securely. Do not use the catheter. Notify the physician.
- Protect the catheter when showering or bathing by covering the entire catheter with transparent dressing or clear plastic wrap. Cover the connections and protect hub connections from water contamination.
- Flush after a blood drawing with 10 to 20 mL of 0.9 percent sodium chloride, using a pulsatile technique.
- Heparin is used to maintain the patency of the catheter, except for the closed-ended catheters such as Groshong® or PASV catheter.
- Change the administration set for continuous infusions every 72 hours. If infusing blood, blood products, or lipids change within 24 hours of initiating therapy.

vena cava. The position is confirmed by fluoroscopy, adjusted if needed, and then sutured to the skin or the incision is closed with Steri-Strips®. These remain in place for 10 to 14 days (Fig. 12–12).

NURSING FAST FACT!

The catheter should be clamped if malfunction is suspected or when catheter breakage occurs.

Flushing Procedure

Flushing procedures vary according to the agency. Generally it is accepted practice to flush the CVTCs with twice the catheter volume of heparinized saline (volumes range from 0.8 to 1.6 mL). After medication administration or daily maintenance, flush the catheter with saline; then follow with heparinized saline. The use of heparinized saline is usually unnecessary in the Groshong® catheter. Refer to Procedures Display 12–5.

NURSING FAST FACT!

Various catheter manufacturers recommend using anywhere from 1 to 10 mL, with concentrations of heparin ranging from 10 to 100 U/mL. The frequency of flushing also varies from daily to once per week. When flushing the catheter, remember that different catheters require different amounts of heparin; always check the manufacturer's recommendations (Hadaway, 2000).

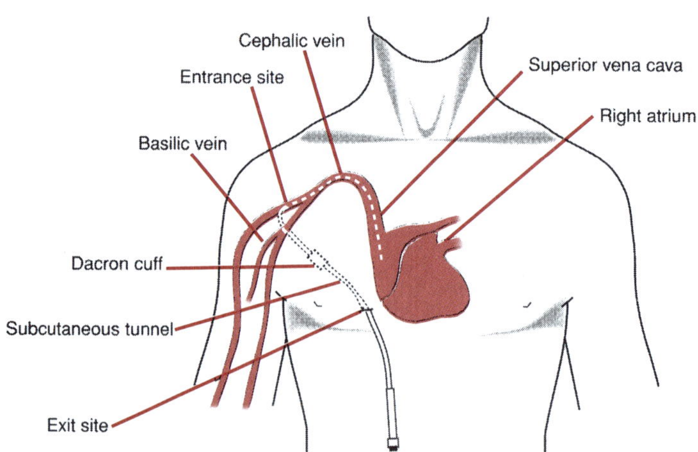

Figure 12–12 ■ Anatomic placement of tunneled catheter. (Courtesy of BARD Access Systems, Salt Lake City, UT.)

PROCEDURES DISPLAY 12–5

Flushing CVTC

Verify the physician's order. Educate the patient on the purpose of the procedure and site observation after discontinuation. Follow hand hygiene procedures. Observe Standard Precautions.

Equipment Needed

- 10-mL syringe
- Preservative-free 0.9% sodium chloride
- Gloves
- Sharps container
- Antiseptic solution
- Prefilled air-locked syringe with 5 mL of heparin 10 to 100 U/mL (or custom-made kits)

Procedure

1. Aseptically prepare sterile supplies.
2. Put on gloves.
3. Prepare air-purged heparin flush.
4. Remove tape holding the catheter to chest wall.
5. Cleanse the cap-catheter connection point with alcohol for 30 seconds.
6. Place on sterile 2 × 2 sponge and allow to dry.
7. Close the clamp.
8. Pick up the catheter hub protected by sterile sponge; do not touch the cleansed connection.
9. Attach syringe containing 0.9% sodium chloride to the injection port via a needleless system.
10. Aspirate to check patency.
11. Instruct the patient to perform the Valsalva maneuver and open the CVC clamp if hub-to-syringe connection (if not accessing through resealable diaphragm).
12. Flush line with 10 to 20 mL of 0.9% sodium chloride using the push–pause method.
13. Attach syringe with air-purged heparinized saline to the injection port.
14. Flush the line with 5 mL of heparin. Clamp the line while infusing the last 0.5 mL of solution. If a three-position pressure-sensitive valve (Groshong®) or pressure-activated safety valve (PASV) is used, heparin is not used and the line does not need to be clamped.
15. Document the procedure on the patient record.

Flush the CVTCs with twice the catheter volume of heparinized saline. After medication administration or daily maintenance, flush the catheter with saline; then follow with heparinized saline. The use of heparinized saline is usually unnecessary for closed valve such as Groshong® or pressure-activated safety valve (PASV®).

FLUSHING A TUNNELED CATHETER WITH CLOSED PRESSURE-SENSITIVE VALVES

Policies and procedures vary from institution to institution. The three-position pressure-sensitive valve (Groshong® catheter) or the pressure-activated safety valve (PASV®) should be flushed every 7 days with 0.9 percent sodium chloride when not in use. Maintain aseptic technique. After administering medications, the catheter should be flushed with 5 mL of sodium chloride using the pulsatile push–pause method. After drawing blood or administering viscous solutions such as lipids, flush briskly with 20 mL of sodium chloride to prevent crystallization of the catheter tip. Manufacturers recommend that the catheter be irrigated with a syringe attached directly to the connection hub of the catheter.

CHANGING THE INJECTION (PRN) CAP

The injection cap must be changed at routine intervals and should be changed no more frequently than every 72 hours or according to the manufacturer's recommendations (CDC, 2002). If the catheter is flushed every other day, cap changing may be coordinated with scheduled flushing. Using an intermittent injection cap that has a very small amount of dead space is recommended.

NURSING FAST FACT!

If you have a multilumen catheter, remember to change all caps, even on unused lumens.

Dressing Management

Dressing management of a CVC dressing and site care is a sterile procedure. Dressing materials for CVC include nonwoven adherent dressing or transparent semipermeable membrane dressing (TSM) dressings. The nonwoven adherent dressing (gauze type dressing) should be changed every 48 hours. Gauze used in conjunction with a TSM dressing should be considered a gauze dressing and changed every 48 hours. The catheter–skin junction site should be visually inspected and palpated for tenderness daily through the intact dressing (INS, 2000, S44). The CDC states that "Transparent dressings reliably secure the device, permit continuous visual inspection of the catheter site, permit patients to bathe and shower without saturating the dressing, and require less frequent changes than do standard gauze dressings. If blood is oozing from the catheter insertion site, gauze dressing might be preferred (CDC, 2002)." Dressings should be changed at least weekly for adult and adolescent patients depending on the circumstances of the individual patient.

Catheter site care should be performed using aseptic technique and observing Standard Precautions and should coincide with all dressing changes. Antimicrobial solutions appropriate for CVC site cleaning include povidone-iodine, alcohol, and 2 percent chlorhexidine gluconate (INS, 2000, S57). The chlorhexidine-based preparations are preferred. Refer to Figure 12–17.

The nurse is required to follow policies and protocols of the agency regarding catheter site care and maintenance procedures.

Repair of the Catheter

The CVTC can tear during reinsertion of the introducer needle, during intermittent therapy when I.V. push therapy is performed, or when scissors are used near the catheter site. When this happens, blood usually backs up and fluid leaks from the site (except with closed pressure–sensitive valves). Air can enter the catheter through the tear, causing an air embolism.

Keeping up to date on repair methods can be difficult. Several types of repair kits are available. CVTCs should always be repaired using the appropriate repair device, according to the manufacturer's instructions for use and after consideration of infection and safety risks to the patient.

To repair the catheter, you need sterile gloves, mask, sterile drapes, sterile scissors, an approved antiseptic agent, extension set, and the appropriate repair kit. Follow the manufacturer's recommendations for external catheter repair.

NURSING FAST FACT!

Avoid serrated clamps on the catheter. External clamps should not be used routinely; they are unnecessary and could damage the catheter.

Blood Sampling from a Tunneled Catheter

See Procedures Display 12–6 for guidance concerning drawing a blood sample from a tunneled catheter.

Complications Associated with Tunneled Catheters

See Table 12–6 for a guide to CVTC catheter complications. Common risks associated with CVTCs include exit site infections, sepsis, thrombosis, nonthrombotic occlusions, catheter migration, torn or leading catheter, and air embolism (Moureau, 2001).

PROCEDURES DISPLAY 12–6

Blood Sampling from Central Vascular Access Device (CVAD)

Verify the physician's order. Educate the patient on the purpose of the procedure and site observation after discontinuation. Follow hand hygiene procedures. Observe Standard Precautions.

Discontinue administration of all infusates into the CVAD before obtaining blood samples.

Equipment Needed

- 10-mL syringe with 5 mL of preservative-free 0.9% sodium chloride
- Gloves
- Sharps container
- Antiseptic solution
- Empty 10-mL or larger syringe
- 20-mL syringe prefilled with 20 mL of sodium chloride
- Prefilled air-purged heparin 10 to 100 U/mL vials, 5 mL (or custom-made kits)

Procedure

1. Confirm order for lab work.
2. Check patient identification.
3. Put on gloves.
4. If injection port is not in use: Prep the valved access port with alcohol; allow to dry. Follow with 2% chlorhexidine gluconate or povidone-iodine.
5. If injection port is in use: Discontinue I.V. tubing and cap end to maintain sterility of tubing.
6. Prep the valved access port with alcohol; allow to dry.
7. Attach the 10 mL syringe prefilled with 5 mL of normal saline, then vigorously irrigate with 5 mL of sodium chloride using the pulsatile, push–pause method.
8. Draw 5 to 10 mL of blood into the attached syringe to discard. Remove the syringe.
9. Attach sterile syringe and withdraw blood sufficient to fill required collection tubes.
10. Attach syringe with sample blood to a Vacutainer and fill collection tubes.
11. Irrigate injection port with at least 20 mL of NS using pulsatile, push–pause method.
12. Reconnect the infusion line and begin infusion; OR attach prefilled air-purged heparinized saline and flush with heparin if catheter does not have a Groshong® valve.

(Continued on following page)

13. Label the collection tubes and deliver the sample to the lab as soon as the integrity of the CVC is ensured.
14. Dispose of used equipment in a sharps container.
15. Document the procedure in the patient record.

NURSING FAST FACTS!

- *If TPN is infusion, stop the infusion for 3 to 5 minutes before obtaining a blood specimen.*
- *Consider obtaining a peripheral venipuncture for coagulation studies in a heparinized catheter with patients receiving aminoglycosides. Blood levels have been shown to be altered when drawn from silicone catheters when concomitant infusions of anticoagulants or aminoglycosides occur (The National Committee for Clinical Laboratory Standards, 1998).*
- *Flushing with positive pressure decreases catheter complications.*

Implanted Ports

Implanted ports, another type of CVC, have been available for venous access since 1983. Originally, implanted ports were targeted to oncology patients who required frequent intermittent venous access. Ports consist of a reservoir, silicone catheter, and central septum (Fig. 12–13).

The implanted port vascular access system provides safe and reliable vascular access; the design provides patients with an improved body image, reduced maintenance, and improved quality of life.

The self-sealing septum of a regular profile can usually withstand 1000 to 2000 needle punctures, with the lower profile ports withstanding

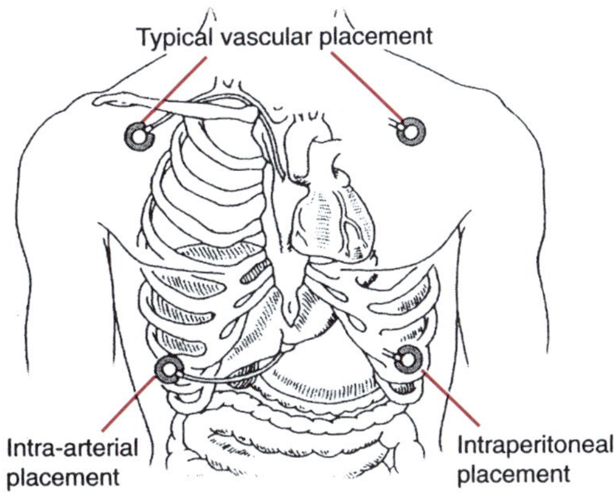

Figure 12–13 ■ Examples of placement sites for vascular access ports. (Courtesy of BARD Access Systems, Salt Lake City, UT.)

around 500 needle punctures. The port is made of stainless steel or titanium and has raised edges to facilitate puncture with a noncoring needle. The Huber Plus (Fig. 12–14) is an example of a noncoring needle that has safety features built in the wings. The port is made of stainless steel or titanium. The septum is connected to a silicone catheter. Many types of implanted VADs are available today and are placed for venous, arterial, and epidural infusion. Figure 12–15 shows various types of implanted ports.

ADVANTAGES

1. Less risk of infection when used intermittently
2. Less interference with daily activities
3. Little site care
4. Needs minimal flushing
5. Easy access for fluids, blood products, or medication administration
6. Less body image disturbance owing to the lack of an external catheter device
7. Few limitations on patient activity

DISADVANTAGES

1. Cost of insertion is high (considerably greater than with other VADs).
2. Postoperative care is 7 to 10 days.
3. Repeated needlesticks cause discomfort.
4. Minor surgical procedure is necessary to remove the device.

Insertion

The port is inserted after a local anesthetic is administered; the entire procedure takes from 30 minutes to 1 hour. An incision is made in the upper

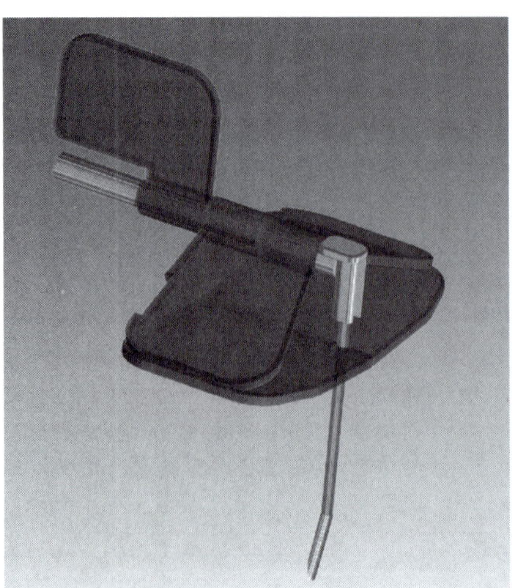

Figure 12–14 ■ Huber Plus Safety Needle. (Courtesy of Now Medical, Chadds Ford, PA.)

Portal Design	Material Composition
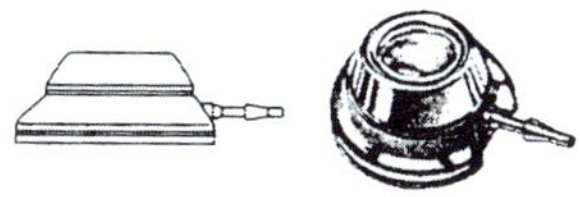 Hickman® Titanium Port	Titanium and Silicone
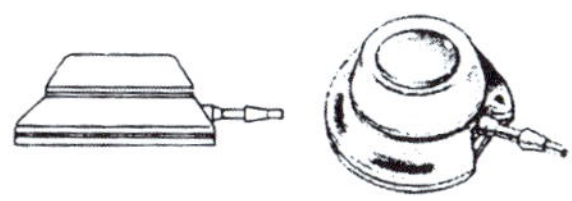 MRI® Port	Thermo Plastic and Silicone
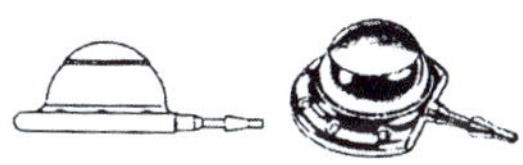 Dome™ Port	Titanium and Silicone
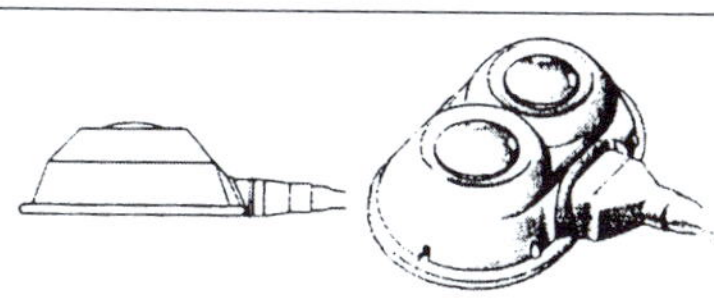 MRI® Dual Port	Thermo Plastic and Silicone

Figure 12–15 ■ Examples of types of port designs. (Courtesy of BARD Access Systems, Salt Lake City, UT.)

to middle chest, usually near the collarbone, to form a pocket to house the port. The silicone catheter is inserted via cutdown into the SVC; the port is then placed in the subcutaneous fascia pocket. The port contains a reservoir leading to the catheter. The incision for the port pocket is sutured closed, and a sterile dressing is applied. The dressing may be removed after the first 24 hours. This area should be monitored until the incision has healed, about 10 days to 2 weeks after insertion.

The subcutaneous port system catheter can be placed in any of the following: SVC, hepatic artery, peritoneal space for intraperitoneal therapy, and epidural space.

Implanted ports are available in single- or dual-septum chambers. Ports designed for peripheral access are also available.

Accessing the Port

To access an implanted port, including how to inject a bolus and inject a continuous infusion, follow the guidelines listed in Procedures Display 12–7 and Figure 12–16.

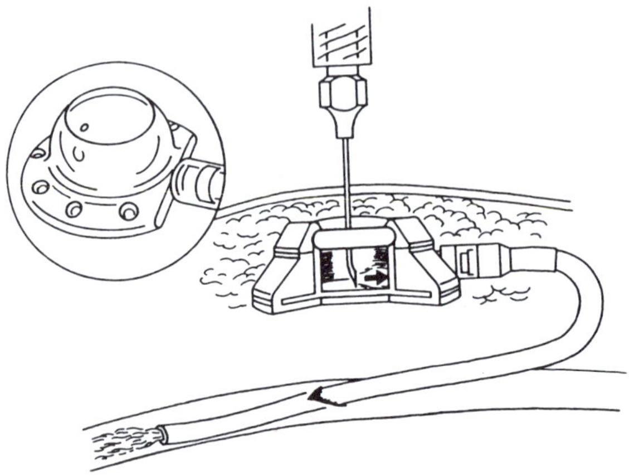

Figure 12–16 ■ Flushing an implanted port. (Courtesy of BARD Access Systems, Salt Lake City, UT.)

PROCEDURES DISPLAY 12–7

Accessing the Port

Verify the physician's order. Educate the patient on the purpose of the procedure and site observation after discontinuation. Follow hand hygiene procedures. Observe Standard Precautions.

Equipment Needed

- Sterile gloves (two pairs)
- Mask
- Gauze pads
- Alcohol swabs
- TSM dressing
- Injection caps
- Povidone-iodine swabsticks or chlorhexidine gluconate swabsticks
- Noncoring needle with clamping extension set
- Flush solutions containing 0.9 percent sodium chloride
- Heparin (100 U/mL)—5 mL
- 10-mL syringes
- Sharps container

Procedure

1. Don gloves and mask.
2. Palpate site to locate septum.
3. Cleanse port access with alcohol, rotating in a circular motion from inside out. Repeat two more times. Let dry.
4. Cleanse access site with 2 percent chlorhexidine gluconate or povidone-iodine, using friction (Fig. 12–17). Repeat two more times, let dry.

(Continued on following page)

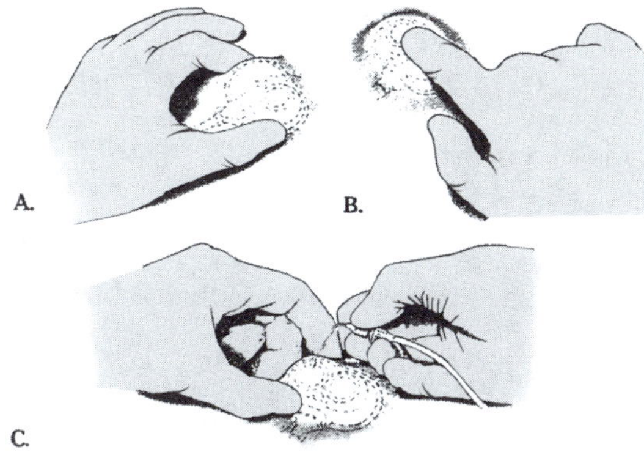

5. Remove and discard gloves.
6. Don a second pair of sterile gloves.
7. Prepare noncoring needle by flushing device, with clamped extension tubing attached, with 10 mL of preservative-free 0.9 percent sodium chloride injection.
8. Relocate the port by palpation and immobilize the device with the nondominant hand.
9. Insert noncoring needle perpendicular to the septum, pushing firmly through skin and septum until the needle tip contacts the back of the port.
10. Aspirate for blood return to confirm patency; flush with attached 10 mL of sodium chloride.
11. Maintain positive pressure when removing syringe from the port by engaging the clamping device.

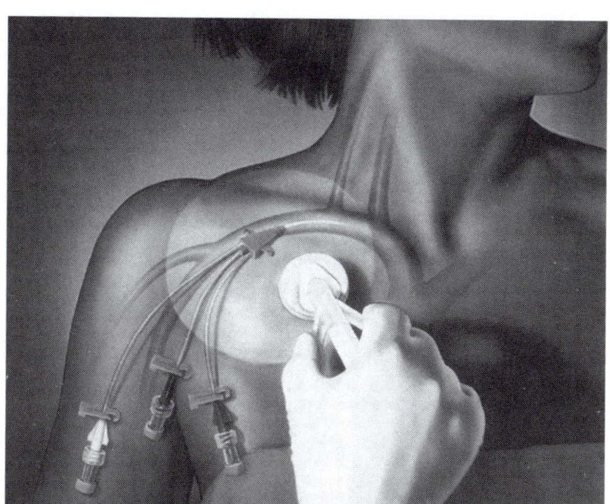

Figure 12–17 ■ Prepping a CVC with 2 percent chlorhexidine, circular scrub, working from center out. (Courtesy of Medi-Flex, Inc., Overland Park, KS.)

(Continued on following page)

PROCEDURES DISPLAY 12–7

Accessing the Port *(Continued)*

12. If port is to remain accessed:
    a. Place sterile gauze under device wing to prevent rocking motion of needle.
    b. Anchor noncoring needle to skin using sterile tape.
    c. Cover the needle and gauze with TSM dressing.
    d. Initiate prescribed therapy.
13. Document in the patient record.

NURSING FAST FACTS!

- *I.V. tubing must be changed every 24 hours.*
- *The dressing and extension tubing must be changed every 7 days (if nonocclusive) and caps changed no more frequently than 3 days (CDC, 2002).*
- *Note use a safety noncoring needle (see Fig. 12–14).*

Deaccessing an Implanted Port

To deaccess an implanted port, loosen the dressing covering the Huber access needle, cleanse the injection cap with alcohol and attach the syringe containing 0.9 percent sodium chloride solution. Flush the catheter.

Withdrawal of the Huber needle requires a two-handed technique. With the nondominant hand, use your thumb and index finger to stabilize the port. Steadily with an upward pull, engage the safety mechanism and remove the needle.

Check the tip integrity and examine the needle for signs of occlusion or clotting. Discard in the sharps container. Cover the site with an adhesive bandage for 30 to 60 minutes (Larouere, 1999).

Safety noncoring needle products are available on the market that are designed for use in implanted venous access devices to prevent inadvertent needlestick injury while deaccessing and should be used to ensure compliance to OSHA standards.

Refer to Procedures Display 12–8 for full instructions on deaccessing an implanted port.

Flushing Procedure

Flushing procedures vary from institution to institution. Flush the system with 5 mL of heparinized saline in a 10-mL syringe. If the port is not being used, flush with heparinized saline every 4 weeks. If the port is

PROCEDURES DISPLAY 12–8

Deaccessing Implanted Port

To deaccess needle from port:

1. Put on gloves.
2. Loosen the dressing covering the noncoring needle. Note discharge/drainage and discard in appropriate biohazard receptacle.
3. Cleanse injection port with alcohol and attach a 10-mL syringe containing sodium chloride.
4. Vigorously irrigate the port using a pulsatile push–pause method.
5. Withdrawing the noncoring needle requires a two-handed technique. With the nondominant hand, use your thumb and index finger to stabilize the port.
6. Steadily with an upward pull (perpendicular to the site) remove the needle with the dominant hand. While withdrawing needle, activate the safety feature on the noncoring needle (Huber–Plus).
7. If bleeding occurs at site, apply direct pressure using a sterile gauze sponge.
8. Apply dressing if needed.
9. Document in the patient record.

used for medication administration or blood component therapy, flush after every infusion with 10 mL of 0.9 percent sodium chloride, followed by 5 mL of sterile heparinized saline. Flush with 20 mL of 0.9 percent sodium chloride, followed by 5 mL of heparinized saline after blood withdrawal.

Complications

The same complications associated with CVTCs can occur with implanted ports. Table 12–6 provides guidelines for dealing with central line complications. Implanted ports can also develop site infection or skin breakdown and port migration. Extravasation of vesicant medications that are infusing into the port can occur if the needle is not in place through the septum of the port and the position is not confirmed. Fluid can extravasate and collect subcutaneously, resulting in burning or swelling around the port during infusion. Patients and nurses must always verify placement, secure the needle before initiating the infusion, and observe for signs of swelling or burning.

Nursing Points-of-Care: Implanted Ports

- Use a noncoring needle with appropriate port.
- Change the needle and extension tubing every 7 days.
- Flush the port with 0.9 percent sodium chloride and heparin every 4 weeks if the port is not in use or after every infusion, following the procedure outlined.
- For continuous infusion, change the dressing every 7 days.
- For continuous infusion, change the tubing every 72 hours. Replace tubing used to administer blood, blood products, or lipids within 24 hours.

Management of Occluded Central Venous Access Devices

Loss of Patency

Vascular access devices can become occluded as a result of mechanical obstruction, thrombotic occlusion, or drug precipitation (nonthrombotic). Loss of patency results from causes as simple as the patient's position to causes as involved as combinations of complex clotting processes juxtaposed on the disease process (Bagnall-Reeb, 1998).

Two criteria define CVC patency: the ability to infuse through the catheter and the ability to aspirate blood from the catheter. Withdrawal occlusion is a subset of catheter occlusions and describes the inability to freely aspirate blood from the catheter (Krzywda, 1999). The treatment must begin promptly; therefore, systematic evaluation of the catheter patency needs to be ongoing. If a VAD occlusion is left untreated, secondary complications can occur, such as loss of venous access, morbidity of recannulation, and risk of catheter infection because of a fibrin sheath for biofilm with bacterial or fungal colonization.

Preventive care of clot formation and subsequent occlusion include careful catheter insertion; routine assessment of dressings, exit sites, tubing, pumps, infusion bags, and clamps; meticulous technique in blood sampling; and avoiding potential drug or solution incompatibilities. Table 12–7 presents a guide to troubleshooting occlusions.

Catheter-related occlusions can be categorized as:

1. Complete occlusions: Total inability to withdraw blood and infuse fluids via the catheter
2. Partial occlusion: Difficulty in withdrawing and infusing fluids via the catheter
3. Withdrawal occlusion: Inability to withdraw blood via the catheter but with a capacity to infuse solutions without difficulty

> Table 12–7 **TROUBLESHOOTING GUIDE FOR OCCLUDED CENTRAL VENOUS CATHETERS**

Purpose of Catheter (Agent Infused)	Cause of Occlusion	Treatment
Prolonged use of catheter	Fibrin sheath or thrombosis	Thrombolytic: tPA (Activase)
Blood draw	Fibrin sheath or thrombosis	Thrombolytic: tPA (Activase)
Transfusions	Fibrin sheath or thrombosis	Thrombolytic: tPA (Activase)
Medication administration	Precipitate	$NaHCO_3$ or HCl
Cold medications or solutions	Precipitate	$NaHCO_3$ or HCl
Stability (pH of medication)	Precipitate	$NaHCO_3$ or HCl
Medication with poor solubility (e.g., Dilantin)	Precipitate	$NaHCO_3$ or HCl
Time elapse since medication mixed	Precipitate	$NaHCO_3$ or HCl
Fat emulsions (or three-in-one TPN)	Lipid aggregation	Ethanol

HCl = hydrochloric acid; $NaHCO_3$ = sodium bicarbonate.

4. Intraluminal obstruction: Obstruction within the catheter lumen that causes complete or partial occlusion
5. Extraluminal obstruction: Obstruction outside the lumen of the catheter, typically causing withdrawal occlusion
6. Intravenous obstruction: An obstruction (usually a thrombus) in the vein that completely or partially stops blood flow; it may or may not affect the catheter's functionality.
7. Mechanical obstruction: An obstruction not related to precipitate or blood that partially or completely occludes the catheter (Mayo, 2001)

Mechanical Occlusion

The mechanical obstruction of a catheter can be either external or internal. External causes of occlusion are a kinked or closed clamp or a tight suture at the catheter exit site. External occlusion of flow may be caused by clogged injection cap, a clogged I.V. filter, an infusion pump that has been turned off, or an empty I.V. bag. Occlusion can also occur at the catheter exit site or vein entry site if the suture used to secure the line constricts the catheter.

Internal obstruction is caused by improper catheter tip placement, as well as catheter kinking or compression. The catheter can be pinched closed as a result of the patient's position by pressure of the clavicle against the first rib (pinch-off syndrome) or it can be obstructed by lodging the catheter tip against the vein wall. Catheter fracture is a partial or complete breaking of the catheter. Pinch-off syndrome is the most common cause when the subclavian vein is used to establish access.

Management

When I.V. flow is occluded, first determine whether the cause is internal or external. Examine the I.V. setup for kinked tubing, closed clamps, an empty infusion bag, and readjustment of the I.V. delivery system. Having the patient change position may correct the problem. Finally, chest radiography may help to confirm catheter tip placement and rule out migration. If pinch-off is documented on radiograph, medical intervention is needed to prevent catheter fracture.

Nursing Points-of-Care: Management of a Suspected Occlusion Caused by Mechanical Forces

- Reposition the patient.
- Have the patient cough.
- Reposition the catheter, if possible.
- Roll the patient's shoulder or raise the patient's arm on the ipsilateral side.
- Use fluoroscopy if indicated to locate a mechanical occlusion.
- Gentle aspiration may dislodge the occlusive material from within the catheter lumen. Thrombolytic agents are the only available drugs to lyse existing clots. They convert plasminogen to plasmin, which acts directly on the clot to dissolve the fibrin matrix.
- Forceful flushing of the catheter to push the clot into the circulation is not recommended.

  The use of a guidewire or snare to manipulate the clot out of the catheter is also not recommended.

Thrombotic Occlusion

Deposits of fibrin and blood components within and around the CVC can impede or disrupt flow. Thrombotic occlusions are caused by intraluminal or extraluminal blood clots, a fibrin sheath totally or partially around the catheter tip, or catheter abutment against the vessel wall. Implanted devices can accumulate fibrin or precipitate within the portal reservoir (Bagnall-Reeb, 1998). Thrombus formation can occur within the first 24 hours after insertion or over a period of time. A variety of thrombotic events can result in catheter occlusion.

An additional factor that can influence the formation of thrombi is blood reflux, which can be caused by needleless injection systems, which leave dead space inside the injection cap once the syringe is removed. Fluid flows back to fill this dead space, pulling blood into the catheter

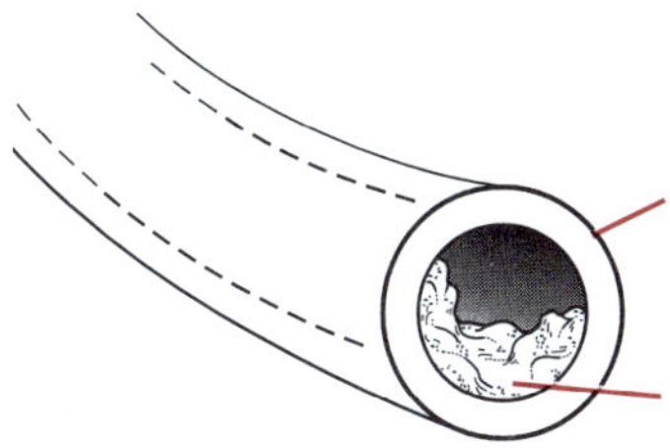

Figure 12–18 ■ Intraluminal occlusion. (From Bagnall-Reeb, Ryder, & Anglim [1994]. Venous Access Device Occlusions Independent Study Module. Abbott Park, IL: Abbott Laboratories.)

lumen (Hadaway, 2000a). Catheter type can affect thrombosis risk; flushing is still the primary method used to prevent thrombotic catheter occlusions (Hadaway, 2000c).

Intraluminal Occlusion

Intraluminal occlusion occurs when the lumen of the catheter is obstructed by either clotted blood or an accumulation of fibrin. Frequently, the cause is blood remaining in the catheter after inadequate irrigation or retrograde flow (Fig. 12–18). Also, poor flushing technique after blood sampling may allow layers of fibrin to accumulate over time, narrowing or obstructing the lumen.

Fibrin Sleeve and Fibrin Tail

Platelet aggregation and fibrin deposition may completely encase the surface of the catheter and form a sac around the distal end of the catheter (Fig. 12–19). The sac causes retrograde flow of infusate up the catheter. The infusate may be observed on the skin (in nontunneled catheters), in the skin tunnel (in tunneled catheters), or in the subcutaneous pocket of implanted ports (Bagnall-Reeb, 1998). A "tail" of fibrin extending off the catheter tip can occur owing to platelet aggregation and fibrin accumulation. The tail usually does not interfere with infusion but may occlude the catheter on aspiration. This is commonly known as the "ball valve effect."

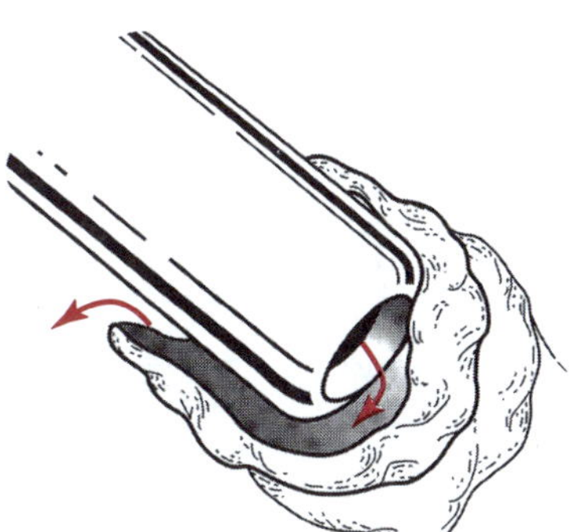

Figure 12–19 ■ Fibrin sleeve. (From Bagnall-Reeb, Ryder, & Anglim [1994]. Venous Access Device Occlusions Independent Study Module. Abbott Park, IL: Abbott Laboratories.)

Venous Thrombosis

Endothelial damage to a blood vessel can result in fibrin deposition at the point of cellular damage. If the thrombus occurs along the wall of the vein, it is a mural thrombus. If the thrombus completely occludes the vein, it is a venous thrombosis.

Portal Reservoir Occlusion

Fluid viscosity or an improper flushing technique can produce fibrin or precipitate deposits within the reservoir of the port (Fig. 12–20). Accumulation of deposits leads to obstruction of the infusion.

Thrombolytic Administration

Alteplase® is a recombinant form of the naturally occurring tissue plasminogen activator (tPA) that enhances the conversion of plasminogen to plasmin in the presence of fibrin. When introduced into the systemic circulation, Alteplase® binds to the fibrin in a thrombus and converts the entrapped plasminogen to plasmin. This action initiates local fibrinolysis.

Cathflo® Activase® (alteplase) is indicated for the restoration of function to central venous access devices as assessed by the ability to withdraw blood. Cathflo Activase is a thrombolytic that works by targeting fibrin (the substance that causes blood to clot), dissolving the thrombus (blood clot) and restoring function to the central venous access device (CVAD). Alteplase is packaged in 50- to 100-mg vials but only 2 mg is needed of catheter clearance (Hadaway, 2000a). It is instilled into a dysfunctional catheter at a concentration of 1 mg/mL. For patients weighing more than 30 kg, instill 2 mg/2 mL into the occluded catheter. For patients

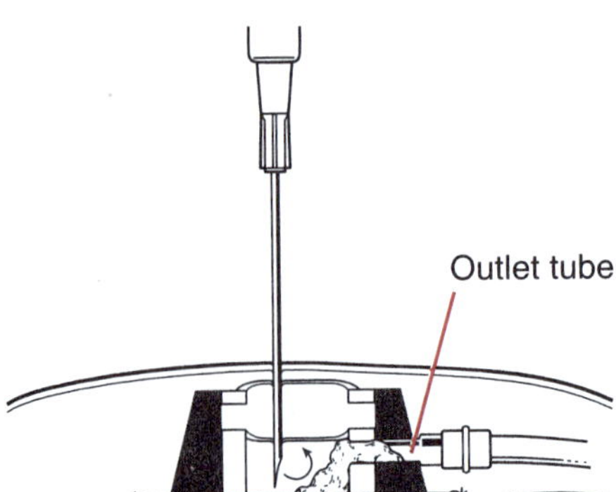

Figure 12–20 ■ Portal reservoir occlusion. (From Bagnall-Reeb, Ryder, & Anglim [1994]. Venous Access Device Occlusions Independent Study Module. Abbott Park, IL: Abbott Laboratories.)

weighing 10 to more than 29 kg instill 110 percent of the internal lumen volume of the occluded catheter not to exceed 2 mg/2 mL. Safety and effectiveness have not been established for patients weighing less than 10 kg (Gahart & Nazareno, 2004).

Contraindications to Thrombolytic Therapy

Patients who have active internal bleeding, intracranial neoplasm, hypersensitivity to thrombolytic agents, liver disease, subacute bacterial endocarditis, or visceral malignancy or who have had a cerebrovascular accident within the past 2 months or intracranial or intraspinal surgery should not receive a thrombolytic agent.

Drug Incompatibilities

Even multiple-lumen catheters may not have enough lumens dedicated to each drug to guarantee that precipitation caused by contact between two or more incompatible drugs, minerals, or electrolytes will not occur. Combinations that commonly lead to precipitation include (Hadaway, 2000b):

1. Phenytoin and most other solutions
2. Vancomycin and heparin
3. Tobramycin and heparin
4. Fluorouracil and droperidol
5. Dobutamine and furosemide
6. Dobutamine and heparin

Complications of Thrombolytic Therapy

BLEEDING

The most frequent adverse reaction associated with all thrombolytics in all approved indications is bleeding. Cathflo Activase has not been studied in patients known to be at risk for bleeding events that may be associated with the use of thrombolytics. Caution should be exercised with patients who have active internal bleeding or who have had any of the following within 48 hours:

- Surgery
- Obstetrical delivery
- Percutaneous biopsy of viscera or deep tissues
- Puncture of noncompressible vessels

In addition, caution should be exercised with patients who have thrombocytopenia, other hemostatic defects (including those secondary to severe hepatic or renal disease), or any condition for which bleeding constitutes a significant hazard or would be particularly difficult to manage because of its location, or who are at high risk for embolic complications (e.g., venous thrombosis).

Death and permanent disability have been reported in patients who have experienced stroke and other serious bleeding episodes when receiving pharmacologic doses of a thrombolytic.

INFECTION

Cathflo Activase should be used in caution in the presence of known or suspected infection in the CVC. Using a thrombolytic with infected catheters may release a localized infection in the systemic circulation. Care should always be taken to ensure aseptic technique.

Nursing Points-of-Care: Thrombolytic Therapy

1. Observe the patient continuously.
2. Do not use force when instilling a thrombolytic agent into a catheter.
3. Attempt to declot the catheter every 15 minutes after dwell time.
4. If using a pharmacologic dose, monitor thrombin time, prothrombin time, or activated partial thromboplastin time.
5. Keep the physician informed.

Nonthrombotic Occlusion

Nonthrombotic occlusions are caused by mineral precipitates. Precipitates result from poorly soluble I.V. fluid components or the interaction of the infusate with other solutions. Crystallization of TPN admixtures and drug-to-drug or drug-to-solution incompatibilities are also causes of catheter occlusions.

Precipitates may occur gradually, causing sluggish flow, or they may be immediate, totally occluding the line. Determining the pH of the medication that has precipitated is the key in attempting to restore patency.

For medications at a low pH (less than 6.0), the instillation of a 0.1 *M* solution of hydrochloric acid (HCl) has been reported to restore catheter function. Sodium bicarbonate ($NaHCO_3$), 1 mEq/mL, has been used to restore patency in catheters occluded by precipitation of medications soluble in a basic state (pH higher than 7.0) (Bagnall-Reeb, 1998).

NURSING FAST FACTS!

- *Use of HCl or $NaHCO_3$ to clear drug precipitates is not FDA approved. Caution should be taken in using either therapy.*
- *As a preventive measure, brisk flushing of the catheter with an appropriate volume of sodium chloride after the infusion of three-in-one solutions may reduce the intraluminal lipid residue.*

Catheter obstruction in patients receiving TPN may be caused by crystallization of calcium phosphate or lipid residue. This precipitation is caused by pH, concentrations of dextrose, amino acid, and calcium as well as by increased temperature. To restore patency in catheters occluded with crystallized calcium phosphate, use 0.1 *M* of HCl in a volume equal to the internal filling capacity and allow it to dwell for 20 minutes before being withdrawn.

Lipid occlusions may occur with three-in-one admixtures of parenteral nutrition. The buildup of lipid residue within the catheter lumen or port reservoir may cause sluggish flow or total obstruction. This residue can be dissolved with a 70 percent solution of ethanol (Hadaway, 1998).

Websites

Intravenous Nurses Society: *www.ins1.org*
National Association of Vascular Access Networks (NAVAN): *www.navannet.org*
Canadian Intravenous Nurses Association (CINA): *web.idirect.com*

Other sites:

Pediatric Central Venous Access

Long-term central venous access is an integral part of managing children with cancer, certain congenital malformations, and gastrointestinal (GI) malfunction as well as for those who need long-term access for medication or blood products.

After a decision is made to use a VAD, the device type must also be patient and disease specific. For children age 3 years and younger, totally implanted devices are used with the least frequency and most frequently in children older than age 15 years (Wiener & Albanese, 1998). The use of peripherally inserted central catheters has become accepted in the pediatric population. Typically with diameters ranging from 20 to 28 gauge, they can be inserted to lengths ranging from 8 to 20 cm. Percutaneous midline catheters have been used in the neonatal patient in 24 to 28 gauge and 8 cm in length, and are used to deliver fluids to the neonate (Dawson, 2002).

Multilumen devices are especially useful in the care of critically ill children or in children who experience continuous multiple-use of the device. Catheter size mirrors the size of the patient. Small-lumen external catheters are commonly placed in children age 3 years or younger.

NURSING PLAN OF CARE

MANAGEMENT OF CENTRAL VENOUS ACCESS DEVICES

Focus Assessment

Subjective

- Assess competency and dexterity of the patient in managing VADs.
- Inspect site for signs of infection. Inspect dressing for integrity.
- Examine PICC and tunneled catheters for integrity.
- Obtain baseline vital signs.

Objective

- Interview regarding present knowledge of illness and VADs.
- Identify learning need and ability.

Patient Outcome/Evaluation Criteria

Patient will:

- Be free of complications associated with insertion and postinsertion of CVCs.
- Describe anxiety and coping patterns.
- Demonstrate progressive healing of tissue.
- Demonstrate a willingness and ability to resume self-care and role responsibilities.
- Verbalize and demonstrate acceptance of appearance.
- Verbalize deficiency in knowledge or skill related to central VAD.

Nursing Diagnoses

- Anxiety (mild, moderate, and severe) related to threat to change in health status or misconception regarding therapy
- Altered tissue perfusion (cardiopulmonary) related to infiltration of vesicant medication

(Continued on following page)

- Body image disturbance related to perceptions of VADs
- Decreased cardiac output related to sepsis or contamination
- Fear related to insertion of catheter; fear of "needles"
- Impaired gas exchange related to ventilation-perfusion imbalance; dislodged VAD
- Impaired skin integrity related to VAD; irritation from I.V. solution; inflammation; infection
- Impaired physical mobility related to pain or discomfort resulting from placement and maintenance of VAD
- Knowledge deficit (VAD and maintenance of I.V. solution) relating to lack of exposure
- Risk of infection related to broken skin or traumatized tissue from the VAD

Nursing Management

1. Assist with insertion of central line.
2. Insert PICC according to agency protocol.
3. Follow standard precautions.
4. Maintain central line patency and dressing according to agency protocol.
5. Monitor for
    a. fluid overload.
    b. infiltration and infection.
    c. vital signs.
    d. daily weight.
    e. intake and output ratios.
6. Maintain occlusive dressing.
7. Maintain sterile technique.
8. Use an infusion pump for delivery of solutions when appropriate.
9. Use 10-mL syringe to flush catheters and obtain blood samples.

Patient Education

Patient instructions for central line devices should include:

- Type of central venous access device, purpose, and length of catheter or port that will be inserted; signs and symptoms to report, such as increased temperature, discomfort, pain, and difficult breathing; site care of PICC, CVTC, or implanted port
- Emergency measures for clamping the catheter if it breaks
- Flushing protocol
- Access line for administering medication, TPN, or fluids

Nurses are instrumental in educating patients and family members that the skin area over a subcutaneously implanted VAD should not be rubbed or manipulated in any way. Twiddler's syndrome, a condition in which a patient manipulates his or her ports by habit, can cause the internal catheter attached to the port to dislodge.

Home Care Issues

Central venous access devices are frequently used in the home for administering TPN, chemotherapy or biologic therapy, blood component therapy, and pain control, and for frequent blood sampling. Home infusion is comprehensive, beginning with principles of asepsis, handwashing, and standard precautions.

It is essential to assess whether or not the patient being considered for using a central venous line at home is interested in and motivated to learn self-care. This procedure requires a certain level of intellectual, emotional, and physical capacity and commitment to comply. If the patient is not physically or emotionally able to self-administer or monitor care, a reliable caregiver must be available.

Pretreatment assessment includes:

1. Taking a health history, including issues relevant to planned therapy
2. Verifying the medication and dosage that the patient is to receive
3. Reviewing complications and side effects of drug therapy and central line management
4. Reviewing the patient's history and past experience, if appropriate, with central lines
5. Assessing the patient's current knowledge of managing central lines
6. Providing written instruction and diagrams of accessing line, site care, and flushing protocol
7. Verifying insurance coverage for home care

The patient and family should have full instructions on how central line devices function and the safety precautions associated with their use. The home infusion patient should have step-by-step written information regarding care and maintenance.

Key Points

- The tip of central venous access devices should be in the SVC; the tip should reside within 3 to 4 cm of the right atrial SVC junction. It must be free floating and lie parallel to the vessel wall without any looping or kinking.
- Central venous access devices and the length of time they may remain include:
  - Percutaneous catheters: 7 days
  - PICCs: 6 weeks to 1 year
  - Midclavicular catheters: 6 weeks
  - CVTCs: 3 years
  - Implanted ports: 3 years
- The patient should be well hydrated if the infraclavicular approach to percutaneous catheterization is used.

- The optimum frequency for changing TSM dressing is unknown, but the dressing should be changed at established intervals (generally every 3 to 7 days) or immediately if the integrity of the dressing is compromised.
- The basilic vein is the preferred insertion site for PICCs.
- After insertion of the central line, verification by chest radiograph must be obtained before any infusion is administered.
- To avoid intravascular malposition of the catheter in the jugular vein, have the patient turn his or her head toward the side of the venipuncture. This changes the angle of the catheter to move downward toward the SVC.
- Syringes with capacities of 10 mL or more must be used to access or irrigate central lines, as excessive pressure from smaller-barreled syringes can cause damage or rupture of the line.
- Nurses managing central lines must be trained in their use, follow manufacturer guidelines, comply with agency protocols and policies, and be fully competent in the assessment, planning, intervention, and evaluation of the patient.
- Use Luer-locking connections on all central lines.
- Immediate complications of central lines include:
  - Bleeding
  - Pneumothorax
  - Hemothorax
  - Chylothorax
  - Brachial plexus injury
  - Extravascular malposition
- Delayed complications of central lines include:
  - Air embolism
  - Catheter migration
  - Local infection
  - Septicemia
  - Thrombosis
  - Thrombolytic occlusions
  - Precipitate occlusions
  - SVC syndrome
  - Pinch-off syndrome
- Implanted ports are available in single- or dual-septum chambers.
- Use the "push–pause" method of flushing central lines.
- Use thrombolytic agent to declot a central line of a thrombus or fibrin sheath. Use HCl for precipitates of drugs that have a low pH. Use $NaHCO_3$ for restoring patency of agents with high pH.
- The first step in troubleshooting an occluded central line is to check for mechanical obstruction.

Critical Thinking: Case Study

As a new graduate, you have been asked to change a complicated abdominal dressing on a patient postoperatively. This patient is receiving chemotherapy via a Hickman tunneled catheter. As you are cutting the dressing off, you accidentally puncture the catheter.

What do you do? How could this have been avoided?

Media Link: Answers to this case study and additional critical thinking exercises are on the enclosed CD–ROM.

Post-Test

1. Implanted ports, when not in use, can be flushed every:
   - a. Week
   - b. 2 Weeks
   - c. 3 Weeks
   - d. 4 Weeks
2. The major complication(s) of short-term central venous access devices include all of the following **EXCEPT:**
   - a. Phlebitis
   - b. Intravascular and extravascular malpositioning
   - c. Air embolism
   - d. Thrombolytic occlusion
3. When tunneled catheters are used, an advantage to the patient is that they:
   - a. Remain patent without flushing procedures
   - b. Can be replaced easily
   - c. Can be used for multiple purposes
   - d. Have minimal associated body image change
4. The majority of central venous access devices are made of:
   - a. Polyurethane
   - b. Silicone
   - c. PVC
   - d. Titanium
5. The blunt catheter tip with a three-way valve is called a:
   - a. PICC
   - b. Dual-lumen catheter
   - c. Groshong® tip
   - d. Hickman® catheter

6. Major complications with the implanted reservoir include all of the following **EXCEPT:**
   a. Displacement of septum
   b. Air embolus
   c. Occlusion
   d. External catheter breakage

7. Which of the following agents is used to declot a thrombus occlusion?
   a. 10 U of heparin
   b. HCl
   c. Activase
   d. $NaHCO_3$

8. The nursing intervention most effective for removing a "stuck" PICC is to:
   a. Stretch the catheter and tape it to the arm for 2 to 4 hours, then remove.
   b. Leave it alone, gently massage or apply moist heat to the area of the upper arm, and reattempt removal in 20 to 30 minutes after the vein relaxes.
   c. Use the guidewire to assist in removal.
   d. Call the physician to remove the catheter under fluoroscopy.

9. The *best* nursing intervention for flushing a central line to prevent fibrin buildup in the catheter is the:
   a. Push–pause technique
   b. Use of positive pressure
   c. Gentle instillation of solution with no pressure or agitation
   d. Instillation of heparin with each flush

10. The choice of syringe barrel capacity for irrigating a central line would be:
    a. 1 cc
    b. 3 cc
    c. 5 cc
    d. 10 cc

11. All of the following are nursing interventions related to dressing management of a PICC **EXCEPT:**
    a. Change gauze dressing after the first 24 hours.
    b. Apply transparent dressing after 72 hours, if no exudate is present at site.

c. Apply transparent dressing after the first 24 hours, if no exudate is present at the site.

d. Document observations of site including the presence of any redness, swelling, or drainage.

12. The nurse inserting a PICC would assess which of the following vein(s) for possible insertion of the catheter?

a. Innominate and jugular

b. Dorsal metacarpal network

c. Antecubital basilic and cephalic

d. Subclavian vein

13. Collection of a blood specimen from a central line that has parenteral nutrition infusing requires that the nurse *first*:

a. Turn off the infusion 3 to 5 minutes prior to obtaining the blood sample.

b. Flush the catheter with 10 mL of 0.9 percent sodium chloride.

c. Use only a Vacutainer system.

d. Withdraw 5 mL of blood and discard.

14. If a PICC needs to be repaired, the nurse should consider using:

a. Any universal repair kit

b. A blunt-end needle and injection cap system

c. Only the manufacturer-specific repair kit

d. Ultrasound to reinsert a new catheter

References

Bagnall-Reeb, H. (1998). Diagnosis of central venous access device occlusion. *Journal of Intravenous Nursing,* 21(5S), S115–S121.

Banton, J., & Banning, V. (2002). Impact on catheter-related bloodstream infections with the use of the Biopatch dressing. *Journal of Vascular Access Devices,* 7(3), 27–32.

Darouche, R., Raad, I., & Heard, S. (1999). A comparison of two antimicrobial-impregnated central venous catheters. Catheter Study Group. *New England Journal of Medicine,* 340, 1–8.

Dawson, D. (2002). Midline catheters in neonatal patients: Evaluating a change in practice. *Journal of Vascular Access Devices,* 7(2), 17–19.

Ellenberger, A. (2002). How to change a PICC dressing. *Nursing 2002,* 32(2), 50–52.

Gahart, B.L., & Nazareno, A.R. (2004). *Intravenous Medications* (15th ed.). St. Louis: Mosby-Year Book.

Gray, H. (1998). *Anatomy, Descriptive and Surgical.* New York: Crown.

Hadaway, L.C. (1998). Major thrombotic and nonthrombotic complications: Loss of patency. *Journal of Intravenous Nursing,* 21(5S), S143–S160.

Hadaway, L.C. (2000a). Managing vascular access device occlusion, Part 1. *Nursing 2000*, 30(7), 20.

Hadaway, L.C. (2000b). Managing vascular access device occlusion, Part 2. *Nursing 2000*, 30(8), 14.

Hadaway, L.C. (2000c). Flushing to reduce central catheter occlusions. *Nursing 2000*, 30(10), 42–55.

Hadaway, L.C. (2003). Skin flora and infection. *Journal of Infection Control*, 26, 44–48

Halerman, F. (2000). Selecting a vascular access device. *Nursing 2000*, 30(11), 59–61.

Intravenous Nurses Society (1997a). Position paper: Peripherally inserted central catheters. *Journal of Intravenous Nursing*, 20(4), 172–174.

Intravenous Nurses Society (1997b). Position paper: Midline and midclavicular catheters. *Journal of Intravenous Nursing*, 20(4), 175–178.

Intravenous Nurses Society (1999). Peripherally inserted central catheter (PICC) education module. Cambridge, MA: INS, Inc.

Intravenous Nurses Society (2000). *Revised Infusion Standards of Practice.* Philadelphia: Lippincott Williams & Wilkins.

Krzywda, E.A. (1999). Predisposing factors, prevention, and management of central venous catheter occlusions. *Journal of Intravenous Nursing*, 22(6S), S11–S17.

Larouere, E. (1999). Deaccessing an implanted port. *Nursing 99*, 99(6), 60–61.

Macklin, D. (2000). Removing a PICC. *American Journal of Nursing*, 100(1), 52–54.

Maki, D.G., & Mermel, L.A. (1998). Infections due to infusion therapy. In Bennett, J.V., & Brachman, P.S. (eds.). *Hospital Infections* (4th ed.). Philadelphia: Lippincott-Raven.

Maki, D., Mermel, L.A., Klugar, D., et al. (2000). The efficacy of a chlorhexidine impregnated sponge (Biopatch) for the prevention of intravascular catheter-related infection – a prospective randomized controlled multicenter study (Abstract). Presented at the Interscience Conference on Antimicrobial Agents and Chemotherapy. American Society for Microbiology, Toronto.

Marx, M. (1995). The management of difficult peripherally inserted central venous catheter line removal. *Journal of Intravenous Nursing*, 18(5), 246–249.

Mayer, T., & Wong, D.G. (2002). The use of polyurethane PICCS an alternative to other catheter materials. *Journal of Vascular Access Devices*, 7(2), 26–30.

Mayo, D.J. (2001). Reflux in venous access devices: A manageable problem. *Journal of Vascular Access Devices*, 6(4), 39–41.

Moureau, N. (2001). Preventing complications with vascular access devices. *Nursing 2001*, 31(7), 52–55.

The National Committee for Clinical Laboratory Standards (1998). *Collection, Transport, and Processing of Blood Specimens for Coagulation Testing and General Performance of Coagulation Assays; Approved Guidelines*, (3rd ed.). NCCLS document H3–A4, Villanova, PA: NCCLS, June 1998.

Perrucca, R. (2001). Intravenous monitoring and catheter care. In Hankins, J., Lonsway, R.A., Hedrick C., & Perdue, M. (eds.). *Infusion Therapy in Clinical Practice* (2nd ed.). Philadelphia: W.B. Saunders, pp. 389–417.

Sansivero, G. (1998). Venous anatomy and physiology. Considerations for vascular access device placement and function. *Journal of Intravenous Nursing, Supplement*, 21(55), S107– S113.

U.S. Centers for Disease Control and Prevention (2002). *Guideline for Prevention of*

Intravascular Device-Related Infections. Atlanta, GA: U.S. Department of Health and Human Services.

Wiener, E.S., & Albanese, C.T. (1998). Venous access in pediatric patients. *Journal of Intravenous Nursing* (Suppl), 21(5S), S123–S131.

Answers to Chapter 12 Post-Test

1. **d**
2. **a**
3. **c**
4. **b**
5. **c**
6. **d**
7. **c**
8. **b**
9. **a**
10. **d**
11. **b**
12. **c**
13. **a**
14. **c**

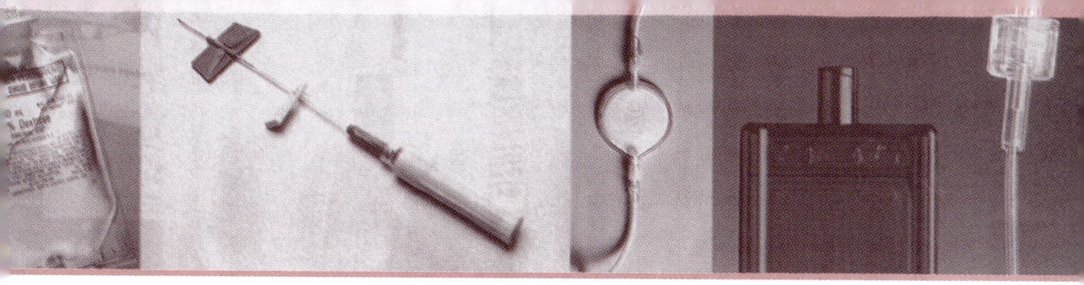

Chapter 13 Transfusion Therapy

Blood—a gift of life
—Author Unknown

Chapter Contents

LEARNING OBJECTIVES

Upon completion of this chapter, the reader will be able to:

1. Define the glossary of terms as related to nursing care of the patients receiving transfusion therapy.
2. Identify the antigens and antibodies in the blood system.
3. Identify the universal red blood cell donor type.
4. Identify the Rh antigens located on the red blood cells.
5. Identify the preservatives used in donor blood storage.
6. Summarize the tests used to screen donor blood.
7. Distinguish between homologous, autologous, and designated blood.
8. Describe each of the blood components, their indications, and key points in administration.
9. Describe the procedure for administration of blood components.
10. Establish a plan of action for a patient exhibiting symptoms of hemolytic transfusion, febrile transfusion, and mild allergic transfusion reactions.

GLOSSARY

ABO system Most important system determining compatibility; human blood groups that are inherited, groups determined according to which antigens are present on the surfaces of red blood cells, and which antibodies are present in the plasma

ADSOL Additive solution of 100 mL containing saline, dextrose, and adenine that is added to packed red blood cells

Agglutinin An antibody that causes particulate antigens, such as other cells, to adhere to one another, forming clumps

Agglutinogen An antigenic substance that stimulates the formation of a particular antibody

Allergic reaction Reaction from exposure to an antigen to which the person has become sensitized

Allogeneic Blood transfused to someone other than the donor

Alloimmunization Development of an immune response to alloantigens; occurs during pregnancy, blood transfusions, and organ transplantation

Antibody Protein produced by the immune system that destroys or inactivates a particular antigen

Antigen Any substance eliciting an immunologic response, such as the production of antibody specific for that substance

Autologous donation Blood donated before needed that is intended for use by the donor

Blood component Product made from a unit of whole blood such as platelet concentrate, red blood cells, fresh frozen plasma, cryoprecipitate

Citrate-phosphate-dextrose (CPD) A preservative for collected blood

Citrate-phosphate-dextrose-adenine (CPDA-1) A preservative that extends the shelf life of stored blood to 35 days

Delayed transfusion reaction Adverse effect occurring after 48 hours and up to 180 days after transfusion

Designated donation Transfer of blood directly from one donor to a specified recipient

Febrile reaction Nonhemolytic reaction to antibodies formed against leukocytes

Hemoglobin Respiratory pigment of red blood cells having the reversible property of taking up oxygen or of releasing oxygen

Hemolysis Rupture of red blood cells, with the release of hemoglobin

Hemolytic transfusion reaction Blood transfusion reaction in which an antigen–antibody reaction in the recipient is caused by an incompatibility between red blood cell antigens and antibodies

Homologous donation Donation of blood by a volunteer donor whose blood structure is similar to that of the selected recipient

Human leukocyte antigen (HLA) Used for tissue typing and relevant for transplant histocompatibility

Hypothermia Abnormally low body temperature

Immunohematology Study of blood and blood reactions

Microaggregate Microscopic collection of particles such as platelets, leukocytes, and fibrin, which occurs in stored blood

Pheresis Derived from the Greek word *aphairesis*, meaning "to take away"; used to denote the removal of blood, the separation into component parts, the retention of only the parts needed, and the return of the rest to the donor (e.g., removal of plasma is plasmapheresis)

Plasma Fluid portion of the blood, composed of a mixture of proteins in solution

Reaction The clinical symptoms that occur when a recipient responds negatively to substances in donor blood

Refractory Not responsive or readily yielding to treatment

Rh system Second most important system determining compatibility; Rh antigens are inherited and found on the surface of red blood cells; classified as positive or negative based on whether D antigen is present

Serum The cells and fibrinogen-free amber-colored fluid that separates from blood or plasma clots after coagulation

Thrombocytopenia Abnormally small number of platelets in the blood

To ensure the delivery of safe transfusion therapy, nurses must possess a knowledge and understanding of the blood system as well as basic immunohematology. Nurses must also be knowledgeable about the theory and practical management of blood component therapy. The first part of this chapter presents fundamental concepts of immunohematology, blood grouping, and the criteria for donor blood, including homologous, designated, autologous, and donation. Fundamental concepts of blood component therapy, administration equipment, administration techniques for each blood component, and management of transfusion reactions are presented in the second part of the chapter.

Basic Immunohematology

Immunohematology is the science that deals with antigens of the blood and their antibodies. The antigens and antibodies are genetically inherited and determine each person's blood group. An **antigen** is a substance capable of stimulating the production of an antibody and then reacting with that antibody in a specific way. Antigens of the blood are called **agglutinogens**. Any substance that can elicit an immunologic response is an antigen, and is located on the cell membrane. The three antigens on the red blood cells (RBCs) that cause problems and are routinely tested for are A, B, and Rh D. The human leukocyte antigen (HLA) is located on most cells in the body except mature erythrocytes. Antibodies are found in the **plasma** or **serum**.

Antigens (Agglutinogens)

ABO System

The most important antigens in the blood are the surface antigens A and B, which are located on the RBC membranes in the ABO system (Table 13–1). The name of the blood type is determined by the name of the antigen on the RBC. Individuals who have A antigen on the RBC membrane are classified as group A; B antigens, group B; A and B surface antigens,

> Table 13–1 **ABO BLOOD GROUPING CHART**

Blood Groupings	Recipient Antigens on RBCs	Antibodies Present in Plasma
A	A	Anti-B
B	B	Anti-A
AB	A and B	None
O	None	Anti-A and Anti-B

group AB; and neither A or B antigens, group O. This **ABO system** was developed in 1901 by Dr. Karl Landsteiner. (Table 13–2 provides an ABO compatibility chart.) Antigens are viewed as foreign substances when they enter the body (AABB, 2002).

Unique to the ABO system is the development of antibody in the serum of persons who lack the corresponding antigen. This phenomenon occurs occasionally in other blood systems but appears to be ubiquitous within the ABO system. As a result, if antigen A is present on the RBC, then antibody to B (anti-B) is present in the serum. If antigens A and B are present, no antibody exists in serum; conversely, if no antigen is present, then both anti-A and anti-B are present in the serum. (Table 13–3 provides ABO compatibility for plasma.)

CULTURAL AND ETHNIC CONSIDERATIONS: BLOOD TYPES AND RH FACTOR 13–1

Blood groups differentiate people in certain racial groups. A prevalence for type O blood has been found among Native Americans, with some incidence of type A blood and virtually no incidence of type B blood. Almost equal incidences of types A, B, and O blood are found in Japanese and Chinese people with the AB blood type found in only about 10 percent of this population.

African Americans and European Americans have been found to have equal incidences of A, B, and O blood types, with predominant blood types of A and O (Giger & Davidhizar, 2004).

Persons with type O blood are at a greater risk for duodenal ulcers, and those with type A blood are more likely to develop cancer of the stomach. The Rh-negative factor is most common in European Americans, much rarer in other racial groups, and absent in Eskimos (Giger & Davidhizar, 2004).

Rh System

After A and B, the most important RBC antigen is the D antigen, which was discovered in 1940 by Drs. Landsteiner and Wiener. The **Rh system** is so called because of its relationship to the substance in the RBCs of the Rhesus monkey. There are approximately 50 Rh-related antigens; the five principal antigens are D, C, E, c, and e. A person who has D antigen is

> Table 13–2 **ABO COMPATIBILITIES FOR PACKED RED BLOOD CELL COMPONENTS**

Recipient	Donor Unit, First Choice	Donor Unit, Second Choice	Donor Unit, Third Choice
A+	A+	O+, A−	O−
B+	B+	O+, B−	O−
AB+	AB+	AB−, A+, B+	O+, A−, B−, O−
O+	O+	O−	—
A−	A−	O−	A+, O+
B−	B−	O−	B+, O+
AB−	AB−	A−, B−, O−	AB+, A+, B+, O+
O−	O−	O+	—

Note: The universal RBC donor is O negative; the universal recipient is AB positive.

classified as Rh positive; one lacking D is Rh negative. A total of 85 percent of the population is classified as D-Rh-positive (AABB, 2002). There are no naturally occurring anti-D antibodies; however, D antibodies build up easily in D-negative recipients when stimulated with D-positive blood. Therefore, typing is done to ensure that D-negative recipients receive D-negative blood. Rh-negative recipients should receive Rh-negative whole blood, and any blood components that might contain RBCs should be Rh negative. Table 13–4 lists the most common blood types.

HLA System

The HLA antigen was originally identified on the leukocytes, but it has been established that **HLA** is present on most cells in the body. It is located on the surface of white blood cells (WBCs), platelets, and most tissue cells. HLA typing, or tissue typing, is important in patients with transplants or multiple transfusions and for paternity testing. The HLA system is very complex and is involved in immune regulation and cellular differentiation.

The HLA system is important in transfusion therapy because HLA antigens of the donor unit can induce **alloimmunization** in the recipient. This alloimmunization has been found to be a major factor in the onset of refractoriness to random donor platelet support. HLA incompatibility is a

> Table 13–3 **ABO COMPATIBILITY FOR FRESH FROZEN PLASMA**

Recipient	Donor Unit
A	A or AB
B	B or AB
AB	AB
O	O, A, B, or AB

> Table 13–4 **MOST COMMON BLOOD TYPES**

Type	Percentage of US Population
O Rh-positive	38
A Rh-positive	34
B Rh-positive	9
O Rh-negative	7
A Rh-negative	6
AB Rh-positive	3
B Rh-negative	2
AB Rh-negative	1

Source: *AABB (2003).*

possible cause of hemolytic transfusion reactions, and HLA antibodies as well as granulocyte- and platelet-specific antibodies have been implicated in the development of nonhemolytic transfusion reactions.

Methods used to decrease HLA alloimmunization include HLA matching and leukocyte depletion of the donor unit (AABB, 2002).

Blood may be depleted of leukocytes during three periods: (1) immediately after collection, (2) 6 to 24 hours after collection, and (3) at the time of infusion (AABB, 2002).

The trend today is for prestorage leukocyte depletion of packed RBCs and platelets. Early removal of leukocytes reduces the development of cytokines that appear to be implicated in many transfusion reactions.

NURSING FAST FACT!

Patients receiving multiple transfusions are at particular risk for developing complications related to leukocytes, such as sensitization to leukocyte antigens, nonhemolytic febrile reactions, transmission of leukocyte-mediated viruses, and graft-versus-host disease (AABB, 2002).

Antibodies (Agglutinins)

Antibodies within the blood system are proteins that react with a specific antigen. Antigens are **agglutinins** in that particulate antigens, such as other cells, adhere to one another in response to a specific antigen. The antibodies anti-A and anti-B are produced spontaneously in the plasma after birth and usually form in the first 3 months of life. An **antibody** has the same name as the antigen with which it reacts. For example, anti-A reacts to antigen A.

The naturally occurring antibodies, similar to those in the ABO system, are blood group antibodies that agglutinate erythrocytes containing corresponding antigens in a saline solution and are called saline antibodies. The naturally occurring antibody in the blood, which occurs within the inherited blood group, is from the class of antibodies called immunoglobulin mu (IgM). Complete antibodies are naturally occurring antibodies. Intravascular hemolysis may occur in vivo with naturally occurring antibodies (IgM).

Immunoglobulins or immune antibodies are a group of glycoproteins (i.e., complex molecules containing protein and sugar molecules) in the serum and tissues of mammals that possess antibody activity. Immunoglobulin molecules are divided into five categories. Some IgM antibodies, and all antibodies of the other four classes (IgG, IgA, IgD, and IgE), are produced by the immune system. These antibodies are produced by the immune system in response to previous exposure to the antigen via previous transfusion or pregnancy; they are not genetically inherited. When these antibodies meet with their corresponding antigen, the cells are affected but not destroyed in the intravascular system. The sensitized cells are removed intact by the reticuloendothelial system, primarily the spleen and liver.

Other Blood Group Systems

In addition to the ABO and Rh blood group antigens, more than 500 other antigens can be found on human RBCs (AABB, 2002). There are 24 known systems associated with RBCs (Weir, 2001).

The following are the most common groups identified: ABO, Lewis, Rh, MNS, Kell, P, Duffy, Lutheran, and Kidd.

Corresponding antibodies to all but ABO and Rh systems are found so infrequently that they do not usually cause common problems in transfusion therapy.

Testing of Donor Blood

At the time of donation, every unit of blood intended for homologous donation must undergo the following tests by the blood bank:

1. The ABO group must be determined by testing the RBCs with anti-A and anti-B serums and by testing the serum or plasma with A and B cells.
2. The Rh type must be determined with anti-D serum. Units that are D-positive must be labeled as Rh-positive.
3. Most blood banks test all donor blood for clinically significant antibodies. If all donors are not tested, then at least blood from donors with a history of previous transfusion or pregnancy should be tested for unexpected antibodies before the crossmatch.
4. All donor blood must be tested to detect transmissible disease. The blood component must not be used for transfusion unless the test results are nonreactive, negative, or within the normal range.

5. Each unit must be appropriately labeled. The label must include the following information: name of the component, type and amount of anticoagulant, volume of unit, required storage temperature, name and address of collecting facility, a reference to the circular of information, type of donor (i.e., volunteer, autologous, or paid), expiration date, and donor number (Fig. 13–1).

NURSING FAST FACT!

The label should also include statements indicating "this product may transmit infectious agents" and "properly identify intended recipient."

6. The facility performing the compatibility testing must do ABO and Rh grouping confirmation tests on a sample obtained from the originally attached segment of all units of whole blood or RBCs (AABB, 2002).

After blood is drawn from a donor, it is tested for ABO group (blood type) and Rh type (positive or negative), as well as for any unexpected RBC antibodies that may cause problems in the recipient. Screening tests are also performed for evidence of donor infection. The specific tests performed are:

- Hepatitis B surface antigen (HBsHg)
- Hepatitis B core antibody (anti-HBc)

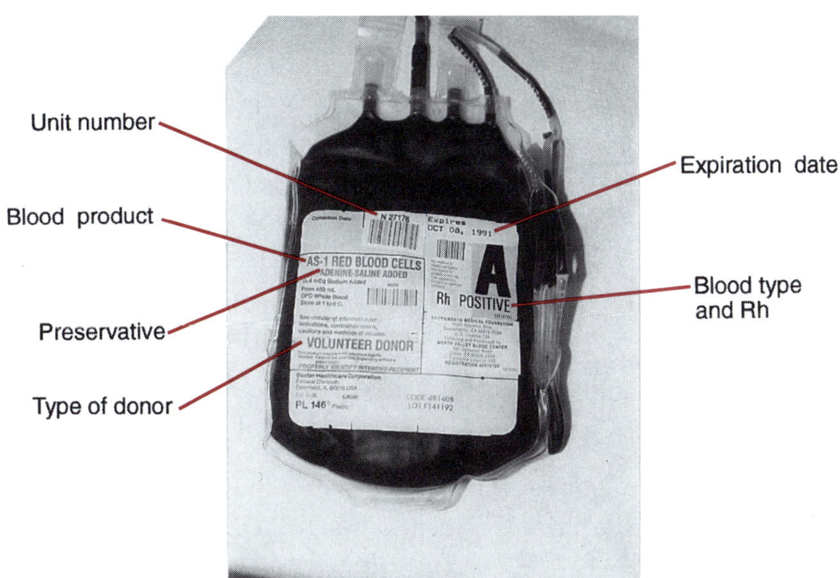

Figure 13–1 ■ Correct labeling of a unit of blood.

- Hepatitis C virus antibody (anti-HCV)
- HIV-1 and HIV-2 antibody (anti–HIV-1 and anti–HTVL-2)
- Serologic test for syphilis
- Nucleic aid amplification testing (NAT) for HIV-1 and HCV
- NAT for West Nile Virus (WNV) (AABB, 2002)

Compatibility Testing

Recipients of transfusions must be tested for ABO and Rh grouping. In addition, antibody screening and compatibility testing must be performed. Previous exposure to an antigen by pregnancy or transfusion may have caused the recipient to develop an antibody against an antigen.

Compatibility testing is performed between the recipient's plasma and the donor's RBCs to ensure that the specific unit intended for transfusion to the recipient is not incompatible. Blood from the donor and recipient are mixed and incubated under a variety of conditions and suspending media. If the recipient's blood does not agglutinate the donor cells, compatibility is indicated. Blood bank personnel are responsible for providing serologically compatible blood for transfusion.

When testing is complete, transfusion therapy can begin. The blood bank has two objectives: (1) to prevent antigen–antibody reactions in the body and (2) to identify antibody that the recipient may have and to supply blood from a donation that lacks the corresponding antigen. The testing of donor blood and recipient blood is intended to prevent adverse effects of transfusion therapy.

Blood Preservatives

There are several available RBC preservatives. Understanding of the RBC preservative is necessary because adverse reactions may occur in some patients as a result of chemicals in the anticoagulant preservative solution. The solutions in the blood collection bag have a dual function: as anticoagulant and as RBC preservative. Citrate is used in all blood preservatives as an anticoagulant. Citrate binds with free calcium in the donor's plasma. Blood will not clot in the absence of free or ionized calcium. Citrate prevents coagulation by inhibiting the calcium-dependent steps of the coagulation cascade. Preservatives provide proper nutrients to maintain RBC viability, function, and metabolism. In addition, refrigeration at 1 to 6°C preserves RBCs and minimizes the proliferation of bacteria (AABB, 2002).

In 1971, citrate-phosphate-dextrose (**CPD**) became a common preservative for blood. Phosphate is added to buffer the decrease in pH. The compound in the RBC that facilitates the transport of oxygen is 2,3-diphosphoglycerate (2,3-DPG). When the pH of the blood drops, there is a decrease in 2,3-DPG and therefore a lowering of the oxygen-carrying capacity of the blood. The 2,3-DPG levels remain higher in blood stored in CPD than in that stored with adenine-citrate-dextrose preservative. The expiration of RBCs preserved in CPD is 21 days stored at 1 to 6°C.

Citrate–phosphate dextrose–adenine (**CPDA-1**) was licensed in 1978, and contains 70 mL of anticoagulant-preservative in 500 mL of collected blood. This preservative contains adenine, which helps the RBCs synthesize adenosine triphosphate (ATP) during storage. Cells have improved viability in this anticoagulant preservative because the energy requirements of the cell are better preserved than with plain CPD. This preservative lengthens the shelf-life of the blood to 35 days at 1 to 6°C (Weir, 2001).

Additive red cell preservative system additive solution (AS) contains sodium chloride, dextrose, adenine, and other substances that support red cell survival and function up to 42 days. The volume of the AS in a 450-mL collection set is 100 mL. AS is added to the red cells remaining in the bag after most of the plasma has been removed. Additives approved by the Food and Drug Administration (FDA) include AS-1 (ADSOL), AS-3 (Nutrice), and AS-5 (Optisol) (AABB, 2002).

NURSING FAST FACT!

RBCs prepared with AS-1, AS-3, and AS-5 have better flow rates and do not require dilution with saline. Hypocalcemia is an adverse reaction that can occur when large amounts of citrated blood are infused in a person with impaired liver function.

Blood Donor Collection Methods

Homologous

The term **homologous** donation describes transfusion of any blood component that was donated by someone other than the recipient. Most transfusions depend on homologous sources and are provided by volunteer donors.

NURSING FAST FACT!

Paid donor blood products are not transfused in the United States. The donor criteria are less limiting than with homologous blood. However, if homologous donation criteria are not followed, the unused units cannot cross over to the volunteer supply.

Guidelines for Homologous Donation

Donor selection for homologous collection is based on a limited physical examination and a medical history to determine the safety of the donated unit. Strict criteria have been established for selection of prospective donors:

1. Brief health history, including illnesses, surgeries, drugs and medications, and immunization information
2. Screening for diseases
3. Stable vital signs
4. Age
5. Weight (smaller volumes should be drawn from donors weighing less than 110 lb)
6. No evidence of skin lesions at site of venipuncture
7. Adequate venous access for venipuncture
8. Has not donated blood or plasma within the last 8 weeks
9. Hemoglobin and hematocrit of at least 12.5 g/dL and 38 percent in males and 12.0 g/dL and 36 percent in females

Autologous

Autologous donation is the collection, storage, and delivery of a recipient's own blood. This option is considered for patients who are likely to receive a transfusion during elective surgery. Patients may be able to donate their own blood before the operation. The use of **autologous** blood avoids the possibility of alloimmunization because it does not contain foreign RBCs, platelets, and leukocyte antigens. The risk of exposure and disease transmission is also eliminated. Because of this, the use of autologous blood is regarded as safer than homologous transfusion. However, risks associated with labeling and documentation are still present. The same precautions used for preparing and administering a homologous **blood component** must be observed.

NURSING FAST FACT!

A significant amount of iron is removed with each autologous donation. When appropriate, iron supplements are prescribed for patients making autologous donations in order to help increase red blood cell count (AABB, 2002).

ADVANTAGES

- Eliminates the risk of isoimmunization (sensitization to RBCs, platelets, and leukocyte antigens).
- Eliminates the risk of exposure to bloodborne infectious agents.
- Expands the blood resources.

- Reduces the need for homologous blood (decreases dependence on the volunteer donor supply).
- Provides an option for patients who find homologous transfusion unacceptable on religious grounds.
- Has a physiologic pH and higher levels of 2,3-DPG than does banked blood; 2,3-DPG increases the oxygen-carrying capacity of **hemoglobin**.
- Contains more viable RBCs than banked blood.

DISADVANTAGES

- Cost; a unit of predeposited autologous blood costs approximately $250 because of increased paperwork and special handling.

Guidelines for Autologous Donation

Autologous transfusion can be accomplished through preoperative collection or from intraoperative or postoperative blood salvage. For preoperative collection, blood is collected into an anticoagulant preservative solution and stored. The 42-day shelf life of RBCs needs to be considered. If necessary, RBCs can be stored frozen. However, frozen storage is not routinely recommended because of the considerable expense and the limitations of some blood banks.

The criteria for patient selection for autologous donation are not as restrictive as with homologous donations. There are no age limits, and underweight patients can have proportionately smaller units withdrawn. Typically, autologous blood is not drawn more often than once a week. The last donation should be at least 72 hours and preferably 1 week before an operation to avoid hypovolemia during surgery. It is best to collect blood as far in advance of the intended date of surgery as is feasible. Except in special circumstances, the hemoglobin should be 11 g/dL and the hematocrit 33 percent or greater before each donation. Oral iron supplementation should be considered to replenish bone marrow iron reserves for autologous donors (AABB, 2002).

Types

Four types of autologous blood are donations currently in use: (1) predeposit or preoperative (PABD), (2) acute normovolemic hemodilution (ANH), (3) intraoperative blood salvage (IBS), and (4) postoperative blood salvage (PBS).

PREDEPOSIT OR PREOPERATIVE AUTOLOGOUS BLOOD DONATION

Predeposit or preoperative autologous blood donation is the collection and storage of the recipient's own blood for reinfusion during or after a later operation. This blood is held for use for elective surgery. Predeposit requires the approval of the donor recipient's physician and the blood bank physician.

Indication
- Elective surgical procedure with realistic possibility of transfusion

Typical uses
- Hip or knee replacement surgery
- Elective cardiac surgery
- Spinal fusion
- Elective major vascular surgery
- Heart–lung transplant

Contraindications
- Hemoglobin less than 11 g/dL
- Bacterial infection
- Severe aortic stenosis
- Unstable angina
- Severe left main coronary artery disease

Advantages
- No age limitations
- Less exclusionary donor criteria

Disadvantages
- Relatively costly
- Risk of clerical error

ACUTE NORMOVOLEMIC HEMODILUTION

Acute normovolemic hemodilution involves the removal of whole blood from the patient, along with simultaneous replacement by a crystalloid solution, such as lactated Ringer's solution. This procedure takes place in the immediate preoperative period, either just before or just after the induction of anesthesia. The purpose of ANH is to decrease the loss of erythrocytes during surgery by decreasing the concentration of erythrocytes in the shed blood.

Indications
- Adequate preoperative hematocrit
- Anticipated intraoperative blood loss of more than 1 L

Typical uses
- Coronary artery bypass graft
- Major vascular surgery
- Spinal fusion
- Arteriovenous malformations

Contraindications
- Anemia
- Decreased renal function
- Significant coronary artery disease (CAD)
- Cerebrovascular disease
- Pulmonary disease
- Hepatic dysfunction

Advantage
- Practical means of obtaining fresh, whole blood

Disadvantages

- Increased potential for critical organ ischemia
- Lowest safe hemoglobin level in humans is unknown

INTRAOPERATIVE BLOOD SALVAGE

Intraoperative blood salvage, or perioperative blood salvage or deposit, involves withdrawal of blood early in a procedure for use as a volume replacement later in the same procedure. Typically, two units of blood are collected early in the surgery. The collected volume is replaced with physiologic solution, and the units are then ready if volume replacement becomes necessary. The logic is that hemoglobin-rich blood is available for immediate reinfusion.

Indications

- Surgical procedure with anticipated major blood loss
- Patient unable to donate preoperatively

Typical uses

- Cardiac surgery
- Major vascular surgery
- Revision hip replacement
- Spinal fusion
- Liver transplant
- Arteriovenous malfunction resection
- Trauma

Contraindications

- Malignancy at operative site
- Bacterial contamination at operative site
- Use of microfibrillar collagen materials

Advantages

- May be acceptable to patients opposed to transfusions for religious reasons.
- May eliminate need for allogeneic transfusion.

Disadvantage

- Risk of air embolism

POSTOPERATIVE SALVAGE

Postoperative salvage involves the salvage of blood from the surgical field in a single-use, self-contained reservoir for immediate return and reinfusion to the patient. This technique is used most often after cardiac surgeries and, recently, with orthopedic surgeries.

Indication

- Substantial bleeding in postoperative period

Typical uses

- Cardiac surgery
- Orthopedic surgery

Contraindication

- Same as IBS

Advantage

- May decrease allogeneic transfusion in some clinical settings.

Disadvantages

- **Febrile reaction** to washed blood
- Cost increases if shed blood is washed

NURSING FAST FACT!

Any autologous blood must be filtered during reinfusion to eliminate the possibility of microclots or debris being infused into the patient.

Designated

Designated donation refers to the donation of blood from selected friends or relatives of the patient. Most blood centers and hospitals provide this service. Designated donations have been requested more frequently because of the concern over the risk of transfusion-transmitted diseases. However, there is no evidence that designated donations are safer than blood provided by transfusion service (AABB, 2002). Relatives or friends who may be members of a risk group may feel forced into donating and hesitate to identify themselves as a risk group member (Fig. 13–2).

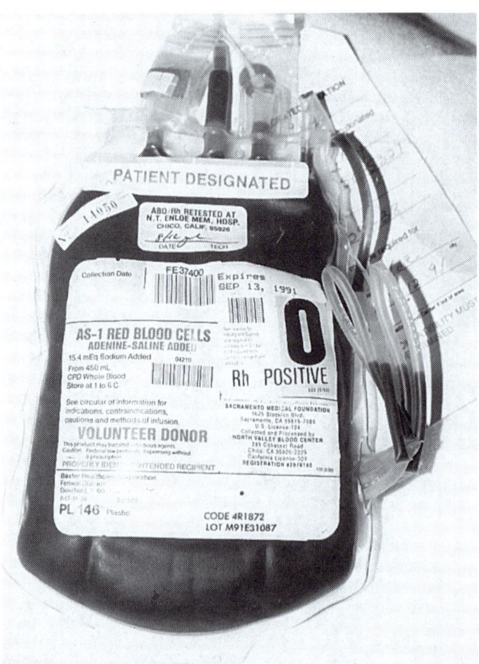

Figure 13–2 ■ Designated donor unit.

Guidelines for Designated Donation

The selection and screening of designated donors are the same as for other homologous donors, except that the units collected are labeled for a specific recipient. The designated donor must pass all the history and screening tests required, and the unit must be compatible with the intended recipient (AABB, 2002).

Blood Component Therapy

Blood is the fluid tissue that circulates through the heart, arteries, capillaries, and veins. It supplies oxygen and food to the other tissues of the body and removes carbon dioxide and the waste products of metabolism from the tissues. Blood is a "liquid organ" with functions as extraordinary and unique as those of any other body organ. A total of 55 percent of blood is plasma (fluid); the remaining cellular portion (45%) is made up of solids: RBCs, WBCs, and platelets.

In the past decade, heightened awareness of the risks and benefits of transfusion therapy has dramatically affected transfusion practices. New methods of testing have lowered the risk of infection transmission; however, the association of blood product administration with virus activation, immunosuppression, increased tumor recurrence, and the increased incidence of bacterial infection has demanded serious consideration. As a result, the administration of **allogeneic** blood components is carefully evaluated. Autologous blood donations have increased substantially and, as an alternative to blood component administration, are evaluated and applied when appropriate.

Whole Blood

Whole blood is composed of RBCs, plasma, WBCs, and platelets. The volume of each unit is approximately 500 mL and consists of 200 mL of RBCs and 300 mL of plasma, with a minimum hemoglobin level of 38 percent. Advances in the use of blood components have made the administration of whole blood unnecessary.

Whole blood is never a "preferred" treatment, but is available for consideration. Fresh frozen plasma (FFP), packed RBCs, and crystalloid and colloids are preferred for treatment of massive hemorrhage over whole blood.

Uses

Most whole blood units are now used to prepare valuable separate RBC and plasma components to meet specific clinical needs. A whole blood unit can be centrifuged and separated into three components: RBCs, plasma, and platelet concentrates. By transfusing the patient with the specific component needed rather than with whole blood, the patient is not exposed to unnecessary portions of the blood product and valuable blood resources are conserved (Fig. 13–3).

Few conditions require transfusion of whole blood. A unit of whole

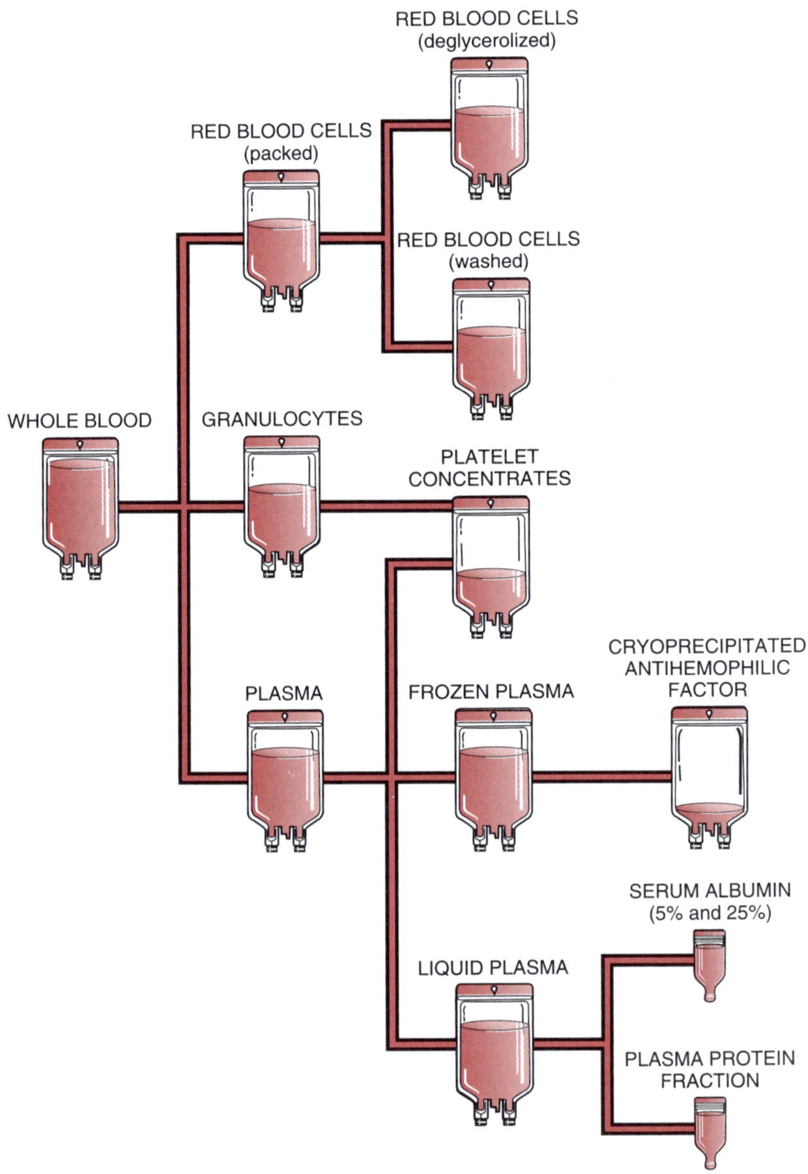

Figure 13–3 ■ Derivation of transfusible blood products.

blood increases RBC mass, which provides oxygen-carrying capacity and provides plasma for blood volume expansion.

When whole blood has been stored for more than 24 hours, degeneration of some of its components occurs, resulting in nonviable platelets and granulocytes. In addition, levels of factor V and factor VIII decrease with storage. Therefore, a whole blood transfusion would not provide a therapeutic platelet transfusion or replace several clotting factors. Stable coagulation factors II, VII, IX, X, and fibrinogen are well maintained throughout the storage period for whole blood units.

NURSING FAST FACT!

In an adult, 1 U of whole blood increases the hemoglobin by about 1 g/dL or the hematocrit by about 3 to 4 percent (AABB, 2002).

Administration

- Amount: Volume of 500 mL
- Catheter size: 20-gauge or larger preferred for rapid flow rates
- Usual rate: 2 to 4 hours
- Administration set: Straight or Y type with 170- to 260-micron filter or microaggregrate recipient set

Compatibility

Whole blood requires type and crossmatching and must be ABO identical.

Red Blood Cells

Red blood cell units are prepared by removing 200 to 250 mL of plasma from a whole blood unit. The remaining packed RBC (PRBC) concentrate has a volume of approximately 300 mL. Each unit contains the same RBC mass as whole blood, as well as 20 to 30 percent of the original plasma, leukocytes, and some platelets. The advantages of RBCs over whole blood are decreased plasma volume in an RBC unit and decreased risk of circulatory overload. Another advantage is that because most of the plasma has been removed, less citrate, potassium, ammonia, and other metabolic byproducts are transfused.

NURSING FAST FACT!

In a normal adult patient, 1 U of RBCs should raise the hemoglobin level approximately 1 g/dL and the hematocrit 3 percent (AABB, 2002).

Uses

Red blood cells are used to improve the oxygen-carrying capacity in patients with symptomatic anemia. The administration of RBCs should be considered only if improvement of the RBC count cannot be achieved by nutrition, drug therapy, or treatment of the underlying disease. A definitive hemoglobin and hematocrit threshold has not been established for when transfusion of RBCs is indicated or above which transfusion would be inappropriate. Criteria for transfusion are based on multiple variables, including hemoglobin and hematocrit levels, patient symptoms, amount and time frame of blood loss, and surgical procedures (AABB, 2002). Patients with chronic anemia should undergo transfusion only if they are symptomatic owing to a decrease in oxygen-carrying capacity: they usually adjust to the lower hemoglobin level and should not be exposed to transfusion-associated risks unless necessary. Even if large volumes of blood are lost, other components (e.g., platelets and plasma coagulation factors) can be provided rather than using whole blood (Cook, 2000).

Administration

Administration of RBCs is used for an operative blood loss of more than 1200 mL. An operative blood loss of less than 1000 to 1200 mL can be replaced by crystalloid or colloid solutions rather than with RBCs (AABB, 2002).

Transfuse RBCs:

- Hypovolemia due to acute blood loss: hypotension and tachycardia not corrected by volume replacement.
- 30 Percent blood loss for otherwise healthy patients, as long as volume is maintained
- Hgb less than 8 to 10 g/dL
- Symptomatic anemia in a euvolemic patient (angina, syncope, congestive heart failure, transient ischemic attacks [TIAs], dyspnea, tachycardia)
- Stable patients with cardiovascular risk factors
- Hgb less than 7 g/dL
- Transfusion patient with no risk factor for ischemia (AABB, 2002)

Do not transfuse RBCs:

- For volume expansion
- In place of a hematinic
- To enhance wound healing
- To improve general well being (AABB, 2002)

ADMINISTRATION SUMMARY

- Amount of component: 250 to 300 mL
- Catheter size: 18- to 20-gauge preferred because the use of a 22-gauge catheter does not always allow free flow and may require an infusion pump
- Usual rate: $1\frac{1}{2}$ to 2 hours; maximum 4 hours

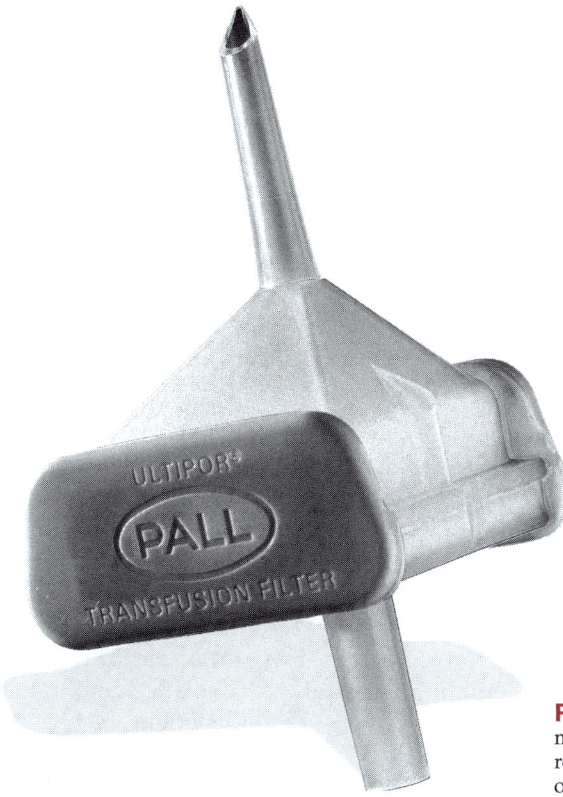

Figure 13–4 ■ Pall SQ40S microaggregate blood filter for red cell transfusion. (Courtesy of Pall Medical, New York.)

- Administration set: Straight or Y type with 170- to 260-micron filter or microaggregate filter (Fig. 13–4).

Compatibility

RBCs require typing and crossmatching before being transfused into a recipient.

NURSING FAST FACT!

The unit of PRBC does not have to be ABO identical, but it must be ABO compatible.

Leukocyte-Reduced Red Blood Cells

Leukocyte-poor RBCs are grouped in a category referred to as modified blood products. A unit of whole blood contains more than 1 to 10 × 10^9 WBCs. Such products are the result of removing the number of leukocytes in whole blood to 5×10^8, while retaining approximately 80 percent of the RBCs. Leukocyte-reduced blood is prepared by filtering blood with a special filter that removes WBCs by sieving and adherence mechanisms. Filtration may be done soon after collection (prestorage), after varying periods of storage in the laboratory, or at the bedside.

NURSING FAST FACT!

The leukocyte-reduced component will have therapeutic efficacy equal to at least 85 percent of that of the original component (AABB, 2002).

Uses

Leukocyte-reduced components are indicated for the prevention of recurrent febrile, nonhemolytic transfusion reactions. These components may be beneficial in preventing HLA alloimmunization and in reducing transfusion-related immunomodulation (Hadaway, 1999).

Safety Concern: On rare occasions patients may develop severe hypotension when leukocyte reduction is performed at the bedside. These reactions are due to the generation of bradykinin in the plasma as it passes over the filter medium. This reaction does not occur when LR is done in the lab because bradykinin has a short half-life and is no longer active or present in the product by the time the patient receives it (Fitzpatrick, 2002).

Deglycerolized Red Blood Cells

Deglycerolized RBCs are prepared to allow for freezing of cells for long-term storage to preserve rare units of RBCs and autologous donor units. The RBCs are frozen after removal of the plasma and glycerol (a cryoprotective agent) is added. The RBCs are stored at –65°C. Glycerol enters the cell and protects the cell from damage caused by cell dehydration and mechanical injury from ice formation. Before transfusion, glycerol is removed by washing to prevent osmotic **hemolysis**. This washing process also has the advantage of removing leukocytes, platelets, and plasma.

Uses

The uses and applications are the same as for washed cells.

NURSING FAST FACT!

Deglycerolization of RBCs extends storage to 10 years or more; a thawed unit is stored at 4°C and must be used within 24 hours (AABB, 2002).

Irradiated Blood Products

When blood products are exposed to a controlled measure of radiation, it causes the donor lymphocytes to become incapable of replication. Products such as cryoprecipitate or fresh frozen plasma do not need to be irradiated.

Uses

- Prevention of graft-versus-host disease (GVHD)
- Patients with acute leukemia and lymphoma (Hodgkin's disease and non-Hodgkin's disease)
- Bone marrow or stem cell transplant recipients
- Patients with immunodeficiency disorders
- Neonates and low-birthweight infants

NURSING FAST FACTS!

- *A label marked irradiated must be placed on the bag containing the product.*
- *Whole blood, red blood cells, platelets, or granulocytes can be irradiated.*
- ***Safety Concern:** The shelf life of irradiated red blood cells is limited to 28 days because irradiation damages the cells and reduces their viability. Platelets and granulocytes are not damaged, so their shelf-life is not affected (Fitzpatrick, 2002).*

Granulocytes

Granulocyte concentrations are prepared by leukapheresis from a single donor. Each unit contains granulocytes and variable amounts of lymphocytes, platelets, and RBCs suspended in 200 to 300 mL of plasma. They are obtained for transfusion by the process of granulocytapheresis.

Hydroxyethyl starch (HES) may be used as a sediment agent; if used, residual HES will be present in the final component. Pheresis should be administered as soon after collection as possible because of the well-documented possibility of deterioration of granulocyte function during short-term storage. If stored, it should be maintained at 20 to 24°C without agitation for less than 24 hours (AABB, 2002).

Uses

- Patients with congenital WBC (granulocyte) dysfunction
- Acquired neutropenia
- Treat patients with severe infections that are unresponsive to conventional antibiotic therapy.

Administration of granulocytes is accompanied by a high frequency of nonhemolytic febrile reactions. These side effects can be managed with the use of diphenhydramine, steroids, and nonaspirin antipyretics and by slowing the transfusion rate. The transfusion should not be discontinued unless severe respiratory distress occurs. The concentrate must be infused within 24 hours after collection; to achieve maximal clinical effect, it should be delivered as soon as possible (AABB, 2002).

Administration

- Amount: 300 to 400 mL suspended in 200 to 300 mL of plasma
- Catheter size: 16- to 20-gauge
- Usual rate: 1 to 2 hours; slower if reaction occurs (maximum of 4 hours)
- Administration set: Straight or Y type with 170-micron filter; microaggregate filter contraindicated

Compatibility

Donor blood must be ABO and Rh compatible because a unit of granulocytes is usually heavily contaminated with RBCs. There is no set standard regarding the amount or duration of granulocyte therapy, but generally transfusion therapy is delivered for at least 4 consecutive days.

Platelets

Platelets are fragments of megacaryocytes, which are particles of a seventh type of leukocyte found in the bone marrow. They are responsible for hemostasis. Platelets live up to 12 days in the blood, do not have nuclei, and are unable to reproduce. They contain no hemoglobin. Normal platelet counts are 150,000 to 300,000/μL. Platelets can be supplied as either random-donor concentrates or single-donor concentrates. Platelet concentrates (random donor) are prepared from individual units of whole blood by centrifugation. The platelets are stored at room temperature 20 to 24°C for 5 days with constant, gentle agitation to maintain the viability of the platelets. Platelets can be stored for up to 5 days, depending on the plastic formation of the storage bag. Single-donor platelet **pheresis** products are collected from a single donor, and all unneeded portions of the donor's blood are returned back to the donor. A single pheresis unit is equivalent to 6 to 8 U of random donor platelets (Fig. 13–5).

The use of a single-donor unit has the obvious advantage of exposing the recipient to fewer donors and is ideal for treating patients who have developed HLA antibodies from previous transfusions and have become **refractory** (unresponsive) to random-donor platelets. HLA typing may be indicated when patients become refractory to platelets after multiple

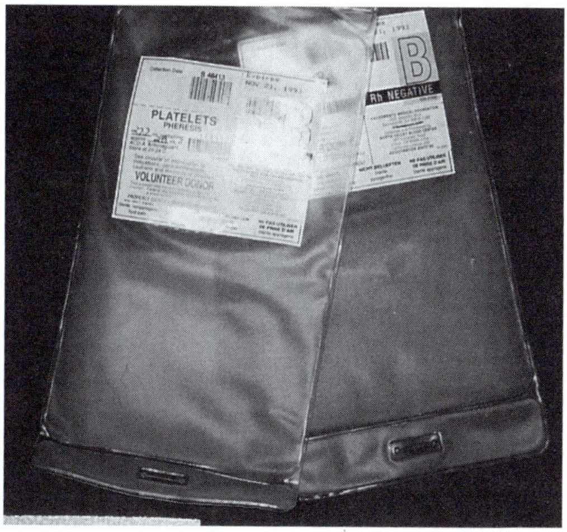

Figure 13–5 ■ Platelets.

transfusions. Platelet crossmatch procedures are also being evaluated for their usefulness with refractory patients.

NURSING FAST FACT!

One platelet concentrate should raise the recipient's platelet count 5000 to 10,000. The usual dose is 6 to 10 U random or 1 unit pheresis (AABB, 2002).

Uses

Platelets are administered to control or prevent bleeding from platelet deficiencies resulting in **thrombocytopenia** or for the presence of functionally abnormal platelets. Indications for platelet transfusion include:

- Platelet count less than 10,000/μL
  - Stable heme-oncology patient
- Less than 20,000/μL
  - Bone marrow aspiration and biopsy
- Less than 50,000/μL
  - Active bleeding, DIC, invasive procedure in cirrhosis, liver biopsy (50 to 100,000/μL)
- Less than 60,000 to 80,000/μL
  - Surgery
- Less than 80,000 to 100,000/μL
  - Neurosurgery or ophthalmic procedures
  - After cardiopulmonary bypass, intra-aortic balloon pump placement
  - Massive transfusions (Rebulla, 2001)

Platelet transfusions at higher platelet counts may be required for patients with systemic bleeding and for those at high risk for bleeding because of additional coagulation defects, sepsis, or platelet dysfunction related to medication or disease. Significant spontaneous bleeding with platelet counts above 20,000/μL is rare. Platelet transfusions are usually not effective in patients with conditions in which rapid platelet destruction occurs, such as those with ITP and untreated disseminated intravascular coagulation (DIC). In patients with these conditions, platelet transfusions should be used only in the presence of active bleeding.

Do NOT transfuse platelets:

- To patients with idiopathic autoimmune thrombocytopenic purpura (ITP) (unless there is life-threatening bleeding)
- Prophylactically with massive blood transfusions
- Prophylactically after cardiopulmonary bypass

Administration

Transfusions may be repeated every 1 to 3 days. The platelets may be infused as rapidly as the patient tolerates, with infusion rates ranging from 1 to 2 mL/min up to 5 min/bag. Platelets should be delivered to infants by means of a syringe-type device and can be transfused at a rate of 1 mL/min.

The effectiveness of platelet transfusions may be altered if fever, infection, or active bleeding is present. To determine the effectiveness of a transfusion, platelet counts may be checked at 1 hour and 24 hours after transfusion. Poor platelet count recovery may also indicate that the patient may be refractory to random donor platelets.

ADMINISTRATION SUMMARY

- Amount: 30 to 50 mL/U; usual dose 6 to 8 U
- Catheter size: 16- to 20-gauge
- Usual rate: 1 U in 5 to 10 minutes as tolerated
- Filter: 170-micron
- Administration set: Component syringe or Y drip set; tubing should be rubber free to prevent platelets from sticking; use 0.9 percent sodium chloride as primer

Platelet concentrates may be pooled before administration or infused individually; after they are pooled, platelets should be transfused within 4 hours

Compatibility

Preferably, platelets should be ABO compatible; however, when ABO-compatible platelets are unavailable, mismatched platelets may be given. Crossmatching is not required. Rh matching is also preferred but not required, especially with pheresed units that have very low RBC concentrations. Standard pretransfusion compatibility testing is not done for platelets.

Plasma and Fresh Frozen Plasma

Plasma is the liquid portion of the blood and lymph in which nutrients are carried to body tissues and wastes are transported to areas of excretion. It is colorless, thin, aqueous solution (91 percent water) that contains chemicals (bile pigments, bilirubin, electrolytes, enzymes, fats, and hormones), protein (7 percent), carbohydrates (2 percent), and serum. Plasma does not contain RBCs.

Fresh frozen plasma (FFP) is prepared from whole blood by separating and freezing the plasma within 8 hours of collection. FFP may be stored for up to 1 year at 18°C or lower. FFP stored at 65°C may be stored for up to 7 years. The volume of a typical unit is 200 to 250 mL. FFP does not provide platelets, and loss of factors V and VIII (i.e., the labile clotting factors) is minimal (Fig. 13–6).

Uses

Liquid plasma is indicated to replace plasma proteins lost from injury. Fresh frozen plasma is primarily used to provide replacement coagulation factors. It is indicated for patients with multiple coagulation factor defi-

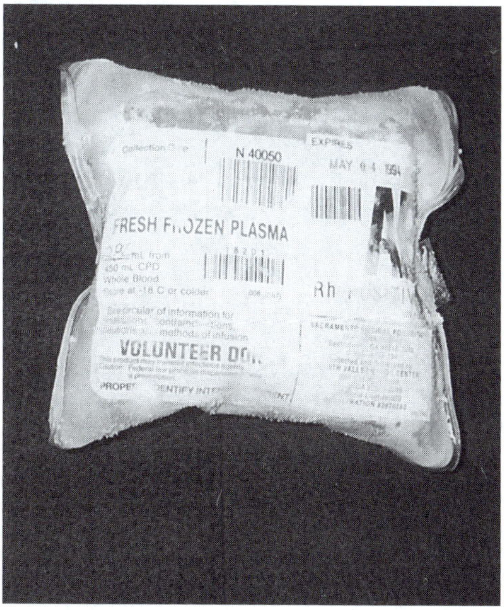

Figure 13–6 ■ Plasma.

ciencies secondary to liver disease, DIC, and the dilutional coagulopathy resulting from massive volume load or volume replacement. FFP is indicated for patients with demonstrated factor deficiencies for which there is no coagulation concentrate available, such as deficiencies of factor V or XI. FFP may also be used for coumarin drug reversal when time does not permit reversal by stopping the drug or administering vitamin K. Patients with other rare deficiencies, such as antithrombin III deficiency and thrombotic thrombocytopenia purpura, may also benefit from FFP.

NURSING FAST FACT!

FFP contains optimal levels of all plasma clotting factors, with approximately 200 U factor activity per bag and 200 to 400 mg fibrinogen per bag (AABB, 2002).

Administration

Plasma is administered at a rate of 200 mL/h, unless there is a potential for fluid volume overload. Medications and diluents must never be added to plasma.

Fresh frozen plasma must be thawed in a 30 to 37°C water bath with gentle agitation or kneading. The thawing process takes up to 30 minutes, and the FFP should be transfused after thawing or within 6 hours. FFP must be delivered through a standard blood filter. It can be infused as fast as the patient tolerates or condition indicates. A rate of 4 to 10 mL/min has been suggested, and most units are generally completed within 1 to 2 hours.

Transfuse FFP:

- PT greater than 19 or PTT greater than 53
  - To correct coagulation factor deficiencies in a bleeding patient with multiple coagulation factor deficits (e.g., liver disease, DIC, massive transfusion)
  - Prior to an invasive procedure
- Warfarin overdose or vitamin K deficiency, when correction of coagulopathy is needed within 12 to 24 hours
  - Bleeding patient or in a patient with high risk of bleeding [International Normalization Ratio (INR) greater than 5.0]
  - Before an invasive procedure
- Replacement fluid in TTP
- Replacement in factor V and XI deficiencies (AABB, 2002)

Do NOT transfuse FFP:

- For volume expansion
- As a nutritional supplement

ADMINISTRATION SUMMARY

- Amount: 200 to 300 mL
- Catheter size: 20- to 22-gauge
- Usual rate: 1 to 2 hours
- Administration set: Straight or Y type with a 170-micron filter, primed with 0.9 percent sodium chloride

Compatibility

Compatibility testing is not required except to identify the recipient's ABO group to ensure that A or B antibodies present in the plasma are compatible with the recipient's RBCs. If the recipient's blood type is not known, group AB can be safely given. Rh matching is not required. The amount of antibody present in a single unit of FFP is not clinically important. If massive transfusion is anticipated, the significance may increase.

Cryoprecipitate

Cryoprecipitate is the insoluble portion of plasma that remains as a white precipitate after FFP is thawed at 4°C under special conditions. The cold-insoluble precipitate is refrozen. Cryoprecipitate has a shelf life of 1 year and contains concentrated factor VIII: C; factor VIII: vWF (von Willebrand factor); fibrinogen; and factor XIII. It is the only concentrated source of fibrinogen.

The frozen component is thawed in a protective plastic overwrap in a water bath at 30 to 37°C up to 15 minutes. It should not be used if there is evidence of container breakage or thawing during storage.

NURSING FAST FACTS!

- *Do not refreeze after thawing.*
- *Good patient management requires that the cryoprecipitate antihemophilic factor (AHF) treatment responses of factor VIII–deficient recipients be monitored with periodic plasma factor VIII: C assays (AABB, 2002).*

Uses

- Hypofibrinogenemia – fibrinogen less than 100 mg/dL
  - Massive transfusion
  - Congenital deficiency
  - Acquired deficiency (e.g., DIC)
- Factor VIII deficiency
- Uremia with bleeding unresponsive to nontransfusion therapy (dialysis, desmopressin)
- Dysfibrinogenemia (dysfunctional fibrinogen) (AABB, 2002)

Administration

Cryoprecipitate is thawed before being transfused and must be used within 6 hours. The inside of the bag should be rinsed with a small amount of saline to maximize recovery. Cryoprecipitate should be administered through a standard blood filter and, as with platelet administration sets, small priming volumes are recommended to decrease loss of the product in the set. The cryoprecipitate units are usually pooled to simplify administration. Cryoprecipitate should be transfused as rapidly as the patient can tolerate. Pooling of cryoprecipitate is not ubiquitously done.

ADMINISTRATION SUMMARY

- Amount: 10 to 15 mL of diluent added to precipitate (3 to 5 mL) unit; usual dose 6 to 10 U
- Catheter size: 18- to 20-gauge
- Usual rate: 1 to 2 mL/min
- Administration set: Component syringe or standard blood component set, with 170-micron filter primed with 0.9 percent sodium chloride

Compatibility

Compatibility testing is not done, but the cryoprecipitate should be ABO compatible with the patient's RBCs because a very small volume of plasma is present. If the patient's blood group is not known, group AB is preferred, but any group can be given in an emergency because the plasma volume is small. Rh matching is not required.

Recombinant Factor VIII

Factor concentrates fall into two broad categories: those that are plasma-derived and recombinant DNA technology–derived products. The second generation of recombinant products provides smaller volume for the patient with hemophilia reducing the risk of fluid overload. Recombinant DNA technology-derived products are growing. Recombinant products are thought to have a safety and purity advantage because human plasma is not used in their manufacture, and DNA technology produces a specific coagulation replacement protein (Schaefer, 2002).

Uses

- Hemophilia (factor VIII or IX deficiency)

Administration

- Usually administered by bolus infusion in home care environment.

- The package contains the vial of lyophilized (freeze dried) product and vial of diluent
- Store in refrigerator or at room temperature; shelf-life up to 2 years.

Complication

- Potential side effect of recombinant products includes any allergic reaction that would be typical of blood transfusion.

Colloid Volume Expanders

Products are available that do not require screening techniques. These products are colloid volume expanders. These include albumin, plasma protein fraction (PPF), dextran, and HES.

Normal human serum albumin is the most widely used colloid solution. It is heat treated for viral inactivation and to become free from hepatitis risk. PPF is also a hepatitis-free plasma derivative and is less expensive than albumin. Dextran is a branched polysaccharide available in low molecular weights: 40,000 (dextran 40) and 70,000 (dextran 70). It is dissolved in either 0.9 percent sodium chloride or 5 percent dextrose. Dextran's use as a volume expander is limited by two factors: (1) it can interfere with coagulation and platelet adhesion and (2) it has been associated with rare anaphylactic reactions (Phillips & Kuhn, 1999).

Hetastarch is an amylopectin derivative marketed in a 6 percent sodium chloride solution. Because of its structural similarity to glycogen, HES is less likely to cause anaphylaxis than dextran.

Albumin

Albumin is a plasma protein that supplies 80 percent of plasma's osmotic activity and is the principal product of fractionation. Administered as PPF and as more purified albumin, albumin and PPF are derived from donor plasma, prepared by the cold alcohol fractionation process, and then subsequently heated. Both products do not transmit viral diseases because of the extended heating process. Normal serum albumin is composed of 96 percent albumin and 4 percent globulin and other proteins. It is available as a 5 or 25 percent solution.

Plasma Protein Fraction

Plasma protein fraction (PPF) is a similar product to albumin except that it is subjected to fewer purification steps in the fractionation process and contains about 83 percent albumin and 17 percent globulins. PPF is available only in a 5 percent solution.

Uses

Plasma protein fraction and 5 percent albumin are isotonic solutions and therefore are osmotically equivalent to an equal volume of plasma. They cause a plasma volume increase, are used interchangeably, and share the same clinical uses. Both are used primarily to increase plasma volume resulting from sudden loss of intravascular volume as seen in patients with hypovolemic shock from trauma or surgery. Their use may also be indicated in individual cases to support blood pressure during hypotensive episodes or induce diuresis in those with fluid overload to assist in fluid mobilization. The plasma derivatives lack clotting factors and other plasma proteins and therefore should not be considered plasma substitutes. Neither component will correct nutritional deficits or chronic hypoalbuminemia.

The 25 percent albumin is hypertonic and is five times more concentrated than 5 percent albumin. The 25 percent albumin is used to draw fluids out of tissues and body cavities into intravascular spaces. This solution must be given with caution. Principal uses for 25 percent albumin include plasma volume expansion, hypovolemic shock, burns, and prevention and treatment of patients with cerebral edema.

NURSING FAST FACT!

Albumin 25 percent must not be used in dehydrated patients without supplemental fluids or in those at risk for circulatory overload.

Administration

Albumin and PPF are supplied in glass bottles. Depending on the brand, albumin in 5 percent concentrations is available in units of 50, 250, and 500 mL, and concentrations of 25 percent are supplied in units of 20, 50, and 100 mL. Manufacturers recommend that the solution be used within 4 hours of opening. Depending on the manufacturer, the solutions are sometimes supplied with an infusion set. Blood transfusion sets and filters are not required for infusion of albumin.

Albumin, 5 and 25 percent, may be given as rapidly as the patient tolerates for reduced blood volumes. When the blood volume is normal or only slightly reduced, rates of 2 to 4 mL/min have been suggested for 5 percent albumin, and 1 mL/min for 25 percent albumin. More caution is used when infusing PPF because hypotension may occur with a rate greater than 10 mL/min (AABB, 2002).

ADMINISTRATION SUMMARY

- Amount: 5 percent solution = 250 mL; 25 percent solution = 50 to 100 mL

- Catheter size: 18- to 22-gauge
- Usual rate: 5 percent solution: 2 to 4 mL/min; 25 percent solution: 1 mL/min
- Administration set: Comes with administration set in package.

Compatibility

ABO or Rh matching and compatibility testing are not necessary for these components because antigens and antibodies are not present in these products.

A summary of blood components is listed in Table 13–5.

Transfusion Alternatives

The research for alternatives for homologous blood continues. This issue has been addressed by alternative therapies to blood components, such as hematopoietic growth factor erythropoietin and desmopressin acetate (DDAVP). Erythropoietin is used for managing chronic anemia in dialysis patients. DDAVP is a synthetic analogue of *l*-arginine vasopressin and is used for increasing factor VIII and vWF and for managing patients with hemorrhagic disorders related to thrombocytopenia. These drugs decrease blood loss and the risk of bleeding, resulting in a reduced need for blood components.

Blood Substitutes

Efforts continue in the search to develop a practical RBC substitute. Several products continue to be evaluated for their ability to serve as oxygen carriers as a substitute for RBCs. One is a synthetic material, a perfluorocarbon emulsion, which was found to not carry enough oxygen under practical conditions. Other preparations being developed include intramolecular crosslinked or polymerized hemoglobin and products containing hemoglobin encapsulated in phospholipid liposomes. (Recombinant human hemoglobin is a cell-free hemoglobin-based blood substitute being investigated for perioperative blood replacement.)

A product currently under development as synthetic blood includes Oxycyte, an oxygen-carrying fluorocarbon, which is a highly effective medium for gas exchange and will be useful in treating stroke, heart attack, and cancer patients and for use as a blood substitute in organ preservation. This product is based on perfluorocarbon technology (Synthetic Blood International, Inc., 2003). In April of 2003, the Costa Mesa Company Synthetic Blood International, Inc., began a three-phase testing program of Oxycyte. If it gains approval from the FDA, Oxycyte is

> Table 13–5 **SUMMARY OF BLOOD COMPONENTS**

Blood Component	Volume	Action and Use	Infusion Guide	Special Considerations
RBCs	250 to 350 mL	Improved oxygen-carrying capacity in patient with symptomatic anemia, aplastic anemia, bone marrow failure caused by malignancy, or chemotherapy	0.9% sodium chloride primer; transfuse in 4 h; use standard 170-micron Y administration set Recommend leukocyte reduction filter	AB and Rh compatible; 1 U raises the hemoglobin 1 g and hematocrit 3 to 4%
Irradiated RBCs	200 to 250 mL	Prevent GFHD in immunocompromised patients	Same as for RBCs	Same as for RBCs
Deglycerolized RBCs (frozen)	200 to 250 mL	Prolonged storage of blood for rare blood types and autologous donations; minimizes allergic reactions	Same as for whole blood; infuse within 4 h	Must be used within 24 hours of being thawed and deglycerolized
Granulocytes (leukapheresis)	300 to 400 mL Note: Suspended in 200 to 250 mL of plasma	For neutropenia, fever, or significant infection unresponsive to antibiotics	Usually administered for 4 consecutive days Standard blood filter; administer slowly over 2 to 4 h as soon as collected or at least within 24 h	ABO-/Rh-compatible; reactions common Check vital signs every 15 min Note: Febrile reactions occur in about two thirds of patients; chills, fever, and allergic reactions common Requires premedication to control reactions
Platelets, random donor	50 to 70 mL/U Usual dose: 6 to 10 U	Control or prevent bleeding associated with platelet deficiencies	Administer as rapidly as patient can tolerate: 1 U/10 min or less Use blood filter, syringe push, or standard Y administration set; leukocyte depletion filter for platelets as ordered Note: RBC leukocyte filters cannot be used with platelets	1 U increases platelet count of 70-kg adult by 5000/gmL Infuse individually or may be pooled; requires 20 minutes' pooling time by laboratory; ABO/Rh preferred but not necessary Prophylactic medication with antihistamines; antipyretics may be needed to decrease the incidence of chills, fever, and allergic reactions

Blood Component	Volume	Action and Use	Infusion Guide	Special Considerations
Platelets, pheresis	Equivalent to 6 U from random donors	Same as for random donor; consider for patients anticipated to receive multiple long-term transfusions to limit exposure to multiple donors and reduce incidence of refractoriness	Same as for random-donor platelets	Same as for random-donor platelets
FFP	200 to 250 mL	Replacement of clotting factors in patients with a demonstrated deficiency or for single-factor deficiency when concentrate not available	Storage is at 18°C for 1 year Standard blood filter; may be infused rapidly: 20 mL over 3 minutes or more slowly within 4 h	Does not provide platelets 1 U (200 U) raises the level of clotting factor 2% to 3%; requires 20 minutes' thawing time by laboratory Must be AB compatible
Cryoprecipitate	Each unit contains factor VIII, vWF, factor XIII, fibrinogen 15 mL plasma (5 to 10 mL U). Usual order is for 6 to 10 U	Controls bleeding associated with deficiency in coagulation factors; treatment of patients with hemophilia A, von Willebrand's disease, hypofibrinogenemia, factor VIII deficiency, DIC associated with obstetric complications	Standard blood filter; administer as fast as patient tolerates	ABO compatible with patient's RBCs; if blood group unknown, use AB blood; Rh matching not required Infuse within 6 h of thawing; saline may be added to bag to facilitate recovery of product
Albumin (5% = 12.5 g/250 mL; 25% = 12.5 g/50 mL)	5% solution is in concentration of 250 mL or 500 mL; 25% solution is in 50 to 100 mL concentration	Plasma volume expander For hypovolemic shock Supports blood pressure during hypotensive episodes; induces diuresis in fluid overload	May be administered as rapidly as tolerated for reduced blood volume Normal rates: 2 to 4 mL/min for 5% solution; 1 mL/min for 25% solution Supplied in glass bottles with tubing for administration	25% albumin is hypertonic and is five times more concentrated than 5% solutions Give with extreme caution; can cause circulatory overload No type and crossmatching necessary; store at room temperature
Plasma protein fraction	Glass bottle with tubing 250 mL	Same as for albumin	Equivalent to 5% albumin	Has fewer purification steps than albumin; no type and crossmatching necessary; has high sodium content

expected to be used for trauma victims, stroke survivors, and other patients who need oxygen in their bloodstream quickly. This synthetic blood could be used with any blood type. It has a two-year shelf life (SYBD, 2003).

Websites

National Institute of Health: *www.nih.gov*
FDA: *www.fda.gov/ola/plasma*
American Association of Blood Banks: *www.aabb.org*
Synthetic Blood International, Inc.: *www.sybd@siscom.net*
Network for Advancement of Transfusion Alternative: *www.nataonline.com*

Other sites:

Administration of Blood Components

The procedure for obtaining a blood component from a hospital blood bank varies from institution to institution. Regardless of the specific institutional procedure, certain essential guidelines must be followed (Table 13–6).

> **INS Standard.** Nurses are responsible for blood product inspection; verification of patent identification, product and expiration date; confirmation of compatibility between recipient and donor; confirmation of informed patient consent; patient education; monitoring during and after administration; identification of immediate and delayed reactions; accountability for initiating appropriate interventions; written documentation; communication of pertinent data to physicians and other healthcare providers involved in patient care; adherence to aseptic technique and standard precautions. (INS, 2000, 75)

Step 1: Verifying the Physician's Order

A physician's order for the blood component is required. The order should specify which component to transfuse and the duration of the transfusion (up to 4 hours). When multiple types of components are transfused, the order should specify the sequence in which they are to be trans-

> Table 13–6 **STEPS IN THE ADMINISTRATION OF A BLOOD COMPONENT**

Step 1: Verifying the physician's order
Step 2: Blood typing and crossmatching the recipient
Step 3: Selecting and preparing the equipment
Step 4: Preparing the patient
Step 5: Obtaining blood product from the blood bank
Step 6: Preparing for administration
Step 7: Initiating transfusion
Step 8: Monitoring the transfusion
Step 9: Discontinuing transfusion

fused and should specify any required modifications to the component (e.g., leukocyte filtration, irradiation, washing, HLA matching). Orders must specify premedications that are to be given before transfusion.

Step 2: Blood Typing and Crossmatching the Recipient

ABO forward typing is the process in which RBCs are mixed with a known antibody (anti-A or anti-B). This process identifies the antigens present in the RBCs by visually apparent agglutination of the cells when the antibody combines with its corresponding antigen.

ABO reverse typing is the testing of serum for the presence of predicted ABO antibodies by adding RBCs of a known ABO type to it.

Rh typing is accomplished by testing the RBCs against anti-D serum. If agglutination occurs, the RBCs possess the D antigen and the blood is Rh positive. If no agglutination is apparent, the RBCs must be tested further to rule out the presence of the weakly expressed D antigen, called weak D (formerly referred to as D). This antigen can be identified most reliably by indirect antiglobulin testing (IAT) after incubating the RBCs with anti-D sera. RBCs that possess the weak D are given to Rh-positive recipients.

Step 3: Selecting and Preparing the Equipment

Selecting the proper equipment involves selecting the catheter and solution selection and obtaining administration sets, special filters, blood warmers, and electronic monitoring devices.

Catheters

An I.V. line should be started according to institution protocol, using the gauge size recommended for the component to be administered. Usually an 18- or 20-gauge catheter is used to provide adequate flow rates. Free flow through a 22-gauge catheter is sometimes difficult with RBC units and may require the use of a pump. A 22-gauge catheter is appropriate for delivering plasma products. After deciding to use a pump, the nurse should make sure that flow is not hindered because of the catheter size or condition (e.g., kinked).

NURSING FAST FACTS!

- *Forcing blood through a tiny or damaged catheter may cause lysis of the cells.*
- *If the patient requires medication or solution administration while the blood component is being administered, a second I.V. site should be initiated.*

Solution

INS Standard. The use of 0.9 percent sodium chloride in transfusion therapy should be established in policies and procedures. (INS, 2000, 75)

The use of dextrose in water can cause RBC hemolysis, and lactated Ringer's solution is not recommended because it contains enough ionized calcium to overcome the anticoagulant effect of CPDA-1 and allows small clots to develop.

Administration Sets

Blood administration sets are available as a two-lead Y-type tubing or as single-lead tubing. Y-type administration sets allow for infusion of 0.9 percent sodium chloride before and after each blood component. A Y-type set also allows for dilution of RBCs that are too viscous to be transfused at an appropriate rate. Platelets and cryoprecipitate should be infused through a filter similar to the standard blood filter but with a smaller drip chamber and shorter tubing so that less priming volume is needed. A syringe device designed specifically for platelets, and cryoprecipitate may also be used to administer these products.

Blood administration sets come with an inline filter. Most routine blood filters have a pore size of 170 to 260 microns designed to remove the debris that accumulates in stored blood.

NURSING FAST FACTS!

- *Blood and blood components should be filtered. The minimum pore size of a standard blood filter is 170 to 260 microns (INS, 2000, 75).*
- *The maximum time for use of a blood filter is 4 hours.*

It is necessary to fill the filter chamber completely to use all the surface area. Filters are designed to filter 2 to 4 U, depending on the manufacturer, the type of filter, the type of blood product, and the age of the cells. Many institutions have a policy of changing sets after every transfusion or limiting their use to several units or several hours in order to reduce the risks of bacterial contamination. As debris in the filter accumulates, the rate of flow through the filter is slowed. In addition, because of the hazard of hemolysis and bacterial contamination, the filter should not be left hanging in place for extended periods and then reused.

Special Filters

Microaggregate filters and leukocyte-depleting filters are also available. These filters are designed to be added to a standard administration set or come already incorporated into the tubing. Microaggregate filters are designed to remove 20- to 40-micron particles, filtering out the microaggregates that develop in stored blood. Microaggregates consist primarily of degenerated platelets, leukocytes, and strands of fibrin. Leukocyte-depleting filters are used for the delivery of RBCs and platelets (see Fig. 13–7A and B).

INS Standard. The use of microaggregate blood filters is recommended in the administration of blood products that have been stored for 5 or more days when administering multiple units (three or more). (INS, 2000, 75)

The filters may be used for leukocyte depletion after blood collection in the blood bank or at the time of administration. HLA immunization (alloimmunization) is directly linked to the number of leukocytes present in a blood product. These filters are capable of removing more than 99.9 percent of the leukocytes present in the unit. These new-generation filters were developed in response to data supporting clinical benefits associated with the administration of leukocyte-poor blood products. The benefits include prevention of nonhemolytic transfusion reactions, HLA alloimmunization, and leukocyte-mediated viral transmission. These filters are more expensive than the standard blood filter and therefore are generally used only per physician order. When using microaggregate or leukocyte-removal filters, follow manufacturer recommendations regarding the number of units that can be filtered through one filter (AABB, 2002).

INS Standard. Consideration may be given to the use of leukocyte-depleting filters for patients with a history of severe febrile transfusion reactions. (INS, 2000, 75)

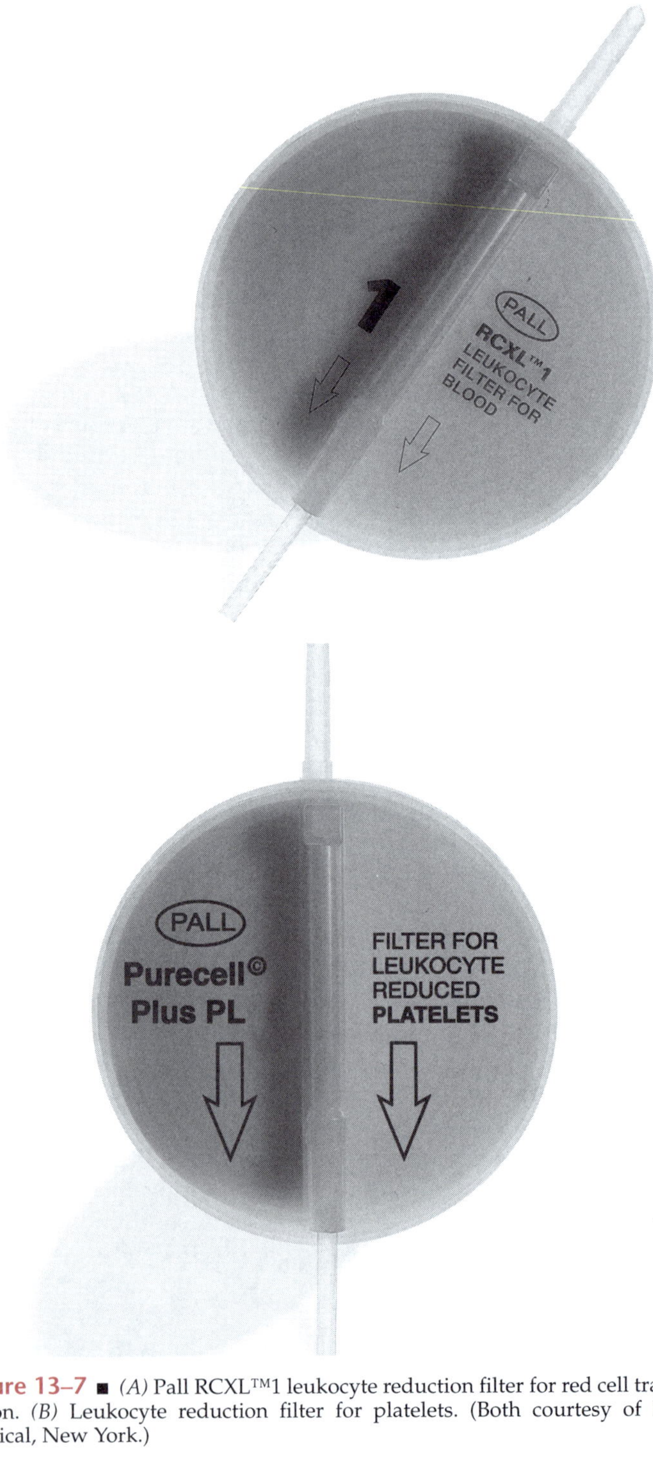

A

B

Figure 13–7 ■ *(A)* Pall RCXL™1 leukocyte reduction filter for red cell transfusion. *(B)* Leukocyte reduction filter for platelets. (Both courtesy of Pall Medical, New York.)

Fluid/Blood Warmers

Specific equipment is also available to warm blood if needed. Most transfusions do not require the use of a blood warmer. Warming of blood toward body temperature is indicated for rapid or massive transfusions, in neonatal exchange transfusions, and for patients with potent cold agglutinins.

The manufacturer's guidelines should be adhered to when using any of the many types of blood and fluid warmers. The temperature control should not warm the blood or fluid above 42°C (AABB, 2002).

> **INS Standard.** Consideration should be given to the use of blood warmers for massive-rapid transfusions, exchange transfusions, and patients with clinically significant cold agglutinins (INS, 2000, 75).

NURSING FAST FACT!

Only temperature devices specifically designed to warm blood should be used. Blood components should NEVER be placed in microwave ovens or hot water baths because of damage to RBCs and the lack of temperature control, which may cause fatal complications for the patient.

Electronic Monitoring Devices

Some transfusions may require an electronic monitoring device to control the blood flow. Only pumps designed for the infusion of whole blood and RBCs may be used because other types of infusion pumps may cause hemolysis. Pumps require the use of special tubing and filters. Little if any increased hemolysis occurs secondary to the use of most infusion pumps. A pump's manufacturer should be consulted for detailed information on the pump's suitability for transfusing blood components.

A pressure bag is a commonly used device for increasing flow rates during transfusion, usually in emergencies or during surgery. This device has a sleeve into which the blood bag is inserted, and the sleeve is inflated by filling it with air from a pressure manometer. As the unit of blood empties, the pressure of the sleeve decreases; therefore, it should be observed frequently and reinflated when necessary. (See Chapter 6 for further information and an illustration of blood administration equipment.)

Step 4: Preparing the Patient

Patient preparation begins when the transfusion of a blood component is anticipated. Urgency factors related to the transfusion may affect the amount of time available to prepare the patient for the transfusion.

The steps of the nursing process are activated, including assessment and the establishment of new goals and interventions related to the transfusion.

Patient/Family Education

The patient's and the patient's family's understanding of the need for blood, the procedure, and related concerns need to be assessed. Concerns are typically expressed regarding the risks of disease transmission; these need to be addressed.

NURSING FAST FACT!

As required by institution-specific protocols, informed consents should be done and a written consent form signed.

The patient should be instructed regarding the length of time for the procedure and the need for the monitoring of his or her physical condition and vital signs. Signs and symptoms that may be associated with a complication of the component to be given should be explained to the patient and his or her family. It is not necessary to offer graphic explanations regarding symptoms; rather, the patient should be asked to report any different sensations after the transfusion has been started along with brief descriptions of possible symptoms. Because transfusions typically take several hours, preparation also includes making the patient physically comfortable.

Assessment

The final step of patient preparation includes a thorough assessment of the patient. Baseline vital signs should be taken. If the vital signs are abnormal, consult with the physician before initiating the transfusion. Assessment of the lungs and kidney function should be documented prior to transfusion. The nurse should review the laboratory data (Hgb, Hct, platelets, clotting times) and anticipate how the component to be administered will impact the patient's laboratory values over the next 24 hours. Premedication with diuretics, antihistamines, or antipyretics may be necessary to help keep the vital signs at an acceptable level. The patient should also be questioned regarding any symptoms he or she may be experiencing that could be confused with a transfusion reaction.

NURSING FAST FACT!

The patient education and assessment should be documented in the chart.

Step 5: Obtaining Blood Product from the Blood Bank

As a rule, except in emergency situations, if blood is obtained from an onsite blood bank, only one product will be issued at a time and must be initiated within 30 minutes or returned to blood bank for proper storage. The blood component should not be obtained until the patient is ready to receive the component. If blood is obtained from an offsite blood bank, multiple units may be issued at one time. These units will be packaged to provide optimum storage conditions, and time limits for safe initiate will be detailed by the blood bank.

No unit of blood is to be placed in a refrigerator after leaving the blood bank. Most refrigerators cannot ensure the rigid temperature controls required to prevent storage lesions. If the transfusion will be initiated within 30 minutes, the blood should be left at room temperature. If a longer period of time will pass (for alternate sites), the blood should be continued to be stored in the container in which it was sent.

NURSING FAST FACT!

Refrigerators on the units may not be used to store blood products.

Proper identification of the blood component and the recipient are essential. Several items must always be verified and recorded before the transfusion is initiated.

- The physician's order should always be verified before the component is picked up.
- When the blood is issued, verification should include the name and identification number of the recipient, which must be recorded on the blood request form.
- The nurse should verify that the transfusion has not already been completed.

The transfusion form becomes part of the patient's permanent record.

- The notation of ABO group and Rh type must be the same on the primary blood bag label as on the transfusion form. This information is to be recorded on the attached compatibility tag or label.
- The donor number must be identically recorded on the label of the blood bag, the transfusion form, and the attached compatibility tag.
- The color, appearance, and expiration date of the component must be checked.
- The name of the person issuing the blood, the name of the person to whom the blood is issued, and the date and time of issue must be recorded. Often this is in a book in the laboratory.

Step 6: Preparing for Administration

Before obtaining the blood component (Step 5), the correct tubing, 0.9 percent sodium chloride, and appropriate catheter should be in place. It is vitally important that the site be checked to ensure that the I.V. line is patent.

Baseline vital signs, including the patient's temperature, blood pressure, pulse, and respirations, should be obtained. The patient should also be assessed for any symptoms that could later be confused as a transfusion reaction (e.g., rash, fever, shortness of breath, lower back pain). A transfusion record and report form are helpful for recording component specifics, vital signs, administration specifics, and reactions (Fig. 13–8).

The transfusion check between two nurses includes:

- *Physician order*: Check the blood or component against the physician's written order to verify that the correct component and amount are being given.
- *Recipient identification:* The name and identification number on the patient's identification band must be identical with the name and number attached to the unit.
- *Unit identification:* The unit identification number on the blood container, the transfusion form, and the tag attached to the unit must agree.
- *ABO and D type:* The ABO and D type on the primary label of the donor unit must agree with those recorded on the transfusion form.
- *Expiration:* The expiration date and time of the donor unit should be verified as acceptable.
- *Compatibility:* The interpretation of compatibility testing must be recorded on the transfusion form and on the tag attached to the unit.

NURSING FAST FACTS!

- *It is helpful if one nurse reads the information for verification to the other nurse; errors can be made if both nurses look at the tags together.*
- *Unless the exact time is given, the component expires at midnight on the expiration date.*
- *Watch for any discrepancies during any part of the identification process; the transfusion should not be initiated until the blood bank is notified and any discrepancies are resolved.*

Step 7: Initiating Transfusion

Use good hand hygiene and follow Standard Precautions when administering blood components. Wear gloves!

BLOOD TRANSFUSION RECORD

Resident's name: ______________________________ ID #: __________

Transfusion visit | Date: ________ Start time: ________ Completion time: ________ Nurse: ____________

Blood component: Unit # ____________ ABO type ________ Rh ________ Exp. date ________

Unit # ____________ ABO type ________ Rh ________ Exp. date ________

Component: ❑ Intact ❑ not intact Transport Temp: At Blood Bank ___ Time ______ At infusion site ___ Time ______

Unit(s) match order: ❑ Yes ❑ No ______________________

Unit(s) match Blood Bank tag: ❑ Yes ❑ No ______________________

Unit(s) match resident identification band: ❑ Yes ❑ No ______________________

Identification band on resident's wrist or ankle: ❑ Yes ❑ No ______________________

Pre-Medication ❑ Yes ❑ No

Drug	Dose	Route	Time

Anaphylaxis kit present: ❑ Yes Exp. Date ________ ❑ No Explain ______________________

Transfusion start: Unit # ____________ Time ______ Unit # ____________ Time ______

Vital signs (15 minute intervals recommended up to 30 minutes post-transfusion)

Time	BP	Temp	Pulse	Resp	Observations

Symptom	Pre-transfusion		During/Post	Time	Observation/Treatment
Fever	❑ Yes	❑ No	❑ Yes		
Chills	❑ Yes	❑ No	❑ Yes		
Hives/rash	❑ Yes	❑ No	❑ Yes		
Itching	❑ Yes	❑ No	❑ Yes		
Dyspnea/SOB	❑ Yes	❑ No	❑ Yes		
Chest pain	❑ Yes	❑ No	❑ Yes		
Hypotension	❑ Yes	❑ No	❑ Yes		
Tachycardia	❑ Yes	❑ No	❑ Yes		
Bradycardia	❑ Yes	❑ No	❑ Yes		
Other	❑ Yes	❑ No	❑ Yes		

Nurse Signature: ______________________ Date/Time: __________

Post transfusion follow-up | Resident's response: ❑ Tolerated without complications ❑ Post-transfusion reaction noted

Remarks: ______________________

❑ Lab tests drawn

Date	Time	Test	Result

Figure 13–8 ■ Transfusion record. (Courtesy of Lynda Cook, CRNI, and Linda Timmons, CRNI.)

To administer whole blood or RBCs, spike the blood container with the Y set and hang it up. Turn off the 0.9 percent sodium chloride and turn on the blood component. It is recommended that transfusions of RBCs be started at 5 mL/min for the first 15 minutes of the transfusion (AABB, 2002).

If the patient shows signs or symptoms of an adverse reaction, the transfusion can be stopped immediately and only a small amount of blood product will have been infused. After the first 15 minutes has safely passed, the rate of flow can be increased to complete the transfusion within the amount of time indicated by the physician or by policy. The rate of infusion should be based on the patient's blood volume, hemodynamic condition, and cardiac status. Gloves should be worn to handle blood products (Fig. 13–9).

Blood should be infused within a 4-hour period (AABB, 2002). When a longer transfusion time is clinically indicated, the unit may be divided by the blood bank and the portion not being transfused can be properly refrigerated.

Step 8: Monitoring the Transfusion

The patient's vital signs should be monitored at the end of the first 15 minutes and then periodically throughout the transfusion. The transfusion should be started slowly at a rate of approximately 2 mL/min except during urgent restoration of blood volume. Careful observation of the

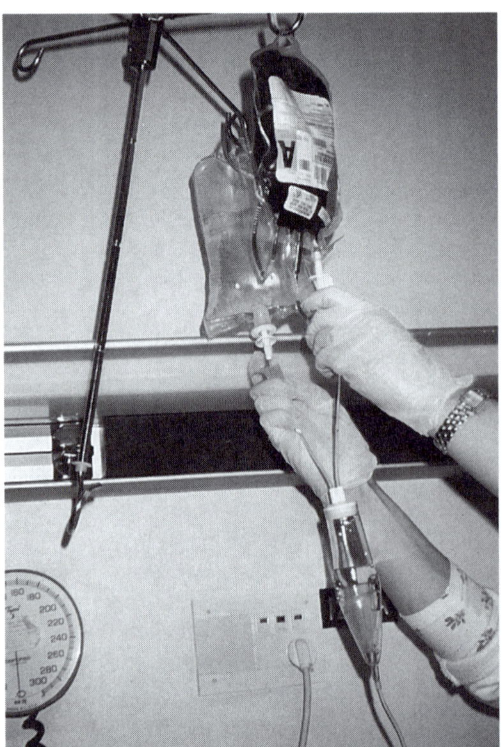

Figure 13–9 ■ Hanging PRBCs with Y administration set. Always wear gloves when handling blood products.

patient during and after a blood transfusion is necessary to provide a more reliable assessment. Vital signs must be recorded before and after the transfusion (AABB, 2002).

NURSING FAST FACTS!

- *Patients should be monitored for 15 minutes after initiation of a blood component (INS, 2000, 75).*
- *Patient education is required for conscious patients. They should be instructed to call if any unusual symptoms or sensations occur during a transfusion.*

A Note on Medications

Drugs should never be mixed with the blood component to be administered. One reason is the indeterminate effect the medication may have on the blood component. Also, if a reaction occurs, it would be difficult to ascertain whether it was the drug or the blood component that was responsible for the adverse effect. Another reason is that if the transfusion needs to be interrupted, it would be impossible to calculate the amount of drug that the patient received. If a patient requires I.V. medications during the course of the transfusion, a separate I.V. site should be started for the blood.

NURSING FAST FACT!

Absolutely no medications or solutions other than 0.9 percent sodium chloride shall be added to blood or blood components (INS, 2000, 75; AABB, 2002).

Step 9: Discontinuing the Transfusion

When the transfusion is complete, flush the tubing with 0.9 percent sodium chloride (except when using leukocyte filters). Because of the sodium and chloride content, a minimal amount should be used to complete the transfusion. At this point, another unit may be infused, the unit and line may be discontinued, the line can be capped with a PRN adaptor, or a new infusion line and solution container may be administered.

NURSING FAST FACT!

Do not save previous solutions and tubing, which were interrupted to give the blood component; they are considered contaminated. Restart with a fresh set and solution.

When the unit of blood has been infused, the time, volume given, and patient's condition should be documented. Some transfusion service departments require that a copy of the completed transfusion form be returned to them. Returning the blood component after an uncomplicated transfusion is not required in all facilities. If disposal is allowed on the unit, use hospital standards in disposing the blood bag in contaminated trash.

Complications Associated with Blood Component Therapy

Despite its numerous and obvious benefits, there are also complications associated with blood component therapy (Table 13-7). The administration of any blood component carries with it the potential of adverse reactions. Most reactions are caused by biologic aspects of blood; however, nonimmune reactions can occur and may be linked to the collection, preparation, or administration of the blood. Table 13-8 lists the complications in a quick-guide format.

INS Standard. INS Standards of Practice (2000, 75) dictate that a transfusion reaction requires immediate intervention. Interventions include but are not limited to:

- Terminating the transfusion
- Maintaining patency of the catheter with 0.9 percent sodium chloride

> Table 13–7 **RISKS OF TRANSFUSION THERAPY**

Viral Infection	Estimated Risks per Unit
HIV-1 and HIV-2	1:1,900,000
HTLV-1 and HTLV-2	1:641,000
HAV	1:1,000,000
HBV	1:63,000
HCV	1:1,600,000
Parvovirus B19	1:40,000
Parasitic infections	
Babesia and malaria	1:1,000,000
Noninfectious risks	
Fatal hemolytic transfusion	
Reactions	1:1,300,000
Febrile nonhemolytic transfusion reaction	1%
Minor allergic reaction	1%
Anaphylaxis	1/20,000
Noncardiogenic pulmonary edema/ transfusion related acute lung injury	1/5,000

Source: *AABB Technical Manual (14th ed.), 2002.*

> Table 13–8 **SUMMARY OF TRANSFUSION REACTIONS**

Transfusion Reaction	Etiology	Signs & Symptoms	Key Interventions	Prevention
Immune Reactions				
Acute hemolytic transfusion reaction	Hemolysis occurs when antibodies in plasma attach to antigens on the donor's RBCs. Cause: infusion of ABO incompatible blood	Burning sensation along vein Lumbar pain Flank pain, flushing of face and chest pain Bleeding Tachycardia, tachypnea Hemoglobinemia Hemoglobinuria, shock, vascular collapse, death	STOP THE TRANSFUSION! Get help immediately. Treat shock. Maintain blood pressure with colloidal solutions. Administer diuretics to maintain blood flow. Monitor for need for dialysis.	Extreme care during the entire identification process Start transfusion slowly and monitor for first 15 minutes.
Delayed hemolytic reaction	Result of RBC antigen incompatibility other than the ABO group. Occur due to destruction of transfused RBCs by alloantibodies not discovered during the process of crossmatching.	Decreased hematocrit and hemoglobin Fever (continual, low grade) Jaundice (mild) Malaise Indirect hyperbilirubinemia	No acute treatment required. Monitor hematocrit level Renal function Coagulation profile Notify physician and transfusion services	Strict attention to crossmatching protocols
Nonhemolytic febrile reaction	Occur due to antibodies direct against leukocytes or platelets. Febrile reactions. Occur immediately or 1 to 2 hours after transfusion completed.	Fever rise of 1° in association with transfusion Chills Headache Nausea and vomiting Chest pain Nonproductive cough Malaise	Stop the transfusion, and start the normal saline. Notify the physician. Monitor vitals Anticipate order for antipyretic agents. If ordered, restart transfusion slowly.	Use of leukocyte-reduced blood component. Filter.

(Continued on following page)

Table 13–8 SUMMARY OF TRANSFUSION REACTIONS *(Continued)*

Transfusion Reaction	Etiology	Signs & Symptoms	Key Interventions	Prevention
Allergic reactions (mild)	Caused by recipient sensitivity to the donor's foreign plasma proteins	Itching Hives (local) Rash, urticaria Facial flushing Runny eyes Anxiety Dyspnea Wheezing	Stop the transfusion. Keep vein open with normal saline. Notify the physician. Monitor vitals. Anticipate antihistamine order. If ordered, restart transfusion slowly. Mild reactions can precede severe allergic reactions. Monitor.	If known mild allergic reaction occur with blood transfusion may receive diphenhydramine (Benadryl) before the transfusion.
Severe allergic reactions: Anaphylaxis	Caused when donor blood with IgA proteins is transfused into an IgA-deficient recipient who has developed IgA antibody.	Anxiety Urticaria Wheezing Hypotension GI distress Shock Cardiac distress Death	Discontinue the transfusion. Keep vein open with normal saline. CPR if necessary. Anticipate order for steroids. Maintain BP.	Use of autologous blood Using blood from donors who are IgA deficient or by administering only well-washed RBCs in which all plasma has been extracted.
Graft-versus-host disease (GVHD)	Delayed reaction associated with donor lymphocytes– leukocyte reaction Highest risk in the immunocompetent patient	Diarrhea Fever Rash Hepatitis Bone marrow suppression Overwhelming infection	No effective therapy Treatment of symptoms Morbidity high	Irradiation of blood products used in immunocompromised patients Use leukocyte reducing filter.

Transfusion Reaction	Etiology	Signs & Symptoms	Key Interventions	Prevention
Acute lung injury	Infrequent Donor-high-titer antileukocyte antibodies and recipient leukocytes. Results in leukoagglutination which is trapped in pulmonary microvascular	Severe respiratory distress Chills Fever Cyanosis Hypotension	Discontinue the transfusion. Provide respiratory support.	
Nonimmune reactions				
Circulatory overload	Administration of blood faster than the recipient's cardiac output.	Hypervolemia Headache Dyspnea Constriction of chest Coughing Cyanosis	Stop the transfusion. Elevate the head of bed. Notify the physician. Rapid-acting diuretics Oxygen Therapeutic phlebotomy may be indicated.	Frequent monitoring of patient Administration of components slowly
Potassium toxicity Hyperkalemia	Administration of blood that has been stored. Related to release of potassium from the RBCs as they go through lysis. Occurs most frequently in multiple transfusions.	Elevated potassium levels Slow, irregular heart rate Nausea Muscle weakness ECG changes Diarrhea Renal failure	Stop or slow the transfusion. Monitor the ECG. Notify the physician. Remove excess potassium: concurrent administration of hypertonic dextrose and insulin or administer polystyrene sulfonate orally or by enema.	In patients receiving multiple transfusions—use only the freshest blood.
Hypothermia	Large volumes of cold blood are infused rapidly.	Drop in core temperature Chills Peripheral vasoconstriction Ventricular arrhythmias Cardiac arrest	Monitor the patient. Use external warming techniques (blankets, lights).	Use blood warmers if possible. Warm blood to 37°C

(Continued on following page)

Table 13–8 SUMMARY OF TRANSFUSION REACTIONS *(Continued)*

Transfusion Reaction	Etiology	Signs & Symptoms	Key Interventions	Prevention
Citrate toxicity	Infrequent High rate infusions, liver unable to keep up with the rapid administration and cannot metabolize the citrate (which chelates calcium), reducing the ionized calcium concentration in the recipient's blood.	Hypocalcemia induced cardiac dysrhythmias Tingling of fingers Muscular cramps Confusions Hypotension Cardiac arrest	Slowing rate of infusion Administration of calcium chloride or calcium gluconate Do not add calcium to infusing blood!	Administer fresh blood. Monitor calcium levels. Monitor patients with liver impairment closer for hypocalcemia.
Bacterial contamination	Occurs at the time of donation or in preparing the component for infusion. Cold-resistant gram-negative bacteria such as *Pseudomonas* species, *Citrobacter freundii*, and *Escherichia coli* are potential causes – release endotoxin	Septic reaction, includes high fever Flushing of skin "Warm" shock Hemoglobinuria Renal failure DIC	Discontinue the transfusion. Aggressively treat shock and anticipate order of steroids and antibiotics. Culture patient's blood, component and all I.V. solutions.	Preventable Bedside transfusion errors Inspection of the unit before administration – Observe for any discoloration of the blood or plasma. Report obvious clots. Ensure the integrity of the system prior to administration.
Coagulation imbalances	Caused by dilutional thrombocytopenia, and altered clotting as a result of transfusing stored blood in which there is a diminished platelet count.	Abnormal bleeding, especially from surgical sites, I.V. sites, or any breaches in skin	Monitoring laboratory reports. Coagulation studies Platelet counts Protect from injury. Anticipate platelet administration.	Administration of fresh blood, less than a week old

Transfusion Reaction	Etiology	Signs & Symptoms	Key Interventions	Prevention
Decreased tissue oxygenation	Oxygen is attracted to hemoglobin in blood, due to a decrease in 2,3-diphosphoglycerate in stored blood. This prevents the oxygen from leaving the blood and getting to the tissues.	Hypoxia Confusion Lethargy Cyanosis Respiratory depression	Respiratory support Monitor and report abnormalities in arterial blood gases.	Use fresh blood or RBCs.
Nonimmune infection related delayed				
Hepatitis-B Hepatitis-C	Viral infection, spread by blood and serum derived fluids and by direct contact with body fluids Average incubation is 90 days.	Elevated liver enzymes Fever Jaundice Malaise Nausea Pharyngitis Dark urine	No specific treatment – nursing care revolves around symptomatic treatment.	Hepatitis B vaccine Pretransfusion testing of donor blood No vaccine for hepatitis C
HIV-1	Viral infection transmitted via bodily secretions from HIV-positive individual.	Six stages by Walter Reed Classification System Positive HIV-flulike syndrome to total anergy with chronic fungal and viral infections	No cure Treatment is symptomatic.	Donor screening New NAT test
Cytomegalovirus	Viral infection, most at risk are low-birthweight neonates, immunosuppressed patients, and recipients of bone marrow and solid organ transplants.	Systemic CMV infection (pneumonia, hepatitis, and retinitis)	No specific treatment	Reduce CMV exposure in specific patient populations use blood from CMV–seronegative donors or depleted leukocytes

(Continued on following page)

> Table 13–8 SUMMARY OF TRANSFUSION REACTIONS *(Continued)*

Transfusion Reaction	Etiology	Signs & Symptoms	Key Interventions	Prevention
Malaria	Parasite infection prevalent in other parts of world. Blood transfusions can transmit malaria parasites.	High fever Organisms present on blood smear		Exclude donors from regions of the world where malaria is prevalent. Donors who have had malaria are deferred for 3 years.
West Nile Virus (WNV)	Viral infection spread by infected mosquito. Incubation period 2 to 14 days following bite	Fever and headache Eye pain Body aches GI complaints	Minimal data available at this time	FDA developing investigation nucleic acid tests to screen blood for WNV. Screening of donors. Donors deferred
Variant Creutzfeldt–Jakob disease (vCJD)	Rare degenerative and fatal nervous system disorder. Occurs when humans eat beef contaminated with bovine spongiform encephalopathy.	There has been no evidence at this time that vCJD has been transmitted through blood transfusion.	Precautions are taken in screening donors.	No screening test currently FDA required deferral policies for anyone who potentially could have been exposed to the disease by eating contaminated beef products.

- Notifying the physician and hospital blood bank or transfusion services
- Implementing other interventions as indicated

Biologic (Immune) Reactions

Acute Hemolytic Reactions

Hemolytic transfusion reactions may be acute or delayed. The most serious and potentially life-threatening reaction is acute **hemolytic transfusion reaction**. This reaction, according to Association of Blood Banks, occurs in 1 in 600,000 transfusions. This type of reaction occurs after infusion of incompatible RBCs. There are two types of RBC destruction. First, intravascular hemolysis, in which the RBCs are destroyed with hemolysis directly in the bloodstream, is usually seen with ABO-incompatible RBCs. Second, extravascular hemolysis, in which the cells are coated with the antibody and subsequently removed by the reticuloendothelial system, is seen in Rh incompatibility. These incompatibilities may lead to an activation of the coagulation system and release of vasoactive enzymes, which can result in vasomotor instability, cardiorespiratory collapse, or DIC. Intravascular hemolysis is the most serious and is usually fatal.

Incompatibilities involving other RBC antigens and IgG antibodies can result in fever, anemia, hyperbilirubinemia, and a positive direct antibody test result. The severity of the reaction can be dose related but can occur with less than 30 mL of blood administered. Most hemolytic reactions are a result of clerical errors, such as incorrect labeling of the blood specimen or errors in identifying the recipient.

SIGNS AND SYMPTOMS

The first symptoms include a burning sensation along the vein in which the blood is being infused. This symptom is quickly followed by lumbar pain, flank pain, flushing of the face, and chest pain. If infusion is allowed to continue, symptoms include fever, chills, hemoglobinemia, oozing of blood at the injection site, shock, and DIC.

INTERVENTIONS

Stop the transfusion. Disconnect the tubing from the I.V. catheter and infuse fresh saline not contaminated by the blood.

NURSING FAST FACT!

In acute hemolytic transfusion reaction, you must not give the recipient another drop of donor blood.

Notify the physician and blood bank or transfusion service *immediately.* Monitor vital signs and maintain intravascular volume with fluids to prevent renal constriction. In addition, diuretics, mannitol, and dopamine can support the renal and vascular systems. This is an emergency situation. The patient's respiratory status may have to be supported.

Interventions that can be anticipated by the nurse include:

- Dopamine 5 mcg/kg per minute may be ordered to increase blood pressure and improve renal blood flow.
- Diuretics, such as 40 to 100 mg of furosemide given I.V. push, may be ordered to maintain urine output above 100 mL/h to decrease the risk of renal damage.
- Other therapies, such as heparin to prevent DIC or mannitol to produce an osmotic diuresis, are controversial but are sometimes used cautiously (Young, 2000).

PREVENTION

Extreme care during the entire identification process is the first step in prevention. The transfusion must be started slowly.

> **INS Standard.** The patient should be monitored the first 15 minutes of the transfusion and throughout the transfusion. (INS, 2000, 75)

Delayed Hemolytic Reaction

Delayed transfusion reaction is a result of RBC antigen incompatibility other than the ABO group. Rapid production of RBC antibody occurs shortly after transfusion of the corresponding antigen as a result of sensitization during previous transfusions or pregnancies. Destruction of the transfused RBCs gradually occurs over 2 or more days or up to several weeks after the transfusion. Most reactions of this type go unnoticed and are common.

SIGNS AND SYMPTOMS

A decrease in hemoglobin and hematocrit levels, persistent low-grade fever, malaise, and indirect hyperbilirubinemia are symptoms that occur with delayed transfusion reaction.

INTERVENTIONS

No acute treatment is usually required. Monitor hematocrit level, renal function, and coagulation profile routinely for all patients receiving transfusions. Notify physician and transfusion services if delayed reaction is suspected.

PREVENTION

Avoid clerical errors.

Nonhemolytic Febrile Reactions

Nonhemolytic febrile reactions are defined as a temperature rise of 1°C or more occurring in association with transfusion and not having any other explanation. These are usually reactions to antibodies directed against leukocytes or platelets. Febrile reactions occur in only 1 percent of transfusions; repeat reactions are uncommon. These reactions can occur immediately or within 1 to 2 hours after transfusion is completed. Fever is the symptom associated with this type of transfusion reaction.

SIGNS AND SYMPTOMS

Signs and symptoms of a nonhemolytic febrile reaction are fever, chills, headache, nausea and vomiting, hypotension, chest pain, dyspnea and nonproductive cough, and malaise.

INTERVENTIONS

Stop the transfusion. Keep the vein open with normal saline and notify the physician. Monitor vital signs. The physician might order antipyretic agents.

NURSING FAST FACT!

In a nonhemolytic febrile reaction, you may turn off the blood and turn on the sodium chloride primer and infuse slowly. Do not take down the blood until notified by the physician; leave the blood hanging but clamp the Y connector to the blood unit.

PREVENTION

This type of reaction can be prevented or reduced by the use of leukocyte-reduced blood components. HLA compatible products may also be indicated.

Allergic Reactions: Mild

In its mild form, **allergic reactions** constitute the second most common type of reaction and are probably caused by antibodies against plasma proteins. The patient may experience mild localized urticaria or full systemic anaphylactic reaction. This can occur immediately or within 1 hour after infusion. Most reactions are mild and respond to antihistamines.

SIGNS AND SYMPTOMS

Signs and symptoms of allergic reactions include itching, hives (local erythema), rash, urticaria, runny eyes, anxiety, dyspnea, and wheezing.

INTERVENTIONS

Stop the transfusion. Keep the vein open with normal saline. Notify the physician. Monitor the vital signs. For mild reaction, administer antihistamines per physician order and continue transfusion if symptoms subside.

PREVENTION

For mild reactions, the patient may receive antihistamines, such as diphenhydramine Benadryl, before the transfusion. With mild reaction, the transfusion may be continued after antihistamines are administered and the symptoms have subsided. Severe reactions may require discontinuation of the transfusion and drug therapy to support the vascular system.

Allergic Reactions – Severe: Anaphylactic Reaction

Anaphylactic reactions are rare, but can occur in patients who are IgA deficient and who have developed anti-IgA antibodies. The two classic signs that an anaphylactic reaction is imminent are symptoms after only a few milliliters of blood or plasma have been infused, in the absence of fever.

SIGNS AND SYMPTOMS

Bronchospasms, respiratory distress, abdominal cramps, and vascular instability accompanied by shock are the characteristic symptoms.

TREATMENT

This is a medical emergency that requires immediate resuscitation of the patient together with administration of epinephrine and steroids.

PREVENTION

Close observation during the first 15 minutes of the transfusion and continuing surveillance throughout and for 1 hour after completion of the transfusion are important to monitor for signs of this reaction.

Transfuse patients who have a history of anaphylaxis with IgA-deficient blood products, washed RBCs, or deglycerolized RBCs.

Alloimmunization and Refractoriness

Alloimmunization is defined as stimulation of antibody development by foreign blood cell antigens. The reaction is delayed and occurs after multiple transfusions. The offending agent can be leukocytes or RBCs.

Alloimmunization directed against RBC antigens creates a more serious issue. The risk however is low: 1.0 to 1.4 percent per unit. After an offending antibody has been recognized, RBC products should be screened for the offending antigen. These units may be labeled "this unit negative for..." to indicate the absence of the offending agent.

Refractoriness is a state in which there is not a reasonable increase in the recipient's platelet count after transfusion. Refractoriness may result from immunization to HLA or to other platelet-specific antigens (Cook, 1997a).

NURSING FAST FACT!

Recipients who are in a refractory state will benefit if future transfusions are with HLA-specific platelets.

Graft-Versus-Host Disease

Transfusion-associated graft-versus-host disease (TA-GVHD) occurs when a recipient is immunocompromised, a fresh blood component containing a sufficient number of viable T lymphocytes is transfused, and the recipient reacts to one of the donor HLA cells. The T lymphocytes become activated, engraft, and proliferate, and begin to attack host tissue cells. The patient will experience tissue dysfunction as the epithelium of various organs such as the liver, gastrointestinal tract, and bone marrow is destroyed. Signs and symptoms include fever, rash, hepatitis, diarrhea, bone marrow suppression, and overwhelming infection. Death due to bleeding or infection normally occurs within 3 weeks. There is no cure for TA-GVHD. Gamma irradiation of all cellular components is the only way to prevent TA-GVHD. Leukoreduction of the products will not prevent TA-GVHD, but it reduces the number of white blood cells requiring irradiation (Harris, 2002).

NURSING FAST FACT!

Immunoincompetent recipients are at risk for TA-GVHD.

Nonimmune Reactions

Circulatory Overload

The rapid administration of any blood product can lead to circulatory overload. RBC products, plasma products and albumin 25 percent are the blood components most commonly associated with overload. Patients at risk for circulatory overload are those of small stature, infants and young children, and frail and elderly individuals. Individuals with compromised cardiac or pulmonary function are also at risk (Cook, 1997b).

SIGNS AND SYMPTOMS

Dyspnea, engorged neck veins, congestive heart failure, and pulmonary edema.

INTERVENTIONS

Stop the transfusion. Elevate the patient's head of the bed and notify the physician. Administer diuretics if necessary.

PREVENTION

Minimize the risk of overload by using RBCs instead of whole blood, infusion at a reduced rate for the high-risk patient, and administering a diuretic when beginning the transfusion in select recipients. Circulatory overload is the easiest reaction to prevent. Monitor vital signs throughout the transfusion.

Recommendations are to administer blood at a rate not to exceed 2 to 4 mL/kg body weight/h, which is about 2 h/U.

Potassium Toxicity (Hyperkalemia)

Potassium toxicity is a rare complication. As the blood ages during storage, potassium is released from the cells into the plasma during RBC lysis. When RBCs have been stored at 1 to 6°C, biochemical changes, known as storage lesions, develop. During the first few weeks of storage, extracellular potassium in the unit may increase by as much as 1 mEq daily (AABB, 1999). As a result of this storage lesion, the recipient receives excessive potassium. Single-unit transfusion is generally not a problem, but individuals who receive multiple units of aged blood may experience this reaction.

SIGNS AND SYMPTOMS

Signs and symptoms of potassium toxicity include immediate onset of hyperkalemia; slow, irregular heartbeat; nausea; muscle weakness; and electrocardiographic changes.

INTERVENTIONS

The goal is to remove the excess potassium. The concurrent administration of insulin and hypertonic dextrose provides a hypokalemic action, which may be effective for 4 to 6 hours. (Refer to Chapter 4 for further treatment modalities for patients with hyperkalemia.)

PREVENTION

Use fresh blood.

Additional Non-Immune Complications

HYPOTHERMIA

When large volumes of blood are administered, hypothermia can occur owing to the consistently cool temperature of the blood. This risk brings about decreased core temperature, chills, peripheral vasoconstriction, ventricular arrhythmias, and cardiac arrest. External warming measures include blankets and warming lights. Internal (core rewarming) warming measures need to be implemented if the core temperature drops to 86°F or 30°C (Emergency Nurses Association, 2002). Use of a blood warmer during transfusions can be helpful to minimize this risk. Time does not always permit the use of these devices in an emergency.

CITRATE TOXICITY: HYPOCALCEMIA

A reaction to toxic proportions of citrate, which is used as a preservative in blood, can cause hypocalcemia. The citrate ion can combine with the recipient's serum calcium, causing a calcium deficiency, or normal citrate metabolism is hindered by the presence of liver disease. Patients at risk for development of citrate toxicity or a calcium deficit are those who receive infusions of blood products at rates exceeding 100/mL per minute, or lower rates in patients who have liver disease. The liver, unable to keep up with the rapid administration, cannot metabolize the citrate, which chelates calcium, reducing the ionized calcium concentration. Hypocalcemia may induce cardiac dysrhythmias. Slow the infusion rate and, based on symptoms and blood values of calcium, administer calcium chloride or calcium gluconate solution. Do not administer calcium via the administration set infusing the blood.

BACTERIAL CONTAMINATION

Bacterial contamination of blood may occur at any time during donation or processing of a unit. Two types of organisms are implicated in contamination: warmth-loving organisms such as *Salmonella* spp. and *Staphylococcus* spp., and cold-loving organisms such as *Pseudomonas* spp., *Citrobacter* spp., *Escherichia coli,* and *Yersinia enterocolitica.* It is difficult to eliminate contaminated units based on visual inspection. However, RBCs that are severely contaminated may have a purplish hue; unsuspended supernatant may be pink, which indicates hemolysis. The recipient may not exhibit symptoms until the transfusion has been completed. Fatality from transfusion-induced septicemia is estimated at 50 to 80 percent (Cook, 1997b). Sudden high fever, marked hypotension, and cardiovascular collapse in an apparently "well" individual characterize septic shock. Endotoxic poisoning causes multiorgan system failure.

Transfusion-Transmitted Diseases

Despite dynamic advances in blood banking and transfusion medicine, there are still risks to blood component therapy. Patients should be told of alternatives to transfusion, including risks to the patient if transfusion is not undertaken. Furthermore, patients need to know about the blood center's autologous transfusion and patient-designated donor programs, without an implication that there is added safety to the latter.

A uniform donor history is designed to ask questions that protect the health of both the donor and the recipient. Questions asked of the donor help determine whether donating blood might endanger his or her health. If a prospective donor responds positively to any of these questions, he or she will be "deferred" or asked not to donate blood. The health history also is used to identify prospective donors who have been exposed to or who may have disease, such as human immunodeficiency virus (HIV), hepatitis, or malaria (AABB, 2002). (Table 13–7 provides the incidence of transfusion-acquired infections.)

Hepatitis

Viral hepatitis, which infects the liver, accounts for only a small proportion of cases of post-transfusion hepatitis. The incidence is low due to screening of donors for behaviors that expose them to viral hepatitis and testing of all donations of HbsAg and anti-HBc. The prevalence of the HbsAg carrier state in blood donations in the United States is approximately 0.02 percent to 0.04 percent (Goodnough et al., 1999). Hepatitis transfusion-transmission fall into two groups: viruses with a chronic course that can readily be transmitted by blood transfusion (hepatitis B and C) and viruses that cause only acute disease and are rarely transmitted by transfusion (hepatitis A and E) (AABB, 2002).

Hepatitis incubation period is approximately 90 days, with symptoms of dark urine, jaundice, malaise, anorexia, headache pharyngitis, and elevated liver enzymes. Treatment is symptomatic.

Cytomegalovirus

Cytomegalovirus (CMV) is a virus belonging to the herpes group that is rarely transmitted by blood transfusion. According to the CDC about 50 to 85 percent of adults in the United States are infected with CMV by the age of 40. CMV infection is usually mild, but may be serious or fall for those who are immunocompromised, and low-birthweight infants, and bone marrow and organ transplant patients. Filtered blood that decreases the number of white blood cells (the cells that carry CMV) will protect patients from getting CMV infection from a transfusion (AABB, 2002).

Human Immunodeficiency Virus

Transfusion transmission of human immunodeficiency virus (HIV) has been almost completely eradicated since blood banks began interviewing donors about at-risk behaviors and blood tests became available in 1985. The HIV antibody tests, used on every blood donation, have undergone continuous improvement. In 1999 nucleic acid amplification testing (NAT) began to be used to directly detect the genetic material of the HIV virus in the blood (AABB, 2003)

West Nile Virus

West Nile virus (WNV) is spread by the bite of an infected mosquito. The virus can infect people, horses, and many types of birds. It was first detected in the United States in 1999, and the first documented cases of WNV transmission through organ transplantation and transfusion were noted in 2002. The most common symptoms of transfusion-transmitted cases of WNV are fever and headache. Screening is by blood bank interview of history of fever and headache. Candidates who will be "deferred" include:

1. A potential donor who has been diagnosed with WNV infection—deferred 28 days from onset of symptoms
2. A potential donor who responds positively to the question. "In the past week, have you had a fever with headache?" —deferred 28 days
3. A donor whose blood or components potentially were associated with a transfusion-related WNV transmission—deferred 28 days (AABB, 2002)

NURSING FAST FACT!

Currently the FDA is developing an investigational nucleic acid test (NAT) to screen blood for WNV.

Creutzfeldt–Jakob Disease

Creutzfeldt–Jakob Disease (CJD) is a rare degenerative and fatal nervous system disorder. Currently, there is no screening test for the disease, and white blood transfusions have never been shown to transmit any form of the disease. As a precaution the FDA prohibits blood donation by individuals who may be at risk. These include potential donors who have received injections of human-derived pituitary hormone, those with a family history of CJD, or those who have had surgeries that involved transplanted dura mater.

Variant Creutzfeldt–Jakob Disease

Similar to CJD, variant CJD (vCJD), commonly known as the human form of "mad cow" disease, is a rare degenerative and fatal nervous system disorder. At this time there is no evidence that vCJD has ever been transmitted through a blood transfusion. The FDA requires donor "deferral" policies for anyone who potentially could have been exposed to the disease by eating contaminated beef products. There is no screening at this time.

Severe Acute Respiratory Syndrome

Severe acute respiratory syndrome (SARS) is a respiratory infection that can develop serious complications. Most cases identified have been in Asia. There has been no evidence this infection is transmitted from blood donors to transfusion recipients, but the virus associated with SARS is present in the blood of people who are sick. Because the risk of contracting SARS through a blood transfusion theoretically exists, anyone who might be at risk of being infected with SARS is "deferred." Questions asked to determine "deferred" status include:

1. "Have you traveled or lived in a SARS-affected area?"—deferred for a period of 14 days after arrival in the United States
2. "Have you had close contact with a person with SARS?"—deferred for 14 days after the last exposure
3. "Have you been ill with SARS?"—deferred 28 days from last date of treatment (AABB, 2002)

Smallpox

Owing to concern that terrorists may have access to the smallpox virus, and may attempt to use it against the American public, the U.S. Department of Health and Human Services (HHS) has been working, in cooperation with the state and local governments, to strengthen to expand the national stockpile of smallpox vaccine.

It is possible that, until the vaccination scab spontaneously separates from the skin, recipients of the vaccine virus could inadvertently infect close contacts who touch the vaccination site or dressing. The scabs themselves contain infectious viruses. Potential donors will be asked by blood collection facilities about history of vaccination or close contact with anyone who has been vaccinated. Donors will be "deferred" until a vaccine recipient has had no complications and the vaccination scab has spontaneously separated, or 21 days after vaccination (AABB, 2002).

Parasitic Infections

A variety of parasitic infections may be transmitted through transfusions: babesiosis (transmitted by tick bites), Chagas' disease (transmitted by reduviid bugs), Lyme disease (bite of certain species of deer tick), and malaria. Blood banking facilities screen for these four parasitic infections and may "defer" the donor or permanently prohibit blood donation from those infected with these parasite infections (AABB, 2003).

Websites

Information on SARS: CDC Website: *www.cdc.gov/ncidod/sars/casedefintion.htm*

Information on West Nile Virus (WNV): *www.cdc.gov/ncidod/dvbid/westnile/citystates.htm*

NURSING PLAN OF CARE

DELIVERY OF BLOOD COMPONENT THERAPY

Focus Assessment

Subjective

- Interview regarding understanding of need for blood component.
- Determine patient's understanding of options: autologous, homologous, and directed donations.

Objective

- Assessment of vital signs (blood pressure, pulse, respiration, temperature)
- Assessment of renal and cardiovascular systems
- Assessment and evaluation of I.V. site before administration of blood component
- Assessment of body weight
- Assessment of level of consciousness
- Review of laboratory test
- Current intake and output

Patient Outcome/Evaluation Criteria

Patient will:

- Receive blood product without untoward effect or complications.
- Display improvement of hemodynamic parameters and urine output of 1/2 m/kg per hour.
- Verbalize an understanding of the reasons for the use of the blood component.
- Verbalize an awareness of anxiety.

Nursing Diagnoses

- Anxiety (mild, moderate, severe) related to threat to or change in health status; misconceptions regarding therapy
- Decreased cardiac output related to sepsis, contamination
- Fear related to homologous blood transfusion and the transmission of disease; fear of needles

(Continued on following page)

NURSING PLAN OF CARE

DELIVERY OF BLOOD COMPONENT THERAPY *(Continued)*

- Hyperthermia related to increased metabolic rate, illness, dehydration
- Hypothermia related to exposure to cool or cold blood
- Impaired physical mobility related to pain or discomfort resulting from placement and maintenance of I.V. catheter
- Impaired skin integrity related to I.V. catheter, irritating I.V. solution, inflammation, infection, infiltration
- Impaired tissue integrity related to altered circulation, fluid deficit or excess, irritating solution, inflammation, infection, infiltration
- Impaired gas exchange related to ventilation perfusion imbalance, decreased oxygen-carrying capacity of the blood
- Knowledge deficit related to purpose of blood component therapy; signs and symptoms of complications
- Risk for infection related to broken skin or traumatized tissue

Nursing Management

1. Verify the physician's orders.
2. Obtain the patient's informed consent.
3. Monitor the
   a. patient's immunologic status.
   b. I.V. site for signs and symptoms of infiltration, phlebitis, and local infection.
   c. vital signs.
   d. fluid overload and physical reactions
   e. and regulate flow rate during infusion.
4. Verify that the blood product matches the patient's blood type.
5. Administer blood products as appropriate.
6. Prime the administration system with 0.9 percent sodium chloride.
7. Prepare an I.V. pump as indicated.
8. Perform venipuncture using the appropriate technique.
9. Refrain from "catching up" blood product administration in cases where the delivery rate was not calculated correctly.
10. Refrain from administering I.V. medication into blood or blood product lines.
11. Change administration set if clogging of the filter occurs.
12. Administer sodium chloride to clear the line after transfusion is complete.
13. Document the timeframe of transfusion and volume infused.
14. Stop the transfusion if blood reaction occurs and keep veins open with 0.9 percent sodium chloride.
15. Obtain the first voided urine specimen after a transfusion reaction.

(Continued on following page)

16. Coordinate the return of the blood container to the laboratory after a blood reaction.
17. Notify the laboratory immediately in the event of a blood reaction.
18. Maintain standard precautions.
19. Evaluate the effect of transfusion on laboratory test within 24 hours.

Patient Education

- Patients who are aware of the steps involved in a transfusion experience less anxiety.
- The nurse should explain how the transfusion will be given, how long it will take, what the expected outcome is, what symptoms to report and that vital signs will be taken.
- The physician has the responsibility to explain the benefits and risks of transfusion therapy, as well as alternatives.
- Informed consent should be obtained.
- Instruct on the need and physiologic benefit of blood product.
- Inform on options: autologous, homologous, or designated donation.
- Instruct on current statistics of transfusion risks, if necessary

Home Care Issues

Transfusion services can be delivered safely and efficiently in the home setting. This is an appropriate alternative for patients who require frequent transfusions but for whom hospitalization is not otherwise indicated. Usually the patient has physical limitations that make travel outside the home difficult (Lonsway, 2001). For non-homebound patients who require transfusions, administration in an outpatient infusion clinic may be a more cost-effective alternative.

Transfusions in the home setting include packed RBCs, modified RBCs, platelets, cryoprecipitate, plasma, plasma derivatives, and factor VIII concentrate. Whole blood is not an alternative in the home setting.

Home blood transfusion carries the same liability risk as hospital transfusion. During the pretransfusion visit, the informed consent and any other company-specific forms should be signed. A complete medical history and thorough physical examination is completed, along with evaluation of vascular access. An identification bracelet with the patient's full name and identification number is attached to the patient's wrist. The home I.V. nurse also obtains blood samples for baseline chemistry.

Guidelines for Home Transfusion Therapy:

1. Transfusion kit and protocol should be available in home during the transfusion.

(Continued on following page)

Home Care Issues *(Continued)*

2. Written physician's order is required.
3. The patient should be:
   a. In stable cardiopulmonary status and medical condition
   b. Alert, cooperative, and able to respond appropriately to body reactions and communicate information to the nurse
4. The following also must be evaluated:
   a. Conducive home environment
   b. Capable adult present during transfusion
   c. Telephone access available
   d. Ready access to emergency medical service and primary physician during transfusion (Lonsway, 2001)
5. Blood components should be transported to the home setting using blood bank standards.
6. Proper blood and patient identification must be carried out.
7. Baseline assessments should be made according to INS Standards for monitoring the infusion.
8. Appropriate blood filter should be used.
9. Electromechanical devices may be used, but the product information should be checked to ensure that the pump is indicated for transfusion delivery and will not cause hemolysis of RBCs.
10. Use only 0.9 percent sodium chloride solutions to prime the administration set.
11. The nurse administering the transfusion must remain in the home setting throughout the transfusion and for an appropriate time after transfusion to check for complications.
12. Blood warming should not be considered for home transfusion because no more than 2 U of blood should be administered at one time in the home setting. Patients with cold agglutinins are not appropriate candidates.
13. A biohazard bag should be brought to the home and all contaminated equipment disposed of according to state regulations.
14. The physician must be immediately available at all times for telephone consultation.
15. Post-transfusion instructions should be left; these include but are not limited to:
   a. Emergency telephone numbers
   b. Information regarding signs and symptoms of delayed reactions
   c. Schedule of the post-transfusion assessment visit
16. Notify the physician of the transfusion completion and the patient's response to therapy.
17. Documentation must include, but not be limited to:
   a. Type of I.V. solution and time started
   b. Type of blood product
   c. Vital signs, skin condition, and appearance

(Continued on following page)

d. Any patient symptoms or complaints
e. The time blood product is discontinued
f. Volume infused
g. Reason for discontinuing the transfusion if done before completion of the infusion
h. Patient reactions to the procedure

Reimbursement: Many carriers will reimburse for this therapy if it is "in lieu of hospitalization." Medicare does not currently reimburse for blood products (Lonsway, 2001).

Key Points

- Immunohematology is the science that deals with antigens of the blood and their antibodies.
- Blood groups are based on the antigens present on the cell surface of RBCs. The two major antigen groups are the ABO and Rh systems. Every human being has two genotypes that, when paired, determine one of four blood types (A, B, AB, or O).
- The universal RBC donor is O negative; the universal plasma donor is AB.
- The majority of people (85 percent) have the Rh antigen D, making them Rh positive. Those without the antigen D are Rh negative.
- ABO incompatibility is the major cause of fatal transfusion reactions.
- The most common preservatives added to blood to extend the shelf life are CPDA-1 (35 days) and ADSOL (42 days)
- Blood donor collection methods include:
  - Homologous: Blood donated by someone other than the intended recipient (allogeneic)
  - Autologous: Recipient's own blood; collected in one of four ways: preoperative blood salvage, intraoperative blood salvage, ANH, postoperative blood salvage
  - Designated (directed): Blood donated from selected friends or relatives of the recipient
- Blood product transfusions are indicated for:
  - Maintenance of oxygen-carrying capacity of the blood
  - Replacement of clotting factors
  - Replacement of vascular volume
- Governmental agencies (i.e., the AABB, INS, and FDA) set standards for responsibilities of nurses in the safe administration of blood products.
- Biologic (immune) reactions include acute hemolytic transfusion reactions, delayed transfusion reactions, nonhemolytic febrile reactions, allergic reactions, GVHD reactions, and alloimmunization and refractoriness.

- Nonimmune complications associated with transfusion therapy include circulatory overload, potassium toxicity, hypothermia, hypocalcemia, bacterial contamination, and infectious disease transmission.
- Key steps in the procedure to delivery of blood transfusion are:
  - Verify physician's order.
  - Type and crossmatch.
  - Select and prepare equipment.
  - Prepare patient.
  - Obtain blood from blood bank.
  - Prepare for administration.
  - Initiate the transfusion.
  - Monitor the transfusion.
  - Discontinue the transfusion.

Critical Thinking: Case Study

At the beginning of your shift, you check on a unit of packed red blood cells that had been hung just prior to your shift. The unit of RBCs is infusing slowly, with approximately 150 mL left. You agitate the bag slightly and discover a pinhole at the top of the bag.

What do you do? What legal factors are involved in this scenario? What are the risks to the patient? What assessments should have taken place prior to hanging this blood component?

Media Link: The answers to this case study and additional critical thinking activities are on the enclosed CD–ROM.

Post-Test

1. All the following statements related to the HLA system are true **EXCEPT:**
   a. HLA is located on the surface of WBCs.
   b. Alloimmunization to HLA antigens is a factor in refractoriness to platelets.
   c. The use of blood typing and crossmatching reduces the alloimmunization to the HLA antigen.
   d. The use of leukocyte-depleted blood can reduce the sensitization to HLA antigens.
2. Antibodies are found in:
   a. RBCs
   b. WBCs
   c. Plasma
   d. Antigens

3. Previous exposure to an antigen by pregnancy or previous transfusion may cause the patient to develop:
   a. An antibody to the antigen
   b. More antigens
   c. Alloimmunization to the antibody
   d. A tolerance to the transfusion
4. A chemical added to donor units to preserve the blood is:
   a. Sodium heparin
   b. Sodium citrate
   c. Sodium phosphate
   d. Dextrose aluminum
5. Blood bank testing for donor blood includes tests for the following diseases **EXCEPT:**
   a. HbsAg
   b. Anti–HIV-1
   c. Anti–HTLV-1
   d. EBV (Epstein–Barr virus)
6. The nurse would anticipate transfusion of platelets in which of the following patients?
   a. Hemorrhage with a platelet count less than 50,000
   b. Nonbleeding patients with a platelet count of 80,000
   c. Preoperative patient with a platelet count of 150,000
7. The nursing intervention for an acute hemolytic transfusion reaction would be to:
   a. Slow the transfusion and call the physician.
   b. Stop the transfusion and turn the saline side of the administration set on at a slow keep open rate.
   c. Stop the transfusion, disconnect the tubing from the I.V. catheter, and initiate new saline and tubing to keep the vein open.
   d. Stop the transfusion and turn the saline side of the administration set on at a rapid rate.
8. The component albumin 25 percent is hypertonic. Caution should be used by nurses when infusing 25 percent albumin because this product can:
   a. Cause circulatory overload
   b. Cause clotting disorders
   c. Increase RBC hemoglobin
   d. Lower the blood pressure

9. Nurses must check all of the following with another nurse before initiating a unit of blood **EXCEPT**:
   a. ABO and Rh
   b. Patient name
   c. Unit number
   d. Expiration date
   e. Preservative

10. The universal recipient is a person with blood type
    a. A-positive
    b. AB-positive
    c. O-negative
    d. AB–negative

11. Which of the following packed red blood cell preparations is considered to prevent transfusion-associated GVHD?
    a. Leukocyte-reduced RBC
    b. Washed RBCs
    c. Irradiated RBCs
    d. Frozen-washed RBCs

12. If a patient receives 2 U of packed red blood cells for a hematocrit (HCT) of 24%, what would the anticipated HCT be in 24 hours postinfusion?
    a. 26 Percent
    b. 28 Percent
    c. 30 Percent
    d. 32 Percent

13. Which of the following adverse effects of transfusion therapy has a potential for a fatal outcome for the patient?
    a. Hyperkalemia
    b. Febrile reaction
    c. Fluid overload
    d. Intravascular hemolysis

14. A patient, group O, may receive which of the following red blood cells?
    a. Group A only
    b. Group O only
    c. Group AB and O
    d. Any blood group

15. A nurse is planning to infuse a unit of packed cells. The order reads to infuse the unit when available. What would be the most appropriate infusion rate?
    a. 250 mL/h
    b. 125 mL/h
    c. 50 mL/h
    d. 25 mL/h

Media Link: Rationales for the answers to these questions, and additional test questions, are located on the enclosed CD–ROM.

References

American Association of Blood Banks (AABB) (2002). *Technical Manual* (14th ed.). American Association of Blood Banks, Bethesda, MD.

American Association of Blood Banks (AABB) (2003). *Facts About Blood*. American Association of Blood Banks, Bethesda, Maryland. Internet: *about blood/faqs*

Brown, M., & Whalen, P.K. (2000). Red blood cell transfusion in critically ill patients: Emerging risks and alternatives. *Critical Care Nursing* (Suppl), 1–14.

Cook, L.S. (1997a). Blood transfusion reactions involving an immune response. *Journal of Intravenous Nursing*, 20(1), 5–13.

Cook, L.S. (1997b). Nonimmune transfusion reactions: When type and cross match aren't enough. *Journal of Intravenous Nursing*, 20(1), 15–22.

Cook, L.S. (2000). A simple case of anemia: Pathophysiology of a common symptom. *Journal of Intravenous Therapy*, 23(5), 271–282.

Emergency Nurses Association (2002). Environmental Emergencies. In Wood, T. (ed.). *Emergency Nursing Core Curriculum* (5th ed.). Philadelphia: W.B. Saunders, p. 179

Fitzpatrick, L. (2002). Blood products: Washing away transfusion risks. *Nursing 2002*, 32(5), 36–41.

Giger, J.N., & Davidhizar, R.E. (2004). *Transcultural Nursing: Assessment and Intervention*.(2nd ed). St. Louis: Mosby, p. 140.

Goodnough, L.T., Brecher, M.E., Kanter, M.H., & Aubuchon, J.P. (1999). Medical progress. *Transfusion Medicine*, 340, 438–445.

Hadaway, L. (1999). Understanding leukocyte reduction in blood transfusions. *Nursing 99*, 29(10), 74.

Harris, D.J. (2002). Immune complications associated with chronic transfusion. *Journal of Infusion Nursing*, 25(5), 316–319.

Infusion Nurses Society (2000). Revised Standards of practice. *Journal of Intravenous Nursing* (Suppl), 23(6S), 75.

Lonsway, R. (2001). Intravenous therapy in the home. In Hankins, J., Lonsway, R.A., Hedrick, C., and Perdue, M. (eds.). *Infusion Therapy in Clinical Practice* (2nd ed.). Infusion Nurses Society and Philadelphia: W.B. Saunders, p. 520.

Phillips, L.D., & Kuhn, M. (1999). *Manual of IV Medications* (2nd ed.). Philadelphia: Lippincott-Raven.

Rebulla, P. (2001). Revisitation of the clinical indications for transfusion of platelet concentrates. *Reviews in Clinical and Experimental Hematology,* 5(3), 288–310.

Schaefer, J. (2002). Advances and dilemmas in recombinant blood products. *Journal of Infusion Nursing,* 25(5), 305–309.

Synthetic Blood International (2003). News Release: Synthetic Blood International's Oxycyte™ Called Promising. Internet Available *www.sybd.com/Synthetic.html* April, 2003

Weir, J. (2001). Blood component therapy. In Hankins, J., Lonsway, R.A., Hedrick, C., & Perdue, M. (eds.). *Infusion Therapy in Clinical Practice* (2nd ed.). Philadelphia: W.B. Saunders, pp. 156–175.

Young, J. (2000). Transfusion reaction. *Nursing 2000,* 30(12), 33.

Answers to Chapter 13 Post-Test

1. **c**
2. **c**
3. **a**
4. **b**
5. **d**
6. **a**
7. **c**
8. **a**
9. **e**
10. **b**
11. **c**
12. **c**
13. **d**
14. **b**
15. **b**

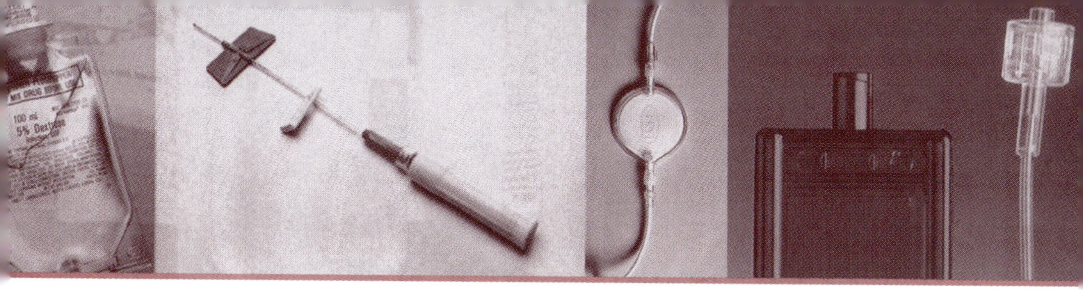

Chapter 14
Antineoplastic Therapy

Pamela Hockett, RN, MSN, CNS, OCN

These seasons of surviving are like the changing seasons of the year. We delight in the fragrant smell of spring, bask in the hot days of summer, then welcome the cool, crisp days of fall. Lest we get too used to it all, the frosty chill of winter is upon us, and when we despair of ever seeing those spring daffodils, violets and tulips again, up they blossom once again to delight us, only in a different way. Enduring seasons in survival give us renewed opportunities to learn more clearly the meaning of living and dying.

—Karen Hassey Dow, RN, MS, Cancer Survivor

Chapter Contents

LEARNING OBJECTIVES

Upon completion of this chapter, the reader will be able to:

1. Define the glossary of terms as related to nursing care of the patient receiving antineoplastic agents.
2. Discuss the principles of cellular kinetics related to delivery of antineoplastic agents.
3. Trace the phases of the cell cycle.
4. Identify the goals of cancer antineoplastic therapy.
5. Define the terms "cell cycle specific" and "cell cycle nonspecific."
6. Identify the role of the clinician in administration of chemotherapy.
7. State the action, drug specificity, and major side effects and specific nursing interventions with alkylating agents, antimetabolites, vinca alkaloids, hormones and hormone antagonists, and biologic response modifiers.
8. State specific nursing interventions that are useful in helping patients deal with alopecia.
9. List the medications available for treating patients who are experiencing nausea and vomiting.
10. Given an extravasated drug, determine the procedure for treatment of extravasation.
11. Identify agents available for oral care of patients receiving chemotherapy to prevent and treat stomatitis.
12. Identify the major toxicities that can occur with antineoplastic therapy.
13. Identify the common routes used for antineoplastic therapy.
14. Use the nursing process in planning care for a patient receiving antineoplastic therapy.
15. List the key areas of patient education for patients receiving chemotherapy.

GLOSSARY

Absolute neutrophil count (ANC) A calculation used to determine the neutrophil status

Adjuvant Addition to primary treatment

Alopecia Loss of hair (scalp, facial, axillary, pubic, and body)

Antineoplastic Medication used for the treatment of patients with cancer

Biologic response modifiers Agents that mimic, stimulate, enhance, inhibit, or alter the host's responses to cancer

Body surface area (BSA) A calculation using body weight and weight to determine drug doses

Cellular kinetics Study of mechanisms and rates of cellular changes; provides the basis for an understanding of the action and side effects of anticancer agents

Chemotherapy Treatment of disease with chemical reagents that have a specific and toxic effect on the disease-causing cells

Curative Successful treatment of a disease

Cytomodulatory Biotherapy agents that cause recognition of tumor-associated antigens

Cytotoxic The degree to which an agent possesses a specific destructive action on certain cells or the possession of such action; antineoplastic agents that kill dividing cells

Desquamation Shedding of the epidermis

Extravasation Leakage of a vesicant or irritant drug into the subcutaneous tissue that is capable of causing pain, necrosis, or sloughing of tissue

Integumentary Cutaneous; dermal

Intraperitoneal (IP) Within the peritoneal cavity

Intraventricular Within a ventricle

Irritant A cancer chemotherapeutic agent capable of producing venous pain at the site and along the vein, with or without an inflammatory reaction

Leukopenia Any situation in which the total number of leukocytes in the circulating blood is less than normal, the limit of which is generally regarded as 5000 cells/mm^3

Mitosis Indirect cell division involving indirect nuclear division and division of the cell body; the process by which all somatic cells of multicellular organisms multiply

Myelosuppression Decrease in function of bone marrow resulting in decrease in the amount of blood cells

Nadir count Point at which the blood counts are the lowest; often 7 to 14 days after the first day of chemotherapy based on the agents used

Neutropenia Diminished number of neutrophils in the blood

Nonstem cells Cells that differentiate
Oncologist Physician involved in the study and treatment of cancers
Palliative Use of procedures to promote client comfort and quality of life without the goal of cure of disease
Peripheral neuropathy Dysfunction of postganglionic nerves ranging from paresthesia to paralysis
Pruritus Itching
Stem cells Mother cells having the capacity for both replication and differentiation
Thrombocytopenia A condition in which there is an abnormally small number of platelets in the circulating blood
Vesicant A drug capable of causing tissue necrosis on skin contact

Nurses participating in administration of antineoplastic agents have a tremendous responsibility. This chapter emphasizes nurses' roles in understanding cellular kinetics, pharmacology of antineoplastic agents, routes of administration, and common side effects of chemotherapy.

> **INS Standard.** The nurse's responsibilities for administering antineoplastic therapy include knowledge of disease process, drug classifications, pharmacologic indications, actions, side effects, adverse reactions, method of administration, rate of delivery, treatment goal, and drug properties (e.g., vesicant, nonvesicant, and irritant). (INS, 2000, 70)

The Role of the Clinician

Administering **antineoplastic** agents and caring for patients with cancer require specific educational preparation and practical experience. The Oncology Nursing Society (ONS) has developed credentialing for oncology nurses.

Nurses practicing in this specialty area are required to be knowledgeable about the biology of cancer, the pharmacology and principles of cancer **chemotherapy**, specific antineoplastic agents, major principles governing the administration of chemotherapy, and patient assessment and management.

Patient Assessment and History

Assessment begins by first determining the patient's knowledge base of the classification of his or her cancer and the symptoms and course of the disease. This is the first step in gathering a history from the client. The information gathered provides a framework for patient education. The history should also include the patient's past medical history; previous organ impairment; or any secondary diagnosis that might influence the toxicities, side effects, and treatment modalities. A record of the total chemotherapeutic agents administered, doses, and any radiation (number of rads) is necessary to complete a cancer history (Table 14–1).

Physical assessment includes the patient's laboratory and diagnostic imaging studies, nutritional status, and psychosocial and spiritual states. Appropriate nursing interventions are based on a complete history and physical assessment.

Treatment Objectives

The role of the clinician also includes an understanding of treatment goals and their rationale. The treatment goal of chemotherapy depends on the situation. Chemotherapy can be **curative** when given as primary treatment. The therapeutic goal is also curative when chemotherapy is given as an adjuvant for surgery or other treatment modalities. Knowledge of the chemotherapy treatment, long- and short-term side effects, symptom management, and lifestyle effects are important because two out of three cancer patients are candidates for chemotherapy at some point in their disease process.

Chemotherapy can also be given to control the disease when cure is not realistic. The goal of **palliative** treatment is symptom management. Chemotherapy can decrease pain caused by a tumor by relieving pressure on nerves, decreasing lymphatic congestion, and relieving organ obstruction (Vandergrift, 2001).

There are few absolute rules related to antineoplastic therapy; however, there are certain basic considerations in chemotherapy treatment:

> Table 14–1 **ONCOLOGY PATIENT ASSESSMENT**

- Interview
  - Cancer history
  - Knowledge of classification of cancer
  - Symptoms
  - Course of disease
  - Past medical history
  - Previous organ impairment
  - Secondary diagnosis
- Physical assessment
- Nutritional status
- Laboratory tests
- Diagnostic imaging studies:
  - Computed tomography
  - Magnetic resonance imaging
  - Radiography
- Psychological state
- Spiritual state

1. The smaller the tumor burden, the easier the patient is to treat.
2. Surgical debulking decreases the tumor burden and recruits resting malignant cells to start dividing, thereby increasing the sensitivity to chemotherapy.
3. The higher the chemotherapy dose, the better the chance for a tumor response.
4. Doses of chemotherapeutic agents are altered based on the degree of toxicity that the patient experiences.
5. The therapeutic margin is the difference between the dose producing the desired benefit and the dose resulting in unacceptable toxicity.
6. The therapeutic margin of antineoplastic agents is narrow compared with that of other types of drugs.

Websites

Oncology Nursing Society (ONS): *www.ons.org*
CancerNet: *www.cancernet.nci.nih.gov*
Cancer Treatment Centers of America: *www.cancercenter.com/home*
Oncology Online Journals: *www.cancerlink.s.usa.com/professional/ journal*
American Cancer Society: *www.cancer.org*
Harvard Center for Cancer Prevention: *www.hsph.harvard.edu/organizations/canprevent/index.html*
National Cancer Institute's CancerNet Cancer Information: *http://cancernet.nci.nih.gov*
American Society of Clinical Oncology: *www.asco.org*

Other sites:

Guidelines for Handling Hazardous Drugs (HDs)

When hazardous drugs (HDs) are used in the workplace, sound practice dictates that a written Hazardous Drug Safety and Health Plan be developed to protect employees from health hazards associated with HDs. The American Society of Hospital Pharmacists (ASHP) has defined hazardous drugs. Hazardous drugs include antineoplastic agents and non-antineoplastic hazardous drugs that have four drug characteristics: (1) genotoxicity; (2) carcinogenicity, (3) teratogenicity or fertility impairment, and (4) serious organ or other toxic manifestation at low doses.

The ASHP recommends that the Hazardous Drug Safety and Health Plan be reviewed and its effectiveness reevaluated at least annually and updated as necessary. The ASHP, along with OSHA, recommends that specific consideration of the following provisions be included:

1. Establishment of a designated HD handling area
2. Use of containment devices such as biological safety cabinets
3. Procedures for safe removal of contaminated waste
4. Decontamination procedures (OSHA, 1999)

NURSING FAST FACT!

For further information on Controlling Occupational Exposure to Hazardous Drugs go to the U.S. Department of Labor Occupational Safety and Health Administration Web site: www.osha.gov/Technical Links. OSHA Technical Manual Section VI: Chapter 2.

Cellular Kinetics

Cellular kinetics is the study of mechanisms and rates of cellular changes. This study is becoming increasingly more useful in planning treatment regimens and scheduling drug administration. Chemotherapy exerts a cytotoxic action by interfering with the reproductive cell cycle. Cancer cells are the intended target of treatment; however, **cytotoxic** action also affects normal cells.

Cell Cycle

Antineoplastic agents act primarily on proliferating cells; therefore, it is important to examine the cell cycle and the growth of normal and malignant cells to understand the rationale for and effects of drug therapy (Fig. 14–1).

Five phases complete the cell growth cycle: G_0, G_1, S, G_2, and M. The letter "G" refers to gap phases or periods when cells are preparing for a more active phase of reproduction (Moran, 2000). Some cells move out of the cell cycle after **mitosis** into G_0, becoming resting and nondividing cells. Other cells enter the first phase, G_1, which is the period between mitosis and the beginning of deoxyribonucleic acid (DNA) synthesis when active ribonucleic acid (RNA) and protein synthesis occurs.

The G_1 phase is the most variable of all phases, and its length influences the rate of cell proliferation. The G_1 phase is called the first growth phase, and it is characterized by the production of RNA, enzymes, and proteins, all of which are essential in later cycles. Whereas cells that are growing slowly have many cells in the G_1 phase, cells that are growing rapidly have few cells in the G_1 phase.

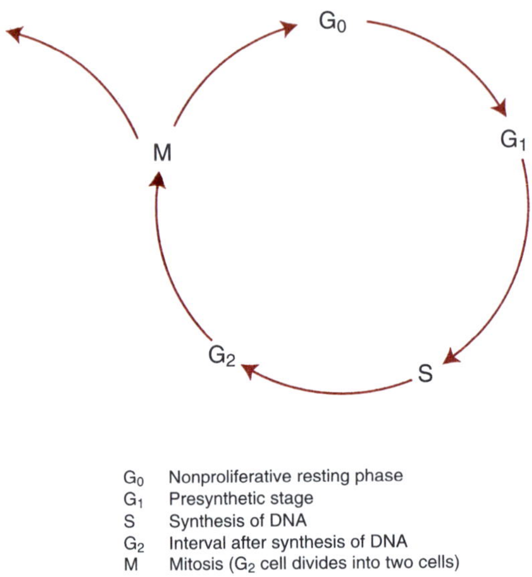

Figure 14–1 ■ Cell cycle.

The cells then emerge from the G_1 phase and enter the S phase, in which enzymes necessary for DNA synthesis increase in activity. Called the synthesis phase, the predominant event in this phase is the creation of DNA, the genetic code of all information needed for cell life. At the end of the S phase, the cell contains twice the original amount of DNA in preparation for the creation of new daughter cells. The duration of this phase ranges from 10 to 20 hours (Moran, 2000).

After the S phase, a resting period called G_2 occurs. During this phase, the RNA and protein necessary for mitosis are synthesized. This phase extends from the end of DNA synthesis to the beginning of mitosis.

The last phase of the cell cycle is the M phase, in which mitosis takes place. This is a brief phase, lasting only about 1 half hour to 1 hour, in which cell division occurs. The formation of the spindle, separation of chromosomes, and the division of the cell into two cells occur, creating a new daughter cell. After mitosis, the cell may resume the cycle at G_1 or move into a dormant state in G_0.

The phases of the cell cycle are correlated to the efficacy of the antineoplastic agents for specific types of cancer. Most agents kill only cells that are actively reproducing, leaving relatively unaffected the cells that are in the G_0 or resting phase. If a tumor mass consists of a large percentage of cells in G_0 at the time of chemotherapy exposure, there will be much less cell kill than would occur in a tumor with a high percentage of cells actively reproducing. The concept of cells in cycle versus resting is essential to understanding tumor growth patterns, or tumor kinetics (Moran, 2000; Oncology Nursing Society, 2001).

Tumor Kinetics

In both normal and malignant tissues, three different cell populations affect growth: cycling cells, nondividing cells, and resting cells called G_0 cells. The cells that are dividing continuously are the *cycling cells.* The group of cells that divide for a time and then complete their life cycle without dividing again are called *nondividing cells.* The third group is made up of G_0, or resting cells, which leave the cell cycle and remain dormant until conditions stimulate them to reenter the cell cycle and divide. Cycling cells and G_0, or resting cells, are further divided into **stem cells** and nonstem cells. Stem cells replenish the stem cell pool, and **nonstem cells** differentiate and enter the maturing groups of cells. As long as G_0 stem cells remain, a damaged cell population can be renewed.

Growth Fraction

Four interrelated factors must be considered during the assessment of normal or tumor cells: the cell cycle time, growth fraction, total number of cells in the population, and rate of cell loss (Skeel & Khleif, 2003). The first factor, the cell cycle time, is the amount of time required for the cell to move from one mitosis to the next. Second, the growth fraction is the percentage of cycling cells in the entire cell population. The third factor is the total number of cells in the population determined at some point in time, which indicates how advanced the cancer is and provides a basis for growth measurement. As the total number of cells increases, so does the number of resistant cells. The fourth factor is the rate of cell loss or the number of cells that die or leave the cell population. Growth depends on the number of cells produced and the number of cells that die. Rate of growth depends on the cell cycle time, the growth fraction, and the rate of cell loss.

Doubling Time

In tumor growth, there is a theory that as the tissue mass increases in size, the doubling time slows. Another factor that affects tumor growth is the decrease in nutrients available for each cell as the total mass increases and blood supply is outgrown. It has been found that some normal cells cycle faster than tumor cells in human beings. Overall, tumor cell cycling times range from 24 to 120 hours. The doubling time of most tumor cells ranges from 5 days to 2 years, with a mean of 1 to 3 months (Moran, 2000). This longer doubling time is caused by several factors. First, the growth fraction of human tumors varies from 0 to 100 percent. Second, many tumor cells die spontaneously. Spontaneous death occurs from inadequate nutrition, cumulative genetic damage in tumor cells, and cell differentiation into nondividing cells.

Cell Kill Hypothesis

The goal of modern chemotherapy is to prevent cancer cells from multiplying, invading, metastasizing, and ultimately killing the host (Skeel & Khleif, 2003). Most active cytotoxic agents are selectively toxic to rapidly proliferating cells; many G_0 or resting cells remain untouched. Resting stem cells can regenerate the tumor cell population. When the tumor mass increases in size, the cell cycle proceeds at a slower rate; therefore, the growth fraction decreases and the cytotoxic effects of the drug diminish. The drugs are not only specific to cancer cells but are also toxic to normal proliferating cells. Normal cells most affected by chemotherapeutic drugs include hematopoietic or bone marrow cells, gastrointestinal (GI) epithelial cells, hair follicle cells, germinal cells, and embryonic cells.

The ability of antineoplastic agents to kill tumor cells comes from research showing that these drugs kill tumor cells according to first-order kinetics. Certain drug doses destroy a constant fraction of tumor cells in the body, rather than a constant number of cells. Also, these drugs follow an exponential, or "log-kill," model. Therefore, cell kill may be expressed as a log-kill of 2, meaning that the body's tumor burdens decreased from 108 to 106 cells (from 100,000,000 to 1,000,000). The maximum cell kill from a single drug dose has been found to be 2 to 5 logs. Treatment must be repeated many times to decrease the number of tumor cells in the body. Because a single dose always kills a fraction of the tumor cells, this hypothesis suggests that chemotherapy can never destroy all malignant cells in the body (Skeel & Khleif, 2003).

The second hypothesis proposes that cell kill caused by antineoplastic drugs is related to the relative growth fraction of the tumor at the time of treatment. Thus, the greatest tumor cell kill occurs when the growth fraction is greatest. The growth fraction is greatest when tumors are of intermediate size; the growth fraction is less when they are very small or very large (ONS, 2001).

The biologic control of normal cells and tumor growth at the modular level has not yet led to improved therapy for patients with cancer; however, it has helped to explain differences in response among populations of patients. Further work in this area may provide a powerful selective means of controlling neoplastic cell growth and lead to effective cancer treatment in the next decade. This is discussed further under Biologic Control Modifiers.

Drug Resistance

Resistance to antineoplastic therapy is a combined characteristic whereby the drug is ineffective in controlling the tumor. Cell resistance to antineoplastic drugs can be natural or acquired (Brown, 2001). Natural resistance results from the initial unresponsiveness of a tumor to a given drug. Acquired resistance is the unresponsiveness that emerges after initially successful treatment (Skeel, 2003).

Factors that influence resistance include the specific drug, number of exposures to the drug, tumor, and the specific host. The first dose of a drug may be effective in treating tumor cells, but administering successive doses at times decreases its efficacy. Many malignant cells develop drug resistance. There appears to be a similarity between cancer cell resistance to drugs and bacterial resistance to antibiotics. Thus, similar approaches such as large initial doses, combination drugs, alternating combinations of drugs, and earliest possible treatment of disease are used to overcome resistance and eventual tumor recurrence (ONS, 2001).

CULTURAL AND ETHNIC CONSIDERATIONS: CANCER 14–1

Because of accumulated genetic damage caused by the Chernobyl nuclear power plant accident, Russians have a 250 percent higher rate of certain cancers than Americans (Giger & Davidhizar, 2004).

Antineoplastic Agents

The goal of antineoplastic therapy is total cell kill by means of selective toxicity. Several principles make this goal difficult to achieve. First, the presence of a single malignant cell may yield sufficient daughter cells to kill the human host. The second factor is the negligible contribution of host immune mechanisms and defenses in augmenting therapy. Administering **chemotherapy** in combination or sequences is a way of dealing with the residual body burden of tumor cells. Other methods include reductive, adjuvant, and intermittent therapy.

Classifications

Antineoplastic agents are classified according to the cell life cycle. This classification has two categories: (1) cell cycle phase–specific (CCS) agents and (2) cell cycle phase–nonspecific (CCNS) agents.

Cell cycle–specific agents kill cells that are actively in cycle, anywhere from G_1 through M. This category is divided into groups that affect specific phases of the cell cycle (Table 14–2). The key to CCS agents lies in tim-

> Table 14–2 **CELL CYCLE PHASE-SPECIFIC AGENTS**

Phase	Agents
G_1	L-Asparaginase, prednisone
S	Cytarabine, 5-fluorouracil (5-FU), hydroxyurea, methotrexate, thioguaine, floxuridine, topotecan, irinotecan
G_2	Bleomycin, etoposide
M	Vinblastine, vincristine, vindesine, paclitaxel

ing. Many CCS regimens employ small divided doses given at repeated intervals or by continuous infusion in an attempt to expose cells during a vulnerable phase. These regimens exploit the fact that 20 percent of reproducing cells are in the S phase at any give time (Moran, 2000).

Agents that are CCNS do not depend on cells' being in a specific phase; rather, they are effective throughout the reproductive cycle and, to a certain extent, in the resting phase. CCNS agents disrupt DNA synthesis in a variety of ways. Cellular contents become unbalanced and the cell dies when it tries to divide. The CCNS drugs do not rely on cycle phase to be effective (Moran, 2000).

The chemical structure also provides a category by which the drugs can be classified; these are alkylating agents, antimetabolites, natural products, hormones and hormone antagonists, and biologic response modifiers.

Chemotherapeutic agents can also be classified according to their potential to cause local tissue reactions. The potential for alteration in skin and tissue integrity ranges from transient local discomfort during administration to severe tissue necrosis. Classification includes **irritants** and **vesicants** (ONS, 2001).

Combination Chemotherapy

Combination regimens are the mainstay today of cancer chemotherapy, and new combinations of old drugs continue to emerge along with the incorporation of new drugs into regimens. The decision to use multidrug regimens is based on cell biology (Moran, 2000):

1. Drugs in the regimen should have at least some cytotoxicity against the target tumor cell.
2. Preferably each drug should have a different mechanism of action to exploit different events occurring in the cell cycle.
3. Each drug should have different potential side effects from the other drugs or at least exert similar side effects at a different time. An example is the MOPP regimen for treating Hodgkin's disease: mechlorethamine, oncovin, procarbazine, and prednisone.

Reductive Therapy

Reductive therapy, also called debulking, decreases the body burden of cancer cells through chemotherapy, surgery, radiotherapy, or other therapy (Chu & DiVita, 2002).

Adjuvant Chemotherapy

Adjuvant chemotherapy is the administration of chemotherapy to destroy micrometastasis and to prevent secondary tumors after the removal or destruction of a primary tumor. This therapy is aimed at reducing residual tumor burden to levels more likely handled by the host's immunologic mechanisms.

Intermittent Therapy

The timing of chemotherapy doses can be critical. Intermittent high-dose (pulse) therapy with CCS and CCNS agents gives better therapeutic results with fewer toxic side effects than more frequent divided doses. Timing drug dose in relation to another drug can allow for cell synchronization to yield greater cell kill (Lilley & Aucker, 2004).

Chemotherapy Dosing

Dose Calculations Using Body Surface Area

Doses of antineoplastic agents used in chemotherapy are calculated according to body surface area (**BSA**). Clinical trials have provided a formula to determine the amount of each drug to be used in a particular regimen.

A nomogram chart is used to calculate the log of the height and weight. Many institutions have computers that are programmed to determine the BSA. The **oncologist** uses weight changes to determine whether an adjustment in the total dosage is necessary to avoid overdosing or underdosing the patient.

The basic formula for determining the chemotherapy dosage is:

$$\text{BSA} \times \text{mg/m}^2 = \text{total dose}$$

NURSING FAST FACT!

It is important to weigh the patient before each course of chemotherapy and it is important to note whether the BSA was determined from ideal body weight or actual weight.

Dose Calculations Using the Calvert Formula

Another formula that attempts to individualize the dose of a drug so that optimal therapeutic response is achieved without toxic effects is the Calvert formula. The formula makes it possible to individualize the drug dose to obtain a maximally effective dose with tolerable side effects (Groenwald & Goodman, 1999). This is usually part of the Carboplatin dosing procedure based on renal function.

$$\text{Carboplatin dose (mg)} = \text{Target AUC (area under the curve)} \times (\text{GFR [glomerular filtration rate]} + 25)$$

Classes of Drugs

Chemotherapeutic agents are divided into several classes. For two of the classes (e.g., alkylating agents and antimetabolites), the names indicate the mechanism of cytotoxic action. The hormonal agents refer to the physiologic type of drug. **Biologic response modifiers** mimic, stimulate, enhance, inhibit, or otherwise alter the host responses to the cancer (Skeel, 2003). Table 14–3 presents commonly prescribed antineoplastic agents and common adverse effects.

> Table 14–3 **ANTINEOPLASTIC AGENTS**

Drug Class	Common Agents	General Adverse Effects
Alkylating agents	Busulfan Carboplatin Carmustine Cisplatin Chlorambucil Cyclophosphamide Dacarbazine Ifosfamide Lomustine Melphalan Oxaliplatin Streptozocin Temozolomide Thiotepa	Pulmonary fibrosis or cardiomyopathy nephrotoxicity, peripheral neuropathy, ototoxicity **Extravasation**
Antimetabolite agents	Azacitidine Capecitabine Cytarabine Cladribine Floxuridine Fluorouracil Fludarabine Gemcitabine Mercaptopurine Methotrexate Pentostatin Thioguanine	Liver, kidney, lung, stomach and heart toxicities

(Continued on following page)

Drug Class	Common Agents	General Adverse Effects
Mitotic inhibitors		All: Hair loss, nausea, vomiting
Vinca alkaloids	Vinblastine Vincristine	Liver toxicities, bone marrow suppression, **extravasation**
Podophyllotoxin derivatives	Etoposide Teniposide	Liver and kidney toxicities, moderate bone marrow suppression, **extravasation**
Pacific yew tree derivatives	Paclitaxel	Severe bone marrow suppression
Cytotoxic antibiotics	Bleomycin Dactinomycin Daunorubicin Doxorubicin Epirubicin Idarubicin Mitomycin Mitoxantrone Plicamycin Valrubicin	Pulmonary fibrosis, pneumonitis, liver toxicities, **extravasation**, cardiovascular toxicities
Topoisomerase-1 inhibitors	Irinotecan Topotecan	Myelosuppression, severe diarrhea during irinotecan infusion
Monoclonal antibodies	Rituximab Trastuzumab	Fever, chills, headache, infection, nausea, vomiting and diarrhea
Miscellaneous agents	Altretamine L-Asparaginase Cladribine Hydroxyurea Mitotane Hormonal agents	Hair loss, nausea, vomiting and myelosuppression. Liver and CNS toxicities Liver, kidney, lung, and CNS toxicities Hematologic toxicities CNS toxicities Genitourinary and lung toxicity
Biotherapy		
Interferons (IFNs)	Interferon-alfa-2a Interferon-alfa-2b Interferon-alfa-n3 Interferon–beta-1a Interferon–beta-1b Interferon-gamma-1b	Flulike effects, fatigue, nausea, vomiting and diarrhea. Capillary leak syndrome, CHF, chills, rash, fatigue
Interleukins (ILs)	Aldesleukin Oprelvekin	Fever, muscle aches, bone pain, and flushing. Hypertension, nausea, vomiting, diarrhea.
Colony-stimulating factors (CSFS)	Epoetin alfa Filgrastim Sargramostim	

Alkylating Agents

Alkylating agents were derived from the sulfur mustard gases used in World War I and II. These agents are a diverse group of chemical compounds capable of forming molecular bonds with nucleic acids, proteins, and many molecules of low molecular weight. The basis for their therapeutic use against cancers is the process of alkylation by which they cause interstrand and intrastrand cross-linkages in DNA, thereby blocking replication.

The alkylating agents are cell cycle–nonspecific (CCNS) because they act on cells at any phase of the cycle. Most of the agents in this group are considered polyfunctional alkylating agents because they contain more than one alkylating group. The nitrosoureas are unique under the class of alkylating agents with respect to being non–cross-resistant with other alkylating agents, being highly lipid soluble, and having delayed myelosuppressive effects. These agents can cross the blood–brain barrier (BBB).

The alkylating agents used as antineoplastic agents consist of three categories (Lilley & Aucker, 2004):

- *Classic alkylators*
  - Busulfan
  - Chlorambucil
  - Cyclophosphamide
  - Ifosfamide
  - Mechlorethamine
  - Melphalan
  - Thiotepa (triethylene thiophosphoramide)
- *Alkylator-like agents*
  - Carboplatin
  - Cisplatin
  - Dacarbazine
  - Procarbazine
- *Nitrosoureas*
  - Carmustine
  - Lomustine
  - Streptozocin

Alkylating agents can cause serious adverse reactions. Major side effects include toxicities to the hematopoietic, GI, and reproductive systems. In addition, all alkylating agents can be carcinogenic.

NURSING FAST FACT!

These agents as a class share common side effects of alopecia, bone marrow depression, nausea and vomiting, and diarrhea.

Antimetabolites

The antimetabolites are a group of low molecular weight compounds that exert their effect because of similarity to naturally occurring metabolites involved in nucleic acid synthesis. This class includes the folic acid antagonists, pyrimidine antagonists, purine antagonists, and immunosuppressant azathioprine (Imuran).

They are structurally similar to vitamins, coenzymes, or normal cell products needed for growth and division of both normal and neoplastic

Nursing Points-of-Care: Alkylating Agents

1. Monitor I.V. sites for infiltration; many alkylating agents cause tissue necrosis with infiltration.
2. Monitor complete blood count (CBC) and platelets and liver enzymes.
3. Administer antiemetic agents, pretreatment.
4. Assess respiratory status and blood pressure with cyclophosphamide and carmustine; monitor for hypotension with busulfan melphalan.
5. Prehydrate for cisplatin.
6. Assess oral cavity for stomatitis.

cells. They interfere with the metabolic pathways of dividing cells and exert their greatest effect in the S-phase of the cell cycle. A drug-induced blockage of DNA synthesis occurs when the antimetabolic agent, rather than the necessary nutrient or enzyme, is taken into the cell. This is the major cause of cell death from antimetabolite therapy (Lilley & Aucker, 2004).

Folic Acid Analogs

Folic acid and its derivatives are critical for the metabolism of proliferating cells. These drugs are potentially nephrotoxic. Methotrexate is an example of a folic acid analog and is nephrotoxic. Side effects include pancytopenia, GI toxicity, skin rash, headache, hepatotoxicity, and pulmonary toxic effects. Methotrexate is used as an immunosuppressive agent to prevent graft-versus-host disease after bone marrow transplantation.

Pyrimidine Analogs

These agents inhibit critical enzymes necessary for nucleic acid synthesis and may become incorporated into the DNA and RNA. Common side effects with pyrimidine agents include GI disturbances, cardiac toxicity, and ataxia. Pyrimidine agents include the following:

- Cytarabine (ARA-C)
- Floxuridine (FUDR)
- Fluorouracil (5-FU)

Purine Analogs

Purine agents interfere with normal purine interconversions and thus with DNA and RNA synthesis. These agents can cause bone marrow suppression, hyperuricemia, and acute hepatic toxicity. They include the following:

- Fludarabine (F-AMP)
- Mercaptopurine (6-MP)
- Thioguanine (6-TG)

NURSING FAST FACT!

Common side effects of antimetabolites are myelosuppression and GI disturbances. Other side effects are stomatitis, esophagitis, elevation in liver function test results, photosensitivity, and severe nausea and vomiting.

Nursing Points-of-Care: Antimetabolite Agents

1. Assess oral mucosa for stomatitis.
2. Monitor complete blood count (CBC), platelets, and liver and renal function.
3. Stop drug if white blood cell (WBC) count drops below 3000/μL.
4. Administer antiemetics, especially with cytarabine and mercaptopurine.
5. High-dose methotrexate requires leucovorin rescue.

Mitotic Inhibitors

The natural products (mitotic inhibitors) include vinca alkaloids, antibiotics, and enzymes. Their modes of action differ significantly. These products are unlike the alkylating and antimetabolite agents, which are classified by their modes of action. Natural products are classified together because their sources are naturally occurring. Although they are classified together, their modes of action differ significantly (Lilley & Aucker, 2004)

VINCA ALKALOIDS

The vinca alkaloids (i.e., vinblastine, vincristine, and vinorelbine) are derivatives of the plant vinca rosea (periwinkle). These agents are CCS, active only when the cell is in the mitotic (M) phase of division. Vinca alkaloids interfere with the microtubule assembly in the mitotic spindle formation (Lilley & Aucker, 2004).

PODOPHYLLOTOXIN DERIVATIVES

The podophyllotoxin derivative (etoposide and teniposide) exert their cytotoxic effects by damaging DNA and thereby inhibiting or altering DNA synthesis. These agents are considered cell-cycle specific (CCS).

YEW TREE

The Pacific yew tree derivative (paclitaxel) works in the late G2-phase and the M-phase of the cell cycle. It is therefore a CCS agent and works by causing the formation of a nonfunctional microtubule (Lilley & Aucker, 2004).

NURSING FAST FACT!

Adverse effects common with use of the plant alkaloids are numbness and tingling of the extremities, loss of deep tendon reflexes, and ataxia. Vinca alkaloids are vesicants and can produce tissue necrosis if I.V. infiltration occurs.

Nursing Points-of-Care: Plant Alkaloid Agents

1. Administer antiemetics 30 to 60 minutes before chemotherapy.
2. Premedication often includes dexamethasone, diphenhydramine, cimetidine, or ranitidine.
3. Monitor vital signs during the first hour.
4. Monitor infusion site for infiltration.
5. Use of 0.22-micron filter is recommended.
6. Do not use PVC bags or sets. Use only glass bottles, polypropylene, polyolefin bags for administration of medication.

Cytotoxic Antibiotics

Cytotoxic antibiotics consist of natural antibiotics produced by the mold *Streptomyces* as well as two synthetic cytotoxic antibiotics not produced by this mold. These antibiotics are used only for treatment of cancer because they are too toxic for the treatment of infections (Lilley & Aucker, 2004).

ANTHRACYCLINE ANTIBIOTICS

Anthracycline agents are derived from fermented products of different *Streptomyces* spp. They are called anthracyclines because the anthracycline portion of their molecules produces the antineoplastic effect. These drugs act by reacting with DNA to form complexes that block DNA-directed RNA and DNA transcription. Current evidence suggests that both drugs are probably effective during all phases of the cell cycle and are therefore CCNS agents.

OTHER CYTOTOXIC ANTIBIOTICS

Other antibiotics are CCS that have their action on the G2 and mitosis phases of the cell cycle. These antibiotics are useful in treating patients with a variety of cancers. These agents are often used in combination with other antineoplastic agents.

Other cytotoxic antibiotics include:

- Bleomycin
- Dactinomycin
- Pentostatin
- Plicamycin
- Mitomycin
- Mitoxantrone hydrochloride

NURSING FAST FACTS!

- *The major side effects of cytotoxic antibiotics are leukopenia, thrombocytopenia, cardiac toxicity, arrhythmias, cardiomyopathy, nausea, vomiting, stomatitis, skin hyperpigmentation, hepatotoxicity, and enhancement of cyclophosphamide-induced bladder injury. Some agents in this class are vesicants. Bleomycin is pulmonary toxic (Lilley & Aucker, 2004).*
- *The drug dexrazoxane (Zinecard) can now be used with doxorubicin to protect the heart from excess cardiotoxicity.*

Nursing Points-of-Care: Cytotoxic Antibiotics

1. Assess for fever and chills.
2. Assess pulmonary status.
3. Monitor CBC prior to and throughout therapy.
4. Monitor baseline and periodic renal and hepatic function.
5. Follow guidelines for handling cytotoxic agents.
6. Prophylactic antiemetics may reduce nausea and vomiting.
7. Observe for signs of infections (Phillips & Kuhn, 1999; Gahart & Nazareno, 2004).

Topoisomerase-1 Inhibitors

A new class of chemotherapy agents isolated from the bush *Camptothecus accuminata* are the topoisomerase-1 inhibitors. These agents have shown significant activity against a broad range of tumors. The new agents are considered CCS antineoplastics. They work by inhibiting the enzyme topoisomerase-1 causing reversible single-strand DNA breaks during the S-phase of the cell cycle. The new agents include topotecan (Hycamtin) and irinotecan (CPT-11, Camptosar) (Lilley & Aucker, 2004).

NURSING FAST FACT!

The main side effect demonstrated by topotecan is suppression of blood cells produced in the bone marrow. Topotecan should not be given to patients with baseline neutrophil counts of less than 1500. Irinotecan has been associated with severe diarrhea. This type of diarrhea is called cholinergic diarrhea and may occur during irinotecan infusion (Lilley & Aucker, 2004).

Miscellaneous Agents

The miscellaneous antineoplastic agents are those that, because of their unique structure and mechanisms of action, cannot be classified into the previously described categories. This is a very diverse group of agents, which includes the following:

- Altretamine
- L-Asparaginase
- Cladribine
- Hydroxyurea
- Mitotane
- Hormonal agents

ALTRETAMINE

Altretamine (Hexalen) is a CCNS agent that is used for the palliative treatment of recurrent, persistent ovarian cancer after the completion of the first-line treatment with cisplatin or alkylating agent-based combination therapy. Side effects include liver and CNS toxicities.

L-ASPARAGINASE

The agent L-asparaginase represents a unique development in the field of cancer chemotherapy. This enzyme was first isolated from *Escherichia coli* and is used primarily in the treatment of patients with acute lymphoblastic leukemia.

Asparaginase destroys the amino acid asparagine, which is needed for protein synthesis, and thus leads to cell death. Many normal cells are not sensitive to the effects of this drug enzyme because they can synthesize their own supply of asparagine, which tumor cells cannot do. Antitumor effects of this drug are primarily in the G_1 phase of the cell cycle.

L-Asparaginase is a foreign protein, and can produce hypersensitivity and anaphylactic reactions. Fever, anorexia, nausea, and vomiting all are signs of acute toxic reaction. Elevated blood urea nitrogen (BUN) and ammonia levels can result from the enzyme action of this agent. Liver function may be impaired and can increase the toxicity of other drugs.

HYDROXYUREA

This agent acts as an antimetabolite, but it cannot be assigned to any of the previous subgroups. Hydroxyurea inhibits DNA synthesis through its action on the enzyme ribonucleotide diphosphate reductase and acts specifically in the S-phase of the cell cycle

Bone marrow depression is the major toxic effect and subsides rapidly after drug is stopped for several days. Other major side effects include GI disturbances; mild dermatologic reactions; and, rarely, stomatitis, alopecia, and neurologic manifestations.

Nursing Points-of-Care: Miscellaneous Agents

1. Monitor patient closely during infusion for possible hypersensitivity reaction.
2. Premedicate with dexamethasone, diphenhydramine, and cimetidine before administering paclitaxel.
3. Assess oral mucosa.
4. Assess infusion site frequently for infiltration; avoid extravasation.
5. Monitor CBC, cardiac enzymes, and electrocardiogram (ECG).
6. Make neurologic assessment to monitor for deviation and severity of peripheral neuropathy.
7. Administer antiemetics.
8. Monitor renal function (Gahart & Nazareno, 2004).

Hormones and Hormone Antagonists

The hormones and hormone antagonists include steroidal estrogens, progestins, androgens, corticosteroids and their synthetic derivatives, nonsteroidal synthetic compounds with steroid or steroid antagonist activity hypothalamic–pituitary analogs, and thyroid hormones. Each agent has diverse effects.

ANDROGENS

Androgens exert their antineoplastic effect by altering pituitary function or directly affecting the neoplastic cells. Nausea, vomiting, anorexia, myalgia, fluid retention, libido changes, and sterilization can result from use of androgens. Synthetic substances exert little or no masculinizing effects.

CORTICOSTEROIDS

Corticosteroids can cause lysis of lymphoid tumors that are rich in specific cytoplasmic receptors and may have other indirect effects as well. Their anti-inflammatory effects help reduce the sequelae of neoplastic activity and nausea and decrease cerebral edema secondary to cranial tumor growth or radiation.

Corticosteroids can cause muscle weakness, diarrhea, nausea, increased appetite, euphoria, hyperglycemia, pancreatitis, and thrombophlebitis. Changes in body fat distribution, increased risk of infection, potassium loss, and, rarely, psychosis may also result.

ESTROGENS

Large doses of estrogens reduce available androgen in men and can alter endocrine-sensitive breast tissue in women. Side effects include headache, nausea, weight changes, thromboembolism, and feminization in men.

PROGESTINS

Progestins act directly at the level of the malignant cell receptor to promote differentiation. Side effects include edema, pulmonary embolism, breast tenderness, hyperglycemia, and increased appetite.

ESTROGEN ANTAGONISTS

Estrogen antagonists act by competing with estrogen for binding on the cytosol estrogen receptor protein in cancer cells and affect the natural growth factors.

NURSING FAST FACT!

Anorexia, nausea, vaginal discharge, bleeding, hot flashes, and a temporary drop in WBCs can result from the use of estrogen protagonist.

Biotherapy

The fourth treatment modality available to treat cancer is referred to as biotherapy (Riegger, 2001). This classification of therapy has advanced over the last 30 years with successful implementation of new therapies. The volume of agents available has increased over the last 10 years and is expected to continue. The term *biologic therapy* describes a variety of

Nursing Points-of-Care: Hormone Agents

1. Assess for mood swings and changes in psychological state.
2. Monitor blood sugar in those taking steroids.
3. Monitor blood pressure.
4. Assess males for signs of feminization with estrogens.
5. Assess for signs of phlebitis at the I.V. site.
6. Assess females for masculinizing effects with androgens.
7. Encourage low-salt diet.
8. Monitor weight (Phillips & Kuhn, 1999; Gahart & Naareno, 2004).

agents and therapeutic approaches derived from the biology of the immune system, the nature of tumor cells, and the relationship between them. Biological agents can augment, modulate, or restore the host's immune response; they can produce direct cytotoxic activity; and they can support the patient's ability to tolerate side effects of other therapy (Rigger, 2001). The goals of biologic response modifying agents are to (1) stimulate immunocompetence by active or passive means, (2) promote tumor-specific immunity, and (3) serve as an adjunct to other treatments to produce tumor regression.

No clear classification system of biotherapeutic agents exists because many are pleomorphic, having multiple immunologic activities against tumors. Early attempts to classify agents used the active and passive delineations typical of vaccines; however, these are not an accurate reflection of the activities of biologic agents used as antineoplastic therapy. Currently, clinicians group agents as (1) antitumor, (2) adoptive, (3) restorative, (4) **cytomodulatory**, and (5) gene manipulative (Rigger, 2001).

Biological Agent Categories

There are six categories of biological agents: cytokines, monoclonal antibodies, differentiation agents; cellular therapies, immunostimulants, and gene therapy (Rigger, 2001). Table 14–3 presents common biotherapy agents and adverse effects. Antitumor biotherapy uses agents that combine active and passive mechanisms to enhance or stimulate the nonspecific and specific host tumor immune responses of the individual. Antitumor biotherapeutic agents include cytokines, vaccines, and monoclonal antibodies (Lilley & Aucker, 2004).

Cytokines are a general classification of cellular proteins that are produced and secreted in response to stimuli by the immune system. Their two main functions are to regulate and differentiate cell growth and to augment cell activities. This class includes the interferons, interleukins, hematopoietic growth factors, tumor necrosis factor. More than 25 cytokines have been isolated.

Antibodies binding to tumor-associated cell surface antigens can result in the destruction of tumor cells through a number of possible mechanisms, such as activation of complement and antibody-dependent, cell-mediated cytotoxicity. These antibodies may be useful as means of targeting cytotoxic radioisotopes, toxins, or drugs to tumors. Monoclonal antibody technology has made important contributions to cancer medicine.

ADOPTIVE BIOTHERAPY

Adoptive biotherapy is based on the assumption that tumor-associated antigens exist that can elicit an autologous antitumor response in the host (patient). Clinical trials using the patient's own genetically altered tumor cells are called tumor infiltrating lymphocytes (TILs) (Lilley & Aucker, 2004).

RESTORATIVE BIOTHERAPY

Restorative biotherapy uses agents that increase the patient's immune response, especially the number of mature, functioning leukocytes. Agents that augment the patient's immune system in this manner are called immunologic stimulants or hematopoietic growth factors.

This category of agents includes natural products such as cyclosporine and tacrolimus used as immunosuppressive agents after solid organ transplantation. These agents exert a variety of immunoproliferative or immunomodulatory functions that are thought to enhance the patient's existing immune defenses. Anticancer agents classed as cytomodulatory include levamisole hydrochloride and retinoids (Lilley & Aucker, 2004).

GENE MANIPULATIVE BIOTHERAPY

Human gene therapy involves a biologic technique to insert a functioning gene into a patient's cells to reverse a defective gene or add functions to an existing cell. Gene therapy has been used investigationally to correct enzyme deficiencies or augment intrinsic antitumor immune responses. This technology is not yet able to remove dysfunctional genes or limit the overproduction of biologic substances (Lilley & Aucker, 2004).

TOXICITIES OF BIOLOGIC RESPONSE THERAPY

The toxicities of biologic agents are related to doses and schedules. Administration of interferons on a daily basis is associated with systemic symptoms, fever, fatigue, and myalgia. The toxicities associated with

Nursing Points-of-Care: Biotherapy

1. Assess emotional status, depression is common.
2. Assess for flu-like symptoms.
3. Assess CBC, electrolytes, and liver function before initiating therapy.
4. Assess for presence of infection.
5. Assess cardiac and pulmonary function.

interleukin-2 (IL-2) are dose dependent and involve significant cardiovascular complications, including hypotension and the development of capillary leak syndrome. Also, with IL-2, some patients develop an erythematous rash that may progress to **desquamation** (Lilley & Aucker, 2004).

Common Side Effects of Chemotherapy

Common side effects associated with chemotherapy include short-term complications, acute side effects, and toxicities (Table 14–4).

> **INS Standard.** Because of the high level of toxicity associated with the administration of antineoplastic agents, a physician or reg-

> Table 14–4 **COMMON SIDE EFFECTS OF CHEMOTHERAPY**

- Short-Term Complications
  - Venous fragility
  - Alopecia
  - Diarrhea
  - Altered nutritional status
  - Anorexia or taste alteration
  - Fatigue
- Acute Side Effects
  - Hypersensitivity or anaphylaxis
  - Extravasation
  - Stomatitis and mucositis
  - Nausea and vomiting
  - Myelosuppression
  - Toxicities
    - Cardiac
    - Neurologic
    - Renal
    - Pulmonary

istered nurse who administers these agents and monitors the patients receiving these therapies must possess specialized knowledge and skills. (INS, 2000, 70)

Short-Term Complications

Venous Fragility

Fragile veins are present in elderly, poorly nourished, and debilitated patients. However, all patients receiving cytotoxic agents have an increased risk of vein fragility. If a patient has fragile veins, the nurse should attempt to cannulate the vein without the use of a tourniquet.

It is imperative that patients receiving chemotherapy and radiation therapy be assessed carefully before a cannula is placed, they are at a higher risk for developing irritation from antineoplastic drugs. They may have thrombocytopenia and therefore depression of platelet production, which increases vascular fragility (Smith & Stutz, 2003). Patients receiving corticosteroid therapy have increased vascular fragility, and bleeding and bruising can occur around their I.V. sites.

Alopecia

The hair follicles are a group of rapidly dividing normal cells that are affected by the action of some chemotherapeutic drugs. Chemotherapy-induced hair loss (**alopecia**) is reported to occur by two mechanisms, depending on the drug and dosage received. Atrophy of the hair bulb occurs from drug insult, and the hair falls out spontaneously or in response to a mechanical action such as combing. If the insult is minimal, a marked constriction of the hair shaft occurs, and the hair breaks off (ONS, 2001).

Nursing Points-of-Care: Alopecia

1. Provide information about hair loss.
2. Provide information about hair and scalp care.
3. Provide information about obtaining a wig if the patient desires. Some sources recommend that patients purchase a wig after therapy because of weight loss and the possibility of poor fit if purchased before therapy.
4. Recommend keeping hair cut short because it is easier to manage.
5. Protect the scalp from sun and cold (ONS, 2001).

Hair loss, if it occurs, from chemotherapy, often occurs 2 to 3 weeks after chemotherapy, is usually temporary, and hair growth returns in about 1 to 2 months after treatment is completed. The new hair may have a different texture or color than its pretreatment characteristics (Tipton, 2003).

Patient education should include information about the loss of body hair in addition to the loss of scalp hair.

Diarrhea

Diarrhea and abdominal cramping most often result from use of antimetabolites. There are many possible causes of diarrhea, such as *Clostridium difficile* infection, other intestinal infections, inflammatory bowel disease, malabsorption syndrome, cancer-related treatments of chemotherapy, and radiation and biologic therapy (Vandegrift, 2001; Yarbro, 2001). Diarrhea can lead to discomfort, severe electrolyte abnormalities, altered social life, and poor quality of life.

The treatment of patients with diarrhea is often symptomatic and may require no alteration in cancer therapy. Diarrhea can be a dose-limiting factor with 5-fluorouracil (5-FU), irinotecan. Agents that decrease bowel motility should not be used for longer than 24 hours unless significant infections have been excluded. Medications commonly used to treat patients with diarrhea are loperamide hydrochloride and diphenoxylate hydrochloride with atropine sulfate.

Nursing Points-of-Care: Diarrhea

1. Educate patients on the importance of early intervention to avoid complications related to diarrhea.
2. Increase fluid intake
3. Tell patients to increase intake of constipating foods such as cheese and eggs; use caution with dairy products; and eat food high in pectin, bulk, and fiber to help slow down peristalsis.
4. Educate patients to avoid spicy, fatty, and greasy foods. Other items to avoid ingesting include raw fruits and vegetables, nuts, caffeine, seeds, popcorn, and alcohol.
5. Establish a baseline history of usual elimination patterns.

Constipation

Managing the constipation of patients with cancer is not the same as that for medical surgical patients. Enemas should be used with caution in myelosuppressed patients that can result in additional complications. In patients with low platelet counts, bleeding can occur; in patients with neutropenia, infection can result.

There are many causes of constipation; along with specific chemotherapeutic agents, narcotics, dietary and fluid deficiencies, decrease in activity, and tumor involvement can result in intrinsic or extrinsic compression. Interventions depend on the underlying cause.

Patients taking narcotics and those receiving vincristine or vinblastine require aggressive bowel regimens.

Nursing Points-of-Care: Constipation

1. Unless contraindicated, the patient should drink 2 to 3 L of fluids per day.
2. Advise the patient to avoid foods known to be constipating (e.g., cheeses, eggs, refined starches, chocolate, candy).
3. Advise the patient to eat a diet high in fiber.
4. Encourage the patient to respond to the urge to defecate immediately and not wait.
5. Use stool softeners, laxatives, cathartics, and lubricants when appropriate; bulk laxatives keep the stool soft and have been found to be gentle (Tipton, 2003). Senna appears to be the safest natural stimulant (Wilkes, Ingwersen, & Barton-Burke, 2003).

Altered Nutritional Status

Malnutrition is reported to occur in 50 to 80 percent of patients with advanced disease. Nutritional management of patients with cancer involves early intervention using a supportive healthcare team. Patients with cancer often experience progressive loss of appetite. This side effect can be a result of therapy or a direct effect of the cancer. Malnutrition can result in a poorer response to therapy, an increased incidence of infections, and an overall worsening of the patient's well being (Tipton, 2003).

Anorexia and Alteration in Taste

Many treatments that patients receive result in taste alterations. Familiar foods may taste different when the gustatory sense is impaired. Patients receiving cisplatin, cyclophosphamide, or vincristine frequently complain that nothing tastes right. Some patients experience a bitter or metallic taste.

Fatigue

Fatigue is the most common and distressing symptom associated with cancer and its therapies (ONS 2001).

Nursing Points-of-Care: Altered Nutritional Status

1. Nutritional assessment: Diet history, nutritional intake, anthropometric measurements, laboratory tests for anemia and serum albumin.
2. Nutritional intervention: Diet, symptomatic treatment of nausea and vomiting, stomatitis and other GI effects of chemotherapy, and supplemental nutrition, which can include creative high-protein and calorie supplements, enteral nutrition, or total parenteral nutrition.
3. Pharmacologic interventions: Pharmacologic appetite stimulation promotes increased weight gain in some patients and decreased rate of weight loss in others. Agents that are in use include megestrol acetate 80 mg four times per day, Dronobinol 2.5 mg before meals or at bedtime (Wilkes, Ingwersen, & Barton-Burke, 2003).

Acute Reactions

Hypersensitivity and Anaphylaxis

Some chemotherapeutic agents have a potential for causing hypersensitivity with or without an anaphylactic response. Nurses should be knowl-

Nursing Points-of-Care: Anorexia and Alterations in Taste

1. Administer antiemetics before meals.
2. Serve foods on glass dishes.
3. Use plastic utensils rather than metal.
4. Use good oral hygiene before meals.
5. Arrange foods attractively on the plate.
6. Provide pleasant, relaxed environment for eating meals.
7. Use pleasant odors, such as cloves and cinnamon.
8. Avoid noxious cooking odors.
9. Serve cold rather than hot foods.
10. Provide small, frequent meals, get help with meal preparation.
11. Add salt or sugar to foods to increase palatability (Vandegrift, 2001).

Nursing Points-of-Care: Fatigue

1. Encourage patient to eat small meals and snacks throughout the day.
2. Encourage patient to take short walks and exercise lightly.
3. Encourage patient to keep a diary of fatigue symptoms, including when they are least and most tolerable.
4. Have patient plan activities to coincide with times when energy level is highest.
5. Have patient take short naps or breaks between activities.
6. Some patients might benefit from antidepressants, antianxiety medications, or psychological counseling.

edgeable about chemotherapy and which agents are prone to evoke hypersensitivity. An allergy history should be documented.

The following are agents for which hypersensitivity reactions may occur:

- Mechlorethamine (topical)
- Melphalan (I.V.)
- Anthracycline antibiotics
- L-Asparaginase
- Bleomycin
- Cisplatin/carboplatin
- Mechlorethamine (topical)
- Melphalan (I.V.)
- Paclitaxel/Taxotere
- Procarbazine
- Teniposide

If a drug is known to cause hypersensitivity reactions, a test dose should be considered. A patient also can be premedicated prophylactically with corticosteroids, histamine antagonists, or both to prevent reactions. Emergency equipment should be immediately accessible, including oxygen, AMBU respiratory assist bag, intubation equipment, and medications (e.g., epinephrine, 1:10,000 solution; diphenhydramine [Benadryl] 25 to 50 mg; methylprednisolone [Solu-Medrol], 30 to 60 mg; hydrocortisone [Solu-Cortef], 100 to 500 mg; dexamethasone, 10 to 20 mg; aminophylline; and dopamine) (Tipton, 2003) (ONS 2001).

Extravasation

Extravasation of a vesicant agent is a major complication of antineoplastic drug administration. As the vesicant escapes the vein, the patient may experience a burning sensation at the insertion site, redness, or swelling. In the days to weeks that follow, the site may become reddened, firm, and necrotic, leading to infection, prolonged illness, and functional as well as cosmetic problems (ONS, 2001; Tipton, 2003). Irritant drugs cause inflammation or pain at the site of insertion.

Commonly used vesicant agents include:

- Plicamycin (Mithramycin, Mithracin)
- Mechlorethamine (nitrogen mustard)
- Dactinomycin (Actinomycin D)
- Daunorubicin (Daunomycin)
- Doxorubicin (Adriamycin)
- Idarubicin (Idamycin)
- Plicamycin (Mithramycin, Mithracin)
- Mitomycin (Mutamycin)
- Mitoxantrone (Novantrone)
- Vinblastine (Velban)
- Vincristine (Oncovin)
- Vindesine (Eldisine)
- Vinorelbine (Navelbine)

Irritant agents include:

- Carmustine (BCNU)
- Cisplatinum
- Carboplatin
- Dacarbazine (DTIC)
- Etoposide (VP-16)
- Ifosfamide
- Paclitaxel (Taxol)
- Teniposide (VM-26)

Large extravasations of concentrated solutions of cisplatin and Taxol may be considered vesicants (ONS 2001).

> **INS Standard.** Decreasing extravasation and associated complications requires technical expertise in cannula placement and immediate recognition of drug extravasation. (INS, 2000, 70)

The management of patients with extravasated vesicants is controversial, with disagreements in the literature on antidotes. Table 14–5 provides the general procedure for patients with suspected extravasation.

NURSING FAST FACT!

The most effective management of extravasation is prevention.

> Table 14–5 **GENERAL PROCEDURE FOR EXTRAVASATION**

1. Stop administration of chemotherapeutic agent.
2. Leave needle in place and immobilize the extremity.
3. Aspirate any residual drug left in the tubing, the needle, or the suspected extravasation site; infiltrate the antidote, if ordered.
4. Remove the needle.
5. Avoid applying pressure to the extravasation site.
6. Inject appropriate antidote drug for the specific chemotherapy drug that extravasated.
7. Photograph the suspected area.
8. Apply warm or cold compresses as indicated.
9. Elevate the arm.
10. Notify the physician.
11. Document the condition of site and treatment of extravasation thoroughly.

A complaint of pain or burning should be considered a symptom of extravasation until proven otherwise. Extravasation kits with the necessary drug antidotes and supplies are helpful (Table 14–6).

INS Standards. Extravasation protocols for vesicants should be established in policies and procedures and administered when a vesicant infiltrates. (INS, 2000, 61)

After extravasation of a vesicant agent occurs, the extremity should not be used for subsequent cannula placement, and alternative interventions should be explored. (INS, 2000, 61)

Stomatitis and Mucositis

The oral mucosa is vulnerable to the effects of chemotherapy. The likelihood of developing stomatitis from a drug depends on the agent, the

> Table 14–6 **RECOMMENDED EXTRAVASATION KIT CONTENTS**

3-mL disposable syringe
5-mL disposable syringe
10-mL disposable syringe
1-mL disposable tuberculin syringe
Several disposable needles: 25-gauge; $^5/_8$ inch (need separate one for each subcutaneous injection)
Luer-Lok caps
Alcohol wipes
Cold and warm packs
Sterile surgical latex gloves
Sterile water for injection in 10-mL vial
Hyaluronidase 150 U/vial
Sodium thiosulfate (25%) for 50-mL vial
Other antidotes per protocol

Source: *Angel, 1995.*

dose, and the schedule of administration. Continuous rather than intermittent administration is more likely to cause stomatitis since there is limited time for healing (Yarbro, 1999).

Specific antineoplastic agents that may cause stomatitis include plant alkaloids (vincristine, vinblastine, etoposide), antimetabolites (methotrexate, 5-FU, cytarabine), antitumor antibiotics (doxorubicin, dactinomycin, mitoxantrone, mitomycin, bleomycin), miscellaneous agents (hydroxyurea), and biologic agents (interleukins, lymphokine-activated killer [LAK] cell therapy).

It is important to implement good oral hygiene before initiating chemotherapy. The primary goal is prevention; however, when oral complications develop, the focus of care should be treatment of symptoms and continued good oral care. Predisposing factors for stomatitis include poor oral hygiene, poor nutritional status, alcohol and tobacco use, head and neck radiation, concurrent corticosteroid therapy, and high doses of chemotherapy (Vandegrift, 2001).

NURSING FAST FACT!

Commercial mouthwashes and lemon glycerin swabs are not recommended for use because of their irritating and drying effects (Tipton, 2003).

Nursing Points-of-Care: Mouth Care

1. Examine mouth at least once daily and report changes.
2. Keep mouth clean and moist
3. Gently massage gums, tongue, and top of mouth with soft toothbrush or oral sponge.
4. Do not floss when platelet count is low (less than 50,000).
5. Keep dentures in only during meals.
6. Keep lips and inside of mouth coated with water-based mouth moisturizer.
7. If mouth is dry, drink water and other fluids frequently.
8. Chew sugarless gum or suck on sugarless hard candy.
9. Avoid irritating foods, alcohol, and tobacco.
10. Use benzocaine or Xylocaine before meals for anesthetic effects. Take pain medication 1.5 to 2 hours before meals.
11. Encourage a well-balanced diet with plenty of protein (ONS 2001).

Nausea and Vomiting

Over the past 10 years, there have been many improvements in the prevention and control of nausea and vomiting in patients undergoing chemotherapy. Nausea and vomiting are major complications of chemotherapy administration. For many patients, nausea and vomiting are the most distressing symptoms that interfere with their quality of life. Studies have shown that approximately 50 percent of all cancer patients receiving chemotherapy experience nausea and vomiting. Uncontrolled nausea and vomiting can lead to severe fatigue and discomfort, fluid and electrolyte imbalances, nutritional problems, and gastroesophageal tears, and it may affect patient compliance with therapy.

Young female patients with a history of motion or morning sickness are more prone to chemotherapy-induced nausea and vomiting. Previous bad experiences related to chemotherapy may stimulate anticipatory nausea and vomiting, especially in younger women. Entering the outpatient waiting room or hearing the sound of an I.V. pole may result in the patient's experiencing nausea. Multiple assessment scales have been used to measure nausea. Because of the subjective element, measurement is not always clear cut (Yarbro, 2001). The goal of therapy is to prevent the three phases of nausea and vomiting: (1) anticipatory (occurring before treatment), (2) acute (occurring the first 24 hours after treatment), and (3) delayed (occurring more than 24 hours after treatment).

Nursing Points-of-Care: Nausea and Vomiting

1. Interventions such as ingesting hard candy and sour or tart foods such as lemons are helpful in controlling nausea.
2. Avoiding fatty foods and foods with strong odor can decrease nausea and vomiting.
3. Acupressure in the form of bracelets positioned on the wrist over the acupressure point that controls nausea is a noninvasive, nontoxic intervention which may be helpful for the patient who is only slightly nauseated or who is reluctant to take antiemetics.
4. Pharmacologic interventions include administration of antiemetics such as anticholinergics, antihistamines, barbiturates, benzodiazepines, benzoquinolizines, butyrophenones, cannabinoids, phenothiazines, corticosteroids, and substituted benzamides (Table 14–7).

> Table 14–7 **ANTIEMETICS COMMONLY USED FOR THE PREVENTION AND TREATMENT OF CHEMOTHERAPY-INDUCED NAUSEA AND VOMITING**

Agent	Route	Dosage (Adult)	Comments
		Phenothiazines	
Prochlorperazine (Compazine)	PO I.V. IM PR	PO/I.V. (slow): 10 mg q 4–6 h IM: 15–30 mg q 12 h PR: 2–10 mg q 8–12 h	Some extrapyramidal reactions; potential for severe postural hypotension when the agent is given I.V.; closely observe the patient and assist when he or she is getting out of bed or sitting up
Thiethylperazine (Torecan)	PO PR IM	PO/PR: 10 mg q 4–6 h IM: 2 mg q 4–6 h	Some extrapyramidal reactions
Trimethobenzamide (Tigan)	PO IM PR	PO: 250 mg q 4–6 h IM/PR: 200 mg q 4–6 h	Some extrapyramidal reactions
		Butyrophenones	
Haloperidol (Haldol)	IM PO	IM/PO: 2–5 mg q 2–4 h	Some extrapyramidal reactions
Metoclopramide (Reglan)	PO I.V.	PO: 10–40 mg q 6 h I.V.: over 20 minutes 1–2 mg/kg at 2-hour intervals	Extrapyramidal reactions common, particularly at higher doses; worse in younger patients; diarrhea may occur
		Benzodiazepine	
Lorazepam (Ativan)	PO I.V.	PO: 1–2 mg q 4–6 h I.V.: 2 mg 30 min before chemotherapy; may be repeated q 4 h prn	Sedation frequent; patients advised not to drive for 24 hours after taking
		Corticosteroid	
Dexamethasone (Decadron)	PO I.V.	PO: 4–8 mg q 4 h I.V.: 4–20 mg q 4–6 h	Similar to ondansetron, for highly emetogenic therapy Potential agitation, delirium
		Serotonin (5HT3) Antagonists	
Ondansetron (Zofran)	I.V. PO	I.V.: 8–32 mg × 1 or 0. 15 mg/kg q 4 h × 3 PO: 8 mg q 8 h	For highly emetogenic therapy; may be a mild headache and mild transient transaminase elevations; lower doses effective for less emetogenic regimens

(Continued on following page)

Agent	Route	Dosage (Adult)	Comments
Granisetron (Kytril)	I.V. PO	I.V.: 10 u/kg × 1 PO: 2 mg before or 1 mg q 12 h	Similar to ondansetron, for highly emetogenic therapy
Dolasetron (Anzemet)	I.V. PO	100 mg before chemotherapy, either PO or I.V.	Similar to ondansetron
		Cannabinoid	
Dronabinol (Marinol)	PO	2.5–10.0 mg PO q 4–6 h	May be habit forming; is a controlled substance; causes sedation

Most of these antiemetics cause sedation or extrapyramidal symptoms. A new class of antiemetics that is selective for serotonin antagonist receptors, ondansetron (Zofran), Granisetron (Kytril) or Dolasetron (Anzemet), given orally or intravenously, has demonstrated its efficacy in alleviating nausea and vomiting without the undesirable side effects of extrapyramidal symptoms. Antiemetics are best used when titrated to the risk profile of the patient and the treatment.

Myelosuppression

Myelosuppression is the most common dose-limiting factor in the administration of antineoplastic therapy. All antineoplastic agents have some effect on blood counts, but certain drugs or dose escalations can result in severe myelosuppression. Patients at risk for prolonged myelosuppression include elderly patients with aplastic marrow, patients with bone marrow involvement, patients with previous radiation to the flat bones, patients heavily pretreated with chemotherapy, and patients with neoplastic infiltrates.

Neutropenia

Neutropenia (diminished number of neutrophils in the blood) predisposes patients to infection. An absolute neutrophil count (**ANC**) of 1500 to 2000/μL puts patients at a moderate risk for infection. Patients who have an ANC lower than 500/μL are at severe risk for infection. They should be started on antibiotics if any signs or symptoms of infection are present. **Leukopenia** is a drop in WBC count below 5000/μL. In patients with neutropenia, the only sign of infection may be an elevated temperature (Lynch, 2002). The risk of infection is also directly related to the rate neutropenia develops and length of time it persists (Yarbro, 1999).

NURSING FAST FACTS!

- *Antipyretic agents should be used with caution in patients with leukopenia so as not to mask infection.*
- *Place the patient in a private room with the door closed at all times. Encourage the patient to be as active as possible.*

Although major medical advances have resulted in an improved survival rate, serious infections continue to place immunocompromised patients at risk. Infection, together with neutropenia, is regarded as an emergency situation. Precautions are usually initiated when the patient's ANC is lower than 1000/μL.

The ANC can be calculated with the following formula:

$$\text{ANC} = \text{total WBC} \times (\% \text{ of segs} + \% \text{ of bands})$$

Nursing Points-of-Care: Neutropenia

1. Place "Neutropenic Precaution" sign on door.
2. Place the patient on a low microbial neutropenic diet (i.e., serve only cooked food; avoid unpeeled fresh fruits, raw vegetables, and garnishes).
3. Upon entering and leaving the patient's room, all persons must consistently and thoroughly wash hands.
4. Prohibit patient contact by staff and visitors with transmissible illness.
5. Avoid contact with persons who have recently been vaccinated with live or attenuated virus vaccines.
6. Avoid exposure to stagnant water (e.g., denture cups, soap dishes, flower vases, water pitchers, respiratory equipment, and irrigation containers); stagnant water provides medium for *Pseudomonas aeruginosa*.
7. Prohibit fresh flowers, plants, or fresh fruit baskets (soil is source of *Staphylococcus marcescens*).
8. Assess patient's oral mucosa every 12 hours for stomatitis and his or her skin for infection breakdown, lesions, and rashes.
9. Prevent rectal trauma by avoiding the use of rectal temperatures, suppositories, and enemas.
10. Assess for changes in neurologic function every 4 hours; central nervous system (CNS) changes are often the first indicators of sepsis.

(Continued on following page)

11. Avoid insertion of indwelling urinary catheters.
12. Assess the I.V. site at least once per shift for signs of phlebitis.
13. Monitor the patient's vital signs every 4 hours around the clock.
14. Use strict sterile technique when performing invasive procedures.
15. Check with physician for the possible use of growth factors (Yarbro, 1999).

Thrombocytopenia

A normal platelet count ranges from 150,000 to 450,000/μL. When the count is below 100,000/μL, there is a concern for the potential of bleeding. Values of 20,000 to 30,000/μL warrant closer watching. Presenting signs of a problem include bleeding gums, petechiae, nosebleeds, and multiple bruises. If the platelet count is lower than 20,000/μL, spontaneous frank bleeding can occur.

Thrombocytopenia places a patient at risk for CNS and GI bleeding. The use of platelet transfusions for nonbleeding patients is controversial. Some authorities recommend holding transfusions until the patient shows signs of bleeding, but others transfuse a patient when the platelet count is lower than 20,000/μL. Interventions include protecting the patient from unnecessary bleeding risks (Smith & Stutz, 2003).

Nursing Points-of-Care: Thrombocytopenia

1. Encourage shaving with an electric razor.
2. Advise the patient to avoid using tampons.
3. Advise the patient to avoid hazardous activity that may cause injury (e.g., contact sports and working with sharp instruments).
4. Avoid invasive procedures such as enemas, rectal temperatures, intramuscular or subcutaneous injections. If injections needed hold site for 5 minutes.
5. Avoid using aspirin-containing products and products with ibuprofen and indomethacin. Use caution with steroids.
6. Avoid dental flossing or use of high pressure water picks (ONS, 2001; Lynch, 2002).

If thrombocytopenia is lower than 100,000/μL, consider:

- Decreased platelet function
- Increased consumption of platelets
- Splenic pooling of platelets (Yarbro, Frogge, & Goodman, 2001)

Anemia

A patient is considered anemic if his or her hemoglobin level is lower than 8 g/dL. Anemic patients may be asymptomatic or may present with headache, dizziness, lightheadedness, shortness of breath, fatigue, pallor, hypothermia, and pale nailbeds and conjunctiva. Blood should be checked for iron deficiencies and treatments with Epogen, vitamin B_{12}, folate, or transfusions may be necessary.

Toxicities

Neurotoxicity

Neurotoxicity can be an acute or chronic encephalopathy of the CNS or a peripheral degeneration. **Peripheral neuropathy** can cause considerable sensory and motor disability. The most common agents that cause neurotoxicity are paclitaxel (Taxol), cisplatin, carboplatin, and vinca alkaloids.

Patients usually complain of numbness and tingling of the hands and feet as beginning symptoms. As toxicity increases, patients complain of muscle pain, weakness, and disturbances in depth perception. Other symptoms are decreased sensation, constipation, and paralytic ileus. The symptoms, depending on severity, may take weeks or months to resolve (ONS, 2001).

Because of the decreased sensation, a patient with neurotoxicity in his or her family must be aware of safety issues. The decrease in sensation causes concern for caution with temperature changes (e.g., hot water, heating pads, electric blankets, hot stoves, and radiators). Exposure to cold is also a concern because these patients are less likely to realize the severity of the temperature.

Cardiac Toxicity (Congestive Cardiomyopathy)

The anthracyclines, especially doxorubicin or daunorubicin, can cause cardiotoxicity. The lifetime dose of anthracyclines is 550 mg/m^2. Certain other chemotherapeutic agents, such as paclitaxel, mitoxantrone, idarubicin, cyclophosphamide, 5-FU, and 5-FU deoxyribonucleoside (FUDR), have also shown potential for cardiac toxicity. Early signs of cardiotoxicity include decrease in voltage of QRS complex and nonspecific ST- or T-wave change. The heart muscle becomes weakened, resulting in a decreased cardiac output with progression to congestive heart failure. These symptoms are difficult to diagnose. Serial ECG monitoring to detect changes in the voltage of the QRS helps to identify early signs of toxicity. A baseline multiple-gated acquisition (MUGA) scan or an echocardiogram with an ejection fraction should be done before administration of the known cardiotoxic chemotherapeutic agent and then repeat these tests periodically throughout the therapy. Toxicity can be acute or chronic (ONS, 2001).

NURSING FAST FACT!

Owing to the large number of women with breast cancer who are treated with doxorubicin as part of an adjuvant chemotherapy regimen, this group is of special concern and warrants ongoing clinical follow-up (Skeel, 2003).

Dexrazoxane (Zinecard) for injection is being used as a cardioprotective agent after administration of cumulative doses of doxorubicin. Because this drug is always given with cytotoxic drugs, patients should be monitored closely. Dextrazoxane may add to the myelosuppression caused by chemotherapeutic agents. The timing of the drug is critical and should be given 30 minutes before the doxorubicin (Chu & DeVita, 2002).

Pulmonary Toxicity

Toxicity to the pulmonary tissue damages the endothelial cells of the lung and results in pneumonitis and interstitial fibrosis. The agents that predispose patients to pulmonary toxicity are bleomycin in doses exceeding 250 U/m^2 or 400 U total dose and carmustine in total doses of 1500 mg/m^2. Other antineoplastic agents known to be responsible for pulmonary toxicity are mitomycin, methotrexate, melphalan, procarbazine, and busulfan. Some combination therapies can increase the risk of pulmonary toxicity.

Symptoms of pulmonary toxicity include dry, hacking cough; complaints of dyspnea; and crackles in the lungs on auscultation. Patients at risk for this complication include those who smoke and those with previous pulmonary conditions or who have previously received Bleomycin. The evaluation of high-risk patients involves a pulmonary function test. The chemotherapeutic drug should be discontinued at the first sign of this complication. Corticosteroids have been used in the treatment of symptomatic relief of pulmonary toxicity (Skeel, 2003).

Renal Toxicity

Renal toxicity is an elevation of the blood urea nitrogen (BUN) and creatinine levels. Agents that cause renal damage are cisplatin, methotrexate, mitomycin, carboplatin, and high-dose carmustine.

Renal toxicity is a life-threatening complication. The risk of renal compromise versus renal toxic agents that could produce a meaningful tumor response must be weighed carefully. Vigorous hydration is required before administering agents that are nephrotoxic.

Mannitol and furosemide (Lasix) may be ordered in an effort to flush the kidneys. Accurate intake and output as well as frequent weights must be recorded.

The risk of **hyperuricemia** from tumor lysis syndrome is another factor that needs to be considered when administering nephrotoxic drugs. Alkalizing the urine prevents the precipitation of uric acid crystals, and the administration of allopurinol helps to prevent their formation. Prophylactic measures begin 12 to 24 hours before chemotherapy.

Chemotherapy: Routes of Administration

Chemotherapy is administered by a variety of routes. The route chosen is an important variable in optimal drug delivery within the body, in minimizing side effects, and in maintaining the person's level of functioning. The oral route is used for drugs that are well absorbed and nonirritating to the GI tract. Table 14–8 summarizes the routes of administration for chemotherapeutic agents.

Systemic Routes

Intravenous Route

The I.V. route is the most common route of chemotherapy administration, and it has two advantages. First, the I.V. route quickly achieves a therapeutic blood level. Second, most chemotherapeutic agents are not absorbed in the GI tract, making the I.V. route more desirable. The subcutaneous and intramuscular routes, used commonly for delivery of other drugs, have limitations with anticancer drug therapy because of the chemotherapeutic drug's irritation of the tissues.

> Table 14–8 **METHODS OF DELIVERING ANTINEOPLASTIC AGENTS**

- Systemic Routes
  - I.V.
  - Indwelling silicone catheters
  - Peripherally inserted central lines
  - Implanted ports
  - Intrathecal catheters
- Regional Routes
  - Intra-arterial
  - Intraperitoneal
  - Cerebrospinal reservoirs

Intrathecal Route

Other routes are used when the delivery of a drug is required to pass the BBB. The intrathecal route allows the drugs to be given directly into the cerebrospinal fluid (CSF). Methotrexate and cytosine arabinoside are most commonly given by this route in treating patients with CNS leukemia and carcinomatosis meningitis (see Chapter 11).

Regional Routes

Some tumors respond better to direct exposure to antineoplastics. An advantage to regional delivery of chemotherapy is that they can "bathe" the affected body cavity or organ without systemically imposing toxic effects.

Intra-arterial Route

Chemotherapy administered through the intra-arterial route allows for high concentrations of antineoplastic agents to be delivered directly into tumor sites by means of arterial catheters or implanted devices. A temporary catheter is placed via percutaneous angiography for carotid, brachial, femoral, or specific limb artery for short-term therapies (from hours to 5 days). This therapy is repeated by means of a new catheter insertion each time for 3 to 6 months of therapy.

An implantable arterial port is placed subcutaneously near the tumor site over a bony surface and sutured in place; the catheter is then threaded into the tumor artery site. The Infusaid Pump (Infusaid Corporation, Norwood, MA) is the most common totally implantable drug-delivery system. The port is accessed via a noncoring needle, covered with a transparent dressing, and connected to a heparinized saline solution via an infusion pump.

Nursing Points-of-Care: Intra-arterial Infusions

1. Intra-arterial drug infusion requires astute clinical observations and interventions.
2. Percutaneous arterial catheters have the potential for restricting tissue perfusion.
3. The insertion site and the affected extremity should be observed every 2 to 4 hours.
4. Monitor vital signs.

(Continued on following page)

Nursing Points-of-Care: Intra-arterial Infusions *(Continued)*

5. Femoral catheter placement requires bedrest with log rolling to maintain catheter alignment.
6. Brachial catheter placement requires immobilizing the affected extremity.
7. All chemotherapy supplies should have Luer Lok connections, and infusion pumps may require a higher PSI (pounds per square inch) setting to overcome arterial flow resistance (ONS, 1999).

Implantable arterial ports must be flushed with heparin weekly to maintain catheter patency if a continuous infusion solution is not being administered.

Intraperitoneal Route

Intracavitary drug administration instills drugs directly into body cavities, such as the bladder, peritoneum, pleura, and pericardium. This technique is used most frequently to control malignant effusions, but it is also used for those with localized malignancies (ONS, 2001). Infusions via the **intraperitoneal** route (IP) involve the administration of therapeutic agents directly into the peritoneal cavity (Fig. 14–2).

The purpose of IP therapy is to increase the concentration of the antineoplastic agent at the tumor site (in this case, the peritoneal cavity) to

Nursing Points-of Care: Intraperitoneal Infusions

1. Follow the procedure for intraperitoneal therapy (Procedures Display 14–1).
2. Assess for complications associated with IP therapy:
   a. Pain or tenderness around the catheter or port
   b. Subcutaneous leakage
   c. Hematoma or bleeding (rare)
   d. Local infection – Fever higher than 100 degrees F, redness around catheter or port
   e. Catheter dislodgement
   f. Obstruction
   g. Colon perforation

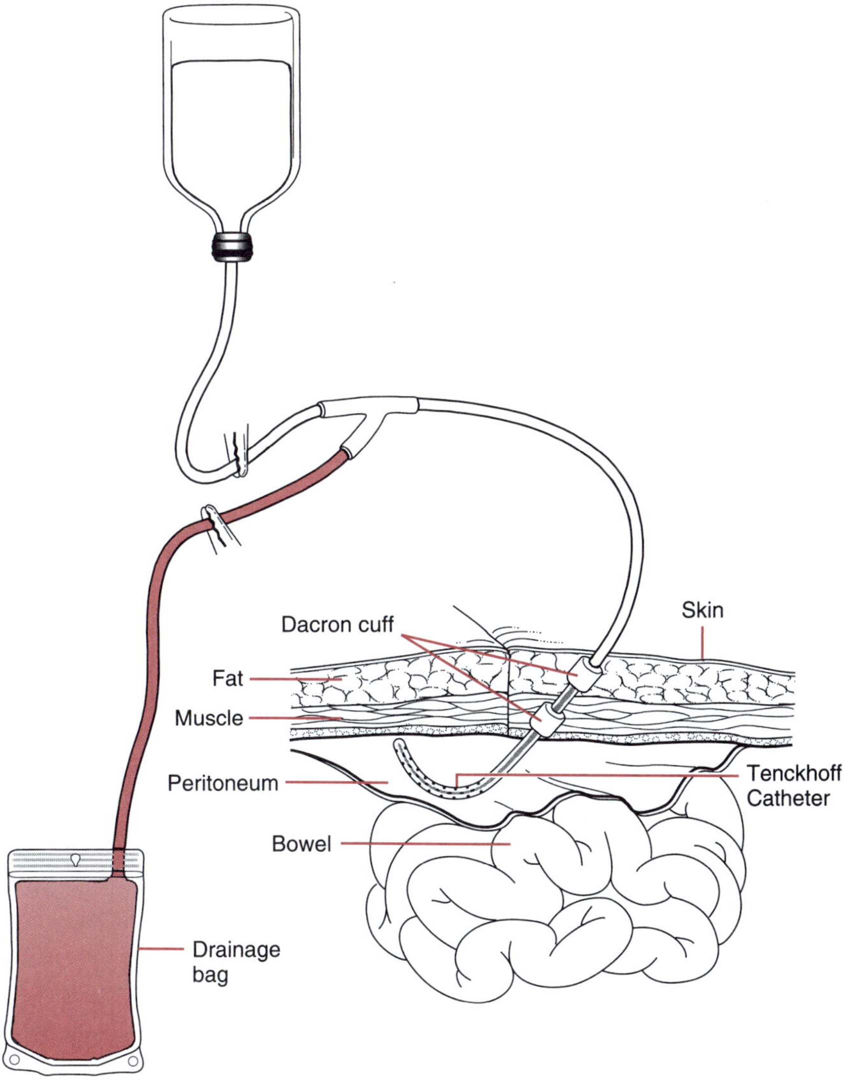

Figure 14–2 ■ Intraperitoneal infusion via Tenckhoff catheter directly into the peritoneal cavity.

enhance its penetration and cell kill while limiting systemic effects. The peritoneal cavity acts as a reservoir for the drug. The goal is to decrease systemic toxic effects and increase the antitumor action of the antineoplastic agent. Chemotherapeutic agents that are delivered via the IP route include cisplatin, carboplatin, cytosine arabinoside, mitoxantrone, calcium folinate, doxorubicin, and 5-FU.

NURSING FAST FACTS!

For IP administration to be effective, the patient must have limited intra-abdominal adhesions.

- *The disease must be limited to the body region in which the antineoplastic agent is administered.*
- *Nursing staff must be well prepared to care for an IP catheter.*
- *The nurse and family must be familiar with the therapeutic effects of antineoplastic agents.*
- *Advantages include:*
  - *When not in use, the IP device is invisible, enhancing a positive body image.*
  - *There is no catheter site care.*
  - *Cytotoxic drugs are administered directly to the tumor area.*
- *Disadvantages include:*
  - *It can be difficult to locate and access the port.*
  - *Catheter infections can occur.*
  - *Build-up of fibrin sheath can occur on the distal catheter tip*
  - *Abdominal adhesions can cause spaces in the cavity, preventing the flow of the infusion into the space and can also prevent the drug from draining out of the space. The fluid is then absorbed by the body.*

PROCEDURES DISPLAY 14–1

Intraperitoneal Therapy

Verify physician's order, provide patient with educational materials, obtain patient written consent, and use good hand hygiene and Standard Precautions during the procedure.

Equipment Needed

- Sterile gloves, mask, and gown
- Gauze pads
- Transparent semipermeable membrane (TSM) dressing
- Warmed infusate
- Povidone-iodine or 2% chlorhexidine
- Drainage bag
- Y-type dialysis administration set
- Large-gauge noncoring needle (if using a port)

Instructions to Patients

Inform patient that a peritoneal dialysis catheter or port is placed to provide access to the peritoneal cavity for instillation of medication.

(Continued on following page)

Explain to patient the need to measure abdominal girth and obtain weight before procedure.

Procedure

ACCESSING PERITONEAL CATHETER: PRETREATMENT AND SITE CARE

1. Maintain strict sterile technique; wash hands with antimicrobial solution before handling system.
2. Prepare infusate and equipment and verify drug order.
3. Assess the area around the catheter or port for redness, edema, warmth, or tenderness.
4. Obtain patient weight and measure abdominal girth.
5. Prepare sterile field and don gloves (and gown if desired).
6. Anesthetize the skin surface before access with 1 percent Xylocaine intradermal or topical anesthetic cream.
7. Clean catheter adapter with 10 percent povidone-iodine or 2 percent chlorhexidine.
8. Connect dialysis administration set, or access implanted port using aseptic technique with a large-gauge, noncoring, 90-degree needle of appropriate length (usually 1 to 15 inches). Secure with tape.
9. Flush the catheter with 10 to 20 mL of nonbacteriostatic sterile saline; catheter should flush easily.
10. Administer antiemetics if ordered.

DRUG ADMINISTRATION

11. Record instillation start time.
12. Position patient comfortably in a semi-Fowler's position
13. Open the clamp on the tubing and infuse the warmed I.P. chemotherapy at the prescribed rate (usually over 30 minutes to several hours). Close clamp when completed; keep solution in cavity for the prescribed time.

NURSING FAST FACT!

Stop infusion immediately if severe pain is experienced and check for catheter migration. Slow the rate of infusion if the patient experiences shortness of breath or discomfort.

14. Close the clamp on the tubing when the infusion is complete and encourage repositioning from side to side every 15 minutes during the indwelling time (usually 2 to 4 hours).
15. Monitor the patient's comfort levels.
16. Repeat as prescribed.

(Continued on following page)

PROCEDURES DISPLAY 14–1

Intraperitoneal Therapy *(Continued)*

17. After the prescribed dwell time, open the clamp to the drainage bag and allow the solution to drain.

NURSING FAST FACT!

Recognize that the volume of drained fluid may be less than that infused and reassure the patient that the fluid will be reabsorbed and metabolized.

18. Clamp tubing on the drainage bag after the fluid has drained (usually 30 min to 2 hours) and send specimen, properly labeled as cytotoxic, to cytology or dispose of in proper hazardous waste container.

POSTADMINISTRATION CARE

19. Flush the catheter or port with nonbacteriostatic sterile saline; if using a port, follow with heparinized saline.
20. Secure the site using the standard technique (e.g., cap and secure the catheter or remove the needle from the port and cover the site with a small dressing, if necessary).
21. Establish I.V. fluids as prescribed or discontinue I.V. needle.
22. Disinfect open hub of catheter and replace with sterile access port.
23. If necessary replace dressing at catheter exit site.

DOCUMENTATION

24. Document in the medical record medication administered, dwell time of the infusion, length of time to drain the infusate, volume and color of drainage, infusion site, and how well the patient tolerated the procedure.

NURSING FAST FACT!

The fluid present in peritoneal catheter should be clear to pale pink in color; if blood is aspirated from device do not use (INS, 2002).

Cerebrospinal Fluid Reservoirs

Intraventricular chemotherapy allows for the administration of antineoplastic agents into the CSF via an Ommaya reservoir (Baxter, IL) (Fig. 14–3). A physician must place the ventricular reservoir. The nurse admin-

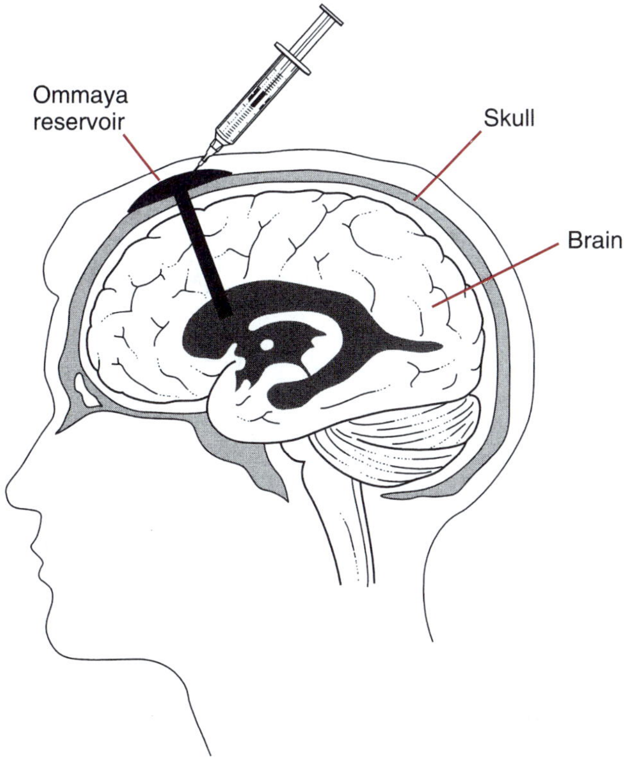

Figure 14–3 ■ The Ommaya reservoir. Intraventricular chemotherapy administration. (From Otto, S.E. [1995]. Advanced concepts in chemotherapy drug delivery regional therapy. *Journal of Intravenous Nursing,* 18[4], 170–176, with permission.)

istering medications into the reservoir must follow the Nurse Practice Act for the state in which he or she practices. An Ommaya reservoir is a silicone rubber device that is implanted surgically under the scalp and provides access to CSF through a burr hole in the skull. Drugs are injected into the reservoir with a hypodermic syringe, and then the domed reservoir is depressed manually to mix drug with the CSF.

Infusion Pumps

Infusion pumps have been widely used in chemotherapy administration to provide continuous or intermittent drug delivery. These pumps are essential in intra-arterial administration, in which the drug must be given against arterial pressure, but they are used in delivery of antineoplastic agents by all routes.

Pumps are available as nonportable and portable. Nonportable pumps are usually designed to clamp onto an I.V. pole and are quite

Nursing Points-of-Care: Delivery of Chemotherapy via a Ventricular Reservoir

1. The patient should be taught the purpose of the reservoir.
2. When accessing the ventricular reservoir, wear sterile gloves and a mask.
3. Use only preservative-free medications.
4. Aspirate to check placement before drug delivery; CSF should be present.
5. Withdrawal of CSF for diagnostic purpose is a medical act.

Advantages include:

- Well tolerated
- Eliminates need for multiple lumbar punctures

Disadvantages include:

- Increased risk of infection to the spinal cord and brain

bulky; these are used in hospital or outpatient clinics. The compact, battery-operated, portable pumps have enabled individuals to receive continuous chemotherapy on an outpatient or home care basis.

AGE-RELATED CONSIDERATIONS: PEDIATRIC ONCOLOGY 14–1

Cancer is the primary cause of death from disease in children who are between 1 and 14 years old (APON, 1998). Pediatric oncology as a nursing specialty has grown rapidly during the past 30 years.

The Children's Cancer Group (CCG) was founded in 1955. It is a cooperative research group that has developed criteria, policies, and procedures to ensure that cooperative clinical trails are conducted uniformly at all participating institutions and to permit the pooling of data from all patients.

The diagnosis of pediatric cancer involves many members of the healthcare team. New techniques to diagnose and stage cancers have facilitated the development of sophisticated plans of treatment. This technique has produced improved patient survival rates, as well as cures for many pediatric malignancies (Apon, 1998).

The selection of antineoplastic agents used in treating a child with cancer is made primarily on the basis of the histology of the tumor and the extent of the disease. The dose and schedule of the drug administered are critical in achieving maximum benefit (Bertolone, 1997).

Websites

American Society of Pediatric Hematology/Oncology: *www.aspho.org*
Association of Pediatric Oncology Nurses: *www.apon.org*

Other sites:

NURSING PLAN OF CARE

ANTINEOPLASTIC THERAPY

Focus Assessment

Subjective

- Interview the patient regarding his or her previous experience with chemotherapy.
- Determine the patient's level of knowledge regarding chemotherapy and cancer.

Objective

- Assess the patient for nausea and vomiting.
- Inspect the patient's oral cavity daily.
- Assess the patient's breath sounds.
- Monitor the patient's vital signs.
- Note the patient's type of cancer, length of illness, prognosis, and previous chemotherapy.
- Assess the patient's nutritional status.
- Review the patient's laboratory data.
- Assess the patient's urinary output and hydration level.

Patient Outcome/Evaluation Criteria

Patient will:

- Demonstrate stable weight or progressive weight gain toward a goal and be free of signs of malnutrition.
- Demonstrate normalization of laboratory values.
- Demonstrate that antinausea medications are effective.
- Comply with dietary restrictions.
- Display adequate fluid balance.
- Display moist mucous membranes.
- Identify techniques to maintain and restore integrity of oral mucosa.

(Continued on following page)

NURSING PLAN OF CARE

ANTINEOPLASTIC THERAPY *(Continued)*

- Identify interventions for specific condition; prevent complications and promote healing as appropriate.
- Demonstrate adequate oxygenation of tissues by arterial blood gas values within patient's normal range.
- Be free of respiratory distress.
- Display appropriate range of feelings.
- Verbalize accurate information about diagnosis and treatment regimen.
- Initiate necessary lifestyle changes and participate in treatment regimen.

Nursing Diagnoses

- Altered nutrition less than body requirements, related to consequences of treatment
- Risk for noncompliance with dietary restrictions of chemotherapy related to no foods high in tyramines while taking procarbazine
- Risk for fluid volume deficit, related to excessive losses through vomiting, diarrhea, wounds, or impaired oral intake
- Oral mucous membrane altered, related to side effects of chemotherapeutic agents (antimetabolites)
- Risk for skin and tissue integrity impaired, related to effects of chemotherapy, immunologic deficit, altered nutritional state or anemia, presence of lesions, or drug extravasation
- Risk for gas exchange, impaired, related to alveolar membrane thickening (pulmonary fibrosis), altered blood flow, or decreased circulation or altered oxygen-carrying capacity
- Fear and anxiety related to situational crisis, threat to or change in health and socioeconomic status, role functioning, interaction patterns, threat of death, separation from family
- Knowledge deficit related to lack of exposure or recall, information misinterpretation, myths, unfamiliarity with resources

Nursing Management

1. Monitor for
   a. side effects and toxic effects of chemotherapeutic agent.
   b. adequate fluid intake, dehydration, and electrolyte imbalance.
   c. effectiveness of measures to control nausea and vomiting
   d. nutritional status and weight.
2. Institute neutropenic and bleeding precautions when necessary.
3. Offer bland, easily digested diet in six small meals a day.
4. Administer antiemetic medication.
5. Administer chemotherapeutic drugs (except urotoxic drugs) in the late evening so the patient may sleep at the time emetic effects are greatest.

(Continued on following page)

6. Assist patient in obtaining a wig or other head covering device as appropriate.
7. Offer six small feedings daily.
8. Ascertain that the I.V. is infusing well; dilute antineoplastic agents.
9. Administer appropriate antidotes per protocol and physician's orders if extravasation occurs.
10. Use mouthwash prepared from warm saline and a dilute solution of hydrogen peroxide or baking soda and water. Avoid using commercial mouthwash products that contain alcohol or phenol and may increase mucous membrane discomfort.
11. Administer analgesics and topical Xylocaine jelly, antimicrobial mouthwash, or both (e.g., nystatin) as needed for stomatitis.
12. Minimize stimuli from noises, light, and odors, especially food.
13. Follow recommended guidelines for safe handling of parenteral antineoplastic drugs during drug preparation.

Patient Education

- Inform the patient and his or her family about how antineoplastic agents work on cancer cells.
- Instruct the patient and his or her family about the effects of chemotherapy on bone marrow functioning.
- Instruct patient and his or her family on ways to prevent infection (e.g., avoiding crowds and using good hygiene and handwashing techniques).
- Instruct the patient on the pretreatment hydration instruction sheet when appropriate.
- Instruct the patient to promptly report fever, chills, nosebleed, excessive bruising, tarry stools, severe headaches, or prolonged vomiting.
- Inform the patient to avoid aspirin products.
- Instruct the patient and his or her family to monitor for signs and symptoms of stomatitis and to perform good oral hygiene.
- Inform the patient that hair loss is expected as determined by the type of chemotherapeutic agent.
- Instruct the patient to avoid hot, spicy foods.
- Instruct the patient and his or her family to monitor for organ toxicity as determined by the type of chemotherapeutic agent used.
- Discuss with the patient the possibility of sterility and other reproductive system impairments.
- Inform long-term survivors and their families of the possibility of second malignancies and the importance of reporting increased susceptibility to infection, fatigue, or bleeding.
- Instruct the patient to avoid scratching his or her skin.

(Continued on following page)

Patient Education *(Continued)*

Websites

Oncolink: *www.cancer.med.upenn.edu*

This site gives extensive information for patients, caregivers, and clinicians. Cancer news, disease-oriented menu, causes and prevention, clinical trails, conferences, and psychosocial support from the University of Pennsylvania Cancer Center.

Home Care Issues

The most common antineoplastic agents given by the I.V. route for chemotherapy prescribed in the home are continuous 5-FU. Many other agents can be administered safely in the home care setting with the appropriate level of specialized clinical oncology support. Common issues of concern in delivery of chemotherapy in the home are as follows.

Patient and Family Education

- Family members must understand the nature of the risk of handling cytotoxic drugs.
- It is the professional healthcare team's responsibility on behalf of the agency to provide education regarding safe practices in handling these drugs.
- Potential risks to persons who come in contact with chemotherapy drugs and associated safety measures should be discussed with patients and their families before the initial home chemotherapy treatment.

Admixture

Antineoplastic agents must be prepared in a biologic safety hood for protection during admixture; this task must be accomplished in a pharmacy.

Transport of Drug

- In the home care situation, the family or nurse often obtains antineoplastic agents. The drugs are labeled as cytotoxic, capped securely, and sealed and packaged in an impervious packing material for transport. The outside of the bags or bottles containing the prepared drug should be wiped with moist gauze. Entry ports should be wiped with moist alcohol pads and capped (OSHA, 1999).
- Transport should occur in sealed plastic bags and in containers designed to avoid breakage. The patient's family should be cautioned to protect the package from breakage and taught the necessary procedures if a spill occurs. Spill kits should be available in the home care setting.

(Continued on following page)

NURSING FAST FACT!

Personnel involved in transporting hazardous drugs should be trained in spill procedures, including sealing off the contaminated area and calling for appropriate assistance (OSHA, 1999).

Administration

- The family member who will administer the drug must be taught safe handling of chemotherapeutic agents, use of latex gloves, and how to handle the tubing or infusion pump during delivery of drug.
- The area of the patient's home designated for preparation of drug should be separate from the family activity area and food preparation.
- Ceiling fans, if present, should be turned off.
- The work surface area should be one that can be cleaned, such as a card table.
- All family members should remain outside the rooms in which the drugs are prepared and administered, if possible. Other young siblings or children should be cared for outside the home on the day of chemotherapy.
- All supplies should be assembled on a disposable, absorbent, plastic-backed pad that is taped over the work surface area. Only syringes, needles, and I.V. sets with Luer Lok fittings are used.
- Administering aerosolized hazardous drugs requires special engineering controls to prevent exposure to healthcare workers and others (OSHA, 1999).

NURSING FAST FACT!

The importance of hand hygiene techniques should be stressed. Peripheral access for administering vesicant agents in the home is discouraged.

Disposal

- Needles, syringes, and breakable items not contaminated with blood or other infectious materials should be placed in a sharps container before being stored in the waste bag. Hazardous drug-related wastes should be handled separately from the trash and disposed of in accordance with the applicable Environmental Protection Agency (EPA) state and local regulations.

Monitoring

- Clinical monitoring of a patient receiving chemotherapy at home demands close attention. Clinical monitoring should include laboratory

(Continued on following page)

Home Care Issues *(Continued)*

values, physical status, fluid status, and drug-related side effects and toxicities (Lonsway, 2001).

Disposal of Excreta

- Cytotoxic activity of drugs and their metabolites can remain active in excreta for 48 hours or more. This special situation means that urine, feces, vomitus, and other excreta should be treated with caution, and the patient's family should wear gloves when handling excreta, linens, or tissues.
- It is suggested that the dilution in most sewer systems is adequate to decrease the risk to both the patient's family and the environment.
- Sheets and other laundry soiled with excreta should be washed twice and kept separate from other family laundry.

Key Points

- The role of nurses in administering chemotherapy includes patient assessment and history, patient education, and knowledge of treatment objectives.
- The cell cycle includes the nonproliferative resting phase (G_0), the presynthetic stage (G_1), the interval after synthesis of DNA (G_2), synthesis of DNA (S), and mitosis (M).
- Classifications of antineoplastic agents are either cell cycle specific (CCS) or cell cycle nonspecific (CCNS).
- Key nursing interventions and assessments with alkylating drugs include monitoring the site for infiltration, CBC, platelets, and liver enzymes; administering antiemetics; assessing respiratory status and blood pressure; and prehydrating and assessing the oral cavity.
- Key nursing interventions and assessments with antimetabolite agents include assessing oral mucosa for stomatitis; and monitoring the CBC, platelets, liver enzymes, and renal function. The drug infusion should be questioned if the WBC count drops below 3000/μL.
- Key nursing interventions and assessments with anthracycline antibiotics include monitoring for possible hypersensitivity reactions; assessing the oral mucosa; assessing the infusion site frequently for infiltration (avoid extravasation); monitoring CBC count, platelets, cardiac enzymes, and ECGs; monitoring renal function; premedicating with dexamethasone, diphenhydramine, or cimetidine before the infusion of paclitaxel; and administering antiemetic agents.
- Key nursing interventions and assessments with hormones and hormone antagonist include assessing for mood swings and changes in

psychological state; monitoring electrolytes when appropriate; monitoring blood pressure; assessing for signs of feminization with estrogens in males; assessing females for masculinizing effects with androgens; assessing for signs of phlebitis; encouraging low-salt diets; and monitoring weight.

- Key nursing interventions and assessments with biologic response modifiers include assessing emotional status; assessing for flulike symptoms; assessing CBC count, differential, platelets, electrolytes, and liver function before initiating therapy; assessing for presence of infection; and assessing cardiac and pulmonary function.
- Common side effects of chemotherapy include:
  - Short-term complications such as venous fragility, alopecia, diarrhea, constipation, altered nutritional status, anorexia or taste alteration, and fatigue
  - Acute side effects such as hypersensitivity or anaphylaxis, extravasation, stomatitis and mucositis, nausea and vomiting, and myelosuppression
  - Toxic side effects involving the cardiac, neurologic, renal, and pulmonary systems
- Neutropenia predisposes patients to infection, and ANC of 1000 to 1500/μL puts patients at moderate risk for infection. An ANC lower than 500/μL places patients at severe risk for infection.
- With a platelet count below 50,000/μL, there is a potential for bleeding. Thrombocytopenia places patients at risk for CNS and GI bleeding.
- Use meticulous sterile technique in accessing vascular devices.
- Assess vein patency with 10 to 20 mL of sodium chloride before infusing cytotoxic agents.

Critical Thinking: Case Study

A 24-year-old man is admitted to the hospital with a diagnosis of acute lymphoblastic leukemia (ALL). His labs are WBC 31.7 mm^3, Hgb 10.1 g/dL, Hct 29 percent, and platelets 16 mm^3. He is scheduled to receive the initial induction combination chemotherapy by I.V. and I.T. (intrathecal) routes. He will be receiving doxorubicin, vincristine and cyclophosphamide IVP, methotrexate I.T., and prednisone P.O. A triple-lumen central venous tunneled catheter (CVTC) is inserted to facilitate chemotherapy and blood product infusions.

What potential adverse effects can the nurse anticipate with this combination chemotherapy?

What nursing care should be implemented for the tunneled catheter, and the intrathecal catheter?

Based on his lab values what other orders can the nurse anticipate?

Media Link: Answers to this case study and additional critical thinking activities are located on the enclosed CD–ROM.

Post-Test

1. The goal of cancer immunotherapy is to:
   a. Produce remission
   b. Promote tumor-nonspecific immunity
   c. Stimulate immunocompetence in cancer patients
   d. Decrease the side effects of traditional chemotherapy
2. A side effect of anthracyclines is:
   a. Photosensitivity
   b. Cardiotoxicity
   c. Psychosis
   d. Neurotoxicity
3. A patient who is considered neutropenic and at risk for infection has an absolute neutrophil count (ANC) below:
   a. 10,000/μL
   b. 4000/μL
   c. 2000/μL
   d. 1000/μL
4. Pulmonary toxicity is associated with which of the following antineoplastic therapies?
   a. Bleomycin
   b. Paclitaxel
   c. Cisplatin
   d. Carboplatin
5. IP antineoplastic therapy delivers the drug directly into a(n):
   a. Artery
   b. Cavity
   c. Vein
   d. Ventricle
6. In a patient receiving doxorubicin (Adriamycin) via peripheral I.V. infusion, the nurse should monitor:
   a. The ECG
   b. The I.V. site
   c. Potassium levels
   d. Abdominal girth
7. When planning nursing care for a patient receiving vincristine intravenously, the following nursing intervention should be considered:

a. Restrict fluids during treatment.
b. Limit the dosage of acetaminophen.
c. Observe the I.V. site for drug infiltration.
d. Place the patient on neutropenic precautions.

8. Which of the following is a major side effect of the alkylating agent carmustine?
   a. Bone marrow depression
   b. Numbness and tingling of extremities
   c. Elevated BUN
   d. Pulmonary toxicity

9. Before administering antimetabolites, the nurse should check the following laboratory data:
   a. Sodium and potassium
   b. BUN and creatinine
   c. Liver enzymes and amylase
   d. WBC count and platelets

10. Cancer patients who experience anemia and thrombocytopenia have traditionally been treated with:
    a. Antibiotic therapy
    b. Blood component therapy
    c. Corticosteroid therapy
    d. I.V. hydration therapy

11. Adverse effects of alkylating agents primarily are related to the:
    a. GI system
    b. Neurologic system
    c. Kidney
    d. Liver

12. All of the following organizations provide nationally established standards that govern nursing practice pertaining to chemotherapy **EXCEPT**:
    a. Oncology Nurses Society (ONS)
    b. Centers for Disease Control and Prevention
    c. American Nurses Association
    d. Infusion Nurses Society (INS)

13. All the following are common nursing diagnoses associated with delivery of chemotherapeutic agents **EXCEPT:**
    a. Altered nutrition less than body requirements
    b. Altered oral mucous membrane

c. Fatigue
d. Alteration in urinary elimination

14. A patient considered neutropenic from bone marrow suppression is at risk for:
    a. Dehydration
    b. Infection
    c. Seizures
    d. Disseminated intravascular coagulation

15. Agents given to increase hematopoiesis are:
    a. Colony-stimulating factors
    b. Interferons
    c. Interleukins
    d. Monoclonal antibodies

Media Link: Additional test questions and rationales are located on the enclosed CD–ROM.

References

Angel, F.S. (1995). Current controversies in chemotherapy administration. *Journal of Intravenous Nursing*, 18(1), 16–23.

Association of Pediatric Oncology Nurses (1998). *Essentials of Pediatric Oncology Nursing*: A Core Curriculum: Glenview: APON.

Bertolone, K. (1997). Pediatric oncology: Past, present, and new modalities of treatment. *Journal of Intravenous Nursing*, 20(3), 136–140.

Chu, E., & DeVita,V. (2002). *Physicians Cancer Chemotherapy Manual*. Boston: Jones & Bartlett.

Gahart, B.L., & Nazareno, A.R. (2004). *Intravenous medications* (20th ed.). St. Louis: Mosby.

Giger, J.N., & Davidhizar, R.E. (2004). *Transcultural Nursing: Assessment and Intervention* (4th ed.). St. Louis: Mosby.

Infusion Nurses Society (2000). Infusion Nurses Standards of practice. *Journal of Intravenous Nursing* (Suppl) 23(6S), 70.

Infusion Nurses Society (2002). *Policies and Procedures for Infusion Nursing*. (2nd ed.). Cambridge, MA: Infusion Nurses Society.

Lilley, L L., & Aucker, R.S. (2004). *Pharmacology and the Nursing Process* (4th ed.). St. Louis: Mosby, pp. 699–723.

Lonsway, R.A. (2001). Intravenous therapy in the home. In Hankins, J., Lonsway, R.A., Hedrick, C., & Perdue, M. (eds.). *Infusion Therapy in Clinical Practice* (2nd ed.). Infusion Nurses Society and Philadelphia: W.B. Saunders.

Lynch, M. (2002). *Oncology Nursing Essentials*. New York: Professional Publishing Co.

Moran, P. (2000). Cellular effects of cancer chemotherapy administration. *Journal of Intravenous Therapy, 23*(1), 44–51.

Oncology Nursing Society (2001). *Chemotherapy and Biotherapy. Guidelines and Recommendations for Practice.* Pittsburgh: Oncology Nursing Society.

OSHA (1999). *Controlling Occupational Exposure to Hazardous Drugs.* U.S, Department of Labor Docket No. CPL 2–2.

Phillips, L.D., & Kuhn, M. (1999). *Manual of Intravenous Drugs* (2nd ed.). Philadelphia: J.B. Lippincott.

Skeel, R.T. (2003). Systematic assessment of the patient with cancer and long-term medical complications of treatment. In Skeel, R.T. (ed.). *Handbook of Cancer Chemotherapy* (6th ed.). Philadelphia: Lippincott Williams & Wilkins, pp. 34–56.

Skeel, R.T., & Khleif, S.N. (2003). Biologic and pharmacologic basis for cancer chemotherapy. In Skeel, R.T. (ed.). *Handbook of Cancer Chemotherapy* (6th ed.). Philadelphia: Lippincott Williams & Wilkins, pp. 3–20.

Smith, M.R., & Stutz, N. (2003). Disorders of hemostasis and transfusion therapy. In Skeel, R.T. (ed). *Handbook of Cancer Chemotherapy* (6th ed .). Philadelphia: Lippincott Williams & Wilkins.

Tipton, J.M. (2003). Side effects of cancer chemotherapy. In Skeel, R.T. (ed.). *Handbook of Cancer Chemotherapy* (6th ed.). Philadelphia: Lippincott Williams & Wilkins.

Vandegrift, K.V. (2001). Oncology therapy. In Hankins, J., Lonsway, R.A., Hedrick, C., & Perdue, M. (eds.). *Infusion Therapy in Clinical Practice* (2nd ed.). Infusion Nurses Society and Philadelphia: W.B. Saunders.

Wilkes, G., Ingwersen, K., & Barton-Burke, M. (2003) *Oncology Nursing Drug Handbook.* Boston: Jones & Bartlett

Yarbro, C., Frogge, M., & Goodman, M. (2001). *Cancer Symptom Management.* Boston: Jones & Bartlett.

Answers to Chapter 14 Post-Test

1. **c**
2. **b**
3. **d**
4. **a**
5. **b**
6. **b**
7. **c**
8. **a**
9. **d**
10. **b**
11. **a**
12. **c**
13. **d**
14. **b**
15. **a**

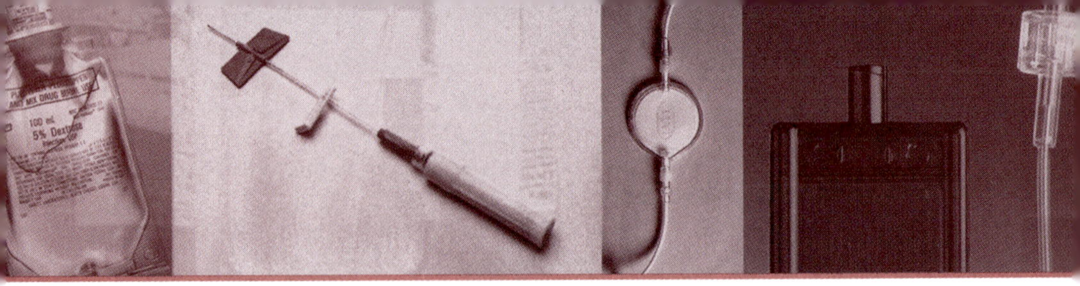

Chapter 15
Nutritional Support

Every careful observer of the sick will agree in this that thousands of patients are annually starved in the midst of plenty, from want of attention to the ways which alone make it possible for them to take food.
—Florence Nightingale, 1859

Chapter Contents

LEARNING OBJECTIVES

Upon completion of this chapter, the reader will be able to:

1. Define the glossary of terms as related to nursing care of the patient receiving nutritional support.
2. Apply the goals of parenteral nutrition to the hospitalized, pediatric and home care client.
3. Identify the key elements of a nutritional assessment.
4. List the key points in administration of glucose, protein, and fat emulsions.
5. Describe the three major classifications of malnutrition.
6. Identify early candidates for nutritional support.
7. Identify the component used to treat essential fatty acid deficiency.
8. Describe the use of the additives heparin, insulin, and H_2 inhibitors to parenteral nutrition.
9. Describe three-in-one solutions.
10. Discuss evidence-based practice for use of cyclic therapy for the home care client.
11. Discuss the TPN point of care plan for patients with renal or liver disease.
12. Discuss the evidence-based practice of peripheral parenteral nutrition.
13. Identify *nursing fast facts* related to the delivery of nutritional support.
14. Assess potential complications related to nutritional support.
15. Implement the steps of the nursing process in caring for a patient with nutritional support.

GLOSSARY

Amino acid Chief organic component of protein

Anergy Lack of immune response to an antigen

Anthropometry measurement Measurement of a part or whole of the body

Basal energy expenditure (BEE) The amount of energy produced per unit of time under "basal" conditions

Essential fatty acid deficiency (EFAD) Compound of carbon, hydrogen and oxygen that combines with glycerol to form fat required in the diet. Essential fatty acids cannot be synthesized by the body, but must be obtained from the diet or intravenous infusion of lipids.

Fat emulsion Natural product consisting of a mixture of neutral triglycerides of predominantly unsaturated fatty acids; permits inclusion of fat calories in the I.V. nutritional regimen

Kwashiorkor Malnutrition characterized by an adequate calorie intake with inadequate amount of protein

Marasmus Malnutrition characterized by decreased intake of calories with adequate amounts of protein intake

Parenteral nutrition Nutrients that are administered intravenously, comprising of carbohydrates, proteins, and/or fats, and additives; such as electrolytes, vitamins and trace elements

Peripheral parenteral nutrition (PPN) Nutritional support via a peripheral vein; glucose limited to 10 percent

Refeeding syndrome Syndrome in which the body, during its bout with starvation, adapts to nutritional deprivation and compensates by decreasing basal energy requirements

Total lymphocyte count (TLC) Integral component of the immune system

Total nutrient admixture (TNA) A three-in-one formula of amino acids, fats, and dextrose in one container

Total parenteral nutrition (TPN) Intravenous nutritional support delivered by central access; supplying glucose, protein, vitamins, electrolytes, trace elements, and sometimes fats to maintain the body's growth, development, and tissue repair

Nutritional Support

Nutritional support nursing is the care of individuals with potential or known nutritional alterations. "Nurses who specialize in nutritional support use specific expertise to enhance the maintenance and/or restoration of an individual's nutritional health" (American Society for Parenteral and Enteral Nutrition [ASPEN], 1999). Nutrition support nursing encompasses all nursing activities that promote optimal nutritional health. Nursing interventions are based on scientific principles. The scope of practice includes, but is not limited to, direct patient care; consultation with nurses and other healthcare professionals in a variety of clinical settings; education of patients, students, colleagues, and the public; participation in research; and administrative functions (ASPEN, 1998).

It is essential for nurses in all settings to respect the importance of adequate nutrition and the adverse effects of malnutrition. The goals of parenteral nutrition include:

1. To provide all essential nutrients in adequate amounts to sustain nutritional balance during periods when oral or enteral routes of feedings are not possible or are insufficient to meet the patient's caloric needs
2. To preserve or restore the body's protein metabolism and prevent the development of protein or caloric malnutrition
3. To diminish the rate of weight loss and to maintain or increase body weight
4. To promote wound healing
5. To replace nutritional deficits

Websites

American Society for Parenteral and Enteral Nutrition: *www.clinnutri.org*

Other sites:

Concepts of Nutrition

Nutritional balance occurs when nutrients are provided in sufficient quantities for the maintenance of body function and renewal of these components. Nutritional balance is based on three factors: (1) intake of nutrients (quantity and quality), (2) relative need for nutrients, and (3) the ability of the body to use nutrients.

Nutritional Deficiency

When nutritional deficiency exists, the body's components are used to provide energy for essential metabolic processes. For example, body stores of carbohydrates, fats, and protein are metabolized as energy sources in nutritional deficiency states. Carbohydrates are stored in the muscle and liver as glycogen. Adipose tissue is the body's long-term energy reserve of fat. Body protein is not stored in excess of the body's needs; therefore, use of body protein without replacement adversely affects total body function (Wilson & Jordan, 2001).

Malnutrition

Malnutrition is a nutritional deficit associated with an increased risk of morbidity and mortality. Death from protein energy malnutrition and other nutritional deficiencies occurs within 60 to 70 days of total starvation in normal weight adults. After total starvation for less than 2 to 3 days in healthy adults the losses are mainly glycogen and water (ASPEN, 1999). Starvation alters the distribution of carbohydrates, fats, and protein substrates. Brief starvation (24 to 72 hours) rapidly depletes glycogen stores and uses protein to produce glucose (gluconeogenesis) for glucose-dependent tissue. Prolonged starvation (longer than 72 hours) is associated with an increased mobilization of fat as the principal source of energy, reduction in the breakdown of protein, and increased use of ketones for central nervous tissue fuel. Stress in the form of pain, shock, injury, and sepsis intensifies the metabolic change seen in those with brief and prolonged starvation. Poor nutrition causes weight loss and generalized weakness, which affects functional ability and quality of life. Three types of malnutrition have been defined and classified by an International Classification of Diseases (ICD) diagnostic code: marasmus, kwashiorkor, and mixed malnutrition. The outcome of nutritional assessment determines the category to which an undernourished person is assigned.

Marasmus

Marasmus is caused by a decrease in the intake of calories with adequate protein–calorie ratio. In this type of malnutrition, a gradual wasting of body fat and skeletal muscle takes place with preservation of visceral proteins. The individual looks emaciated and has decreased **anthropometric** measurements and **anergy** to common skin test antigens.

NURSING FAST FACT!

Marasmus may be seen in chronic illness and prolonged starvation, as well as the elderly, and the patient with anorexia nervosa (McGinnis, 2002).

Kwashiorkor

Kwashiorkor is characterized by an adequate intake of calories along with a poor protein intake. This condition causes visceral protein wasting with preservation of fat and somatic muscle. It is seen during a period of decreased protein intake as seen with liquid diets, fat diets, and long-term use of I.V. fluids containing dextrose. Loss of body protein is caused by depleted circulating proteins in the plasma. Individuals may appear obese and have adequate anthropometric measurements but decreased visceral proteins and depressed immune function.

Mixed Malnutrition

Mixed malnutrition is characterized by aspects of both marasmus and kwashiorkor. The person presents with skeletal muscle and visceral protein wasting, depleted fat stores, and immune incompetence. The affected person appears cachectic and usually is in acute catabolic stress. This mixed protein–calorie disorder is associated with the highest risk of morbidity and mortality.

Effects of Malnutrition

The hazards of malnutrition on bodily function are decreased protein stores, albumin depletion, and impaired immune status. Without protein stores in the body, a deficiency of total body protein results first in decreased strength and endurance (loss of muscle mass) and ultimately in decreased cardiac and respiratory muscle function. Skeletal muscle wasting occurs in a ratio of about 30 to 1 compared with visceral protein loss. The loss of gastrointestinal (GI) function follows skeletal muscle wasting and is associated with hypoalbuminemia. Protein–calorie malnutrition is one of the most common causes of impairment of immune function. Both B- and T-cell–mediated immune functions are impaired, causing enhanced susceptibility to infections.

Nutritional Assessment

A nutritional assessment of high-risk patients supplies the physician and nurse with invaluable information regarding a patient's nutritional status (Table 15–1). The nutritional assessment encompasses routine history taking with emphasis on dietary history, anthropometric measurements, diagnostic testing, and a complete physical examination. The nutrition assessment combines the patient history with physical and biochemical markers to define the nutritional health.

> **INS Standard.** The nurse's responsibility before administration includes review of the patient's height, weight, nutritional status, and diagnosis and current laboratory values. (INS, 2000, 14)

The Joint Commission on the Accreditation of Healthcare Organizations (JCAHO) standards for both hospital and home care mandated screening and nutritional assessment as part of the specific nutritional care standards. The standards emphasize an interdisciplinary approach. Nutritional screening is "the process of using characteristics

> Table 15–1 **COMPONENTS OF A NUTRITIONAL ASSESSMENT**

History

- Medical
- Social
- Dietary

Anthropometric measurements

- Skinfolds
- Height and weight
- Midarm circumference
- Midarm muscle circumference

Biochemical assessment

- Serum albumin and transferrin levels
- Serum electrolytes
- Total lymphocyte count
- Urine assays (creatinine, height index)

Energy requirements
Physical examination
Other Indices

- Nitrogen balance
- Indirect calorimetry
- Prognostic Nutritional Index (PNI)

known to be associated with nutrition problems in order to determine if patients are malnourished or at high nutrition risk for malnourishment" (JCAHO, 1999).

History

The history is divided into four major components: medical, weight changes, social, and dietary. The medical history should include a specific history of weight; chronic diseases; surgical history; presence of increased losses, such as from draining wounds and fistulas; and factors such as age and drug, alcohol, and tobacco use. The social history affecting nutrient intake includes income, education, ethnic background, and environment during mealtime, along with religious considerations. The dietary history often provides clues as to the cause and degree of malnutrition. The components of a dietary history include appetite, GI disturbances, mechanical problems such as ill-fitting dentures, food allergies, medications, and food likes and dislikes.

AGE-RELATED CONSIDERATIONS: ELDERLY ADULTS 15–1

It is estimated that one in four elderly people is malnourished. Elderly people who are malnourished tend to have a longer and more expensive hospital stay.

Inadequate dietary intake in elderly people is multifaceted and includes physiologic changes in the GI tract, social and economic factors, drug interactions, disease, and excessive alcohol abuse. Poor dental health and missing teeth contribute to the malnutrition problem (Smeltzer & Bare, 2004).

CULTURAL AND ETHNIC CONSIDERATIONS: NUTRITION 15–1

Culture can determine the foods a patient eats and how they are prepared and served. Culture and religion together often determine if certain foods are prohibited and if certain foods and spices are eaten. When taking a dietary history, the nurse must be sensitive to culture and religious beliefs related to foods (Smeltzer & Bare, 2004).

Anthropometric Measurements

Anthropometry is the measurement of a part or whole of the body. It is a method of determining body composition. To estimate the size of the body fat mass, a skinfold test is done on the triceps of the nondominant arm using a caliper. Along with the skinfold measurement, a midarm circumference and midarm muscle circumference evaluation are performed. The height and weight are also part of this evaluation, with serial weights providing helpful information related to the protein–calorie status of the person. To calculate the current weight as a percentage of the usual weight, use the following calculation:

$$\text{Percent ideal body weight (IBW)} = (\text{Current weight} \div \text{IBW}) \times 100$$

Weight loss is important because it reflects inadequate calorie intake. Weight loss indicates an increased loss of protein from the body cell mass in individuals who are malnourished. Current weight does not provide information about recent changes in weight; therefore, patients are asked about their usual body weight (UBW) (Smeltzer & Bare, 2004).

$$\text{Percent of UBW} = (\text{Current body weight} \div \text{UBW}) \times 100$$

NURSING FAST FACT!

A loss of 10 percent of the usual weight or a current weight less than 90 percent of IBW is considered to be a risk factor of nutrition-related complications (Wilson & Jordan, 2001).

Mild malnutrition = 85 to 95 percent IBW
Moderate malnutrition = 75 to 84 percent IBW
Severe malnutrition = less than 75 percent IBW

In simple starvation, 20 percent loss of body weight is associated with marked decreases in muscle tissue and subcutaneous fat, giving the patient an emaciated appearance. Gross loss of body fat can be observed not only from appearance but also by palpating a number of skinfolds. When the dermis can be felt between the fingers on pinching the triceps and biceps skinfolds, considerable loss from body stores of fat has occurred. Protein stores can be assessed by inspection and palpation of a number of muscle groups, such as the triceps, biceps, and subscapular and infrascapular muscles. The long muscles in particular are profoundly protein depleted when the tendons are prominent to palpation.

Biochemical Assessment

Several tests are available to assess patients' biochemical nutritional status. The anergy test is recommended for assessing immunologic response and involves the intradermal injection of antigens. Proper nutrition is a key to an intact immune system, and a lack of response to antigens is considered anergic and possibly indicates malnourishment.

Biochemical assessment reflects both the tissue level of a given nutrient and any abnormality of metabolism. Studies of serum protein, albumin, globulin, transferrin, retinol-binding protein, hemoglobin, serum vitamin A, carotene, and vitamin C can reflect the utilization of nutrients. Total lymphocyte count is also measured for the body's response immunologically.

Serum Albumin and Transferrin Levels

Albumin is a major protein synthesized by the liver. Approximately 40 percent of protein mass is in the circulation. The serum albumin concentration is normally between 3.5 and 5.0 g/dL. An albumin level of 2.8 to 3.2 g/dL represents mild protein depletion, 2.1 to 2.7 g/dL reflects moderate depletion, and less than 2.1 g/dL indicates severe depletion.

Serum transferrin is a beta globulin that transports iron in the plasma and is synthesized in the liver. Transferrin is present in the serum in concentrations of 250 to 300 mg/dL. The serum levels are affected by nutritional factors and iron metabolism. Levels lower than 100 mg/dL indicate severe depletion (Smelzter & Bare, 2004).

Prealbumin and Retinol-Binding Protein

Prealbumin functions in thyroxine transport and as a carrier for retinol-binding protein. Normal serum concentrations range from 15.7 to 29.6 mg/dL. Levels of 10 to 15 mg/dL reflect mild depletion, those of 5 to 9.9 mg/dL reflect moderate depletion, and a level lower than 5 mg/dL indicates severe depletion.

Total Lymphocyte Count

Immunologic testing is designed to assess nutritional deficiencies. The most commonly used test for the assessment of immunocompetence is the **total lymphocyte count (TLC)**. The TLC is derived from the routine complete blood count (CBC) with differential. The TLC is calculated by means of the following formula:

$$\text{TLC} = \text{Percent lymph} \times \text{WBC} \div 100$$

A TLC between 1200 and 2000/µL indicates mild lymphocyte depletion; a TLC between 800 and 1199/µL indicates moderate lymphocyte depletion; and a TLC lower than 800/µL indicates severe lymphocyte depletion.

TLC must be interpreted with caution because many other nonnutritional factors may contribute to decreased lymphocyte counts.

Serum Electrolytes

Serum electrolyte levels provide information about fluid and electrolyte balance and kidney function. The creatinine/height index calculated over a 24-hour period assesses the metabolically active tissue and indicates the degree of protein depletion, comparing expected body mass for height and actual body cell mass (Smeltzer & Bare, 2004).

NURSING FAST FACT!

Many nutrition teams have incorporated a Subjective Global Assessment into their practice. A disadvantage to the Subjective Global Assessment is that it is a subjective data collection and depends on the experience of the clinician collecting and interpreting the data.

Energy Requirements

Energy requirements are dependent on a number of factors, which include the body surface area (derived from height and weight), age, and gender. Total daily energy expenditure has three components: (1) **basal energy expenditure** (**BEE** or BMR); (2) energy expenditure related to an activity; and (3) specific dynamic action of food. Determination of energy needs can be determined from the BEE or resting metabolic expenditure. The BEE accounts for 65 to 75 percent of energy expenditure and may be measured or estimated. The traditional method used to estimate BEE is the Harris–Benedict equation, which takes into consideration influence of patient's weight in kilograms, height in centimeters, age, and gender.

NURSING FAST FACT!

A simpler, widely accepted method used to estimate daily adult caloric requirements is to use 30 to 35 cal/kg.

Physical Examination

The final phase of the nutritional assessment is a complete physical examination. Findings from a physical examination can reflect protein–calorie malnutrition along with vitamin and mineral deficiencies. The physical examination should include evaluation of the patient's hair, nails, skin, eyes, oral cavity, glands, heart, muscles, and abdomen, along with a neurologic evaluation and evaluation of delayed healing and tissue repair (Table 15–2). The physical examination should also include objective measurements of wound healing, grip strength, skeletal muscle function, and respiratory muscle function (Burnett, 2000).

> Table 15–2 **PHYSICAL FINDINGS ASSOCIATED WITH DEFICIENCY STATES**

Area Assessed	Physical Findings	Associated Deficiencies
Hair	Flag sign (transverse depigmentation of hair)	Protein, copper
	Hair easily pluckable	Protein
	Hair thin, sparse	Protein, biotin, zinc
Nails	Nails, spoon shaped	Iron
	Nails, lackluster, transverse riding	Protein-calorie
Skin	Dry, scaling	Vitamin A, zinc, essential fatty acids
	Flaky paint dermatosis	Protein
	Follicular hyperkeratosis	Vitamins A, C; essential fatty acids
	Nasolabial seborrhea	Niacin, pyridoxine, riboflavin
	Petechiae, purpura	Ascorbic acid, vitamin K
	Pigmentation, desquamation (sun-exposed area)	Niacin (pellagra)
	Subcutaneous fat loss	Calorie
Eyes	Angular blepharitis	Riboflavin
	Corneal vascularization	
	Dull, dry conjunctiva	Vitamin A
	Fundal capillary microaneurysms	Ascorbic acid
	Scleral icterus, mild	Pyridoxine
Perioral	Angular stomatitis	Riboflavin
	Cheilosis	
Oral cavity	Atrophic lingual papillae	Niacin, iron, riboflavin, folate, vitamin B_{12}
	Glossitis (scarlet, raw)	Niacin, pyridoxine, riboflavin, vitamin B_{12}, folate

(Continued on following page)

Area Assessed	Physical Findings	Associated Deficiencies
	Hypogeusesthesia (also hyposomia)	Zinc, vitamin A
	Magenta tongue	Riboflavin
	Swollen, bleeding gums (if teeth present)	Ascorbic acid
	Tongue fissuring, edema	Niacin
Glands	Parotid enlargement	Protein
	Sicca syndrome	Ascorbic acid
	Thyroid enlargement	Iodine
Heart	Enlargement, tachycardia, high output failure	Thiamine ("wet" beriberi)
	Small heart, decreased output	Calorie
	Sudden heart failure, death	Ascorbic acid
Abdomen	Hepatomegaly	Protein
Muscles, extremities	Calf tenderness	Thiamine, ascorbic acid (hemorrhage into muscle)
	Edema	Protein, thiamine
	Muscle wastage (especially temporal area, dorsum of hand, spine)	Calorie
Bones, joints	Bone tenderness (adult)	Vitamin D, calcium, phosphorus (osteomalacia)
Neurologic	Confabulation, disorientation (Korsakoff's psychosis)	Thiamine
	Decreased position and vibratory senses, ataxia	Vitamin B_{12}, thiamine
	Decreased tendon reflexes, slowed relaxation phase	Thiamine
	Ophthalmoplegia	Thiamine, phosphorus
	Weakness, paresthesias, decreased fine tactile sensation	Vitamin B_{12}, pyridoxine, thiamine
Other	Delayed healing and tissue repair (e.g., wound, infarct, abscess)	Ascorbic acid, zinc, protein

Other Indices

Nitrogen Balance

A sensitive indicator of the body's gain or loss of protein is its nitrogen balance. An adult is said to be in nitrogen equilibrium when the nitrogen intake from food equals the nitrogen output in urine, feces, and perspiration. The nitrogen balance is a measure of daily intake of nitrogen minus the excretion. It is used to assess protein turnover. A positive nitrogen balance indicates an anabolic state with an overall gain in body protein for the day. A negative nitrogen balance indicates a catabolic state with a net low of protein.

Negative nitrogen balance indicates that tissue is breaking down faster than it is being replaced. In absence of protein, the body converts protein to glucose for energy. This occurs with fever, starvation, surgery, burns, and debilitating diseases.

NURSING FAST FACT!

Each gram of nitrogen loss in excess of intake represents the depletion of 6.25 g of protein or 25 g of muscle tissue (Smeltzer & Bare, 2004).

Indirect Calorimetry

The indirect calorimetry is a technique used in measuring the resting energy expenditure based on oxygen consumption and carbon dioxide production.

Prognostic Nutritional Index

The prognostic nutritional index (PNI) is an assessment technique that is based on four measures selected by analysis and computer-based stepwise regression that are then incorporated into a linear predictive model. The clinically important factors as determined by this analysis include the serum albumin concentration, serum transferrin, triceps skinfold thickness, and delayed hypersensitivity. This predictive model relates the risk of morbidity to nutritional status.

Nutritional Requirements

Nutritional requirements are based on a basic formula that must contain all essential macro- and micronutrients for adequate energy production, support of synthesis, replacement, and repair of structural or visceral proteins; cell structure; production of hormones and enzymes; and maintenance of immune function. The basic design contains carbohydrates, protein, fat, electrolytes, vitamins, trace elements, and water.

Carbohydrates

The I.V. source of carbohydrates is predominately dextrose. Glycerol, sorbitol, or fructose can provide other sources of carbohydrate calories. These are considered nondextrose carbohydrates and do not require insulin for metabolism. The nondextrose carbohydrates may require more energy in the metabolism process. Invert sugar and xylitol provide other sources of carbohydrate calories.

NURSING FAST FACTS!

- *1 g carbohydrate = 4 kcal*
- *Dextrose increases the metabolic rate, which in turn raises ventilatory requirements.*

Glucose

The major function of carbohydrates is to provide energy. Glucose provides calories in parenteral solutions. Carbohydrates also spare body protein. When glucose is supplied as a nutrient, it is stored temporarily in the liver and muscle as glycogen. When glycogen storage capacity is reached, the carbohydrate is stored as fat. When glucose is provided parenterally, it is completely bioavailable to the body without any effects of malabsorption.

When dextrose is administered rapidly, the solution acts as an osmotic diuretic and pulls interstitial fluid into the plasma for subsequent renal excretion. The nurse must be aware that when infusing 20 to 70 percent dextrose solutions, the rate must be kept within 10 percent of the prescribed order. (Table 15–3 provides a list of dextrose solutions, osmolarity, and kcal/L.) The pancreas secretes extra insulin to metabolize infused glucose. If 20 to 70 percent dextrose is discontinued suddenly, a temporary excess of insulin in the body may cause symptoms of hypoglycemia (Metheny, 2000).

Dextrose is usually administered concurrently with lipids for two reasons: (1) to prevent hyperglycemia and avert the need for extra insulin and (2) to reduce respiratory demands.

The number of dextrose calories in parenteral preparation may vary considerably, depending on the needs of the patient. The range may be from 400 to 5000 cal/day and depends on the age, weight, and clinical status of the patient along with laboratory determinations.

For peripheral infusions, a 10 percent or less dextrose concentration must be maintained at an isotonic or mildly hypertonic osmolarity to prevent vein irritation, damage to the vein, and thrombosis. Hypertonic concentrations of 20 percent and above must be administered through a central venous catheter (CVC) placed in the superior vena cava.

Dextrose Substitutes

When a patient has allergies to corn derivatives, invert sugar, alcohol sugars (sorbitol and xylitol), or fructose may be used in place of dextrose.

> Table 15–3 **DEXTROSE SOLUTIONS FOR TOTAL PARENTERAL NUTRITION**

Solution (%)	g/L	kcal/L	mOsm/L
5	50	170	252
10	100	340	505
20	200	680	1010
30	300	1020	1515
40	400	1360	2020
50	500	1700	2525
60	600	2040	3030
70	700	2380	3535

Fructose and alcohol do not require insulin for peripheral utilization, but they have potentially dangerous side effects that are not associated with dextrose use. Severe toxic effects can occur with alcohol sugars, including lactic acidosis, hepatic failure, hyperuricemia, and depletion of liver adenosine triphosphate and inorganic phosphate.

Fats

Fat is a primary source of heat and energy. Fat provides twice as many energy calories per gram as either protein or carbohydrate. Fat is essential for the structural integrity of all cell membranes. Linoleic acid and linolenic acid are the only fatty acids essential to humans. These two acids prevent essential fatty acid deficiency (**EFAD**). Linoleic acid is necessary as a precursor of prostaglandins. It regulates cholesterol metabolism and maintains the integrity of cell walls. Signs and symptoms of EFAD include desquamating dermatitis, alopecia, brittle nails, delayed wound healing, thrombocytopenia, decreased immunity, and increased capillary fragility.

Lipid Administration

When fat is used as a calorie source in parenteral nutrition, there are fewer problems with glucose homeostasis, carbon dioxide (CO_2) production is lower, and hepatic tolerance to I.V. feedings may improve. Primarily, I.V. fats are supplied by safflower or soybean oil, with egg yolk phospholipids and glycerol to provide tonicity. Fat emulsions provide 1.1 kcal/mL (10 percent solution) or 2.0 kcal/mL (20 percent solution) (Metheny, 2000).

The initial rate of **fat emulsions** should be 1 mL/min for the first 15 to 30 minutes of the infusion. The rate may be increased to 2 mL/min subsequently.

NURSING FAST FACTS!

- *1 g of fat = 9 kcal*
- *Use of fat can help control hyperglycemia in stress states.*
- *Twenty percent (20 percent) fat emulsions are better utilized by the body.*

Complications associated with EFAD include impaired wound healing, platelet dysfunction, increased susceptibility to infection, and development of fatty liver. In patients with respiratory failure, the administration of fat can help decrease carbon dioxide excretion. The primary purpose of fat emulsions in patients with TPN is to prevent or

> Table 15–4 **LIPID EMULSIONS FOR TOTAL PARENTERAL NUTRITION**

Manufacturer	Emulsion/Percentage	Available	Osmolarity (mOsm/L)
Abbott	Liposyn II 10%	50/50 Safflower oil, soybean oil	10% (1.1 kcal/mL) 276
	Liposyn II 20%	50/50 Safflower oil, soybean oil	20% (2.0 kcal/mL) 258
	Liposyn III 10%	Soybean oil	10% (1.1 kcal/mL) 284
	Liposyn III 20%	Soybean oil	20% (2.0 kcal/mL) 292
	Liposyn III 30%	Soybean oil	30% (3.0 kcal/mL) 305
Clintec	Intralipid 10%	Soybean oil	10% (1.1 kcal/mL) 280
	Intralipid 20%	Soybean oil	20% (2.2 kcal/mL) 330
	Intralipid 30%	Soybean oil	30% (3.0 kcal/mL)
B. Braun	NutriLipid 10%	Soybean oil	10% (1.0 kcal/mL) 280
	NutriLipid 20%	Soybean oil	20% (2.0 kcal/mL) 330

Source: *Gahart B.L., & Nazareno, A.R. (2004). Intravenous Medications (20th ed.). St. Louis: Mosby.*

treat EFAD with infusion of two or three 500-mL bottles of 10 or 20 percent fat emulsions per week (Table 15–4 provides a listing of lipid emulsions for TPN.)

To prevent EFAD, 2 to 4 percent of the total calorie requirement should come from linoleic acid (25 to 100 mg/kg per day). Ten percent of calories from soy or safflower oil emulsions should provide adequate linoleic acid to prevent EFAD.

A 1.2-micron filter must be used when infusing total nutrient admixtures (TNA). This filter was found to remove *Candida albicans* and to prevent passage of particulate and precipitates.

Administration sets that contain di(2-ethylhexyl) phthalate (DEHP) plasticizers extract lipids from the set. It is recommended to use a separate administration set, glass infusate containers, or special non–polyvinyl chloride (non-PVC) bags.

It is very important to carefully inspect fat emulsions for "breaking-out" (or "oiling out"), which is the separation of an emulsion visually. Do not use if there is an identifiable yellowish streaking or the accumulation of yellow droplets in the admixed emulsion.

Protein

Protein is a body-building nutrient that functions to promote tissue growth and repair and replacement of body cells. Protein is also a component in antibodies, scar tissue, and clots. **Amino acids** are the basic units of protein. There are eight essential amino acids needed by adults that must be supplied by the diet: isoleucine, leucine, lysine, methionine, phenylalanine, threonine, tryptophan, and valine.

AGE-RELATED CONSIDERATIONS: NEWBORN INFANTS 15–2

Newborn infants require another amino acid, histidine. Premature infants also require cystine and tyrosine.

Parenteral proteins are elemental, providing a synthetic crystalline amino acid that does not cause an antigenic reaction. These proteins are available in concentrations of 3 to 15 percent and come with and without electrolytes. (Some amino acid solutions are presented in Table 15–5.) An increased need for protein by the body is usually reflected by an increase in excretion of urinary nitrogen, as evidenced by laboratory values.

NURSING FAST FACT!

Protein requirements for healthy adults are 0.8 percent g/kg per day; in critical illness states, the requirements are 1.2 to 2.5 g/kg per day. Protein sparing can be accomplished by administration of 100 to 150 g of carbohydrate daily.

Electrolytes

Electrolytes are infused either as a component already contained in the amino acid solution or as a separate additive. Electrolytes are available in several salt forms and are added based on the patient's metabolic status.

> Table 15–5 **AMINO ACID SOLUTIONS FOR TOTAL PARENTERAL NUTRITION**

Manufacturer	Protein Solution	Concentration (%)	Nitrogen (%)	Osmolarity mOsm/L (g/100 mL)
Abbott	Aminosyn	3.5	0.55	357
	Aminosyn II	3.5	0.55	308
	Aminosyn II	4.25	0.65	894
	Aminosyn	5	0.786	500
	Aminosyn II	5	0.786	438
	Aminosyn	7	1.10	700
	Aminosyn II	7	1.10	800
	Aminosyn	8.5	1.33	850
	Aminosyn II	8.5	1.3	742
	Aminosyn	10	1.57	875
	Aminosyn II	10	1.57	1000
	Aminosyn III	15	2.3	1300
	Stress formulation: Aminosyn-HBC	7	1.12	665

(Continued on following page)

Manufacturer	Protein Solution	Concentration (%)	Nitrogen (%)	Osmolarity mOsm/L (g/100 mL)
Clintec Nutrition	Travasol	3.5	0.591	450
	Travasol with electrolytes	3.5	0.591	450
	Travasol	5.5	0.924	575
	Travasol	8.5	1.42	890
	Travasol	10	1.68	970
	Travasol with electrolytes	8.5	0.924	575
	Novamine	15	2.37	1388
	Stress formulation: BranchAmin	4	0.443	316
B. Braun	FreAmine III	3	0.46	300
	FreAmine III	8.5	1.42	810
	FreAmine III	10	1.57	950
	FreAmine III with electrolytes	3	0.46	405
	TrophAmine	6	0.93	5.25
	TrophAmine	10	1.55	875
	ProcalAmine	3	0.46	735
	Stress formulation: FreAmine HBC	6.9	0.97	620
	Hepatic formulation: HepatAmine	8	1.2	785
Baxter	Clinimix (SF)	2.75	0.40	297
	Clinimix E (SF) with electrolytes and calcium	2.75	0.40	297
	Clinimix (SF)	4.75	0.65	480
	Clinimix E (SF) with electrolytes and calcium	4.25	0.65	490
	Clinimix E with electrolytes and calcium	5	0.786	550
Baxter (Pediatric) New Preservative Free	PREMASOL	6	0.93	525
	PREMASOL	10	1.57	950

Source: *Gahart, B. & Nazareno, A. (2004). Intravenous Medications (20th ed.). St. Louis: Mosby.*
SF = sulfate free

The electrolytes necessary for long-term TPN include potassium, magnesium, calcium, sodium, chloride, and phosphorus. Potassium is needed for the transport of glucose and amino acids across cell membranes. Approximately 30 to 40 mEq of potassium is necessary for each 1000 calories provided by the parenteral route. Potassium may be given as potassium chloride, potassium phosphate, or potassium acetate salt. Serum potassium levels must be closely monitored during TPN administration.

NURSING FAST FACT!

Patients with impaired renal function may need decreased amount of potassium.

Other electrolytes included in nutritional support include:

- Magnesium sulfate at 10 to 20 mEq every 24 hours
- Calcium gluceptate, gluconate, or chloride at 10 to 15 mEq in 24 hours
- Sodium chloride, acetate, lactate, or phosphate at 60 to 100 mEq in 24 hours (as needed to maintain acid–base balance)
- Phosphorous sodium or potassium at 20 to 45 mmol in 24 hours
- Chloride is provided based on acid–base status

Electrolytes must be individually compounded and can be highly variable in the patient receiving TPN. Choice of each of the above salts depends on renal and cardiac functioning, disease-specific needs, acid–base balance, and any abnormal losses during the course of illness.

Vitamins

Vitamins are necessary for growth and maintenance, as well as for multiple metabolic processes. The fat- and water-soluble vitamins are needed for patients requiring TPN. Controversy exists over the exact parenteral vitamin requirements for patients receiving TPN. Certain disease states can alter vitamin requirements, and the sequelae of vitamin deficiency can be catastrophic to very ill patients. Vitamin K is not a component of any of the vitamin mixtures formulated for adults. Maintenance requirements can be satisfied by administering vitamin K, 5 mg per week, intramuscularly (McGinnis, 2002).

NURSING FAST FACT!

Sufficient vitamin K is found in lipids; if a patient receives daily lipid supplementation, vitamin K injections are not needed.

Trace Elements

Trace elements (also called microelements) are found in the body in minute amounts. Basic requirements are very small, measured in milligrams. Each trace element is a single chemical and has an associated deficiency state. The many functions of trace elements are often synergistic (Metheny, 2000).

Zinc contributes to wound healing by increasing the tensile strength of collagen; copper assists in iron's incorporation of hemoglobin. The other trace elements (i.e., selenium, iodine, fluorine, cobalt, nickel, and iron) all have been identified as beneficial.

Parenteral Nutrition Medication Additives

In addition to combining amino acids, dextrose, fats, electrolytes, vitamins, and trace elements, medications such as insulin, heparin, and histamine 2 (H_2) inhibitors are commonly added to TPN solutions. A variety of other medications are compatible with TPN solutions, including some anti-infective agents. Adding medications with TPN solutions depends on various factors, including the physical compatibility of the admixed components, the chemical stability of the drug, the retention of drug concentration over time, and the bioactivity of the components after admixture.

When there has been habitual alcohol ingestion or a suspected alcohol habit before initiation of nutritional support, thiamine should be given to help prevent Wernicke–Korsakoff syndrome and other potential problems. Thiamin often is administered as 100 mg/day for 3 days or more, and can be given in the parenteral nutrition formula (McGinnis, 2002).

Compatibility is always an issue whenever two agents are combined. Parenteral solutions should be used immediately after mixing or else refrigerated. Stability of the admixed component dictates the appropriate length of time that the solution may be refrigerated. The parenteral solutions must be infused within 24 hours or discarded (INS, 2000, 42).

NURSING FAST FACTS!

- *Always check current information about drug compatibility with TPN solutions.*
- *Piggybacking medications directly into TPN solutions is generally not recommended because of the guidelines that a designated port be used only for nutritional support.*
- *Only regular insulin is appropriate for I.V. administration.*

Insulin

Hyperglycemia is the most common complication of TPN therapy. Hyperglycemia is caused by the high concentration of glucose in the TPN solutions. Insulin is considered to be chemically stable in parenteral nutrition. By adding regular insulin to the parenteral admixture, some patients benefit from the enhanced blood glucose levels. Insulin is responsible for adequate metabolism of carbohydrates. Insulin also has a lipolytic effect and an increased muscle uptake of amino acids.

Heparin

Heparin in doses of 1000 to 3000 U/L is sometimes added to parenteral nutrition solutions to decrease potential formation of a fibrin sleeve, which may lead to venous thrombosis. Concerns related to the possibility of heparin-induced thrombocytopenia have decreased this practice.

Histamine 2 (H_2) Inhibitors

Cimetidine, Pepsid, Reglan, or Zantac can be added to the TPN solution as a prophylactic measure against development of stress ulcers.

Admixture Complications

Admixture complications involve the formation of precipitates in the formula. Caution should be taken to ensure that precipitates have not formed in any parenteral nutritional admixtures.

The FDA (1994) suggests the following steps to decrease the risk of precipitate formation:

1. The amounts of phosphorus and calcium added to the admixture are critical. The solubility of the added calcium should be calculated from the volume at the time the calcium is added and should not be based on the final volume.
2. Some amino acid injections for TPN admixtures contain phosphate ions. These phosphate ions and the volume at the time the phosphate is added should be considered.
3. The line should be flushed between additions of any incompatible components.
4. A lipid emulsion in a TNA admixture obscures the presence of a precipitate. Add calcium before the lipid solution.
5. A filter should be used when infusing either central or peripheral parenteral nutrition (PPN). Standards of practice vary, but the following is suggested: 1.2-micron air-eliminating filter for lipid containing admixtures or a 0.22-micron air-eliminating filter for nonlipid-containing admixtures.
6. Parenteral nutrition admixture should be administered within the following time frames:
   a. If stored at room temperature, start within 24 hours after mixing.
   b. If stored at refrigerated temperatures, start within 24 hours of rewarming.
7. If symptoms of acute respiratory distress, pulmonary embolus, or interstitial pneumonitis develop, stop the infusion immediately and thoroughly check solution for precipitates.

Modalities for Delivery of Nutritional Support

Modalities for nutritional support include enteral nutrition, peripheral parenteral nutrition (PPN), total parenteral nutrition (TPN), total nutrition admixture (TNA), and cyclic therapy. There are also specialized parenteral formulas that can be used for patients in renal or liver failure or in stress formulas. Figure 15–1 provides an algorithm for determining the choice of nutritional support.

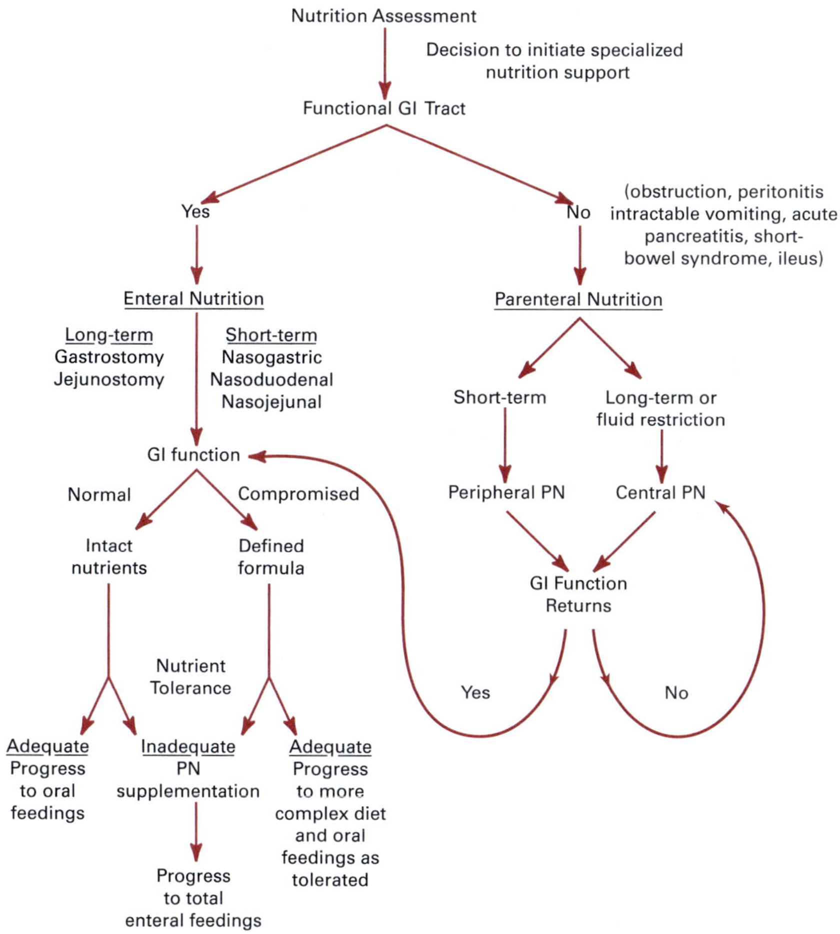

Figure 15–1 ■ Routes to deliver nutritional support to adults: Clinical decision algorithm. This clinical decision algorithm outlines the selection process for choosing the route of nutritional support in adult patients. Major considerations for selecting the feeding route and nutritional support formula include gastrointestinal function, expected duration of nutritional therapy, aspiration risk, and the potential for or actual development of organ dysfunction.

Nutritional Support Candidates

Patients who are good candidates for nutritional support are those who suffer from a multiplicity of problems. Their clinical course can be complicated by malnutrition and depletion of body protein (Fig. 15–2).

The indications for TPN in adults include a 10 percent deficit in preillness body weight; an inability to take oral food or fluids within 7 days after surgery; and hypercatabolic situations, such as major infections with fever and burns. Other conditions that have shown an efficacy for nutritional support include short gut syndrome, enterocutaneous fistulas, renal failure, and hepatic failure (Table 15–6).

Candidates for TPN within the home care environment include patients (1) whose intake is insufficient to maintain an anabolic state; (2) whose ability to ingest food orally or by tube is impaired; (3) who are uninterested in ingesting or unwilling to ingest adequate nutrients; (4) who have underlying medical conditions that preclude their being fed orally or by tube; and (5) whose preoperative and postoperative nutritional needs are prolonged (Smeltzer & Bare, 2004).

AGE-RELATED CONSIDERATIONS: PEDIATRICS 15–3

The leading use of nutritional support in the pediatric population is for the support of infants with inadequate absorptive surface owing to congenital defect or loss from necrotizing enterocolitis.

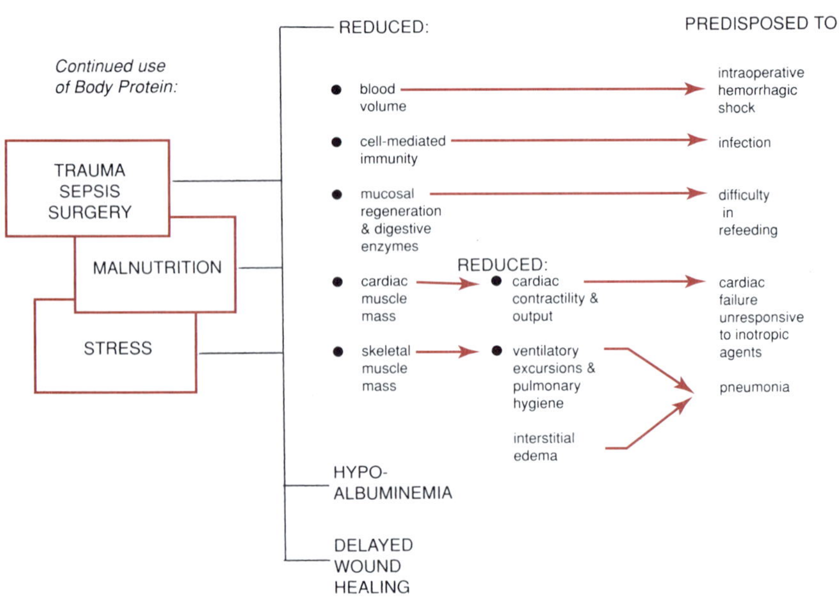

Figure 15–2 ■ Body protein depletion.

> Table 15–6 **CANDIDATES FOR TOTAL PARENTERAL NUTRITION**

Chronic weight loss

- Malnutrition
- Anorexia nervosa
- Anorexia of cancer
- Cancer malabsorption syndrome
- Chronic vomiting and diarrhea
- 10% of preillness weight loss

Serum albumin below 3.5 g/dL

- Bowel surgery
- Short-bowel syndrome
- Massive bowel resection

Conditions requiring bowel rest

- Acute pancreatitis
- Bowel fistulas
- Inflammatory bowel disease
- Obstruction
- Paralytic ileus
- Peritonitis

Malabsorption of enteral therapy
Excessive nitrogen loss

- Abscesses
- Fistulas
- Infections
- Wounds

Hypermetabolic states

- Burns
- Critical illness

Multiple trauma
Hepatic or renal failure
Coma

Enteral Nutrition

Enteral nutrition includes the ingestion of food orally and the nonvolitional delivery of nutrients by tube into the GI tract. Patients who are good candidates for enteral tube feeding are those who will not, should not, or cannot eat but who have a functional GI tract.

Advantages of enteral tube feeding include the following:

1. Maintenance of GI structure and functional integrity
2. Enhanced utilization of nutrients
3. Ease and safety of administration
4. Lower cost

Disadvantages include:

1. Contraindicated for patients with diffuse peritonitis, intestinal obstruction, intractable vomiting, paralytic ileus, or severe diarrhea that makes metabolic management difficult.

2. Not recommended during the early stages of short bowel syndrome or presence of severe malabsorption (ASPEN, 1999).

NURSING FAST FACTS!

- *For enteral nutrition, the GI tract must be functioning!*
- *Enteral tube feeding is considered safer than parenteral nourishment because mechanical, infectious, and metabolic complications are usually less severe than those encountered with parenteral nutrition.*
- *Use the parenteral route only when a patient is at risk of malnutrition from not eating, a trial of enteral nutrition has failed, or when a patient has severely diminished intestinal function because of underlying diseases or treatment is anticipated.*

Complications Associated with Enteral Nutrition

1. Incorrect tube placement
2. Occlusion of feeding tube
3. Pulmonary aspiration of feeding
4. Tracheoesophageal fistula
5. Acute sinusitis
6. Otitis media
7. Diarrhea
8. Metabolic imbalances: hypoglycemia, hyperglycemia, hyperosmolar nonketotic dehydration, EFAD

Nursing Points-of-Care: Delivery of Enteral Nutritional Support

1. The nutrition program should be tailored to meet lifestyle needs.
2. Potential candidates for enteral tube feeding should be evaluated by a multidisciplinary team of healthcare professionals.
3. The patient must be monitored for:
   a. Formula intolerance (gastric residuals every 4 to 8 hours)
   b. Stools (frequency and consistency)
   c. Tube tolerance (placement and maintenance checks)
   d. Effectiveness (weight gain, nutrient intake)
   e. Laboratory tests (CBC, chemistry panel)

Peripheral Parenteral Nutrition

Parenteral nutrition support is used to nourish patients who either are already malnourished or have the potential for developing malnutrition and who are not candidates for enteral nutrition (ASPEN, 1999). PPN was first proposed in the early 1970s as a "nitrogen-sparing" therapy.

The ASPEN (1998) practice guidelines may be used to provide partial or total nutritional support for up to 2 weeks in selected patients who cannot ingest or absorb oral or enteral tube-delivered nutrients or in those for whom central vein parenteral nutrition is not feasible.

> **INS Standard.** Peripheral Parenteral Nutrition provides dextrose in percentages not to exceed 10 percent in final concentrations and/or 5 percent protein or lower, with 500 mL of amino acids and fat emulsions, via a peripheral line should not be infused for longer than 7 to 10 days unless supplementation with oral or enteral feeding is provided concurrently to ensure adequate nutrition. This therapy maintains the nutritional state in patients who can tolerate relatively high fluid volume, those who usually resume bowel function and oral feeding within a few days, and those who are susceptible to catheter-related infection of central venous TPN. PPN can be delivered by an over-the-needle catheter. Osmolarity factors of the solution must be considered when delivering PPN. (INS, 2000, 74)

Prolonged infusions should be limited to solutions that are lower than 900 mOsm/L. Reports have shown that with the use of three-in-one solutions, a higher osmolality may be tolerated. No greater than 10 percent final concentration of dextrose should be infused peripherally (ASPEN, 1999).

The delivery of PPN involves both advantages and disadvantages. Advantages of PPN include:

1. Avoids insertion and maintenance of a central catheter.
2. Delivers less hypertonic solutions than central venous TPN.
3. Reduces the chance of metabolic complications from that of central venous TPN.
4. Increases calorie source, along with fat emulsion.

Disadvantages of PPN include:

1. Cannot be used in nutritionally depleted patients.
2. Cannot be used in volume-restricted patients because higher volumes of solution are needed to provide adequate calories.
3. Does not usually increase a patient's weight.
4. May cause phlebitis owing to the osmolarity of the solution.

A standardized ordering sheet is used to specify the protein, calories, and electrolyte content of each solution tailored to the client. Standard PPN includes the following basic formula:

- 100 to 150 g of dextrose with 1.0 to 1.5 g amino acids/kg (final concentrations of 1.75 to 3.5 percent amino acids and 5 to 10 percent dextrose), along with 500 mL of 10 or 20 percent lipids and electrolytes, trace elements, and vitamins.

Nursing Points-of-Care: Peripheral Parenteral Nutrition

1. PPN is mildly hypertonic and should be delivered into a large peripheral vein
2. Midline catheters are used more frequently for PPN.
3. Phlebitis is a complication of PPN; the catheter site should be observed and the condition of peripheral vein and site documented frequently.
4. PPN is most commonly used for short-term therapy for fairly stable patients whose normal GI functioning will resume within 3 to 4 weeks.

Total Parenteral Nutrition

Parenteral nutrition via central vein is used to provide nutrients at greater concentrations and smaller fluid volumes than is possible with PPN. Central venous access can be maintained for prolonged periods (weeks to years) with a variety of catheters that must be surgically placed and maintained. Central I.V. nutrition support is referred to as TPN. It reverses starvation and adequately achieves tissue synthesis, repair, and growth.

TPN solutions infused through a central vein are highly concentrated and range from 1800 to 2000 mOsm/kg with final additives compared with 300 mOsm/kg in plasma. TPN is usually administered at rates of no more than 200 mL/h.

The delivery of TPN involves both advantages and disadvantages. Advantages include:

1. Dextrose solution of 20 to 70 percent administered as a calorie source.
2. Beneficial for long-term use (usually longer than 3 weeks).
3. Useful for patients with large caloric and nutrient needs.
4. Provides calories; restores nitrogen balance; and replaces essential vitamins, electrolytes, and minerals.
5. Promotes tissue synthesis, wound healing, and normal metabolic function.
6. Allows bowel rest and healing.
7. Improves tolerance to surgery.
8. Is nutritionally complete.

Disadvantages include:

1. May require a minor surgical procedure for insertion of a tunneled catheter or implanted port.
2. May cause metabolic complications, including glucose intolerance, electrolyte imbalances, and EFAD.
3. Fat emulsions may not be used effectively in some severely stressed patients (especially burn patients).
4. Risk of pneumothorax or hemothorax with central line insertion procedure

INS Standard. Administration of Parenteral Nutrition

- Once parenteral nutrition solutions are prepared, they should be used immediately or refrigerated. The length of time that the solution may be refrigerated is based on stability of the admixed components.
- After they are hung, parenteral nutrition solutions must be infused or discarded within 24 hours.
- All parenteral nutrition solutions should be filtered during administration with a 0.2-micron filter. When lipid emulsion is added to these solutions, a 1.2-micron filter should be used during administration.
- Parenteral nutrient lines, whether central or peripheral, should be dedicated to these solutions. With the exception of lipid emulsions, it is preferred that no I.V. push or piggyback medication be added to these lines.
- Solutions should be compounded in the pharmacy using aseptic technique under a horizontal laminar flow hood.
- Parenteral nutrition solutions should be removed from refrigeration 1 hour prior to infusion in order to reach approximate room temperature.
- Parenteral nutrition an electronic infusion device for administration. (INS, 2000, 74)

NURSING FAST FACT!

Because of the high dextrose content in TPN, it is an ideal medium for microbial growth. For this reason, the CDC recommends that parenteral nutrition catheters not be used for anything other than the infusion of TPN (CDC, 2002).

Total Nutrient Admixtures

Total nutrient admixtures (TNAs) are systems that are combinations of dextrose, amino acids, and fat emulsions in one container. Referred to as total nutritional admixture, all-in-one solutions, or three-in-one solutions,

Nursing Points-of-Care: Total Parenteral Nutrition

1. TPN must be administered through a central line because of its hypertonic nature.
2. Strict aseptic technique must be maintained when performing site care, cap or dressing changes.
3. The container of TPN must not infuse beyond a 24-hour period of time.
4. TPN should be initiated slowly, increasing at a rate of 25 mL/h increments until the desired rate of infusion is achieved.
5. Vital signs and blood glucose should be monitored every 4 to 6 hours until stable.
6. Daily weights track patterns of weight gain.
7. An electronic infusion device (EID) should be used to infuse the TPN.
8. The rate of infusion should be kept within 10 percent of the prescribed rate.

Appropriate hand hygiene should be used when caring for the client with TPN.

or trimix solutions, this product combines fat, amino acids, and dextrose in one container. The formula is provided in a large container that infuses over 24 hours. Lipids are mixed with dextrose and amino acid solution in the pharmacy. This solution is usually a milky white and opaque, although a faint yellow hue may be evident with the addition of vitamins. These admixtures have been shown to be stable and well tolerated by patients via central line administration. Compounding of lipids, amino acids, and dextrose solutions raises the pH of the formula.

The TNA solutions offer a significant advantage in the ability to provide cost-effective, patient-specific nutritional support. Nursing time is saved by having only one solution container to hang each day. Pharmacy admixing is simplified by the use of computerized automixing systems, which also allow for more patient-specific formulations.

Total nutrient admixtures must be administered through a 1.2-micron filter because of the mean particle size of fat droplets (Fig. 15–3). The stability of TNA is affected by many factors, including admixture contents, storage time and conditions, addition of non-nutrient drugs, pH of the solution and variability in temperature. The FDA strongly advises pharmacists to use care in the compounding order of nutrients, and advocates the use of a 1.2-micron filter during infusion to avoid problems with calcium and phosphate precipitation (National Advisory Group, 1998).

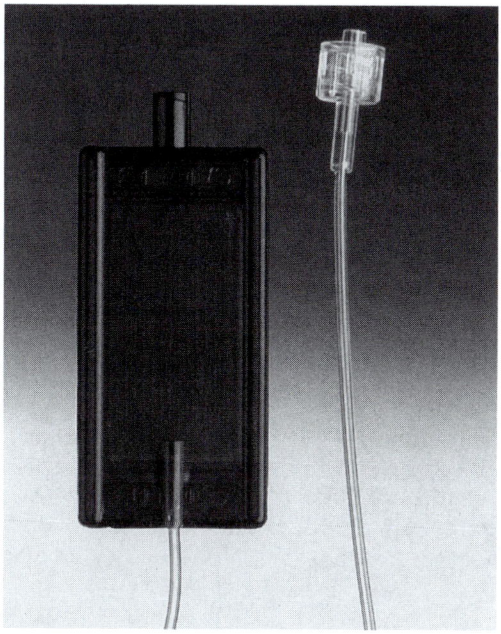

Figure 15–3 ■ Lipipor TNA filter set for total nutrient admixture administration with 1.2-μm air-eliminating filter. (Courtesy of Pall Corporation, Port Washington, NY.)

There is a potential that cholestasis may develop and that long-chain triglycerides may depress the immune system. Catheter occlusion resulting from fat deposits has been reported with long-term use of this therapy.

NURSING FAST FACT!

Most microorganisms grow rapidly in commercial 10 percent lipid emulsions. Infections with Malassezia fufur have been associated with administration of lipids. Use of TPN supplemented with lipids has been shown significantly to increase the risk of blood stream infection by coagulase-negative staphylococci. Candida albicans can grow in the synthetic amino acid and glucose solutions used for TPN (Maki & Mermel, 1998).

Bacterial or fungal growth may be enhanced by admixture of fat emulsions with dextrose and amino acid solutions. The solutions should be observed for pink discoloration and for separation of oils in the three-in-one admixture.

Cyclic Therapy

For patients requiring long-term parenteral nutritional support, cyclic TPN (C-TPN) is widely used. This therapy delivers concurrent dextrose, amino acids, and fat over a regimen of reduced time frame, usually 12 to

Nursing Points-of-Care: Total Nutrient Admixtures Administration

1. The nurse should examine the solution for any signs of instability before hanging and periodically thereafter.
2. The nurse should be aware of physical or chemical phenomena which may occur with TNA solutions and include:
   a. Aggregation (stratification)—rare white "streaks," which is an early stage of creaming. It is not harmful to the patient
   b. Creaming—dense white color at top of solution ("cream") layer. Reverses with gentle agitation and is not harmful. If creaming reappears in 1 to 2 hours it may indicate an unstable emulsion.
   c. Chemical Phenomena ("oiling")—Oil globules on the surface of creamed emulsion fuse and form larger oil droplets. This is irreversible, and cannot be dispersed. Do not hang the container, or take the container down and return it to the pharmacy.

18 hours, versus a 24-hour continuous infusion. Cyclic therapy is indicated for patients who have been stable on continuous TPN, and require long-term parenteral nutrition, for those receiving home TPN; for those patients who can handle total infusion volume in a shortened time period; and those who require TPN for only a portion of their nutritional needs (Wilson & Jordan, 2001).

Dehydration can occur when fluid requirements are not met. Monitoring should include pulse, orthostatic blood pressures, examination of mucous membranes, skin turgor, and laboratory tests such as blood urea nitrogen (BUN), creatinine, hematocrit, and albumin.

Symptoms of excess fluid administration should be monitored, such as weight gain resulting in edema or infusion-related shortness of breath. If too much fluid is administered during the cyclic period, the time frame should be extended. Using the C-TPN regimen requires twice the manipulations as continuous TPN; therefore, the risk of sepsis associated with central line manipulation must be considered.

Advantages include:

1. Prevents or treats hepatotoxicity induced by continuous TPN.
2. Prevents or treats EFAD in patients on fat-free TPN.
3. Improves quality of life by encouraging normal daytime activities and enhances psychological well-being.

Disadvantages include:

1. Patients must be observed for symptoms of hypoglycemia, hyperglycemia, dehydration, excessive fluid administration, and sepsis associated with central-line manipulation.

2. Hyperglycemia can develop during the peak C-TPN flow rate. Blood glucose levels should be checked whenever the patient displays symptoms of nausea, tremors, sweating, anxiety, or lethargy.

NURSING FAST FACT!

The patient who is septic or metabolically stressed is not a good candidate for C-TPN.

Nursing Points-of-Care: Cyclic Total Parenteral Nutrition

1. Initially, until the patient is stable, blood glucose should be checked 1 hour after tapering off C-TPN.
2. This therapy is indicated for patients stabilized on continuous TPN.
3. This therapy is indicated for long-term parenteral nutrition.
4. The patient's cardiovascular status must be able to accommodate large fluid volume during the cyclic phase.
5. For patients without complications such as glucose intolerance or a precarious fluid balance, a 12-hour cycling regimen can be used.

Specialized Parenteral Formulas

Some parenteral formulas are designed to meet the needs of patients with specific disease states such as renal and liver failure and general stress conditions such as trauma, burns, and sepsis.

Renal Formulas

Patients in renal failure who are in need of parenteral nutrition minimal quantities of essential amino acids enhance urea utilization and improve nephron repair. The amino acid L-histidine enhances amino acid utilization in those with uremia. Formulas used for patients in renal failure should not contain nonessential amino acids. Standard crystalline amino acid solutions contain both essential and nonessential amino acids.

Renal preparations decrease the rate of blood urea nitrogen formation and minimize deterioration of serum potassium, magnesium, and phosphorus.

Common preparations include Aminess 5.2 percent, Aminosyn-RF 5.2 or 5.4 percent, and NephrAmine. These formulas are contraindicated in the presence of severe, acid–base and electrolyte imbalances or hyperammonemia.

Hepatic Formulas

Solutions high in branched-chain amino acids (BCAA) are designed for liver disease. Patients with chronic liver disease have elevated levels of aromatic amino acids and depressed levels of **BCAA**. Most commonly these formulas are limited to patients with encephalopathy. The administration formulas high in BCAA would seem to be beneficial; however, as with formulas for renal failure, controversy exists.

Common preparations include BranchAmin, HepatAmine, and Novamine 15 percent. These formulas are contraindicated in patients who are anuric.

Stress Formulas

Patients with infection; sepsis; and the trauma of burns, surgery, shock, and blunt or penetrating injuries often become hypercatabolic. In this situation, an increase in nitrogen excretion caused by altered protein metabolism occurs. Severely stressed patients need more protein to meet increased nutritional needs, so high metabolic stress formulas, which are similar to hepatic formulas, are available for this patient population. This group of patients has a predilection to break down BCAA in the muscles. Formulas with high BCAA replenish those depleted in the stressed patient. Examples of stress formulas include Aminosyn-HBC, BranchAmin, FreAmine HBC, and Novamine 15 percent.

Parenteral Nutrition in the Pediatric Patient

Pediatric patients receiving PPN or TPN usually fall into two major categories:

- Those with congenital or acquired anomalies of the GI tract
- Those with intractable diarrhea

Total parenteral nutrition must be monitored in the pediatric patient to meet the demands of growth and development. Children have a high basal metabolic rate per unit of body weight, an increased evaporative fluid loss, and immature kidneys. Infants and young children need additional amino acids, which are nonessential in adults. The amino acids required for infants and children include histidine, tyrosine, cystine, and taurine. Special amino acid formulas are available to meet these needs (Wilson & Jordan, 2001).

Assessment

Nutritional assessment of pediatric patients uses standard growth curves. Calculation of the ratio of weight to height indicates wasting, and calculation of the ratio of height to age indicates stunting of growth. Anthropometric measurements are used as gauges of somatic protein and fat stores. Visceral protein stores are evaluated by determining serum albumin, serum transferrin, prealbumin, and retinol-binding protein levels.

Pediatric requirements for intravenous nutrition follow general guidelines and are based on protein, calorie, and fluid needs per kilogram of body weight. The nurse must monitor the child's physical status, including reporting abnormal findings of temperature spikes, inappropriate glucose spills, chills, rashes, irritability, and decreased level of consciousness. Serum level of various chemistry and hematology tests are assessed daily for the first week and then decreased to a weekly schedule for the stable hospitalized or home TPN patients.

Another area of assessment includes psychological support. Most TPN patients are infants who are acutely ill and deprived of maternal warmth and comfort. Cuddling and holding the child should be encouraged, along with allowing the parents to participate in their child's care.

Monitoring

Many children require long-term support at home. Monitoring includes many of the same parameters as for adults. The monitoring during initiation of parenteral nutrition includes daily weight, strict intake and output, daily electrolytes until stable, serum glucose measurements every 8 to 12 hours, serum triglycerides and free fatty acid levels weekly, and liver function test biweekly.

In addition, children require evaluation of growth determinations including weight, height, head circumference, and anthropometric measurements for the duration of the therapy.

When a child if first started on TPN, the percentage of dextrose infused is gradually increased from 5 percent to a maximum of 20 to 25 percent via a central line, according to caloric needs and tolerance of the child. Depending on caloric expenditure based on stress levels, lipids may be provided biweekly or daily.

NURSING FAST FACTS!

The predominant complication associated with parenteral nutrition in infants is cholestasis.

Because of the high-risk behaviors of children, catheter sepsis rate in children may rise as high as 10 percent because of increased risks (e.g., teething children have been known to bite the TPN catheter).

Complications Associated with Total Parenteral Nutrition

Complications associated with parenteral nutrition are divided into four groups: (1) mechanical or technical (involving catheters, pumps, and other apparatus for administration), (2) infections, (3) metabolic, and (4) nutritional (Table 15–7). Complications may be minimized by appropriate monitoring and nursing interventions.

Mechanical or Technical (Catheter-Related) Complications

PNEUMOTHORAX

Pneumothorax results when injury occurs during catheter placement. Blood, air, or infusion of fluid collects in the pleural cavity. Care must be taken to assess catheter placement before infusion of TPN. Assess for sharp chest pain, decreased breath sounds, changes in vital signs, and respiratory status. If pneumothorax has occurred, it is evident on a chest radiogram.

AIR EMBOLISM

Passage of air into the heart can occur during insertion of the central line or during catheter maintenance. All connections should be taped and procedures strictly followed for tubing changes along with dressing management techniques. Change tubing during patient's expiratory respiratory phase. Apply an occlusive dressing over the site after the catheter has been removed.

VEIN THROMBOSIS

Long-term central catheterization can cause vein thrombosis in the superior vena cava or its tributaries. Use of a silicone catheter decreases the risk of thrombogenic factors. Pulmonary emboli can be a secondary complication of vein thrombosis. Thrombolytic therapy is of benefit when flow rates are affected owing to thrombus formation, as is the use of heparin added to the infusate to prevent thrombosis. The physician should be notified if thrombosis is suspected.

CATHETER MALPOSITION

This complication can occur during introduction of the catheter. If there is difficulty in passage of the catheter, cardiac arrhythmias during insertion along with irregularities of flow of infusate could indicate malposition of the catheter. Check dressing at least every 4 hours for signs of inadvertent displacement. Report suspected catheter malposition to the physician promptly.

CARDIAC DYSRHYTHMIAS

During insertion various cardiac dysrhythmias can be precipitated by the guidewire or the catheter, causing irritation to the myocardium or carotid

Table 15–7 COMPLICATIONS ASSOCIATED WITH NUTRITIONAL SUPPORT

Complication/Etiology	Symptoms	Treatment	Prevention
Mechanical/Technical Complications			
Air embolism Cause: When line is interrupted and air is inspired while the line is open	Cyanosis, tachypnea, hypotension churning heart murmur (classic sign)	Immediately place patient on left side and lower the head of the bed; this may keep the air within the apex of the right ventricle until it is reabsorbed; administer oxygen	Line placement by appropriately trained personnel; use care in injection cap changes; do not use scissors near catheter
Vein thrombosis Causes: Mechanical trauma to vein, TPN osmolarity, hypercoagulopathy	Swelling or pain in one or both arms, shoulders, or neck; increased anterior chest venous pattern, external jugular distension; or fluid leaking from arm May be asymptomatic	Diagnosis may be made by arm venography, contrast studies, MRI, and radionucleotide study Treatment is controversial and depends on extent of thrombus Conservative treatment without removal consists of anticoagulants Discontinuation of catheter	Tip placement in SVC not upper arm or subclavian Early recognition of symptoms
Catheter malposition Cause: Catheter inadvertently advanced into an incorrect vein during placement Can occur spontaneously after insertion caused by coughing or vomiting	Swelling of arm or neck, pain, difficulty flushing catheter, difficulty infusing TPN Ear gurgling sound	Reposition with guidewire under fluoroscopy or remove Reposition the patient before flushing line	Not always possible to prevent Follow techniques to prevent malposition Always use radiography to confirm tip placement
Metabolic Complications			
Altered glucose metabolism Hypoglycemia: Rebound Cause: Abrupt cessation of TPN	Diaphoresis, irritability, nervousness, shakiness	Administer dextrose or decrease insulin Maintain I.V. at constant rate	Maintain steady rate of infusion; wean gradually

(Continued on following page)

Table 15–7 COMPLICATIONS ASSOCIATED WITH NUTRITIONAL SUPPORT *(Continued)*

Complication/Etiology	Symptoms	Treatment	Prevention
Hyperglycemia Cause: Carbohydrate intolerance, insulin resistance, rapid TPN delivery, diabetes, sepsis, traumatic stress	Increased serum glucose, acetone breath, anxiety, confusion, dehydration, polydipsia, polyuria, malaise	Decrease dextrose TPN concentration or decrease rate administer insulin per sliding scale	Accurate glucose monitoring, gradual TPN rate, increase stable TPN infusion rate
Hyperammonemia Cause: Liver disease where ammonia is shunted past the liver and accumulates in blood	Asterixis (flapping tremor), lethargy, neurologic changes, altered ECG, vomiting, coma	Limit protein intake, enemas and antibiotics to revert growth of ammonia-producing bacteria in intestines	Accurate monitoring of serum ammonia level, monitoring of protein intake for patients with liver disease
Hypernatremia Cause: Water deprivation or loss, excessive TPN administration, profuse diaphoresis, diabetes insipidus, vomiting, diarrhea	Serum Na elevated to 145 mEq/L; urine specific gravity elevated to 1.015; thirst; elevated temperature; dry, swollen tongue; sticky mucous membrane; lethargy	Gradually decrease serum sodium levels to prevent cerebral edema Administration of water	Monitor serum electrolytes I and O, assess for insensible losses
Hypokalemia Cause: Alkalosis caused by shift of K into cells, GI losses, diuretic therapy, TPN, steroid administration, osmotic diuresis, anorexia	Serum K below 3.5 mEq/L, anorexia, fatigue, muscle weakness, decreased gastric motility, postural hypotension, ECG changes	TPN supplementation; replace GI losses	Monitor serum potassium, strict I and O, assess for digitalis toxicity
Hyperkalemia Cause: Renal impairment, iatrogenic-induced, TPN, metabolic and respiratory acidosis, tissue damage	Serum K elevated above 5.5 mEq/L ECG changes, cardiac arrest, muscular weakness, flaccid muscles, intestinal colic, diarrhea	Reduce TPN volume of K, cation exchange resins, dialysis	Accurate monitoring of K, accurate I and O
Hypomagnesemia Cause: GI losses, refeeding after starvation, renal disease, TPN administration	Apprehension, depression, apathy, neuromuscular hyperexcitability, tremors, PVCs, tachycardia, ventricular fibrillation	Parenteral supplementation	Monitor serum Mg, assess for neuromuscular changes

Complication/Etiology	Symptoms	Treatment	Prevention
Hypophosphatemia Cause: TPN supplementation without adequate phosphorus replacement, burns, malabsorptive states, and starvation	Apprehension, irritability, seizures, decreased RBCs, muscle weakness, insulin resistance	I.V. supplementation in the TPN	Monitor serum Mg levels
Hypocalcemia Cause: Vitamin D deficiency, insufficient calcium or magnesium intake, malabsorption, pancreatitis	CNS irritability, confusion, muscle cramps in extremities, muscle spasms, laryngeal spasms, seizures, tetany	Supplement TPN with calcium or I.V. calcium, correct magnesium or phosphate deficiencies	Accurate serum chemistry levels, avoid calcium-depleting medications, maintain adequate calcium intake
Infections			
Sepsis Cause: Skin contamination at insertion site, hub, and tubing junction from hands of healthcare professionals; homogeneous seeding from other sources	Chills, fever, malaise, elevated WBC count, diarrhea, tachycardia, tachypnea, flushing hypotension	Remove catheter or replace catheter over guidewire Antibiotics Administer oxygen Prepare to treat for septic shock	Maintain aseptic technique Aseptic dressing changes Use 0.22-micron filter
Nutritional Alterations			
Refeeding Syndrome Cause: Occurs during initial phase of TPN Body during its bout of starvation has adapted somewhat to nutritional deprivation: decreased basal energy requirements Causes electrolyte shift	Cardiorespiratory complications, edema, hypernatremia, hypokalemia, hypomagnesemia, hypophosphatemia	Can be averted by starting TPN gradually and gradually increasing rate	Monitor patient response to TPN

(Continued on following page)

Table 15–7 COMPLICATIONS ASSOCIATED WITH NUTRITIONAL SUPPORT *(Continued)*

Complication/Etiology	Symptoms	Treatment	Prevention
Essential Fatty Acid Deficiency Cause: Deficient intake	Minimal symptomatology until long term, soft tissue calcification, hypocalcemia, and tetany Numbness and tingling of the mouth and fingers	Fat emulsion supplementation in TPN or with intermittent infusions	Accurate calculation of protein and fat and CHO ratios to maintain a positive nitrogen balance
Altered Mineral Balance Cause: Result of deficiencies caused by malnourishment or starvation	Chromium: elevated serum lipid levels, insulin resistance, glucose tolerance Copper: hypochromic microcytic anemia, neutropenia Iron: fatigue, glossitis, hypochromic microcytic anemia Manganese: CNS changes Selenium: Cardiomyopathies Zinc: Alopecia, apathy, confusion, poor wound healing	Supply adequate supplementation in TPN	Monitor for abnormal laboratory values
Altered vitamin balance Cause: Disease processes can alter vitamin requirements TPN must supply the needed fat- and water-soluble vitamin supplements	Vitamin A: Dry, scaly, rough, cracked skin; decreased saliva; impaired digestion; diarrhea Vitamin D: Decreased serum calcium or phosphorus levels Vitamin E: RBC hemolysis Vitamin K: Delayed clotting Vitamin B_1: Increased serum and urine lactate or pyruvate levels, anorexia, confusion, fatigue, painful calf muscle Vitamin B_2: Glossitis, stomatitis, dermatitis, photophobia Vitamin B_3 (Niacin): Dermatitis, glossitis, diarrhea, dementia Vitamin B_{12}: Anorexia, depression dyspnea, memory lapses, delirium, hallucinations Folic acid: Macrocytic anemia, diarrhea, glossitis Vitamin C: bleeding gums, petechiae, depression	Provide vitamin supplements in TPN	Monitor for symptoms and assess for deficits

sinus. Retracting the guidewire during insertion or repositioning the catheter after insertion corrects this complication.

NERVE INJURY

Both the brachial plexus and the phrenic nerves may be inadvertently damaged during insertion because of their proximity to the central veins. The phrenic nerve can be damaged in both internal jugular and subclavian insertions by the needle or a malpositioned catheter.

Metabolic Complications

Complications associated with metabolic imbalances when administering TPN are either avoidable or controllable.

ALTERED GLUCOSE METABOLISM: REBOUND HYPOGLYCEMIA

Rebound hypoglycemia condition is caused by abrupt cessation of TPN. Maintain a steady rate of infusion, and wean gradually when discontinuing usually prevents with condition. The patient exhibits diaphoresis, irritability, nervousness, and shaking. The infusion rate can be decreased by one half the rate for 1 to 2 hours if needed. This usually is not necessary if the patient is eating (Lyman, 2002).

ALTERED GLUCOSE METABOLISM: HYPERGLYCEMIA

Hyperglycemia is a common metabolic occurrence with TPN because of the high dextrose concentrations included in the admixture. Other factors that put the patient at risk for hyperglycemia are the presence of overt or latent diabetes mellitus, older age, sepsis, hypokalemia, and hypophosphatemia.

Conditions of stress result in decreased glucose tolerance and hyperglycemia in up to 25 percent of patients on TPN. Infusion of large amounts of glucose can also unmask latent diabetes, making hyperglycemia one of the most common complications encountered with parenteral nutrition. Other considerations when infusing formulas containing high concentrations of glucose is the potential effect of carbohydrate metabolism on respiration. Metabolism of carbohydrates results in increased production of carbon dioxide that must be compensated for by increased minute ventilation. This could precipitate respiratory failure in patients with preexisting respiratory disease or interfere with weaning from mechanical ventilation.

Factors that predispose a patient to glucose intolerance include:

- Presence of overt or latent diabetes mellitus
- Older age
- Pancreatitis
- Hypokalemia
- Hypophosphatemia
- Thiamine or B_6 deficiency

- Some antibiotics
- Steroids
- Conditions of stress, such as sepsis or surgery, result in decreased glucose tolerance and hyperglycemia in as many as 25 percent of TPN patients

Nursing Points-of-Care: Monitoring Metabolic Needs

1. Begin TPN infusion at a slow rate (40 to 60 mL/h).
2. Gradually increase the rate 25 mL/h until the maximal infusion rate is achieved.
3. Maintain a steady state of infusion (TPN must stay within 10 percent of prescribed rate).
4. Use a rate control device to monitor the infusion.
5. Monitor serum blood sugar every 6 hours, particularly during the first week of infusion.
6. Record fluid intake and output accurately every 8 hours.
7. Measure hourly urine output if urinary losses are above 250 mL/h.
8. Check body weight daily using the same scale. The ideal weight gain for patients receiving TPN is approximately 2 lb per week.
9. Monitor vital signs at regular intervals. Look for signs of hypovolemia.

ESSENTIAL FATTY ACID DEFICIENCY

Lipid administration is important for delivery of essential fatty acids. If the regimen for nutritional support does not include a calorie source from fats, the patient is at risk for EFAD. Fats may be administered in amounts that supply 30 to 50 percent of the calories. By adding fats to the nutritional support, CO_2 production can be decreased and other metabolic complications may be avoided.

HYPERAMMONEMIA

Ammonia accumulates in the blood in those with liver disease. An elevated blood ammonia level is a common finding in infants and children receiving TPN. High protein intake may lead to elevated ammonia levels. Arginine is important in the urea cycle, and a deficiency of this amino acid may contribute to the development of hyperammonemia.

Limiting protein intake, administration of enemas, and use of antibiotics to prevent growth of ammonia-producing bacteria in the intestines may help. Monitor the serum ammonia levels and limit the essential protein in the TPN solution (Sherliker, 2000).

NURSING FAST FACT!

In adults, the most common laboratory finding is that of elevated transaminase levels; the most common abnormality is liver steatosis. Cholestasis and gallbladder disease are potential complications of long-term TPN.

ELECTROLYTE IMBALANCES

Major electrolyte imbalances associated with TPN can occur if excessive or deficient amounts of electrolytes are supplied in the daily fluid allowance. These include imbalances of sodium, potassium, magnesium, phosphate, or calcium.

- Sodium: Hypernatremia: To maintain homeostasis, the sodium ion is driven from the intracellular space into the extracellular space. This compensatory mechanism tries to combat the extracellular anion loss (Metheny, 2000). This shift can cause hypernatremia.
- Potassium: Hypokalemia: Potassium is also driven into the intracellular space during TPN. Serum potassium can become depleted with an inadequate supply of this electrolyte along with the use of insulin in the TPN solution. Insulin administration further intensifies intracellular potassium.
- Potassium: Hyperkalemia: A high potassium blood level can occur with renal impairment, iatrogenic-induced, or with metabolic and respiratory acidosis when potassium shifts out of the cells. Interventions include reducing the amount of potassium ion in the TPN solution.
- Magnesium: Hypomagnesemia: The magnesium electrolyte also is driven into the intracellular space during TPN administration. This condition is less common than hypophosphatemia or hypokalemia in patients receiving TPN (Metheny, 2000). This electrolyte should be included in TPN solution compounding. Hypomagnesemia is a common imbalance in critically ill and less acutely ill patients. This condition is often overlooked.
- Phosphate: Hypophosphatemia: Adenosine triphosphate (ATP) is required for all cell energy production. Protein synthesis begins when TPN is administered and phosphate is driven into the intracellular space as a component of ATP. Therefore, a deficiency of phosphate can occur. Include phosphate in TPN supplementation.
- Calcium: Hypocalcemia: Because of the fact that most patients receiving parenteral nutrition are malnourished and have low serum albumin levels, their total serum calcium levels are usually also below normal. The hypocalcemia is not physiologically

significant and does not usually result in paresthesias or other signs of tetany. The usual TPN solution contains 5 to 10 mEq/L of calcium.

Nursing Points-of-Care: Monitoring Electrolyte Balance

1. Observe for signs and symptoms of hypophosphatemia, hypokalemia, hypomagnesemia, and hypernatremia. (See Chapter 4 for a review of signs and symptoms.)
2. Chemistry panel should be drawn every 3 days to check electrolyte levels.

Infectious and Septic Complications

When TPN is provided by a central line, there are concerns related to the contamination of the CVC, as discussed in Chapter 12. Catheter-related sepsis is a serious complication of central TPN therapy. This complication is preventable with strict aseptic techniques.

Patients undergoing TPN are often immune compromised as a result of malnutrition; these patients are highly susceptible to infection. The origin of TPN catheter-related sepsis is most often the site itself; infection related to contaminated infusates is rare because of meticulous admixing protocols.

CATHETER-RELATED SEPSIS

Catheter-related infections or sepsis may result from skin contaminants at the insertion site, hub and tubing/device junction contamination, from the hands of healthcare professionals, and homogeneous seeding from other sources (e.g., lungs, urine, abdomen, wounds).

Options for management of catheter-related sepsis include exchange of the catheter over the guidewire and removal of the catheter. The decision is determined by the patient's clinical status, culture results, and the nature of the offending organism.

Nutrition Alterations

REFEEDING SYNDROME

Refeeding syndrome is a complication that can occur during the initial phases of TPN. This occurs when the body, during its bout with starvation, adapts to nutritional deprivation and compensates by decreasing basal energy requirements. This initiation of nutritional support, especially if it is undertaken too aggressively, can result in an electrolyte shift from the plasma to the intracellular fluid. Cardiorespiratory complications can occur. The result of refeeding syn-

Nursing Points-of-Care: Prevention of Infection

1. Maintain aseptic technique in catheter maintenance and administration of TPN.
2. Aseptic dressing changes should be done every 48 to 72 hours if nontransparent occlusive dressing is used; every 4 to 7 days, depending on institutional policy, if transparent dressing is used. (See Chapter 12 for dressing management.)
3. Use of a 0.22-micron inline antimicrobial filter is recommended for TPN lines, except when lipid emulsion is added to these solutions, at which time a 1.2-micron filter should be used (INS, 2000, 30).

drome is manifested by edema, hypernatremia, hypokalemia, hypomagnesemia, and hypophosphatemia.

After the body has reestablished normal albumin and electrolyte balances, the refeeding processes are reversed. Refeeding syndrome can be avoided by initiating TPN slowly, then gradually increasing the rate while carefully monitoring the patient's response and serum electrolyte levels.

ALTERED MINERAL BALANCE

Mineral imbalances are usually the result of deficiencies, the cause being malnourishment or starvation and insufficient supplementation in the parenteral nutrition source. The most common deficiencies include chromium, copper, iron, manganese, selenium, and zinc.

ALTERED VITAMIN BALANCE

Vitamin requirements can be altered by disease processes. The parenteral nutrition must supply the needed fat-soluble and water-soluble vitamin supplements. During illness, vitamin deficiencies can produce serious consequences for which the nurse must assess.

Discontinuation of Nutritional Support

Before discontinuation of parenteral or enteral nutritional support, one of the following criteria should be applicable:

- Parenteral nutrition should not be discontinued until nutrient requirements can be met by enteral or oral nutrients.
- Enteral nutrition should not be discontinued until nutrient requirements can be met by oral nutrients.
- Parenteral or enteral nutrition support should be discontinued whenever the patient's medical condition, especially complications, indicates.

- Parenteral or central nutrition support should be terminated when the physician judges that the patient no longer benefits from the therapy. The decision to discontinue support must be made according to accepted community standards of medical care and in compliance with applicable law (ASPEN, 1998).

Standards of Practice for Nutritional Support

Standards of practice related to nutritional support have been addressed by ASPEN (1998) and the INS (2000). Presented here are the accepted Standards of Practice related to nutritional support. Parenteral nutrition volume is based on patient tolerance.

Implementation Standard

Parenteral formulations shall be prepared according to established guidelines for safe and effective nutritional therapy (Fig. 15–4).

1. Parenteral formulations shall be sterile.
2. Parenteral formulations should be stored at 4°C.
3. Policies should be established limiting additions to the parenteral feeding formulations after they are infusing.
4. Patients or responsible persons shall receive education and demonstrate competence in access route care in home care situations.
5. The TPN catheter or CVC lumen is not to be used for anything other than the delivery of parenteral nutrition.
6. A container of TPN must not infuse beyond a 24-hour period of time.
7. TPN should be removed from the refrigerator 1 hour prior to administration to reach approximate room temperature.
8. TPN should be administered using an electronic infusion pump (EID).
9. The flow rate should be monitored at 30- to 60-minute intervals even if an EID is used.
10. The infusion must be maintained at the prescribed rate. Should it get behind schedule, do not "catch up," as this may precipitate hyperglycemia and metabolic complications. The infusion may be adjusted within a 10 percent margin of the original rate to compensate for any deviation of the infusion schedule.

Monitoring Standards

Patients should be monitored for therapeutic efficacy, adverse effects, and clinical changes that might influence specialized nutritional support. The potential for serous complications with TPN is unacceptably high unless careful monitoring is conducted by experienced clinicians. Protocol for monitoring TPN is included in Table 15–8 (ASPEN, 1998).

ADULT TAILORED TPN SOLUTION ORDERS

TAILORED SOLUTION
- 1000 ml -

A 24 hour supply of TPN solution compounded by pharmacy will reflect changes with the next bottle made unless otherwise noted.

Amino Acids
_____% ❑ Aminosyn _______% Final concentration
❑ Aminosyn RF_____ml
❑ Heptamine _____ml

Dextrose _______ % Final concentration
_______ cc

	Additions	PHARMACY USE
Na Chloride	mEq	
Na Acetate	mEq	
Na Phosphate°	mM*	
K Chloride	mEq	
K Acetate	mEq	
Mg Sulfate	mEq	
Ca Gluconate	mEq	
Insulin, regular	Units	
Adult Tace-Element Solution° Multivitamin Infusion° Famotidine	_____ _____ _____	To be added per 24 hours

TAILORED SOLUTION: FLOW RATE __________ ml/hr.

FAT EMULSION _____% Volume _____ml Frequency _____ Flow Rate _____ ml/hr.

* Monitoring Note
Na Phosphate contains (per ml):
Na+ 4.4 mEq, and P 3 mM
K Phosphate contains (per ml):
K+ 4.4 mEq, and P 3 mM

° Recommended Dosage:
MVI-12 . . . . .1 unit/day
Adult Trace Element Solution. . . . . . .5 ml/day

Physician Signature ______________________ M.D. Date __________

Figure 15–4 ■ Adult-tailored TPN solution orders. (Courtesy of Enloe Medical Center, Chico, CA.)

> Table 15–8 **SUMMARY OF MONITORING PARENTERAL NUTRITION THERAPY**

Before initiation of therapy by central line:

- Check placement of catheter tip by radiography

After initiation of TPN:

- Start TPN infusion slowly.
- Check temperature and vital signs every 6 hours.
- Monitor blood sugar every 6 hours initially, then once a day.
- Maintain strict intake and output.
- Check weight daily.
- Decrease TPN solutions gradually.
- Change TPN and lipid administration sets every 24 hours.

Metabolic monitoring

- Liver function: Periodically monitor liver enzyme, bilirubin, triglyceride, and cholesterol levels.
- Electrolyte profile daily, then twice a week
- Serum profiles weekly at first calcium, AST, ALT, alkaline phosphatase, BUN and creatinine, PT, PTT; and then monthly
- Trace elements initially, then every 3 months with long-term TPN

Nutritional monitoring

- Serial weight daily until stable
- Serum albumin twice a week
- Assess nitrogen balance with a 24-hour urine collection.
- Check albumin, transferrin, prealbumin, or retinol-binding protein.
- Check total lymphocyte count and anergy panels.
- Check creatinine height index to monitor protein.

1. Protocols shall be developed for periodic review of the patient's clinical and biochemical status.
2. Routine monitoring should include nutrient intake; review of current medications; signs of intolerance to therapy; weight changes; biochemical, hematologic, and other pertinent data, including clinical signs of nutrient deficiencies and excesses; adjustment of therapy; changes in lifestyle; psychosocial problems; and changes in home environment.
3. Assessment of patient's major organ functions should be made periodically
4. Blood glucose levels should initially be monitored every 6 hours.
5. Vital signs should be monitored every 4 hours or more frequently.
6. Strict intake and output record monitoring should be done daily.
7. Patients must be weaned off TPN once it is discontinued to prevent rebound hypoglycemia. This is usually done over a 24 to 48 hours period by gradually decreasing the volume of TPN while monitoring patient response.

Nutritional Standards

1. Weigh the patient daily (may be decreased to two to three times per week in stable patients).

2. Evaluate nitrogen balance weekly (or as needed to determine adequacy of protein intake).
3. Albumin, transferrin, transthyretin (prealbumin), or retinol-binding protein may be measured as needed to assess visceral protein status.
4. Total lymphocyte count and anergy panels may be used to monitor changes in immune function.
5. Creatinine height index may be used to monitor somatic protein status.

NURSING PLAN OF CARE

ADMINISTRATION OF TPN

Focus Assessment

Subjective

- History of weight loss
- History of disease and malnourished state
- Biographic data
- Past health history
- Allergies and medications

Objective

- Vital signs, especially temperature
- Level of consciousness
- Skin turgor
- Weight gains or losses
- Tissue edema
- Ratios of urinary output to intake
- Oral mucous membranes
- Serum blood glucose levels

Patient Outcome/Evaluation Criteria

Patient will:

- Stabilize weight and gradually increase to within 10 percent of ideal weight
- Be free of infection; afebrile.
- Gain weight at a rate of 1 lb every 3 weeks, increasing to 1 lb every 2 weeks.
- Display moist skin and mucous membranes, stable vital signs, individually adequate urinary output, and no edema.
- Verbalize understanding of condition or disease process and individual nutritional needs.

(Continued on following page)

NURSING PLAN OF CARE

ADMINISTRATION OF TPN *(Continued)*

- Correctly perform necessary procedures and explain reasons for the actions.
- Demonstrates skill in managing the TPN regimen.

Nursing Diagnoses

- Altered nutrition less than body requirements related to chewing or swallowing difficulties; anorexia; nausea; vomiting; difficulty or inability to procure foods
- Altered health maintenance related to poor dietary habits, with perceptual or cognitive impairment
- Altered nutrition (greater than body requirement) related to imbalance of intake versus activity expenditure
- Altered tissue perfusion (peripheral) related to infusion of irritating solution

Nursing Management

1. Assist with insertion of central line.
2. Insert peripheral I.V. central catheter per agency protocol.
3. Ascertain correct placement of I.V. central catheter by radiography before beginning TPN.
4. Maintain central line patency and dressing per agency protocol.
5. Monitor for
   a. infiltration and infection.
   b. daily weight.
   c. intake and output.
   d. serum albumin, total protein, electrolyte, glucose and chemistry profile.
   e. vital signs.
   f. blood sugar every 6 hours.
6. Check the PPN or TPN solution to ensure correct nutrients are included as ordered.
7. Maintain sterile technique when preparing and hanging TPN solution.
8. Keep infusion within 10 percent of prescribed rate.
9. Use an electronic infusion pump for delivery of TPN solutions.
10. Avoid rapidly replacing lagging TPN solutions.
11. Administer insulin as ordered, to maintain serum glucose in the designated range as appropriate.
12. Report abnormal signs and symptoms associated with TPN to the physician and modify care accordingly.
13. Maintain standard precautions.

Patient Education

The patient receiving enteral nutrition, PN, or TPN will need education, periodic assessment, and retraining as needed.

- Inform the patient about the purpose and duration of the projected nutritional support.
- Instruct the patient on the product hang time.
- Educate the patient and caregiver about management of the access device.
- Instruct the patient receiving enteral feedings about clean techniques for handling the tube, maintaining the access site, and flushing the tube to maintain patency.
- Inform the patient about complications associated with TPN administration, including:
  - Metabolic complications such as hypoglycemia and electrolyte imbalances (recognize and respond to these complications)
  - Mechanical or procedural problems (catheter or tube occlusion, leakage, breakage, or dislodgement)
  - Equipment malfunction or breakage
  - Infusion contamination precipitate or in homogeneity (recognize and report signs and symptoms of localized or systemic infectious process)
- Provide 24-hour phone numbers for home care agency or physician so that patient or caregiver can access professional help.

NOTE > Refer to Home Care Issues for further educational information for the home care patient.

Home Care Issues

Home parenteral nutrition (HPN) has been well established and should be instituted and supervised by a multidisciplinary team with knowledge and expertise (ASPEN, 1998). Patients and their families can be taught to safely administer I.V. admixtures, and they can be monitored in a home setting. Hospital to home transition can be a difficult task. Keep in mind that the day of discharge is usually physically and emotionally stressful; the home care nurse should be in attendance for starting the TPN infusion at home.

Before home therapy for nutritional support is initiated, a baseline electrolyte chemistry panel, magnesium and phosphorus levels, and a CBC should be obtained within 7 days of discharge. Home safety must be determined before discharge from the hospital. Successful home therapy depends on several factors:

- Medical stability
- Emotional stability
- Patient's lifestyle

(Continued on following page)

Home Care Issues *(Continued)*

- Intellectual ability (client or primary caregiver)
- Visual acuity
- Manual dexterity
- Home environment
- Dry storage space for supplies
- Refrigerator large enough to store admixtures
- Clean low-traffic area for procedure preparation
- Electronic outlets for any electronic equipment

The patient or caregiver and home environment should be suitable for safe delivery and monitoring of HPN (ASPEN, 1998).

Advantages of home treatment for nutritional support are that it involves lesser expense than treatment in the hospital; it allows the patient to remain in a familiar, comfortable surrounding, thereby decreasing the confusion associated with age-related environment changes; in many cases, it allows the patient to return to normal activities; and it is associated with a lower risk of acquiring a nosocomial infection. HPN is usually cycled or given over a 12- to 16-hour period, and most of the administration occurs during the sleeping hours (Lonsway, 2001). In addition, a person's control over his or her body and the self-care responsibility increase self-esteem

The home education process should include but not be limited to:

- Verbal and written instructions of appropriate procedures
- Demonstration and return demonstration of procedures by primary caregiver
- Evaluation and documentation of competency
- Self-monitoring instruction
- Limitations of physical activity
- Emergency intervention and problem-solving techniques
- Care of infusion equipment, solutions, and supplies
- Disposal of supplies
- Expectations of home care and medical and nursing follow-up

Home care training must be individually designed according to the individual's capabilities. Assessment of the patient's physical and emotional status before each teaching session aids in determining goals for that session. A minimum number of people should be involved with each teaching session to limit distractions and anxiety.

Because complex treatments such as ventilators, I.V. infusions and chemotherapy are being administered in home and outpatient settings, nutritional assessment of the patient in these settings is important (Smeltzer & Bare, 2004).

The patient or caregiver shall receive education and demonstrate competence in the preparation and administration of home parenteral nutrition support.

Instruction should be given on:

- Proper storage of formulated and admixed parenteral feeding formulations

(Continued on following page)

- Inspection of home parenteral nutrition containers and contents
- Aseptic technique required for the admixture procedure and administration via access device
- Use of parenteral infusion equipment
- Proper disposal of used containers, tubing, and needles
- Drug–nutrient and nutrient–nutrient interactions
- Medication information and administration
- Educational material tailored to the patient and the therapy is provided to the patient/caregiver for use at home.
- Patient or caregiver education should include periodic reassessment and retraining as needed.
- Patient or caregiver should receive education and demonstrate competence in recognition and riptide response to complications.
- Able to recognize and respond to indications of potential metabolic complications.
- Should be able to recognize mechanical and procedural problems that include, but are not limited to, catheter or tube occlusion, leakage, breakage or dislodgement; equipment malfunction or breakage; infusate or precipitate contamination or in homogenicity.
- Able to recognize and report signs and symptoms of a localized or systemic infectious process.
- State when and whom to contact when complications occur.

Key Points

- Candidates for nutritional support include those with:
  - Altered catabolic states
  - Chronic weight loss
  - Conditions requiring bowel rest
  - Excessive nitrogen loss
  - Hepatic or renal failure
  - Hypermetabolic states
  - Malabsorption states
  - Malnutrition
  - Multiple trauma
  - Serum albumin levels below 3.5 g/dL
- Nutritional deficiencies fall into three categories: marasmus, kwashiorkor, and mixed malnutrition
- Effects of malnutrition include a decrease in protein stores, albumin depletion, and impaired immune status.
- Nutritional assessment includes:
  - History (medical, social, and dietary)
  - Anthropometric measurements (weight, skinfold tests, midarm circumference)

- Biochemical assessments (serum albumin, serum transferrin, prealbumin and retinol-binding protein, total lymphocyte counts, serum electrolytes)
- Energy requirements
- Physical examination
- Other indices (nitrogen balance, indirect calorimetry, prognostic nutritional index)

- Parenteral nutrition is an admixture of water, carbohydrates, amino acids, lipids, electrolytes, multivitamins, and minerals formulated to meet an individual patient's needs
- Modalities for delivery of nutritional support include:
  - Enteral nutrition
  - Peripheral nutrition
  - Parenteral nutrition
  - TPN
  - TNA
  - Cyclic therapy
- Peripheral parenteral nutrition, delivered into a peripheral vein, is indicated for patients who need a complete nutrient source but are not depleted; consist of a 2 to 5 percent amino acid solution in combination with 5 to 10 percent dextrose. Fat emulsions of 10 to 20 percent may be combined or administered separately. This therapy is delivered for a limited time, usually 2 weeks.
- Total parenteral nutrition, delivered by central line, is the I.V. administration of hypertonic glucose (20 to 70 percent) and amino acids (3.5 to 15 percent), along with all additional components required for complete support.
- Nutritional support must be filtered with a 0.22-micron filter, except for when lipids are added to TNAs, which must have a 1.2-micron filter.
- Complications of parenteral nutrition include:
  - Mechanical or technical complications
  - Metabolic complications
  - Complications associated with infections
  - Nutritional complications

Critical Thinking: Case Study

A 45-year-old man is admitted with severe abdominal pain. He is 6 feet 1 inches tall and weighs 132 pounds, and has experienced a 45-pound weight loss in the past 3 months (25 percent). He is weak and pale, has dry mucous membranes, a red beefy tongue, and cracks at the sides of his mouth. His abdomen is distended and somewhat firm. He reports decreased appetite with diminished oral intake during the past 4 months. He has been drinking 6 or more beers per day over the past 6 months. He is diagnosed with pancreatitits with pseudocyst formation. He is placed NPO and total parenteral nutrition is ordered. He is to receive a solution of 20 percent dextrose, 50 g of protein/L with standard electrolytes and daily multiple vitamin/trace elements. The goal is 2 L of this solution per day. With lipids, this will provide an average of 2260 calories per day, 100 g of protein, and 21/4 L of fluid per day. The solution is initiated at 1 L/day and increases according to patient tolerance. Thiamine is added to the regimen (100 mg/day for 3 days). The TPN will be infused through a peripherally inserted central line.

What are the points-of-care in monitoring this patient?
Why is the patient receiving thiamine?
What potential complications related to TPN is this patient at risk for?

Media Link: Answers to this case study and additional critical thinking activities are located on the enclosed CD–ROM.

Post-Test

1. H_2 Inhibitors are added to parenteral nutrition to:
   a. Decrease incidence of vein thrombosis
   b. Act as a prophylactic measure against development of stress ulcers
   c. Increase muscle uptake of amino acids
   d. Increase the tensile strength of the collagen
2. Insulin is added to parenteral nutrition for:
   a. Enhancing blood glucose levels
   b. Metabolism of carbohydrates
   c. Lipolytic effect
   d. All of the above
3. Which of the following key concepts is true of TNAs?
   a. Solution must be changed every 8 hours.
   b. Precipitation may be difficult to observe.
   c. Solution must be administered through a 0.22-micron filter.
   d. Risk of contamination increases because of twice the manipulations of the system.
4. The nursing points of care in delivery of PPN would include all of the following **EXCEPT**?
   a. PPN is mildly hypertonic and should be delivered into a large peripheral vein
   b. A 20 percent dextrose solution is appropriate for PPN in a large peripheral vein.

c. Phlebitis is a complication of PPN, the catheter site should be observed with frequent documentation of the condition of the peripheral vein and site.

d. PPN is most commonly used for short-term therapy for fairly stable patients whose normal GI functioning will resume within 3 to 4 weeks.

5. The advantage(s) of home care nutritional support include:

   a. Increased control of one's body

   b. Decreased risk of acquiring a nosocomial infection

   c. Continuation of normal routine

   d. All of the above

6. The type of malnutrition that most commonly occurs in the acutely ill hospitalized patient is:

   a. Kwashiorkor

   b. Marasmus

   c. Mixed malnutrition

   d. Anorexia nervosa

7. How many kilocalories does a 20 percent lipid emulsion provide?

   a. 1.0

   b. 1.1

   c. 2.0

   d. 2.2

8. All of the following are metabolic complications associated with TPN administration **EXCEPT:**

   a. Hypoglycemia

   b. Hypocalcemia

   c. Hyperkalemia

   d. Refeeding syndrome

9. Which of the following are the three essential nutrients included in parenteral nutrition required for anabolism and tissue synthesis?

   a. Trace elements, protein, and fats

   b. Protein, carbohydrates, and fats

   c. Fats, electrolytes, and carbohydrates

   d. Vitamins, electrolytes, and protein

10. All of the following are considered anthropometric measurements **EXCEPT:**
    a. Midarm muscle circumference
    b. Weight
    c. Skinfold thickness
    d. Serum transferrin
11. Which of the following filters should be used with TNA solutions?
    a. 0.22-Micron filter
    b. 0.45-Micron filter
    c. 1.2-Micron filter
    d. 170-Micron filter
12. To treat or prevent essential fatty acid deficiency which of the following should be included in parenteral nutrition?
    a. Trace elements
    b. Transferrin
    c. Crystalline amino acids
    d. Lipids
13. Which of the following visceral proteins is most useful in monitoring the effectiveness of parenteral nutritional support?
    a. Albumin
    b. Transferrin
    c. Prealbumin
    d. Total protein
14. Refeeding syndrome is associated with which of the following electrolyte abnormalities?
    a. Hyponatremia
    b. Hypercalcemia
    c. Hypophosphatemia
    d. Hypermagnesemia
15. Common components of the nutritional assessment include all of the following **EXCEPT**?
    a. Social history
    b. Dietary history
    c. Physical examination
    d. Anthropometric measurements
    e. Laboratory diagnostic evaluation

Media Link: Additional test questions and rationales are located on the enclosed CD–ROM.

References

American Society for Parenteral and Enteral Nutrition (ASPEN) (1998). *The A.S.P.E.N. Nutrition Support Practice Manual.* American Society for Parenteral and Enteral Nutrition, Silver Spring, MD.

American Society for Parenteral and Enteral Nutrition (ASPEN) (1999). Guidelines for the use of parenteral and enteral nutrition in adult and pediatric patients. Internet. Available: *www.clinnutri.org* (1999/2000).

American Society for Parenteral and Enteral Nutrition (ASPEN) Board of Directors (1998). Standards for home nutrition support. *Nutrition in Clinical Practice,* 14(96), 151–161.

Burnett, C. (2000). Patient assessment. In Hamilton, H. (ed.). *Total Parenteral Nutrition: A Practical Guide for Nurses.* Philadelphia: Churchill Livingstone Harcourt.

Infusion Nurses Society (2000). *Revised Standards of Practice.* Philadelphia: Lippincott Williams & Wilkins.

Joint Commission on Accreditation of Healthcare Organizations (JCAHO) (1999). *Comprehensive Accreditation Manual for Hospital and Home Care. Improving Organization Performance.* Oakbrook Terrace, IL, pp. 267–294.

Lonsway, R. (2001). Intravenous therapy in the home. In Hankins, J., Lonsway, R.A., Hedrick, C., & Perdue, M. (eds.). *Infusion Therapy in Clinical Practice* (2nd ed.). Philadelphia: W.B. Saunders, pp. 505–534.

Lyman, B. (2002). Metabolic complications associated with parenteral nutrition. *Journal of Infusion Nursing*, 25(1), 36–44.

Maki, D., & Mermel, L.A. (1998). Infection due to infusion therapy. In Bennett, J.V., & Brachman, P.S. (eds.). *Hospital Infections* (4th ed.) Philadelphia: Lippincott-Raven.

McGinnis, C. (2002). Parenteral nutrition focus: Nutritional assessment and formula composition. *Journal of Infusion Nursing*, 25(1), 54–64.

Metheny, N.M. (2000). *Fluid and Electrolyte Balance: Nursing Considerations* (4th ed.). Philadelphia: Lippincott, Williams & Wilkins.

Sherliker, L. (2000). Complications. In Hamilton, H. (ed.). *Total Parenteral Nutrition: A Practical Guide for Nurses.* Philadelphia: Churchill Livingstone Harcourt.

Smeltzer, S.C., & Bare, B.G. (2004). Health assessment. In *Brunner & Suddarths's Textbook of Medical-Surgical Nursing* (10th ed.). Philadelphia: Lippincott, pp. 71–75.

Wilson, J.M., & Jordan, N.L. (2001). Parenteral nutrition. In Hankins, J., Lonsway, R.A., Hedrick, C., & Perdue, M. (eds.). *Infusion Therapy in Clinical Practice* (2nd ed.). Philadelphia: W.B. Saunders, pp. 219–245.

Answers to Chapter 15 Post-Test

1. **b**
2. **b**
3. **b**
4. **b**
5. **d**
6. **a**
7. **c**
8. **d**
9. **b**
10. **d**
11. **c**
12. **d**
13. **c**
14. **c**
15. **a**

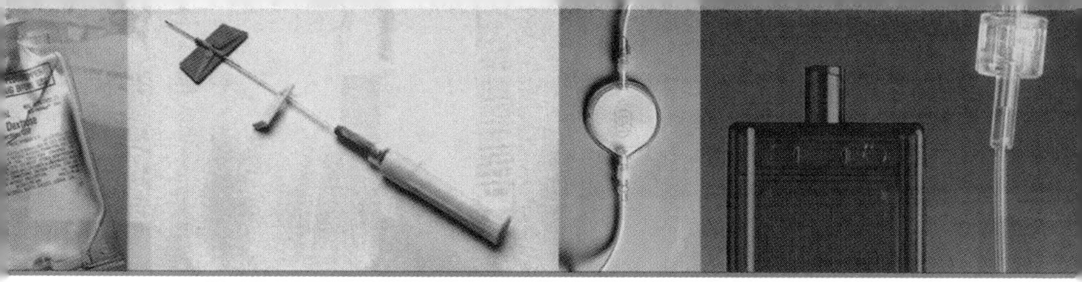

Appendix A
Summary of Recommended Procedures for Maintenance of Intravascular Catheters, Administration Sets, and Parenteral Fluids

Catheter	Replacement and relocation of device	Replacement of catheter site dressing	Replacement of administration sets	"Hang Time" for parenteral fluids
PERIPHERAL VENOUS CATHETERS	In adults, change catheter and rotate site at 72- to 96-hour intervals. Replace catheter inserted in emergency conditions within 24 hours. For pediatric patients, do not replace peripheral catheters unless clinically indicated.	Replace dressing when the catheter is removed or replaced, or when the dressing become damp, loosened, or soiled. Replace dressings more frequently in diaphoretic patient. Visually inspect the catheter if a large bulky dressing that prevents palpation or direct visualization has been used. Inspect the catheter at least daily.	Replace intravenous tubing including add-on devices, no more frequently than at 72-hour intervals unless clinical indicated. Replace tubing used to administer blood components or lipid emulsions every 24 hours. No recommendation for replacement of tubing used for intermittent infusions.	No recommendation for the hang time of intravenous fluids. Complete infusion of lipid containing parenteral nutrition (3 in 1) fluids within 24 hours of hanging. Complete infusion of lipid emulsions alone within 12 hours of hanging. Complete infusions of blood products within 4 hours.
MIDLINE CATHETERS	No recommendation for frequency of catheter change (often in place 7–49 days)	As above	As above	As above
CENTRAL VENOUS CATHETERS INCLUDING PICC AND HEMODIALYSIS CATHETERS	In adults, do not replace catheters routinely to prevent catheter-related infection. No recommendation for the frequency of catheter replacement. Replace disposable or reusable transducers at 72 hour intervals. Replace continuous flush device at the time the transducer is replaced	Replace gauze dressing every 2 days and transparent dressings every 7 days on short-term catheters. Replace the dressing when the catheter is replaced, or when the dressing becomes damp, loosened, or soiled, or when inspection of the site is necessary. Healed CVC in the home setting may not need a dressing.	Replace intravenous tubing and add on devices no more frequently than at 72-hour intervals. Replace tubing used to administer blood products or lipid emulsions within 24 hours of initiating the infusion.	No recommendation of the hand time of intravenous fluids. Including non-lipid containing parenteral nutrition fluids. Complete infusion of lipid containing fluids within 24 hours of hanging the fluid

Catheter	Replacement and relocation of device	Replacement of catheter site dressing	Replacement of administration sets	"Hang Time" for parenteral fluids
PULMONARY ARTERY CATHETERS	Do not routinely replace catheters	As above	As above	As above
PERIPHERAL ARTERIAL CATHETERS	No recommendation for the frequency of the catheter replacement	Replace dressing when the catheter is replaced, or when the dressing becomes damp, loosened, or soiled, or when inspection of the sit is necessary	Replace the intravenous tubing at the time the transducer is replaced (i.e., 72 hours)	Replace the flush solution at the tine the transducer is replaced (i.e., 72 hours)
UMBILICAL CATHETERS	Do not routinely replace	Not applicable	Replace intravenous tubing and add on devices no more frequently than at 72-hour intervals. Replace tubing used to administer blood products or lipid emulsions within 24 hours of initiating the infusion	No recommendations for the hang time of intravenous fluids. Complete infusion of lipid containing fluids within 24 hours of hanging the fluid, includes nontunneled chatter, tunneled catheters, and totally implanted devices.

Source: *Centers for Disease Control and Prevention (2002). Guidelines for the Prevention of Intravascular Catheter Related Infections. Atlanta GA: U.S. Department of Health and Human Services.*

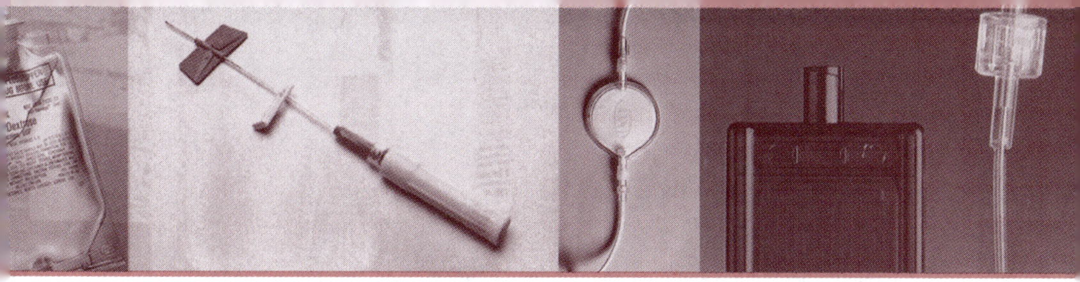

Appendix **B**

Competency SkillChecks

SkillChecks are presented here for the following Competency Criteria:

Name__________________Date__________Evaluator__________________

COMPETENCY SKILLCHECK

Competency Criteria: Implementing infection control standards
Competency Statement: The competent nurse will be able to use CDC guidelines for infection control practices in the delivery of client care.

Performance	S	NS	Evaluator Comments
Critical Action Statements			
1. **Demonstrates hand hygiene techniques using antimicrobial soap.** Stands in front of skin, keeping hands and uniform away from skin surface. Wets hands and wrists thoroughly under *warm* running water. Keeps hands and forearms lower than elbows during washing. Applies a small amount of antimicrobial soap, lathering thoroughly. Washes hands using plenty of lather and friction for 15 seconds. Rinses hands and wrists thoroughly. Dries hands thoroughly from fingers to forearms with paper towel. Turns off hand faucet using clean dry paper towel avoid touching handles with hands. Turns off water with foot or knee pedal if applicable. 2. **Uses alcohol-based agent between hand washing.** Prewashes hands and forearms with non-antimicrobial soap and dry hands. Applies alcohol-based product to palm of one-hand and rubs hands together until hands are dry. 3. **Applies principles of standard precaution to all clients.** Does not wear artificial fingernails or extenders when having direct contact with patients at high risk. Wears gloves when contact with blood or other potential infectious materials, mucous membranes and non-intact skin. Removes gloves after care for a client. Washes hands after removal of gloves. Does not wear the same pair of gloves for care of more than one patient. Changes gloves during client care if moving from contaminated body site to clean body site.			

S= Satisfactory NS = Not Satisfactory – needs comment

Name________________Date__________Evaluator________________

COMPETENCY SKILLCHECK

Competency Criteria: Performing assessments to monitor for fluid balance

Competency Statement: The competent nurse will be able to perform physical assessment to monitor clients in all settings for signs and symptoms of fluid volume disturbances.

Performance	S	NS	Evaluator Comments
Critical Action Statement			
Performs physical assessment directed at identifying fluid volume disturbances. 1. **Cardiovascular system assessment** Assesses radial and apical pulses. Uses edema scale to rate peripheral edema. Measures blood pressure. Assesses for jugular vein distension. Assesses hand vein filling (3–5 second variance). 2. **Pulmonary system assessment** Observes complete respiratory cycle. Auscultates lung sounds. 3. **Skin assessment** Assesses turgor back of hand, chest or forehead. Inspects skin surfaces for moisture or excessive dryness. Pediatric—assesses fontanels. 4. **Special senses** Inspects condition of conjunctiva. Inspects condition and characteristics of mucous membranes. Inspects for tongue turgor. 5. **General data collection** Performs serial weight. Performs specific gravity on urine using a refractometer. Correlates intake and output data. Records all assessments on appropriate document forms.			

S= Satisfactory NS = Not Satisfactory – needs comment

Name__________________Date__________Evaluator__________________

COMPETENCY SKILLCHECK

Competency Criteria: Performing assessments and monitoring for electrolyte balance

Competency Statement: The competent nurse will be able to perform physical assessment to monitor clients in all settings for signs and symptoms of electrolyte disturbances.

Performance	S	NS	Evaluator Comments
Critical Action Statements			
1. **Sodium balance** Interprets lab report for sodium deficit or excess. Assesses skin turgor. Assesses orientation/mentation. 2. **Potassium balance** Interprets lab report for potassium deficit or excess. Reviews ECG for electrical changes indicating K+ deficit or excess. Assesses deep tendon reflexes. 3. **Calcium balance** Interprets lab report for calcium deficit or excess. Assesses for Trousseau's sign. Assesses for Chvostek's sign. Assesses deep tendon reflex. Assesses orientation/mentation. 4. **Magnesium balance** Interprets lab report for magnesium deficit or excess. Observes circulation, motion and sensation of extremities. Assesses respirations. Observes and questions client about muscle cramps. Assesses Trousseau's sign. Assesses Chvostek's sign. Assesses for tachydysrhythmias. Observes for seizures. 5. **Chloride balance** Interprets lab report for chloride deficit or excess. Interprets ABG to assess for metabolic alkalosis or acidosis. Assess for tetany or hypertonic reflexes. Assess respirations. 6. **Documentation** Records all assessments on appropriate document forms.			

S= Satisfactory NS = Not Satisfactory – needs comment

Name__________________Date__________Evaluator__________________

COMPETENCY SKILLCHECK

Competency Criteria: Initiating peripheral infusion therapy with over-the-needle catheter.
Competency Statement: The competent nurse will be able to initiate an over-the-needle catheter using Phillips 15 steps.

Performance	S	NS	Evaluator Comments
Critical Action Statement			
Step 1 Verifies physician order.			
Step 2 Uses principles of hand hygiene.			
Step 3 Inspects all I.V. equipment for integrity.			
Step 4 Identifies the patient by checking the wristband and asking the patient to state his/her name. Informs patient about procedure, and interview regarding previous I.V. experiences.			
Step 5 Inspects both arms for appropriate I.V. site.			
Step 6 Chooses appropriate size catheter. Inspects catheter tip for burrs, and integrity.			
Step 7 Dons gloves before site preparation.			
Step 8 Performs site preparation with 2% chlorhexidine or povidone-iodine for 20 seconds. If allergy, use 70% alcohol for 30 seconds.			
Step 9 Performs venipuncture technique using aseptic technique. Inserts stylet/catheter through skin at 30–45 degree angle with bevel up. Lowers angle of catheter once through the skin. Establishes blood return before threading catheter. Threads catheter to the hub. Removes the stylet. Connects hub to locking device or administration set. Uses only one catheter per attempt.			

(Continued on following page)

Competency Criteria: Initiating peripheral infusion therapy with over-the-needle catheter.

Performance	S	NS	Evaluator Comments
Critical Action Statement			
Step 10 Stabilizes the catheter with tape using Chevron, U or H taping methods. Applies dressing over the site. ▪ 2 × 2 gauze with tape ▪ TSM dressing **Step 11** Labels site, tubing, and solution according to agency policy and procedures. **Step 12** Provides patient education. **Step 13** Disposes of equipment in biohazard containers and sharps containers. **Step 14** Calculates rate accurately. Uses EID appropriately, sets rate correctly. **Step 15** Documents initiation of peripheral I.V. therapy based on institution policy and procedure. Includes: ▪ Assessment of catheter site ▪ Number of attempts ▪ Size and length of catheter ▪ Location of catheter ▪ Use of equipment (EID, inline filters, extension sets, resealable lock) ▪ Solution infusing and rate ▪ How well patient tolerated procedure			

S= Satisfactory NS = Not Satisfactory – needs comment

Name________________Date__________Evaluator________________

COMPETENCY SKILLCHECK

Competency Criteria: Initiating secondary infusion (piggyback)
Competency Statement: The competent nurse will be able to administer medications via a secondary infusion (piggyback).

Performance	S	NS	Evaluator Comments
Critical Action Statement			
1. **Checks the physician order.** ■ Identifies the patient by checking the wristband and asking the patient to state his/her name. ■ Verifies the allergy status of the patient. ■ Explains the purpose of the medication to the patient. 2. **Obtains medication.** ■ Verifies it is correct and compatible with the current infusate. ■ If necessary, removes the medication from refrigerator 20–30 minutes before administration. 3. **Dons gloves.** 4. Opens the sterile container and spikes the container with the secondary administration set. 5. **Primes the secondary administration set with medication just until all air is removed from set, then clamps set.** 6. **Swabs the injection port directly below the check valve on the primary tubing with alcohol.** 7. Attaches the secondary set to the cleansed injection port with needleless system. ■ Attaches the hanger included in the secondary set and attaches it to the primary infusate container. The primary container hangs lower than the secondary set. ■ Slowly opens the clamp on the secondary administration set and lets infusate begin to flow. 8. **Sets the appropriate flow rate.** ■ Assesses the patient response to the medication. 9. **Documents the amount of medication infused, time, and patient's response on appropriate patient record.**			

S= Satisfactory NS = Not Satisfactory – needs comment

Name__________________Date__________Evaluator__________________

COMPETENCY SKILLCHECK

Competency Criteria: Administering intravenous push medication.
Competency Statement: The competent nurse will be able to administer medication by the intravenous push method.

Performance	S	NS	Evaluator Comments
Critical Action Statement			
1. **Checks the physician order.** ■ Identifies the patient by checking the wristband and asking the patient to state his/her name. 2. **Verifies the allergy status of the patient.** 3. **Explains the purpose of the medication to the patient.** 4. **Uses appropriate hand hygiene.** 5. **Draws up medication in a syringe.** ■ Draws up 2 to 3 mL of sodium chloride (0.9%) in each of two separate syringes or uses prefilled sodium chloride syringes. ■ Checks for patency by drawing back on syringe plunger. 6. **Dons gloves.** 7. **Swabs lowest injection port or locking device with alcohol.** 8. **Flushes catheter with 2 mL of sodium chloride after checking for patecy.** 9. **Connects syringe to resealable lock or injection port and slowly administers medication over a minimum of 1 minute.** 10. **Observes patient for response to medication.** 11. **Flushes catheter with 2 mL of sodium chloride, using push–pause pulsatile method.** 12. **Disposes of sharps in sharps container.** 13. **Documents medication administration and patient responses.**			

S= Satisfactory NS = Not Satisfactory – needs comment

Name__________________Date__________Evaluator__________________

COMPETENCY SKILLCHECK

Competency Criteria: Discontinuing intravenous infusion or locking device.
Competency Statement: The competent nurse will be able to discontinue an intravenous catheter.

Performance	S	NS	Evaluator Comments
Critical Action Statement			
1. **Checks the physician order.** 2. **Gathers supplies:** 2 × 2 gauze, alcohol swab and Band-Aid. 3. **Identifies the patient** by checking the wristband and asking the patient to state his/her name. 4. **Explains the procedure to the patient.** 5. **Uses appropriate hand hygiene.** 6. **Clamps administration set,** and turns off EID if appropriate. 7. **Dons gloves.** 8. **Removes all tape** and loosens the TSM dressing using stretch method, or rubs alcohol over dressing to loosen. 9. **Removes dressing and catheter as one unit.** 10. **Applies gentle pressure over venipuncture site** once dressing and catheter are removed. 11. **Places catheter on paper towel.** 12. **Elevates extremity** and applies firm gentle pressure to site for 60 seconds. 13. **Assesses site** and applies 2 × 2 gauze and tape or Band-Aid over site. 14. **Examines the removed catheter for integrity.** 15. **Documents the procedure,** how well the patient tolerated, patient education regarding post infusion site care, and integrity of removed catheter.			

S= Satisfactory NS = Not Satisfactory – needs comment

Name__________________Date__________Evaluator__________________

COMPETENCY SKILLCHECK

Competency Criteria: Changing the central venous catheter dressing and performing site care.
Competency Statement: The competent nurse will be able to aseptically perform site care and change a central venous catheter dressing using standards of practice.

Performance	S	NS	Evaluator Comments
Critical Action Statement			
1. Checks the physician order. **2.** Identifies the patient by checking the wristband and asking the patient to state his/her name. **3.** Uses appropriate hand hygiene. **4.** Gathers equipment: dressing kit and injection cap if necessary. **5.** Explains the procedure to the patient. ▪ Elevates the bed. **6.** Dons mask. **7.** Dons clean, disposable gloves. **8.** Gently removes soiled dressing, maneuvering the skin from the dressing in the direction toward the catheter insertion site. Uses stretch method if dressing is TSM. **9.** Does not touch catheter site. **10.** Examines the dressing for purulent drainage or foul odor. **11.** Removes disposable gloves and uses good hand hygiene. **12.** Examines the catheter site. **13.** Removes outer plastic wrap from dressing kit. **14.** Aseptically open the supplies. **15.** Dons sterile gloves. **16.** Cleans the CVC site slowly using friction and moving from the insertion site outward in a concentric circle covering the area that will be covered by dressing. ▪ First cleans with alcohol swab sticks to remove all debris. Uses all three swab sticks using cleansing procedure. ▪ Allows the alcohol to dry. ▪ Cleans with 2% aqueous chlorhexidine gluconate or povidne-iodine using cleansing procedure. Allows to dry.			

(Continued on following page)

Performance	S	NS	Evaluator Comments
Critical Action Statement			
17. Applies agency-approved dressing, TSM or occlusive dressing, making sure it molds around the catheter and junction of the hub. **18.** Secures the CVC pigtails to the skin above the dressing site. **19.** Applies label to the side of the dressing with date, time, and nurse's initials. **20.** Documents in the patient record the condition of the removed dressing, site inspection, and patient's response to procedure.			

S= Satisfactory NS = Not Satisfactory – needs comment

Name__________________Date__________Evaluator__________________

COMPETENCY SKILLCHECK

Competency Criteria: Irrigating the central venous catheter
Competency Statement: The competent nurse will be able to irrigate the central venous catheter using standards of practice.

Performance	S	NS	Evaluator Comments
Critical Action Statement			
1. Checks the physician order. 2. Uses proper hand hygiene. 3. Gathers equipment: 0.9% sodium chloride and heparinized saline (if indicated). 4. Identifies the patient by checking the wristband and asking the patient to state his/her name. 5. Explains the procedure to the patient. 6. Cleanses the central venous catheter injection cap (port) with 70% isopropyl alcohol. Allows solution to air dry. 7. Attaches syringe containing 0.9% sodium chloride to the injection port via needleless system. 8. Flushes the line with 0.9% sodium chloride using the push–pause method. 9. Attaches the syringe with the heparinized saline to the injection port (if indicated). 10. Flushes the line with heparin. Clamps the line while infusing the last 0.5 mL of solution. 11. Documents the procedure on the patient record.			

S= Satisfactory NS = Not Satisfactory – needs comment

Name__________________Date__________Evaluator__________________

COMPETENCY SKILLCHECK

Competency Criteria: Collecting venous sample from central venous access device

Competency Statement: The competent nurse will be able to collect blood samples from the central venous catheter for lab analysis.

Performance	S	NS	Evaluator Comments
Critical Action Statement			
1. Checks the physician order. **2.** Confirms the orders for lab work. **3.** Verifies the patient by checking the wristband and asking the patient to state his/her name. **4.** Uses appropriate hand hygiene. **5.** Gathers equipment, including collection tubes, Vacutainer 10-mL syringe with 5 mL of normal saline, empty 10-mL or larger syringe, 20-mL syringe prefilled with 20 mL of normal saline. **6.** Dons gloves. **7. Turns off EID if infusion is running.** ■ *For multilumen devices:* Turns off **ALL** infusates prior to specimen collection. ■ *If injection port is not in use:* Preps the valved access port with alcohol. ■ *If the access port is in use:* discontinues I.V. tubing and caps end to maintain sterility. Preps the valved access port with alcohol. **8.** Attaches a 10-mL syringe prefilled with 5 mL of normal saline, then vigorously irrigates with 5 mL of sodium chloride using the pulsatile, push–pause method. **9.** Draws 5–10 mL of blood into the attached syringe to discard. Removes syringe. **10.** Attaches sterile syringe and withdraws blood sufficient to fill required collection tubes. **11.** Attaches syringe with sample blood to Vacutainer and fills collection tubes. **12.** Discards syringe and Vacutainer in appropriate biohazard container. **13.** Irrigates injection port with at least 20 mL of normal saline using pulsatile, push–pause method. **14.** Reconnects the infusion line and begins infusion. **15.** Labels the collection tubes and delivers the sample to the lab as soon as blood draw is completed and the integrity of the CVC is ensured. **16.** Disposes of used equipment in biohazard containers. **17.** Documents the procedure in the patient record.			

S= Satisfactory NS = Not Satisfactory – needs comment

Name__________________Date__________Evaluator__________________

COMPETENCY SKILLCHECK

Competency Criteria: Initiating blood component therapy
Competency Statement: The competent nurse will be able to initiate and monitor the client receiving blood components using standards of practice.

Performance	S	NS	Evaluator Comments
Critical Action Statements			
1. Verifies order for blood component. 2. Obtains informed consent. 3. Performs preinfusion assessment. 4. Verifies the patient by checking the wristband and asking the patient to state his/her name. 5. Assesses the patient's understanding of the purpose and risks of blood transfusion. 6. Assesses previous responses to blood component therapy; allergies. 7. Obtains baseline vital signs. 8. Assesses lungs and kidney function. 9. Reviews Hgb, Hct, platelet counts. 10. Premedicates, if ordered (antihistamines, antipyretics, or diuretics). 11. Initiates I.V. access with 18 g catheter, or verifies patency of catheter prior to obtaining blood product. 12. Obtains blood component from blood bank 13. Verifies blood component with blood bank: ▪ Component type ▪ ABO and Rh ▪ Unit number ▪ Expiration date ▪ Patient identification number 14. Verifies blood component with another nurse on patient care unit, and records on blood component record: ▪ Component type ▪ ABO and Rh ▪ Unit number ▪ Expiration date ▪ Patient identification number 15. Uses good hand hygiene. 16. Hangs Y blood administration set with 0.9% sodium chloride at keep open rate. 17. Dons gloves 18. Turns off sodium chloride			

(Continued on following page)

Performance	S	NS	Evaluator Comments
Critical Action Statements			
19. Spikes and primes Y set pigtail with blood component. **20.** Starts transfusion slowly **21.** Monitors patient for signs and symptoms of transfusion reaction for 5 –15 minutes based on agency policy. **22.** Reassesses vital signs and patient tolerance to transfusion every 30 minutes until transfusion completed. **23.** Reports any adverse effects to physician. **24.** Disposes of blood components bag in appropriate biohazard container. **25.** Documents the component administered, the volume of sodium chloride and blood infused, and how the patient tolerated the procedure in the patient record.			

S= Satisfactory NS = Not Satisfactory – needs comment

Name__________________Date__________Evaluator__________________

COMPETENCY SKILLCHECK

Competency Criteria: Administering chemotherapy agents
Competency Statement: The competent nurse will be able to administer and monitor the client receiving chemotherapeutic agents using standards of practice.

Performance	S	NS	Evaluator Comments
Critical Action Statements			
1. Verifies physician order. 2. Verifies the patient by checking the wristband and asking the patient to state his/her name. 3. Obtains informed consent if required. 4. Performs preinfusion assessment ■ Assesses previous responses to drug therapy ■ Reviews laboratory data (CBC, AGC, platelet, chemistry panel) ■ Performs physical assessment ■ Calculates body surface area or dose based on height and weight 5. Provides patient education regarding chemotherapy's expected risks and benefits. 6. Prepares the drug using Hazardous Drugs protocol. 7. Ensures chemo-spill kit is available. 8. Identifies correct dose, administration route, and rationale for administration with another nurse. 9. Administers antineoplastic agent following set protocols. ■ Inspects medication or infusate container for leaks, cracks, or particulate matter. ■ Gathers supplies needed for drug administration. ■ Uses good hand hygiene. ■ Dons chemotherapy gloves. ■ Checks patency of catheter by instilling 10–20 mL of sodium chloride. ■ Use Luer Lok connectors. 10. Administers drug at prescribed rate. 11. Checks IV site frequently for signs and symptoms of adverse reactions. 12. If more than one drug is to be administered, flushes the catheter on completion of one drug before administering second drug. 13. Identifies the frequency of IV patency checks. 14. Disposes of equipment using receptacle marked "HAZARDOUS WASTE." 15. Documents the drugs administered, the dose and volume of medication, and how well the patient tolerated the drug.			

S= Satisfactory NS = Not Satisfactory – needs comment

Name________________Date__________Evaluator________________

COMPETENCY SKILLCHECK

Competency Criteria: Initiating total nutritional support via central line
Competency Statement: The competent nurse will be able to initiate and monitor the client receiving nutritional support using standards of practice.

Performance	S	NS	Evaluator Comments
Critical Action Statement			
1. Verifies physician order. **2.** Verifies the patient by checking the wristband and asking the patient to state his/her name. **3.** Obtains informed consent if required. **4.** Educates patient on type of parenteral fluid, route of administration, monitoring parameters, and potential complications. **5.** Obtains baseline vitals and weight and reviews laboratory tests (BUN, creatinine, chemistry, and blood sugar). **6.** Obtains nutritional support from the pharmacy. ▪ If 3 in 1 solution, checks for separation of emulsion. **7.** Verifies the TPN solution to the physician order. **8.** Obtains equipment, filter (0.2 or 1.2) and administration set. **9.** Uses good hand hygiene. **10.** Verifies placement of central line. **11.** Maintains aseptic technique while initiating TPN solution. **12.** Maintains infusion rate within 10% of prescribed rate. ▪ Uses EID. **13.** Monitors patient's blood sugar every 6 hours. **14.** Performs serial weights daily. **15.** Monitors vital signs every 4–6 hours (especially temp) **16.** Documents procedure in the patient record, including solution administered, rate, vitals, blood sugars, weights, and how well the patient is tolerating procedure.			

S= Satisfactory NS = Not Satisfactory – needs comment

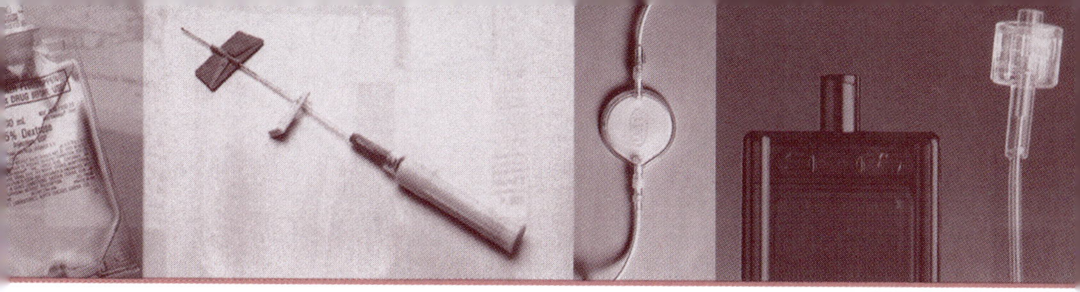

Index

Note: Page numbers followed by f refer to figures; page numbers followed by t refer to tables.

D

M